CRITICAL CARE of the OBSTETRIC PATIENT

CRITICAL CARE of the OBSTETRIC PATIENT

Edited by

Richard L. Berkowitz, M.D.
Professor
Department of Obstetrics and Gynecology
The Mount Sinai School of Medicine
Director
Division of Maternal-Fetal Medicine
The Mount Sinai Hospital
New York, New York

CHURCHILL LIVINGSTONE
New York, Edinburgh, London, and Melbourne 1983

Acquisitions editor: *William R. Schmitt*
Copy editor: *Peggy Brigg*
Production editor: *Karen Goldsmith Montanez*
Production supervisor: *Nina R. West*
Compositor: *Bi-Comp, Inc.*
Printer/Binder: *The Murray Printing Co.*

Distributed in the United Kingdom by Churchill Livingstone, Robert Stevenson House, 1-3 Baxter's Place, Leith Walk, Edinburgh EH1 3AF and by associated companies, branches and representatives throughout the world.

First published 1983

Printed in USA

ISBN 0-443-08195-6

7 6 5 4 3 2 1

Library of Congress Cataloging in Publication Data

Main entry under title:

Critical care of the obstetric patient.

Includes bibliographical references and index.
1. Pregnancy, Complications of. 2. Critical care medicine. I. Berkowitz, Richard L. [DNLM: 1. Critical care—In pregnancy. 2. Obstetrics. 3. Pregnancy complications. WQ 240 C934]
RG573.C67 1983 618.3'028 83-14285
ISBN 0-443-08195-6

To Trudy, Michael, and Laura

Contributors

Fernando Arias, M.D., Ph.D.
Professor, Department of Obstetrics and Gynecology; Director, Division of Maternal-Fetal Medicine, Washington University School of Medicine, Saint Louis, Missouri

Paul G. Barash, M.D.
Professor, Department of Anesthesiology, Yale University School of Medicine, New Haven, Connecticut

Ronald M. Becker, M.D.
Associate Professor, Department of Surgery, Albert Einstein College of Medicine, New York, New York

Richard L. Berkowitz, M.D.
Professor, Department of Obstetrics and Gynecology, The Mount Sinai School of Medicine; Director, Division of Maternal-Fetal Medicine, The Mount Sinai Hospital, New York, New York

George L. Blackburn, M.D., Ph.D.
Associate Professor, Department of Surgery, Harvard Medical School, Boston, Massachusetts

Glen Z. Brooks, M.D.
Assistant Professor, Departments of Anesthesiology and Obstetrics and Gynecology, Yale University School of Medicine, New Haven, Connecticut

Burton V. Caldwell, M.D.
Associate Professor, Departments of Obstetrics and Gynecology and Internal Medicine, Yale University School of Medicine, New Haven, Connecticut

Donald R. Coustan, M.D.
Associate Professor, Department of Obstetrics and Gynecology, Brown University Program in Medicine; Director, Division of Maternal-Fetal Medicine, Women and Infant's Hospital of Rhode Island, Providence, Rhode Island

Dwight P. Cruikshank, M.D.
Associate Professor, Department of Obstetrics and Gynecology; Director, Perinatal Section, Medical College of Virginia, Virginia Commonwealth University, Richmond, Virginia

Alan H. DeCherney, M.D.
Associate Professor, Department of Obstetrics and Gynecology; Director, Division of Reproductive Endocrinology, Yale University School of Medicine, New Haven, Connecticut

Alexander M. Dlugi, M.D.
Endocrine Fellow, Department of Obstetrics and Gynecology, Yale University School of Medicine, New Haven, Connecticut

James O. Donaldson, M.D.
Associate Professor, Departments of Neurology and Internal Medicine, University of Connecticut School of Medicine, Farmingdale, Connecticut

Patrick Duff, M.D.
Clinical Assistant Professor, Department of Obstetrics and Gynecology, University of Texas Health Sciences Center, San Antonio, Texas

Ronald S. Gibbs, M.D.
Professor, Department of Obstetrics and Gynecology, University of Texas Health Sciences Center, San Antonio, Texas

Morton G. Glickman, M.D.
Professor, Department of Diagnostic Radiology; Chief, Vascular and Interventional Radiology, Yale University School of Medicine, New Haven, Connecticut

John P. Hayslett, M.D.
Professor, Department of Medicine, Chief, Section of Nephrology, Yale University School of Medicine, New Haven, Connecticut

David J. Hirsch, M.D.
Postdoctoral Fellow in Nephrology, Department of Medicine, Yale University School of Medicine, New Haven, Connecticut

Mark M. Jacobs, M.D.
Postdoctoral Fellow, Maternal-Fetal Medicine, Department of Obstetrics and Gynecology, University of California, San Francisco, School of Medicine, San Francisco, California

J. Robert Keefer, M.D.
Assistant Professor, Department of Anesthesiology, Yale University School of Medicine, New Haven, Connecticut

Ramón Martin, M.D.
Clinical Fellow in Nutrition, Massachusetts Institute of Technology, Cambridge, Massachusetts

Steven J. Mason, M.D.
Assistant Clinical Professor, Department of Medicine, Yale University School of Medicine, New Haven, Connecticut

Richard A. Matthay, M.D.
Associate Professor of Medicine; Associate Director, Pulmonary Section, Department of Internal Medicine, Yale University School of Medicine, New Haven, Connecticut

Denis Miller, M.D.
Associate Professor, Department of Medicine, Yale University School of Medicine, New Haven, Connecticut

Jennifer R. Niebyl, M.D.
Associate Professor, Department of Obstetrics and Gynecology, The Johns Hopkins University School of Medicine; Director, Division of Maternal-Fetal Medicine, The Johns Hopkins Hospital, Baltimore, Maryland

Michael S. Niederman, M.D.
Postdoctoral Fellow, Department of Medicine, Yale University School of Medicine, New Haven, Connecticut

Terence D. Rafferty, M.D.
Associate Professor, Department of Anesthesiology, Yale University School of Medicine, New Haven, Connecticut

Roberto Romero, M.D.
Assistant Professor, Department of Obstetrics and Gynecology, Yale University School of Medicine, New Haven, Connecticut

Peter E. Schwartz, M.D.
Associate Professor, Department of Obstetrics and Gynecology; Director, Gynecologic Oncology, Yale University School of Medicine, New Haven, Connecticut

Frank R. Witter, M.D.
Instructor, Department of Obstetrics and Gynecology, The Johns Hopkins University School of Medicine; Fellow, Division of Clinical Pharmacology, The Johns Hopkins Hospital, Baltimore, Maryland

Preface

Today's specialists and subspecialists are hard-pressed to stay abreast of developments in their own fields. The extraordinary scientific advances which have been made over the past 20 years have occurred in virtually all areas of patient care. Furthermore, the rate of increase in medical knowledge is itself rapidly accelerating. Paradoxically, the subspecialty groups which were created to cope with this problem have themselves generated much more information, thereby compounding the intellectual overload. The result of all this is that our most valued consultants are often people who have an enormous fund of knowledge which is narrowly focused on restricted areas of interest. It has become virtually impossible to be up to date on the current "state of the art" in fields which are not directly and intimately related to one's area of primary practice.

Obstetrics has more than shared in the benefits and burdens of this transforming information explosion. One of the major changes over the last 2 to 3 decades has been the recognition of the special nature of medical complications superimposed on pregnancy. The subspecialty of maternal-fetal medicine was created, in large part, because of an awareness that the physiologic alterations which accompany pregnancy may have profound effects on a variety of pathologic conditions. In addition, of course, the fetus may be adversely affected by a maternal disease or its therapy, and this consideration is unique to the obstetric patient. Successful perinatologists must, therefore, understand the pathophysiologic consequences of medical disorders on pregnant women as well as their fetuses. They are then challenged to provide therapy which is designed to maximize maternal and fetal outcome while at the same time minimizing the risks to both patients.

High-risk obstetricians have done a remarkably good job in responding to the challenges associated with being internists to pregnant women. They have learned to manage common diseases such as diabetes, asthma, and chronic hypertension with great sophistication in regard to the special needs of their patients. They have also learned to choose as consultants subspecialists in various fields who have a particular interest in pregnancy. Nevertheless, regardless of the medical sophistication of the perinatologist or the obstetrical orientation of the consultant, life-threatening emergencies during pregnancy challenge the knowledge and skills of anyone who works with these patients. Fortunately, these conditions are rare, but unfamiliarity increases their danger since expertise based on experience is usually not available.

Considerable information exists about the management of critically ill obstetric patients, but it is disseminated in fragmented disarray throughout the medical literature. This book has been written in an attempt to correct that situation. We have tried to create a reference work which assembles relevant material from a variety of sources relating to the modern assessment and therapy of potentially fatal conditions which can arise during pregnancy. The authors are subspecialists in a number of different disciplines and are all clinicians who actively practice in the area of their academic expertise.

Much of the information in this book can be found by performing an arduous search of unrelated subspecialty journals. Some of it, however, has been derived from previously unpublished data. An example of this is the results of a survey sent by Dr. R. Baker to 2,000 members of the Society of Thoracic Surgeons in order to evaluate their cumulative experience with cardiac surgery during pregnancy (Chap. 4). Furthermore, in each chapter the authors have been asked to make specific recommendations for evaluating and treating the conditions being considered. Whenever this is done the author's opinion is clearly identified and, when necessary, separated from the consensus wisdom as expressed in the literature. Physicians in academic medicine are often loath to make recommendations based on speculation, but in these chapters they were asked to do so when published data are so limited that optimal proven strategies are simply not available.

It would be wonderful if none of our patients ever needed the diagnostic or therapeutic interventions described in this book, but, unfortunately, some of them will. It is hoped that this volume will provide some guidance for those obstetricians and their consultants who on rare occasions are called upon to treat a pregnant woman who is critically ill.

I would like to thank all the contributors to this book for their outstanding efforts. I am exceedingly grateful to them for putting up with my badgering at a time when the problems associated with a move from one institution to another complicated the task of being an editor. I would also like to acknowledge the tireless support of Inge Venus, Kathy Potter, Terry Miller, and Patti Lincoln of the Perinatology Unit at the Yale University School of Medicine. Finally, I would like to express my appreciation to Bill Schmitt and Peggy Brigg at Churchill Livingstone for being such a pleasure to work with and for making this entire undertaking possible.

Richard L. Berkowitz, M.D.

Contents

1

The Swan-Ganz Catheter and Colloid-Osmotic Pressure Determinations

Richard L. Berkowitz, M.D.

PULMONARY ARTERY FLOW-DIRECTED (SWAN-GANZ) CATHETERS

In 1970, Swan, Ganz et al.[55] described the use of a balloon-tipped double-lumen pulmonary-arterial catheter which has revolutionized the bedside care of hemodynamically unstable patients. This device, subsequently modified in a number of ways, has become accepted as an integral part of the continuous monitoring of individuals with acute myocardial infarction. It has also proved to be a valuable guide to fluid management in pulmonary edema, adult respiratory distress syndrome, and shock. Other major uses include the evaluation of therapeutic interventions with mechanical ventilation, vasoactive drugs, and assisted circulation.[36]

Because of the unique cardiovascular demands of pregnancy, especially during labor and delivery, these devices are proving to be particularly useful in the critically ill parturient. Any discussion of the modern care of critically ill pregnant women would be incomplete without defining the role of Swan-Ganz (SG) catheters.

The Structure and Placement of Swan-Ganz Catheters

The catheter is made of polyvinylchloride. The original model has a small lumen in the wall, which parallels a single major lumen. A latex balloon with a

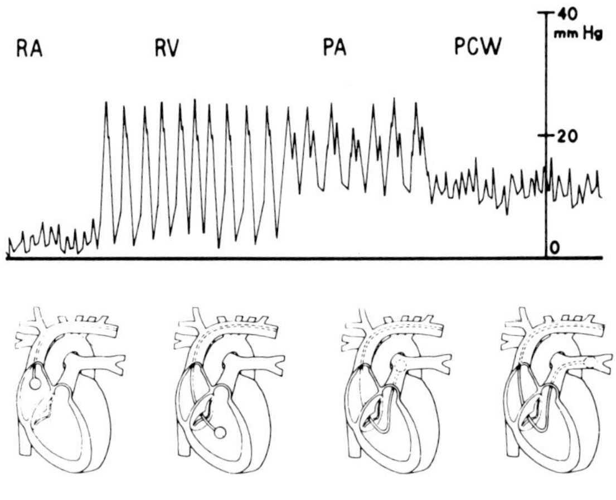

Fig. 1-1 Pressure waves in relation to catheter position from right atrium to pulmonary capillary wedge position. (From Dizon, C.T. and Barash, P.G.: The value of monitoring pulmonary artery pressure in clinical practice. Conn. Med., *41*:622, 1977 Fig. 2 Copyright 1977, Connecticut Medicine.).

bursting volume of 3 cc is placed approximately 1 mm from the tip of the catheter and connects via a side hole in the shaft to the minor lumen. The major lumen extends to an opening at the tip of the catheter.[55]

The device can be introduced via percutaneous insertion into the internal or external jugular, subclavian, femoral, or proximal basilic veins. Placement involves following the progress of the catheter tip by means of continuous pressure monitoring with electronic transducers and an oscilloscopic display.[9] When the catheter tip enters the thorax, respiratory fluctuations appear on the pressure trace. At this point the balloon is inflated and the catheter advanced. Movement of blood through the heart floats the inflated balloon through the right atrium (RA) and ventricle (RV) into the pulmonary artery (PA). As the catheter passes through each of these locations, characteristic pressure traces are displayed on the oscilloscope. Once in the pulmonary artery, the catheter is advanced until the tracing converts to that of a pulmonary capillary wedge pressure (PCWP) (Fig. 1-1). When the balloon is deflated, a typical PA trace should reappear. At this point the catheter is secured and the position of the tip confirmed by chest x-ray.

A major modification of this device over previous models of right heart catheters is the placement of the latex balloon at the catheter's distal end. This permits rapid and reliable entry into the pulmonary artery and minimizes arrhythmias as the catheter traverses the right ventricle. The utilization of an oscilloscope display makes it possible to introduce the device at the bedside without the use of fluoroscopy.

Pulmonary Capillary Wedge Pressure

When a Swan-Ganz (SG) catheter is resting in a small pulmonary artery radicle, inflation of the balloon occludes the vessel lumen and permits free communication of the opening at the tip with the pulmonary venous circulation. This, in turn, is an accurate reflection of left atrial (LA) pressure.[31] Comparative readings with conventional right heart catheters, which do not have balloons on the tips, give identical PCWP values.[36] An important difference between these devices is that while the conventional catheters must be manually advanced and then withdrawn each time a PCWP is measured, the SG catheters will float forward into the appropriate position by simply inflating the balloon.

The original criteria cited for verification of a true wedge pressure were: (1) blood withdrawn from the wedge position should be fully saturated with oxygen; (2) the PA trace should convert to one resembling the LA trace on wedging and; (3) mean PCWP should be less than mean PA pressure.[36] It has subsequently been noted that patients with significant pulmonary shunts who require positive end-expiratory pressure (PEEP) may not fulfill the first criterion, and consequently only the latter two are now required.

Pulmonary capillary wedge pressure is an important variable for two basic parameters of cardiopulmonary function. First, it reflects pulmonary venous pressure and consequently capillary hydrostatic pressure, which is a critical factor in the development of pulmonary edema.[54] Second, PCWP is closely related to LA pressure, which, in the absence of mitral valve disease, reflects left ventricular end-diastolic pressure (LVEDP). The pulmonary wedge pressure therefore provides considerable insight into the functional status of the left ventricle.

Central Venous Pressure and Pulmonary Artery Diastolic Pressure

The central venous pressure (CVP) reflects right ventricular function and systemic vascular compliance. It has been used for years to monitor the relative relationship of blood volume to vascular capacity.[54] However, LV failure and pulmonary congestion may occur without an elevation of this variable. Conversely, patients with high CVPs may have no evidence of pulmonary edema. In a study of 27 critically ill surgical patients, Toussaint et al.[56] found that CVP provided a reliable assessment of PCWP only when cardiopulmonary disease was absent. In patients with dissociated right and left heart function, absolute CVP values correlate poorly with left-sided filling pressures, and even changes in this modality may be misleading.[16,17]

In many cases pulmonary artery diastolic (PAD) pressure is an excellent index of PCWP. However, when pulmonary vascular resistance is increased, the PAD pressure may significantly exceed pulmonary venous and LA pressures. This can occur in association with cor pulmonale, pulmonary embolization, pulmonary fibrosis, primary pulmonary hypertension, and a variety of other conditions. Whenever the PAD-PCWP gradient exceeds 8 mmHg, an increase in pulmonary vascular resistance is present.[54]

Mixed Venous Oxygen Saturation

Mixed venous oxygen saturation (MVO_2) is measured in blood aspirated from the PA. When arterial oxygen content and oxygen consumption remain constant, the

MVO_2 is an excellent index of systemic flow since it is directly proportional to cardiac output under those conditions.[44] Knowledge of the MVO_2 also permits accurate calculations of arteriovenous oxygen content [$(a - v)O_2$] differences and intrapulmonary shunt fractions. These measurements have been reported to be helpful in determining the relative contributions of cardiac and pulmonary dysfunction to respiratory failure.[51,52] When the $(a - v)O_2$ difference is abnormally elevated, it reflects increased tissue extraction of oxygen from circulating blood. This parameter is therefore an excellent index of effective tissue perfusion, which in turn reflects adequate cardiac performance.

Scheinman and colleagues[44] have shown that in healthy patients central venous oxygen saturation (CVO_2) measured from an intrathoracic vein accurately reflects the MVO_2. Patients in heart failure and shock, however, showed a poor correlation between individual values of CVO_2 and MVO_2. Furthermore, there was a poor correlation between changes in these variables over a period of hours to days. In contrast, right atrial oxygen saturation (RAO_2) correlated excellently with corresponding values of MVO_2. It is therefore apparent that blood obtained from a central venous pressure line with its tip in an intrathoracic vein cannot be substituted for right atrial or pulmonary artery samples in determining the true MVO_2 of a critically ill patient.

Swan-Ganz Catheter Modifications

The original SG catheter was limited to continuous monitoring of PA pressures, with intermittent determinations of PCWP whenever the balloon was inflated. Since the initial report, a family of balloon-tipped catheters has been developed. The potential of these devices includes in vivo oximetry, His bundle electrocardiography transvenous cardiac pacing, pulmonary angiography and, perhaps most importantly, cardiac output (CO) determination by thermodilution.

Measurements of CO are performed with a triple-lumen catheter which has a thermistor on the tip. In addition to lumens for the balloon and catheter tip, these devices have a lumen leading to a proximal port opening into the right atrium. The principle employed by this catheter is that net blood flow can be calculated when a known quantity of cold solution is adequately mixed with the circulation and a cooling curve is derived at a downstream site. In practice the determinations are made by injecting 5 or 10 ml of sterile saline at room temperature or 0°C through the proximal port into the RA. The thermistor at the catheter tip measures baseline PA blood temperature and the subsequent decline in temperature following the injection. A bedside computer integrates the area under the cooling curve generated and calculates the CO.[9]

The thermodilution method of cardiac output determination averages over 4 to 10 heartbeats, while the Fick method averages over 2 to 3 min.[36] Therefore, this method is not only efficient and simple to perform and to repeat but is also inherently extremely accurate.

Cardiac Output Determination during Pregnancy

Cardiac hemodynamics during pregnancy have been studied by a variety of techniques during this century. The earliest work utilized an indirect application of the Fick principle and was dependent on measured blood levels of inhaled foreign gases such as nitrous oxide, ethyl iodide, and acetylene.[10,20,47] The introduction of right heart catheterization permitted sampling of RA and PA blood, and thereafter direct application of the Fick principle became possible.[22] Other investigators used a pulse pressure method to study cardiac output during labor.[24] Dye dilution studies using Evans blue[1,42] or indocyanine green[28,59] made more refined investigations possible. Most of the work in this field during the 1970s has utilized the latter technique.

Cardiac output is the product of heart rate and stroke volume. Fick's principle states that the difference between arterial and mixed venous (RA) oxygen concentrations reflects oxygen uptake per unit of blood as it flows through the lung.[45] This principle can be used to calculate cardiac output as follows:

$$\text{CO (ml/min)} = \frac{O_2 \text{ consumption (ml/min)}}{\text{arterial } O_2 \text{ content (vol \%)} - \text{mixed venous } O_2 \text{ content (vol \%)}}$$

The determination of O_2 consumption requires the time-consuming and tedious collection of expired air and the subsequent measurement of its PO_2 and PCO_2. Since oxygen consumption is primarily a reflection of metabolic status, some investigators estimate this value by multiplying a basal state constant (125 ml/min) by the patient's body surface area. Other assumptions can be made to simplify this technique, but each additional shortcut makes it increasingly less accurate. Some of the major problems with this method of cardiac output determination are that: the patient should be in a steady state; arterial and mixed venous samples are required; patient cooperation is necessary to collect expired air; two investigators are needed for the simultaneous collection of expired air and blood samples; and oxygen administration alters the results.[45]

The dye dilution technique of calculating CO is based on the principle that the quantity of fluid in a reservoir can be determined by adding a known amount of indicator to the fluid and then analyzing a sample for the concentration of the indicator after adequate mixing has occurred. In practice, dye is rapidly injected into the venous system while arterial blood is steadily withdrawn through a photodensitometer, which plots a time-concentration curve as the dye passes through one circulation of the body. The CO is calculated from the amount of blood which has diluted the known amount of dye over a measured period of time. The problems associated with this technique are that venous and arterial catheters are necessary; rapid recirculation may affect the calculation; arterial blood must be withdrawn for each determination; an accurate recording device is essential; and tedious hand measurements and calculations of time-concentration curves are necessary unless computer analysis is used.[45] While not as accurate as the Fick method in patients with low COs, valvular insufficiencies, and shunts, this technique can be rapidly performed, and serial outputs are easier to determine. Furthermore, the results are not directly influenced by oxygen administration and are immediately available if a bedside computer is used.

The thermodilution technique of CO determination employs the same principle as the dye dilution method. The advantages of using a thermistor-tipped, triple-lumen SG catheter to obtain this measurement are that only one catheter is needed; blood withdrawal is not necessary; determinations are rapid and readily reproducible; recirculation has little if any effect; only one person is needed to do the study; and oxygen administration does not affect the results.[45] The problems with this method include the complications associated with passage and maintenance of pulmonary artery catheters; the necessity for an accurate recording device and bedside computer; and inaccuracy in very low CO states or in the presence of intracardiac shunts or right-sided valvular insufficiencies.

Starling Curves and Hemodynamic Tracking

During periods of significant stress rapid changes may occur in cardiovascular parameters. In these circumstances sequential observations of hemodynamic variables are of critical importance in unstable patients. By measuring mean PCWP, CO, heart rate, and mean arterial pressure ($\overline{BP}$), the cardiac index (CI), stroke volume index (SVI), and left ventricular stroke work index (LVSWI) can be calculated (Table 1-1). Body surface area (BSA) is a function of the patient's height and weight and can be obtained from standard tables.[8] When cardiac output, stroke volume, and left ventricular stroke work are divided by BSA, these variables are expressed as indices (CI, SVI, and LVSWI, respectively). Because they eliminate the influence of large variations in body size, indices are usually preferable to uncorrected values.

The Starling law of the heart states that within physiologic limits an increase in diastolic cardiac volume results in the stretching of myocardial fibers, which re-

Table 1-1. Hemodynamic Formulas

$$CO = HR \times SV \text{ (L/min)}$$

$$CI = \frac{CO}{BSA} \text{ (L/min/m}^2\text{)}$$

$$SVI = \frac{SV}{BSA} \text{ (cc/beat/m}^2\text{)}$$

$$LVSWI = SVI \times (BP - PCWP \times 0.0136 \text{ (g} \cdot \text{m/m}^2\text{)}$$

Key to abbreviations:

CO = Cardiac output
HR = Heart rate
SV = Stroke volume
CI = Cardiac index
BSA = Body surface area
SVI = Stroke volume index
LVSWI = Left ventricular stroke work index
BP = Mean systemic arterial pressure
PCWP = Mean pulmonary capillary wedge pressure

spond with an increased energy of contraction.[48] Along with an increase in left ventricular end-diastolic volume there is a concurrent rise in LVEDP, which reflects the increase in myocardial tension. When indices of left ventricular work are plotted against measurements of LVEDP, a Starling curve is generated.

In 1964 Ross and Braunwald[41] performed left heart catheterizations on 18 individuals with varying degrees of cardiac compromise. Cardiac output was determined by the indicator dilution method. The LVSWI was plotted against LVEDP as afterload was increased with an infusion of angiotensin II. Three different groups were identified according to their performance in response to the infusion. In patients without significant disease, the ventricular function curves exhibited steep ascending limbs, with large increases in stroke work occurring in association with relatively small elevations of LVEDP. In contrast, the patients with significant cardiac disease had plotted curves which either were flat (i.e., small changes in LVSWI associated with large increases in LVEDP) or exhibited descending limbs. Prior to the infusion of angiotensin many of these patients had comparable LVEDP and LVSWI values despite markedly differing responses when afterload was subsequently increased. This work, therefore, confirmed earlier studies on animals[43] and demonstrated that hemodynamic deterioration in association with cardiac stress cannot necessarily be predicted by values obtained during a basal state.

At the Yale–New Haven Hospital, utilization of a ventricular function graph based on the work by Ross and Braunwald is currently a routine part of the intra- and postoperative management of critically ill patients (Fig. 1-2). The only modification of the original graph is the use of PCWP values instead of direct LVEDP measurements for the abscissa. Holub et al.[25] have shown that it is possible to easily perform instantaneous in-depth hemodynamic evaluation at the bedside. By utilizing a programmable hand calculator, ventricular function curve determinations can rapidly be generated from data obtained via a thermistor-tipped SG catheter and a sphygmomanometer or arterial pressure line. When these are sequentially plotted, evolving responses to rapidly changing hemodynamic stresses can be followed with precision. Group I values represent normal cardiac activity, while those of groups II and III, respectively, indicate mild and marked depression of ventricular function. A hemodynamic tracking profile therefore permits an ongoing evaluation of cardiac function and allows therapeutic intervention to be initiated prior to clinically obvious deterioration. This type of monitoring also provides objective evidence of the effectiveness of both prophylactic and therapeutic manipulations. It has obvious applicability to the critically ill pregnant patient during labor and delivery.

Complications of Swan-Ganz Catheters

The reported incidence of complications with these devices is low. This is partly due to the flexibility of the polyvinylchloride catheter shaft and the protective influence of the inflated balloon during placement. The most frequently detected problem is pulmonary infarction secondary to undetected wedging in the distal pulmonary tree. This can also occur if the balloon is kept inflated for excessive periods of time. The infarcts are usually small and totally asymptomatic. Swan states that most

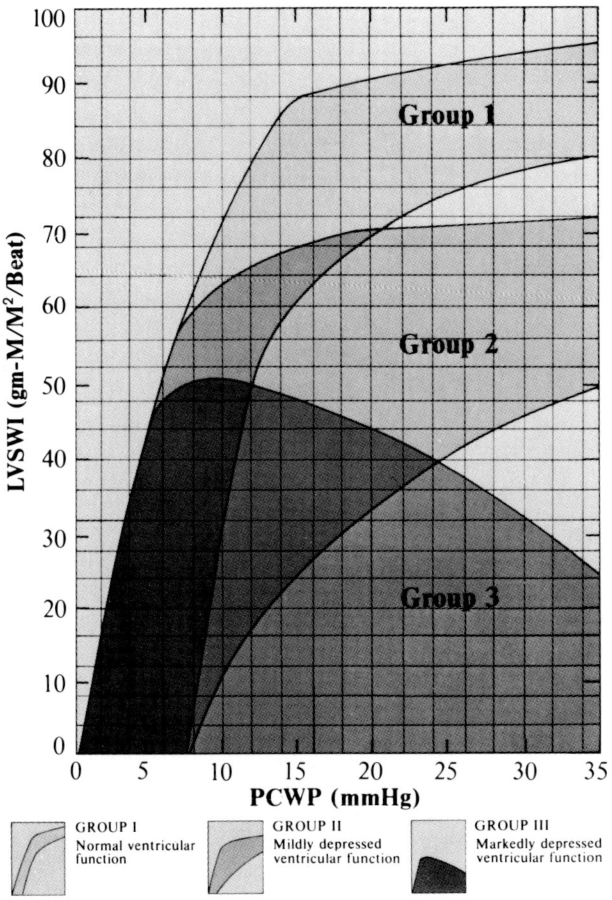

Fig. 1-2 Graphic illustration of hemodynamic tracking profile used at Yale-New Haven Hospital. (Modified from Ross, J., Jr. and Braunwald, E.: The study of left ventricular function in man by increasing resistance to ventricular ejection with angiotensin. Circulation, 29:739, 1964. By permission of the American Heart Association, Inc.)

of these lesions are only detectable on close scrutiny of pre- and postplacement chest x-rays.[54]

A serious but uncommon complication is pulmonary artery rupture, resulting in massive hemoptysis and death. This has been associated with the use of saline instead of air for balloon inflation and with maintenance of the catheter in situ for periods exceeding one week. Unfortunately, PA rupture has also occurred without warning in some patients who did not have these extenuating circumstances. It has therefore been recommended that inflation of the balloon be performed slowly and stopped immediately when the pressure trace changes from a PA to a pulmonary capillary wedge configuration.[9] Barash et al.[3] reported six cases of pulmonary artery perforation associated with the use of SG catheters in a series of approximately 1,700 patients, who were catheterized intraoperatively or in the surgical intensive care unit. Four of these patients died and postmortem examinations suggested that one or more of three separate mechanisms were responsible for vascular perforation: (1) the inflated balloon directly caused disruption of the artery; (2) eccentric or distorted balloon inflation caused the catheter tip to be propelled through the vessel wall; (3) with the balloon deflated the catheter tip was advanced too far distally and perforated the vessel. These investigators recommend taking PCWP measurements only when absolutely necessary and relying on PAD pressure as an indirect measurement of LA pressure when significant pulmonary artery hypertension is not present. They also advise using no more than 1.5 cc to inflate the balloon and if an "overwedge" pattern is observed on inflation, immediately withdrawing the catheter 2 to 3 cm. Since these guidelines were instituted, there have been no further cases of PA perforation in over 1,000 additional catheterized patients at their institution. It should be pointed out that the population studied by Barash et al. is not comparable with an obstetric population. Those authors felt that the most significant risk factors for perforation of the pulmonary artery in their patients were advanced age, pulmonary hypertension, and anticoagulation.

Balloon rupture is not uncommon when the catheter is left in place for several days or has been subjected to many PCWP determinations. The introduction of 0.8 to 1.5 cc of air into the circulation normally has no detectable adverse sequelae.[9] When the possibility of a right-to-left shunt exists, however, CO_2 should be used to inflate the balloon instead of air in order to prevent the occurrence of cerebral or coronary air embolization.

Ventricular arrhythmias may complicate SG catheter use. These are usually noted during insertion or are associated with displacement of the catheter tip from the main trunk of the pulmonary artery into the RV. In the latter situation inflation of the balloon may cause the tip to be propelled forward into the PA or, alternatively, the catheter can easily be pulled back into the right atrium. Sprung et al.[46] have reported a high incidence of SG-associated ventricular irritability in a group of 40 critically ill patients. Of these patients, 27 (68 percent) had evidence of catheter-induced ventricular ectopic beats and 19 (48 percent) developed ventricular tachycardia. Most of the arrhythmias were short-lived, but sustained ventricular tachycardia developed in 3 patients and ventricular fibrillation in 1, who died. This series, however, contained a group of seriously ill patients in whom the overall mortality rate was 60 percent.

Thrombosis of the catheter tip can be clinically significant in hypercoagulable patients, and in these cases anticoagulation therapy may be required if long-term monitoring is necessary.[9] A recent French study[11] found that 66 percent of 33 critically ill patients who required SG monitoring had venographic or autopsy evidence of internal jugular vein thrombosis on the side of catheter placement. There were no significant differences between the group with thrombosis and those without this finding with regard to initial hemodynamic status, age, indications for monitoring, concurrent infection, renal failure, hospital mortality, number of attempts to insert the catheter, duration of catheterization, drugs used to treat the circulatory defect, or clotting indices at the time of insertion. Fifteen of the patients with demonstrable thrombosis had been treated with low-dose or therapeutic levels of heparin. None of the patients in this series had clinical evidence of thrombosis. The authors point out that the clinical implications of their findings are unclear. While no sequelae of the thrombosis were evident in this study, pulmonary emboli and septic phlebitis are certainly potential complications of thrombus formation along the length of the catheter.

O'Toole and colleagues[35] have reported two cases of pulmonary valve damage with resultant insufficiency occurring with catheterization. Dalen[14] mentions tricuspid valve injury in his discussion of catheter-related complications. Aseptic endocarditis has also been reported.[19] Finally, knotting of the catheter is a potential problem. If this occurs, the device should be gently withdrawn to the site of insertion and then removed by venotomy if necessary. This complication can be essentially eliminated if attention is paid to the length of catheter introduced prior to obtaining identifiable RV and PA traces. Standard maximum figures are available, which are dependent, of course, upon the initial site of venipuncture.[9] Stiffening of the catheter by the injection of 10 to 20 ml of a sterile cold solution may facilitate entry into the PA and avoid coiling in the RV.

Katz et al.[26] reported that in a series of 392 critically ill patients undergoing intraoperative SG catheterization over a 17-month period, no deaths were caused by the device. Immediate complications included cardiac arrhythmias (primarily premature ventricular contractions (PVCs) during passage through the RV), inadvertent carotid artery puncture during internal jugular percutaneous puncture (without cardiovascular or neurologic sequelae), and one episode of pneumothorax in a patient with severe bullous emphysema who had been mechanically ventilated for 6 h before the problem was noted. Pulmonary artery embolization which may have been related to the presence of the catheter was indicated by x-ray evidence in 4 percent of the patients. Positive blood cultures, most of which could not be attributed to the catheter, were obtained in 5.4 percent of the cases. It should be noted that routine prophylactic antibiotic coverage has not been recommended for patients undergoing continuous SG monitoring. In a series of 21 obstetric patients in whom SG catheters had been used, the only complications were a ruptured balloon, a positive culture of the catheter tip, and, in 2 cases, transient PVCs at the time of insertion.[37]

Swan-Ganz Catheters in the Obstetric Patient

Despite their limitations, the various techniques employed prior to the introduction of SG monitors have generated a great deal of valuable knowledge about hemodynamics in the normal obstetrical patient. Excellent reviews by Kerr[29] and Metcalfe and Ueland[33] summarize the relevant accumulated data. The family of flow-directed PA catheters has provided superb investigational tools to further study maternal cardiovascular adjustments to complicated pregnancy, labor, and delivery. In addition, of course, they have made sophisticated clinical management possible in a variety of complex situations.

Berkowitz and Rafferty[6] reviewed the literature on this subject up until April 1979 and described the published cases in which SG catheters were used in the management of pregnant women. Conditions in which these devices had been inserted include severe toxemia, abruptio placenta with disseminated intravascular coagulation (DIC), amniotic fluid embolus, various forms of cardiac disease with and without pulmonary hypertension, and adult respiratory distress syndrome (ARDS). Studies performed on healthy elective first-trimester abortion patients following intravenous injections of prostaglandin $F_2\alpha$ ($PGF_2\alpha$), oxytocin, and methyl ergometrine, along with those on third-trimester patients with pregnancy-induced hypertension and others with heart disease, were also described. Since the appearance of this review, additional studies of obstetrical patients with severe toxemia,[5,38,53] noncardiogenic pulmonary edema,[2,27] and molar pregnancies[13] have been published. The use of SG catheters in pregnant women was the major emphasis of two additional articles[7,12] and a review of the experience with these devices in gynecologic patients was the subject of a third.[23] A discussion of some of the studies cited above are included in relevant chapters of this book.

Indications for the Use of SG Catheters

Dalen has pointed out that while the incidence of complications associated with the use of flow-directed PA catheters may be low, some of them have proved to be fatal. Furthermore, he estimated that the direct cost of inserting one of these catheters was between $400 and $500 in 1979. He concludes that hemodynamic monitoring "should only be used when precise hemodynamic data are needed to determine therapy, and when such data cannot be derived from noninvasive, clinical, or radiological evaluation."[14] I agree with this statement entirely. It is not necessary, for example, to prophylactically insert these catheters in class 1 or 2 cardiac patients during labor, or even in all pregnant women with pulmonary edema. Using the guidelines outlined by Dalen, a busy tertiary care obstetrical service should probably only require the use of these devices a few times each year unless they are using them in clinical research. In the latter instance, of course, informed consent should be obtained.

When indicated, however, SG catheters may provide unparalleled insight into the pathophysiology of a complex clinical picture and serve as a guide to rational therapy. Cotton and Benedetti[12] have suggested the following indications for SG insertion in pregnant women:

1. Hypovolemic shock unresponsive to initial fluid therapy
2. Septic shock requiring volume resuscitation or vasopressor therapy
3. Surgery and/or labor and delivery in class 3 or 4 cardiac patients
4. Severe preeclampsia, or eclampsia complicated by marked oliguria, hypovolemia, or pulmonary edema

I agree with the first three items on this list and the fourth with regard to toxemic women who develop pulmonary edema. My specific recommendations for the use of SG catheters in women with pregnancy-induced hypertension are discussed in Chapter 11, Hypertensive Crisis in Pregnancy. I would add the following conditions to the above list:

1. Adult respiratory distress syndrome severe enough to require intubation

2. Known pulmonary hypertension, regardless of the New York Heart Association classification, at the time of labor and delivery
3. Respiratory insufficiency presumed to be caused by amniotic fluid embolization
4. Pulmonary edema not quickly responsive to medical management in an undelivered patient

COLLOID OSMOTIC PRESSURE

Physiologic Effects of Colloid Osmotic Pressure

Under normal circumstances the vascular endothelium functions like a semipermeable membrane. The minipores which are present are so small that molecules of plasma protein are retained within the vascular lumen while fluid can freely move to and from the interstitial space. This results in differences in the concentration of protein within these two compartments, which in turn is responsible for differences in colloid osmotic pressure (COP). In a system in which a semipermeable membrane separates two compartments containing fluids of different COP, the forces of hydrostatic pressure oppose those of COP on each side of the membrane. Within a capillary, hydrostatic pressure tends to move fluid from the lumen into the intravascular space, while COP pulls fluid from the interstitium into the vessel lumen. The same forces are at work within the interstitial space, and as a result net movement of fluid depends on the balance between these two hydrostatic and two osmotic pressures. This complex interaction was originally described by Starling in 1896 and can be expressed as[49]:

$$Q = k(P_c - P_i) - k\sigma(\pi_c - \pi_i)$$

where
Q = net transvascular flow of fluid
k = filtration coefficient
P_c = hydrostatic pressure in the capillary
P_i = hydrostatic pressure in the interstitial space
σ = reflection coefficient
π_c = osmotic pressure in plasma
π_i = osmotic pressure in interstitial space

Normally there is a net outward filtration of fluid, which is carried off by the pulmonary lymphatics at a rate that has been estimated to be 10 to 20 cc/h in adults. If, however, the balance of the Starling forces is significantly changed or capillary permeability is altered, the efflux of fluid may exceed the lymphatic capacity to remove it and pulmonary edema will result.

Cardiogenic pulmonary edema is caused by an increase in hydrostatic pressure within pulmonary capillaries while noncardiogenic pulmonary edema results from an increase in capillary wall permeability. Regardless of the etiology of the pulmonary edema, however, the relationship of the Starling forces will have a major influence on the rate and quantity of fluid movement across pulmonary capillary walls. Currently, there are no clinically useful ways to measure interstitial fluid hydrostatic and colloid osmotic pressures. However, it is possible to obtain accurate estimates of pulmonary capillary pressure with the SG catheter, and COPs can be measured with commercially available oncometers.

Principles of Measuring COP

In a steady state at physiologic pH, the COP can be calculated from serum protein values. In pathologic sera, however, the derived value is sufficiently unreliable to make it necessary to directly determine plasma COP in any situation where this parameter is considered to be important.[34] The oncometer is an instrument designed for measuring COP in small samples of serum or plasma. In this instrument two chambers are separated by a semipermeable membrane, which is usually impermeable to molecules with molecular weights greater than 30,000. The lower chamber is connected to a pressure transducer and is filled with a colloid-free isotonic saline solution. The upper chamber is filled with the sample to be measured. After zeroing and calibrating the system, a sample of the unknown solution is placed in the upper chamber. The colloid osmotic force of the sample being tested draws water into the upper chamber, which results in a negative pressure in the chamber below the membrane. This pressure is transmitted to a digital readout, where it is expressed in millimeters of mercury. After equilibration between the two chambers is achieved, the readout stabilizes and the pressure displayed corresponds to COP.

In nine subjects in whom COP was measured on both plasma and serum obtained from the same blood sample, Weil et al. found that the mean values for the plasma were 0.13 torr higher than those for serum.[58] This was not statistically significant. Furthermore, the same investigators found that 25 paired samples of arterial and venous plasma obtained from simultaneously drawn samples from the femoral and pulmonary arteries showed no significant difference in COP between the two groups. Ladegaard-Pedersen,[30] on the other hand, found that the COP of plasma was 0.32 torr higher than that of serum. Although this difference was small, it was statistically significant.

When 19 healthy, ambulatory, nonpregnant volunteers had plasma COP values determined following a 12-h fast, the range varied from 21.7 to 28.7 (mean 25.4 ± 2.3) torr.[58] Samples from 14 healthy hospitalized patients prior to elective minor surgery were also studied. These patients were at bed rest and fasting for 12 h prior to drawing the plasma and their COP values ranged from 15.2 to 26.4 (mean 21.6 ± 3.6) torr. The mean difference between the supine and ambulatory subjects was highly significant at 14.8 percent. This confirmed the findings of Ladegaard-Pedersen,[30] who had previously found the COP to be 5 to 24 percent lower in patients at bed rest than in those who were ambulatory. The latter author felt that patients should be confined to bed when the sample is taken but that fasting is not necessary.

The Rationale for Measuring COP

In early reports of patients with myocardial infarction who were followed with central monitoring, pulmonary edema was said to occur when PCWPs exceeded 17 torr[17] or 22 to 25 torr.[32] In general, subsequent series reported a good correlation between the level of PCWP and the presence or absence of pulmonary edema; however, occasional patients developed pulmonary edema with lower wedge pressures, while some did not with persistently elevated values for 6 to 24 h.

In 1959 Guyton and Lindsey[21] found that dogs with normal plasma albumin levels developed pulmonary edema when left atrial pressures exceeded 24 torr. When, however, the albumin concentration was reduced by plasmaphoresis to an average of 47 percent of the control values, pulmonary edema was produced when LA pressures exceeded 11 torr. In 1974 da Luz et al.[15] used COP and PCWP measurements to define a simplified version of the net intravascular fluid filtration pressure and then compared these data with x-ray evidence of pulmonary edema in 26 patients with acute myocardial infarctions. The COP-PCWP gradient was derived by simply subtracting the pulmonary artery wedge pressure from the plasma COP. In the absence of pulmonary edema the gradient averaged 9.7 ± 1.7 torr, while in those patients who developed pulmonary edema the gradient was reduced to 1.2 ± 1.3 torr. Furthermore, only 3 of the 14 patients who developed pulmonary edema had gradients exceeding 3 torr, and none had values in excess of 9 torr. In a subsequent paper[50] investigators from the same group reported that the vigorous infusion of crystalloid fluids to treat hypovolemia could be associated with pulmonary edema in patients with no underlying heart disease and with only modest elevations in PCWP. In that study the presence of pulmonary edema in 11 patients with left ventricular filling pressures (LVFP) of 18 torr or less was associated with COP-LVFP gradients of 6 torr or less.

In normal supine individuals the COP-PCWP gradient reportedly ranges from 9 to 17 torr. The reports cited above suggest that a reduction in this gradient may be associated with the development of pulmonary edema, even at relatively low PCWP values. Other authors, however, have not been able to demonstrate such a clear-cut relationship. Virgilio et al.[57] were unable to find a correlation between decreases in COP-PCWP gradients secondary to reduced COP and increases in intrapulmonary shunting or evidence of pulmonary edema in 43 patients undergoing abdominal aortic surgery. In this series one patient had a negative gradient (−10 torr) secondary to hemodilution with crystalloid infusion (COP 8 torr) and showed no clinical or x-ray signs of pulmonary edema in spite of marked peripheral edema and weight gain. Goodlin[18] reported that in a study of 35 obstetrical patients with "edema-proteinuria-hypertension gestosis" the COP-PCWP gradient was not predictive of pulmonary edema since the value was sometimes −5 to −8 torr with no x-ray evidence of edema. Rafferty et al.[39] studied 17 consecutive patients admitted to their surgical intensive care unit following cardiothoracic, peripheral vascular, or general surgical procedures. No significant relationship between the COP-PCWP gradient and either roentgenographic evidence of pulmonary edema or percent venous admixture was found. These authors concluded that the gradient may be a poor predictor of pulmonary edema because of "the multiplicity of variables involved in its genesis."

COP During Pregnancy

Robertson and Cheyne[40] serially measured the serum COP of 83 healthy ambulatory pregnant women on 10 occasions between 12 and 38 weeks of gestation. They found that the COP fell from mean prepregnant values of 27.6 ± 2.3 torr to 22.4 ± 1.9 torr at term. A progressive decline in COP was noted until 26 weeks when a plateau was reached, which was maintained until term. Interestingly, this pattern virtually paralleled a decline in serum albumin levels, which fell from 4.04 ± 0.3 g/100 ml in the prepregnant state to 3.42 ± 0.3 g/100 ml at term.

Benedetti and Carlson[4] studied antepartum COP values in 23 normal ambulatory pregnant women when they presented in labor at term. Postpartum values were then obtained from these patients in the supine position 6 and 24 h after delivery. Mean values were 22.0 ± 0.48 torr prior to delivery and 18.2 ± 0.46 torr postpartum. The authors felt that the following three mechanisms might account for this decline in COP after delivery: patients being in the supine position for several hours, blood loss at the time of delivery, and administration of crystalloid infusions. These investigators also found that 22 women with pregnancy-induced hypertension had significantly lower COP values than controls in both the antepartum and postpartum periods. The actual values obtained are not necessarily relevant to other patients with PIH because of possible variations in fluid administration and gestational age, but it is not unreasonable to expect to find reductions in COP below normal pregnant levels in women with significant proteinuria. In one hypertensive patient in this series, pulmonary edema developed with a PCWP of 18 torr. The COP was only 13 torr at that time and the COP-PCWP gradient was consequently −5 torr. This patient was simply treated with fluid restriction and the pulmonary edema resolved within 24 h of delivery.

CONCLUSIONS

The flow-directed pulmonary artery catheters developed by Swan, Ganz and coworkers have made bedside monitoring of central hemodynamic fluctuations a reality. The low incidence of serious complications and the value of the information made available by these devices have made them an integral part of the modern management of critically ill medical and surgical patients. Their use permits rational therapeutic decisions to be made on the basis of continuously evolving objective data.

During the second half of pregnancy obstetrical patients have markedly elevated blood volumes and cardiac outputs. They also have major alterations in cardiac preload caused by positional changes of the gravid uterus relative to the inferior vena cava. Labor and especially delivery cause major increases in intravascular volume and place further demands on the heart. Postpartum fluid shifts are significant and take several days before stabilizing. When cardiac function is compromised or other factors place unacceptable burdens on the cardiovascular system, these additional stresses of pregnancy may become overwhelming. The hemodynamically unstable obstetrical patient, therefore, is an ideal candidate for accurate central monitoring, especially during labor and delivery.

Regardless of the precise accuracy of the COP-PCWP gradient as a prognosticator of pulmonary edema, there is no question that abnormally low intravascular COP values may increase the potential for pulmonary edema to occur in patients with modestly elevated pulmonary capillary hydrostatic pressure. It is therefore recommended that serial COP determinations be performed in pregnant women who are sick enough to require SG catheterization. This is particularly true of patients with significant hypoalbuminemia. Measurement of COP may help to diagnose the nature of an ongoing pathophysiologic event and may also be useful in determining the type and quantity of infusion to be administered.

Rapidly evolving knowledge concerning care of the critically ill patient has made intensive care medicine an established subspecialty. In my opinion the ideal team for the management of hemodynamically unstable obstetrical patients is a perinatologist and an intensive care unit specialist. When this type of expertise is pooled, the appropriate utilization of SG catheterization and COP determinations should help to improve survival for both the mother and the fetus. In addition, these tools may be expected to provide insight into the hemodynamic complexities accompanying some types of obstetrical disasters.

REFERENCES

1. Adams, J.Q.: Cardiovascular physiology in normal pregnancy: Studies with the dye dilution technique. Am. J. Obstet. Gynecol., *67:*741, 1954.
2. Andersen, H.F., Lynch, J.P., and Johnson, T.R.B.: Adult respiratory distress syndrome in obstetrics and gynecology. Obstet. Gynecol., *55:*291, 1980.
3. Barash, P.G., Nardi, D., Hammond, G. et al.: Catheter-induced pulmonary artery perforation: Mechanisms, management, and modifications. J. Thorac. Cardiovasc. Surg. *82:*5, 1981.
4. Benedetti, T.J., and Carlson, R.W.: Studies of colloid osmotic pressure in pregnancy-induced hypertension. Am. J. Obstet. Gynecol. *135:*308, 1979.
5. Benedetti, T.J., Cotton, D.B., Read, J.C., and Miller, F.C.: Hemodynamic observations in severe preeclampsia with a flow-directed pulmonary artery catheter, Am. J. Obstet. Gynecol. *136:*465, 1980.
6. Berkowitz, R.L and Rafferty, T.D.: Invasive hemodynamic monitoring in critically ill pregnant patients: Role of Swan-Ganz catheterization. Am. J. Obstet. Gynecol. *137:*127, 1980.
7. Berkowitz, R.L. and Rafferty, T.D.: Pulmonary artery flow-directed catheter use in the obstetric patient. Obstet. Gynecol., *55:*507, 1980.
8. Boothby, W.M. and Sandiford, R.B.: Nomographic charts for the calculation of the metabolic rate by the gasometer method. Boston Med. Surg. J. *185:*337, 1921.
9. Buchbinder, N. and Ganz, W.: Hemodynamic monitoring: invasive techniques. Anesthesiology, *45*(2):146, 1976.
10. Burwell, C.S., Strayhorn, W.D., Flickinger, D. et al.: Circulation during pregnancy. Arch. Intern. Med. *62:*979, 1938.
11. Chastre, J., Cornud, F., Bouchama, A., et al.: Thrombosis as a complication of pulmonary-artery catheterization via the internal jugular vein. N. Engl. J. Med. *306:*278, 1982.

12. Cotton, D.B. and Benedetti, T.J.: Use of the Swan-Ganz catheter in obstetrics and gynecology. Obstet. Gynecol., *56:*641, 1980.
13. Cotton, D.B., Bernstein, S.G., Read, J.A. et al.: Hemodynamic observations in evacuation of molar pregnancy. Am. J. Obstet. Gynecol. *138:*6, 1980.
14. Dalen, J.E.: Bedside hemodynamic monitoring (editorial). N. Engl. J. Med., *301:*1176, 1979.
15. da Luz, P. L., Shubin, H., Weil, M. H. et al.: Pulmonary edema related to changed in colloid osmotic and pulmonary artery wedge pressure in patients after acute myocardial infarction. Circulation, *51:*350, 1975.
16. De Laurentis, D.A., Hayes, M., Matsumoto, T., and Wolferth, C.C.: Does central venous pressure accurately reflect hemodynamic and fluid volume patterns in the critical surgical patient? Am. J. Surg., *126:*415, 1973.
17. Forrester, J.S., Diamond, G., McHugh, T.J., and Swan, J.J.: Filling pressures in the right and left sides of the heart in acute myocardial infarction. A reappraisal of central-venous pressure monitoring. N. Engl. J. Med., *285:*190, 1971.
18. Goodlin, R.C.: Pulmonary edema in pregnant patients treated for hypertension (Letter to the editor). Am. J. Obstet. Gynecol., *136:*1087, 1980.
19. Greene, J.F., Fitzwater, J.E., and Clemmer, T.P.: Septic endocarditis and indwelling pulmonary artery catheters. JAMA *233:*891, 1975.
20. Grollman, A.: The Cardiac Output of Man in Health and Disease. Bailliere, Tindall and Cox, London, 1932.
21. Guyton, A.C. and Lindsey, A.W.: Effect of elevated left atrial pressure and decreased plasma protein concentration on the development of pulmonary edema. Circ. Res., *1:*649, 1959.
22. Hamilton, H.F.H.: The cardiac output in normal pregnancy. J. Obstet. Gynaecol. Br. Empire, 56:548, 1949.
23. Helmkamp, B.F., Civetta, J.M., Girtanner, R. et al.: The Swan-Ganz catheter and its application in the gynecologic patient. Am. J. Obstet. Gynecol., *139:* 628, 1981.
24. Hendricks, C.H. and Quilligan, E.J.: Cardiac output during labor. Am. J. Obstet. Gynecol., *71:*953, 1956.
25. Holub, D.A., Fugua, J.M., Igo, S.R. et al.: Utilization of hand-held programmable calculators for rapid bedside computation of physiologic-pharmacologic variables and prognostic indices during mechanical circulatory support. Cardiovasc. Dis. Bull., Tex. Heart Inst., 5:271, 1978.
26. Katz, J.D., Cronau, L.H., Barash, P.G., and Mandel, S.D.: Pulmonary artery flow-guided catheters in the perioperative period. JAMA, *237:*2832, 1977.
27. Keefer, J.R., Strauss, R.G., Civetta, J.M., and Burke, T.: Noncardiogenic pulmonary edema and invasive cardiovascular monitoring. Obstet. Gynecol., *58:*46, 1981.
28. Kerr, M.G.: Maternal cardiovascular adjustments in pregnancy and labor. p. 395. In: Goodwin, J.W., Godden, J.O., and Chance, G.W., Eds.: Perinatal Medicine. William & Wilkins, Baltimore, 1976.
29. Kerr, M.G.: Cardiovascular dynamics in pregnancy and labour. Br. Med. Bull., *24:*19, 1968.
30. Ladegaard-Pedersen, H.J.: Measurement of the colloid osmotic pressure in patients. Scand. J. Clin. Lab. Invest., *20:*79, 1967.
31. Lappas, D., Lell, W.A., Gabel, J.C. et al.: Indirect measurement of left-atrial pressure in surgical patients—pulmonary-capillary wedge and pulmonary-artery diastolic pressures compared with left-atrial pressure. Anesthesiology, *38:*394, 1973.
32. McHugh, T.J., Forrester, J.S., Adler, L. et al.: Pulmonary congestion in acute myocardial infarction: Hemodynamic and radiologic correlations. Ann. Intern. Med., *76:*29, 1972.

33. Metcalfe, J. and Ueland, K.: Maternal cardiovascular adjustments to pregnancy. Prog. Cardiovasc. Dis., *16*:363, 1974.
34. Morissette, M.P.: Colloid osmotic pressure: its measurement and clinical value. Can. Med. Assoc., J. *116*:897, 1977.
35. O'Toole, J.D., Wurtzbacher, J.J., Wearner, N.E., and Jain, A.C.: Pulmonary valve injury and insufficiency during pulmonary-artery catheterization. N. Engl. J. Med., *301*:1167, 1979.
36. Pace, N.L.: A critique of flow-directed pulmonary arterial catherization. Anesthesiology, *47*:455, 1977.
37. Rafferty, T.R. and Berkowitz, R.L.: Complications of pulmonary artery catheterization in obstetric patients. Int. J. Gynaecol. Obstet., *18*:133, 1980.
38. Rafferty, T.D. and Berkowitz, R.L.: Hemodynamics in patients with severe toxemia during labor and delivery. Am. J. Obstet. Gynecol., *138*:263, 1980.
39. Rafferty, T.D., Ljungquist, R., Firestone, L. et al.: The plasma colloid oncotic pressure–pulmonary artery occlusion pressure gradient—a poor predictor of pulmonary edema in surgical intensive care unit patients. Arch. Surg. (in press).
40. Robertson, E.G. and Cheyne, G.A.: Plasma biochemistry in relation to oedema of pregnancy. J. Obstet. Gynaecol. Br. Commonw., *79*:769, 1972.
41. Ross, J., Jr. and Braunwald, E.: The study of left ventricular function in man by increasing resistance to ventricular ejection with angiotensin. Circulation, *29*:739, 1964.
42. Rovinsky, J.J. and Jaffin, H.: Cardiovascular hemodynamics in pregnancy. I. Blood and plasma volumes in multiple pregnancy. Am. J. Obstet. Gynecol., *93*:1, 1965.
43. Sarnoff, S.J. and Berglund, E.: Ventricular function. I. Starling's law of the heart studied by means of simultaneous right and left ventricular function curves in the dog. Circulation, *9*:706, 1954.
44. Scheinman, M.M., Brown, M.A., and Rapaport, E.: Critical assessment of use of central venous oxygen saturation as a mirror of mixed venous oxygen in severely ill cardiac patients. Circulation, *40*:165, 1969.
45. Schroeder, J.S. and Daily, E.K.: Techniques in Bedside Hemodynamic Monitoring. The C.V. Mosby Co., St. Louis, 1976.
46. Sprung, C.L., Jacobs, L.J., Caralis, P.V., and Karpf, M.: Hazards of pulmonary-artery catheterization (letter to the editor). N. Engl. J. Med., *302*:807, 1980.
47. Stander, H.J. and Cadden, J.F.: The cardiac output in pregnant women. Am. J. Obstet. Gynecol., *24*:13, 1932.
48. Starling, E.H.: The Linacre lecture on the law of the heart, Cambridge, 1915; Longmans Green and Co., London, 1918.
49. Staub, N.C.: Pulmonary edema—Physiologic approaches to management. Chest, *74*:5, 1978.
50. Stein, L., Beraud, J.J., Morissette, M. et al.: Pulmonary edema during volume infusion. Circulation, *52*:483, 1975.
51. Stevens, P.M.: Assessment of acute respiratory failure: cardiac versus pulmonary causes (editorial). Chest, *67*:1, 1975.
52. Stevens, P.M., Friedman, G.K., and Nicotra, M.B.: The value of flow directed intravascular catheters in cardiorespiratory failure. Am. Rev. Respir. Dis., *107*:1111, 1973.
53. Strauss, R.G., Keefer, R., Burke, T., and Civetta, J.M.: Hemodynamic monitoring of cardiac pulmonary edema complicating toxemia of pregnancy. Obstet. Gynecol., *55*:170, 1980.
54. Swan, H.J.C.: The role of hemodynamic monitoring in the management of the critically ill. Crit. Care Med., *3*:83, 1975.
55. Swan, H.J.C., Ganz, W., Forrester, J. et al.: Catheterization of the heart in man with use of a flow-directed balloon-tipped catheter. N. Engl. J. Med., *283*:447, 1970.

56. Toussaint, G.P.M., Burgess, J.H., and Hampson, L.G.: Central venous pressure and pulmonary wedge pressure in critical surgical illness. Arch. Surg., *109*:265, 1974.
57. Virgilio, R.W., Smith, D.E., Rice, C.L. et al.: Effect of colloid osmotic pressure and pulmonary capillary wedge pressure on intrapulmonary shunt. Surg. Forum, *27*:168, 1976.
58. Weil, M.H., Morissette, M., Michaels, S. et al.: Routine plasma colloid pressure measurements. Crit. Care Med., *2*:229, 1974.
59. Winner, W., and Romney, S.L.: Cardiovascular responses to labor and delivery. Am. J. Obstet. Gynecol., *95*:1104, 1966.

2

Ventilator Therapy and Care of the Patient with ARDS

Terence D. Rafferty, M.D.
Michael S. Niederman, M.D.

Respiratory distress syndrome is a well-known fetal complication of pregnancy. In 1967, Ashbaugh, Bigelow, and Petty described an adult disease "remarkably similar to the infantile respiratory distress syndrome" which they termed adult respiratory distress syndrome (ARDS).[5]

This syndrome is a clinical pathophysiologic consequence of a variety of acute lung injuries occurring in both obstetric and nonobstetric patients with previously normal lungs. Clinically, patients present with marked respiratory distress, tachypnea, hypoxemia refractory to oxygen therapy, "stiff" lungs that require high pressures to achieve inflation, and diffuse interstitial and alveolar infiltrates on chest radiograph.[51] This "final common pathway" of pulmonary response results from a direct injury to the alveolar-capillary membrane or from damage to this membrane via mediators delivered by the pulmonary vasculature. Generally, the injury is an acute catastrophic event such as massive aspiration, trauma, or circulatory shock. In making the diagnosis of ARDS, chronic pulmonary disease and left heart failure must be excluded. The physiologic abnormalities of ARDS are in part responsible for its high mortality of approximately 50 percent.[18] These abnormalities include severe hypoxemia resulting from both increased shunting of unoxygenated blood and impaired ventilation and perfusion matching in the alveoli. These features are summarized in Table 2-1.[50]

Table 2-1. Criteria for Diagnosing Adult Respiratory Distress Syndrome

A. Clinical setting
   1. Catastrophic event
      a. Pulmonary
      b. Nonpulmonary, e.g., shock
   2. Exclusions
      a. Chronic pulmonary disease
      b. Left heart abnormalities
   3. Respiratory distress (judged clinically)
      a. Tachypnea > 20, usually greater
      b. Labored breathing
B. X-ray: diffuse pulmonary infiltrates
   1. Interstitial (initially)
   2. Alveolar (later)
C. Physiologic
   1. $PAO_2 < 50$ with $FIO_2 > 0.6$
   2. Overall compliance < 50 cc/cm—usually 20 to 30 cc/cm
   3. Increased shunt fraction $\dot{Q}S/\dot{Q}T$ and deadspace ventilation $\dot{V}D/\dot{V}T$
D. Pathologic
   1. Heavy lungs, usually > 1000 g
   2. Congestive atelectasis
   3. Hyaline membranes
   4. Fibrosis

Reprinted from Bone, RC (ed): Clinics in Chest Medicine. Vol. 3. Philadelphia, W. B. Saunders, 1982, p. 5.

PATHOLOGY

Injury to the alveolar capillary membrane (shown in Fig. 2-1) results in increased endothelial cell permeability and noncardiogenic pulmonary edema.[50,51] This capillary leak is the earliest finding in ARDS and results in the accumulation of protein-rich fluid in the extravascular space of the lung.[22] Initially fluid appears in the interstitium, but then it floods the alveolar sacs. Alveolar type I epithelial cells are injured, the alveolar basement membrane is denuded, and the alveolar space fills with red blood cells, leukocytes, macrophages, and cell debris. Damage to the epithelium results in loss of surfactant and alveolar collapse. Early hyaline membranes composed of protein, fibrin, and cellular debris can be seen.[6] Morphologically, epithelial cell injury is more obvious than endothelial cell injury, although the presence of increased capillary permeability points to the endothelial injury which must be present.[22,6] After 24 to 96 h, the early exudative phase of injury is followed by a cellular proliferative phase, with repopulation of the alveolar basement membrane by alveolar type 2 cells (Fig. 2-2). The hyaline membrane begins to organize, and morphologic evidence of endothelial injury is more obvious.[6] This phase is present from the third to the tenth day and is then followed by a fibrotic proliferative phase as the hyaline membranes undergo fibrosis. Patients may not enter these more advanced stages of injury if their disease resolves rapidly. However, even after reaching a fibrotic stage, resolution and repair of alveolar injury can occur.[6,18]

The physiologic consequences of this injury pattern can best be understood by

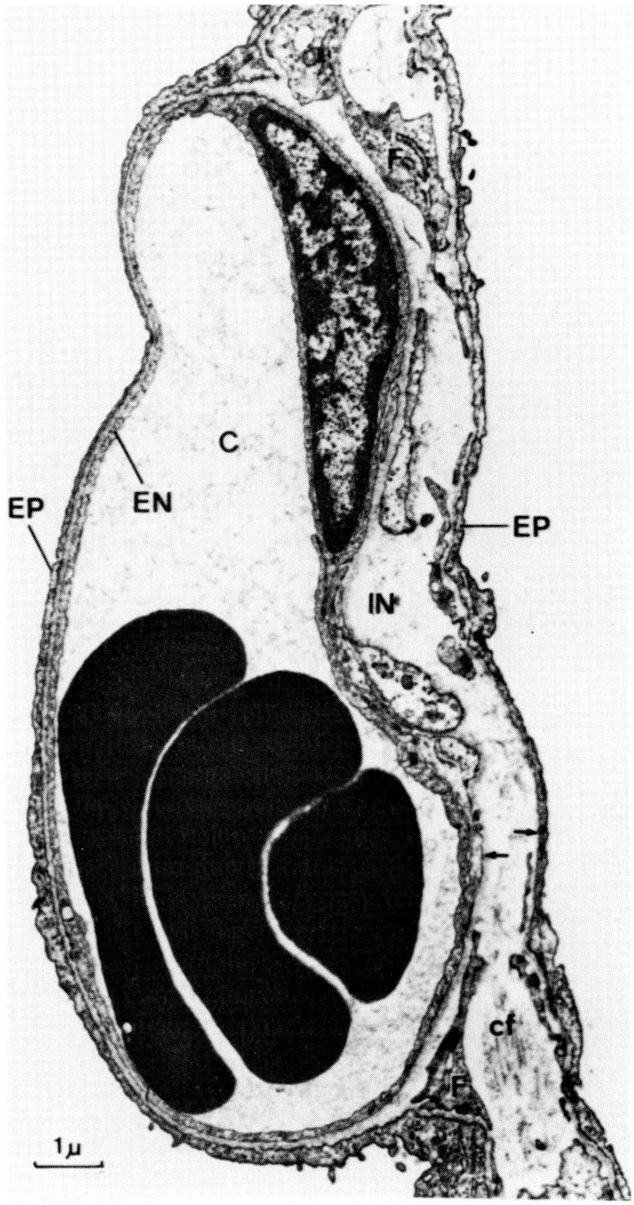

Fig. 2-1 Transmission electron micrograph of the alveolar capillary membrane in the human lung. In part of the interface alveolar epithelial cells (EP) are fused with capillary endothelial cells (EN) and the interstitial space is absent. In other areas a free interstitial space (IN and arrows) is present and contains connective tissue fibers (cf). (Reprinted with permission from Fishman, A.P. and Renkin, E.M., Pulmonary Edema, American Physiological Society, Bethesda, Md., 1979.)

keeping the pathologic picture in mind. Increased capillary permeability leads to exudation of protein-rich fluid into the alveoli. Suction of airway secretions from patients with ARDS produces fluid with a high protein content, and as this fluid fills the alveoli, it contributes to the hypoxemia commonly seen.[22] Alveolar epithelial injury and loss of surfactant leads to alveolar collapse and consequently perfusion of nonventilated alveoli. Shunting of this unoxygenated blood through the lung then

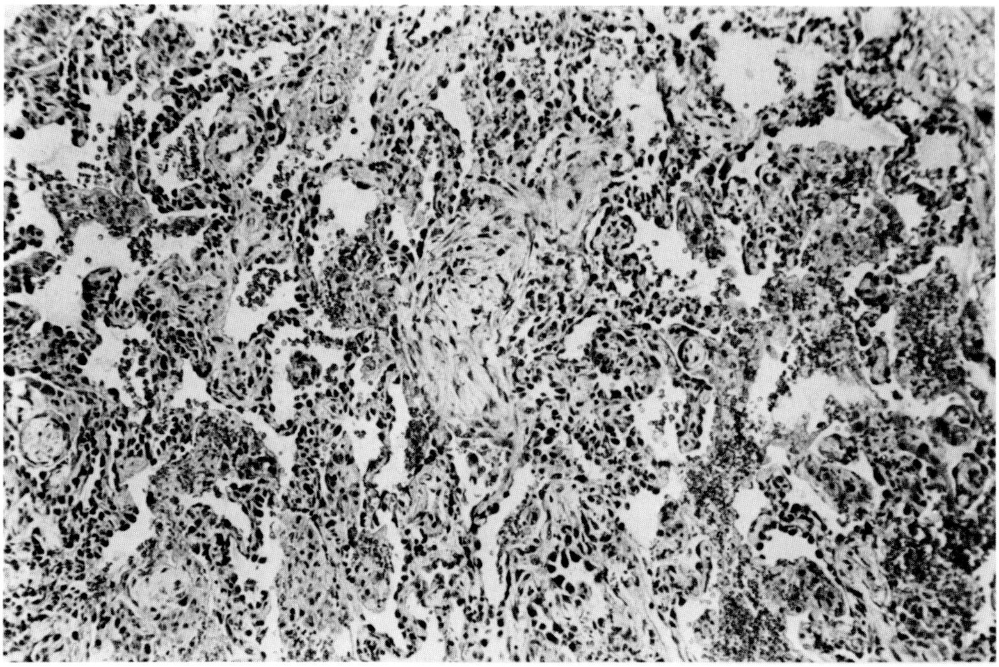

Fig. 2-2 Lung biopsy specimen from a patient with adult respiratory distress syndrome (100 × magnification). This section shows features of both cellular proliferative and fibrotic proliferative phases. Alveolar walls are thickened and infiltrated with inflammatory cells. At 5 o'clock in the lower portion of the slide, hyperplastic type 2 cells (dark nuclei— are repopulating an alveolus. At 2 o'clock and in the right-hand corner of this section, alveoli filled with proteinaceous exudate are evident. In the center of this section, an early fibrotic pattern is present. (Micrograph courtesy of G.J. Walker Smith, Department of Pathology, Yale University School of Medicine.)

results in hypoxemia. Some evidence also suggests that the injured pulmonary vascular bed is unable to constrict in response to local alveolar hypoxia, and this loss of hypoxic vasoconstriction accentuates any existing shunt effect.[47] The pulmonary inflammatory response can also lead to airway injury and thus an increase in the resistance to air flow. In addition, the lung becomes "stiff" and pulmonary compliance, defined as the change in lung volume achieved by an applied transpulmonary pressure, has been shown to be reduced when autopsy specimens from patients dying of ARDS are studied.[52] These changes in airway resistance and lung compliance lead to an inhomogenous distribution of alveolar gas, and further mismatching of pulmonary ventilation and perfusion can result.

In one study, the pathologic findings of ARDS correlated with the patient's physiologic abnormalities.[39] In that study patients with minimal alveolar edema, exudate, and hyaline membrane formation with intact and open alveoli had the best oxygenation. Those with only fibrosis were more hypoxemic, and the most severely hypoxemia patients were those with marked alveolar edema, exudation, intra-alveolar hemorrhage, and consolidation.

ETIOLOGY

The list of diseases that can cause ARDS is continually expanding. One such list appears in Table 2-2. The value of "lumping" such a variety of diseases together lies in common management features for all cases of ARDS, and similarities of disease mechanisms in many instances. However, this lumping should never deter the physician from searching for the specific inciting factor in each patient. If this initiating factor is detected, it can often be treated, and such specific therapy may prevent further pulmonary injury.

As described in the pregnant patient ARDS can be associated with many of the factors that complicate pregnancy and delivery. These include septicemia, amniotic fluid embolism, aspiration of gastric contents, eclampsia, intra-abdominal sepsis, septic abortion, air embolism, abruptio placenta, blood transfusion (with white cell agglutination in the pulmonary circulation), dead fetus syndrome (with disseminated intravascular coagulation), drug overdose (narcotics, barbiturates, aspirin), fat embolism (after long bone fracture), hemorrhagic shock, seizures, and certain forms of pulmonary infection.[3,33] In the pregnant patient with ARDS, undiagnosed sepsis and aspiration pneumonitis must be ruled out because both of these conditions may benefit from early institution of steroid therapy.[58,75]

The incidence of ARDS in pregnancy is unknown, but in one general hospital respiratory care unit 9.5 percent of patients carried this diagnosis, and it is estimated that at least 150,000 cases occur annually in the United States.[11]

Table 2-2. Disorders Associated with (Causing) Adult Respiratory Distress Syndrome

Blood-borne or Vascular Source of Injury	
*Trauma	Drug overdoses
*Sepsis	heroin, methadone
Fat embolism	ethchlorvynol, acetylsalicyclic acid, propoxyphene
Pancreatitis	Drug idiosyncratic reaction
Shock	Thrombotic thrombocytopenic purpura
Multiple transfusions	Leukemia
microemboli	Venous air embolism
leukoagglutinin reaction	Head injury
Disseminated intravascular coagulation	Paraquat
Surface burns	Cardiopulmonary bypass/hemodialysis
Miliary tuberculosis	
Inhalation of Airway Source	**Direct or Physical Source**
*Aspiration of gastric contents	Lung contusion
*Diffuse infectious pneumonia	Radiation
viral, mycoplasma,	High altitude
Legionnaires', pneumocystis	Hanging
*Near-drowning	Reexpansion
Irritant gas inhalation	
NO_2, Cl_2, SO_2, NH_3	
Smoke inhalation	
O_2 toxicity	

* common cause of ARDS

From Bone, RC (ed): Clinics in Chest Medicine. Vol. 3. Philadelphia, W. B. Saunders, 1982. p. 196.

Mechanisms of Lung Injury

By activating similar inflammatory pathways, multiple seemingly unrelated catastrophic events may lead to ARDS. With an understanding of these pathways, the physician can often anticipate clinical situations in which this disease complication can occur. Such an awareness may allow early diagnosis and appropriate therapy of the life-threatening hypoxemia that is so deleterious to fetal and maternal well-being.

Although all the mediators of this syndrome are not known, observations in humans and animals have supported a role for certain specific agents. Because components of the complement system can be activated by the same types of etiologic events leading to ARDS, their role has been investigated.[31] The C5a component of activated complement can lead to leukocyte aggregation and stasis, and several investigators have hypothesized that complement-mediated leukostasis could play a role in lung injury. They proposed that a systemic insult might lead to C5a generation and leukocyte aggregation. Since the pulmonary vasculature is the first filtration bed for aggregated leukocytes, the stasis would be evident at that site. The many toxic products of activated leukocytes could then initiate pulmonary endothelial and epithelial cell injury. In support of this concept, Hammerschmidt found C5a activity to be elevated in a small subset of patients at risk to develop ARDS. When followed prospectively, those with elevated C5a levels often did develop ARDS.[31]

Activated granulocytes may cause lung injury by releasing superoxide and other free radicals along with lysosomal products. Neutrophilic proteases not only can destroy lung tissue, but they may cleave other inflammatory mediators into an activated form and amplify the lung injury already present. Leukocyte-derived elastase, a destructive protease which may cause emphysema, has been detected in the lung lavage fluid of ARDS patients, which supports a role for leukocyte products in causing lung injury.[41] In addition, leukocytes may produce arachidonic acid metabolites, which can mediate the inflammatory process themselves.

In addition, ARDS can be associated with a wide variety of coagulopathies, which in turn may contribute to the lung injury. Thrombocytopenia caused by a decreased platelet survival time, platelet aggregation, and disseminated intravascular coagulation is a common concomitant of the disease[55] and can result in a bleeding diathesis. Conversely, disseminated intravascular coagulation can lead to widespread pulmonary vascular thromboses in as many as 48 percent of ARDS patients.[55]

The products of arachidonic acid metabolism have been studied in animal models of ARDS, but their role in human disease is unknown. Arachidonic acid, present in cell-membrane phospholipids, may be released with cell injury. This substance can then be converted to cyclooxygenase or lipoxygenase prostaglandin metabolites. The cyclooxygenase products include prostacycline and thromboxane. In one animal study endotoxin induced a vasodilator, possibly prostacycline, which blocked hypoxic pulmonary artery vasoconstriction.[73] This effect could permit continued pulmonary artery blood flow to poorly oxygenated alveoli and contribute to the hypoxemia of ARDS. In the experimental animal, cyclooxygenase inhibitors prevented the loss of hypoxic vasoconstriction. The thromboxane cyclooxygenase products in turn may lead to airway narrowing and leukocyte stasis, both of which could result in abnormalities of gas exchange.[8,73] The lipoxygenase products of arachidonic acid metabolism may also be important because they can attract leukocytes to the ARDS lung, and this may mediate further injury.

The action of these mediators could well explain the pathophysiologic events in ARDS. They can cause endothelial cell injury and increased vascular permeability; altered vascular reactivity (either excessive vasoconstriction or inappropriate local vasodilation in hypoxic lung regions); and altered airway function with increased airway resistance. These defects can account not only for the pathologic features which are present but also, as will be described, the gas exchange abnormalities that are the hallmark of ARDS.

In addition, the proposed disease mechanisms have several therapeutic implications.[55] Corticosteroids may inhibit complement-induced granulocyte aggregation and prostaglandin synthesis. Oxygen therapy may add to further superoxide radical–mediated lung injury, thus emphasizing the need to improve gas transport by means other than high oxygen concentrations alone. Positive end-expiratory airway pressure (PEEP) not only can reduce the oxygen concentration required for successful therapy but also may partially prevent the surfactant defect observed in this syndrome.[76]

Physiology of Gas Exchange

The impairment of arterial oxygenation that accompanies ARDS can result in dysfunction of nonrespiratory organs by causing a reduction in tissue oxygen delivery. It is this factor, tissue oxygen delivery, which must be kept in mind when considering the gas exchange abnormalities in ARDS.

Oxygen delivery can be calculated as follows:

$$\begin{aligned}\text{Oxygen delivery (ml/min)} &= \text{cardiac output (ml/min)}\\ &\quad \times \text{hemoglobin (g)} \times 1.34 \text{ ml oxygen}\\ &\quad \times \text{percent arterial oxygen saturation}\end{aligned}$$

This equation shows that the delivery of oxygen is determined not only by arterial oxygen saturation but also by cardiac output and hemoglobin concentration. This is especially important because often these nonrespiratory factors can be manipulated in patients when severe lung injury precludes adequate arterial oxygenation.

The impaired arterial oxygenation present in ARDS may be due to several factors. As has been described, extravascular lung water increases owing to endothelial and epithelial cell injury. This fluid first accumulates in the connective tissue around the airways and pulmonary arteries and then spreads to the interstitial space and finally the alveolar space. In animal studies[48] gas exchange has been found to be impaired only when alveolar flooding occurs. If fluid fills the alveoli, they cannot be ventilated and such alveoli have a ventilation/perfusion ($\dot{V}/\dot{Q}$) ratio of zero. As a result, the blood that flows past these alveolar capillary membranes is not oxygenated and when it is mixed with oxygenated blood in the left atrium, the final arterial oxygen content is lowered. Blood that has gone past flooded alveoli is in effect shunted from the right side of the heart to the left (as would occur in congenital cyanotic heart disease through cardiac shunt pathways). Such a shunt cannot be eliminated by changing the inspired oxygen concentration because even if oxygen tension in the lung increases, flooded alveoli will not be affected by the increase and desaturated blood will continue to enter the left atrium. If the nonshunted blood is already greater than 90 percent saturated, increasing alveolar oxygen will not greatly improve the oxygen content of this blood either (Fig. 2-3).

A patient's shunt fraction ($\dot{Q}s/\dot{Q}T$) can be calculated by using the method described in Appendix 1.[23] Although these calculations allow the physician to estimate the extent of a shunt, they do not indicate how nonrespiratory variables affect it. In both animal and human studies, calculated shunt fraction may decrease with decreases in cardiac output and increase with increases in that parameter.[43] These studies have suggested that shunt vessels undergo a greater change in flow when cardiac output changes than do nonshunt vessels. Thus, if the shunt calculation demonstrates a patient to have a decreased shunt, this may mean a deterioration in cardiac output and not an improvement in lung function. For this reason, shunt fractions are best evaluated in association with a knowledge of cardiac function.

Although shunt fraction may decrease as cardiac output falls, arterial oxygenation often does not improve in this situation. To understand this observation, one must consider the concept of mixed venous oxygenation (MVO_2).[70] Referring to the equation for oxygen delivery, it can be seen that if cardiac output falls, tissue oxygen delivery declines. The tissues must then extract more oxygen from the blood that reaches them, and this decreases the whole body's MVO_2. If MVO_2 decreases, any shunted blood that enters the left atrium will do so with a lower oxygen content than if cardiac output and MVO_2 were normal. Therefore, if a decline in MVO_2 occurs in a patient with a large shunt fraction, arterial oxygenation (PaO_2) may deteriorate. In this case, the arterial oxygen content decreases because of a nonrespiratory factor

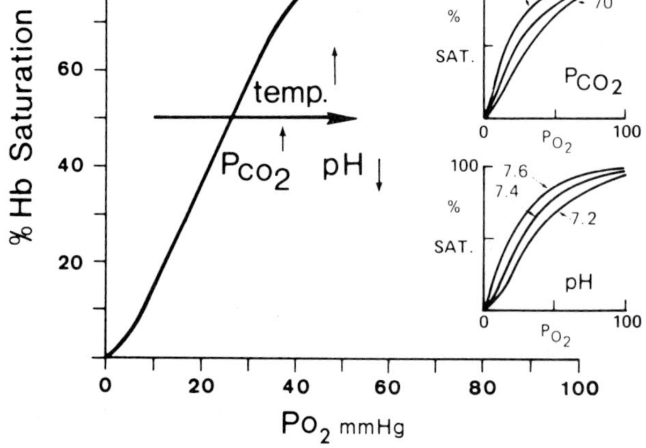

Fig. 2-3 The oxyhemoglobin dissociation curve can be used to measure the saturation of hemoglobin (in percent) for any oxygen tension (in millimeters of mercury). As shown, pH, temperature, and PCO_2 can shift the position of the curve and must be accounted for when estimating hemoglobin saturation. (Reprinted with permission from West, J.B., Respiratory Physiology—the Essentials, Williams & Wilkins, Baltimore, 1974. © 1974 The Williams & Wilkins Co., Baltimore.)

even though the calculated shunt fraction appears to improve as the cardiac output falls.

Similarly, a decrease in hemoglobin may reduce oxygen delivery and PaO_2 without directly changing respiratory function. Again, the tissues will try to extract more oxygen from the anemic blood that reaches them, decreasing MVO_2. With a reduction in MVO_2, arterial oxygenation may decline if the patient has a fixed intrapulmonary shunt.

Since MVO_2 is a measure of oxygen extraction by the tissues, it can be useful in the management of patients with ARDS. Mixed venous blood can be obtained by slowly withdrawing pulmonary artery blood from the distal tip of a Swan-Ganz catheter. A low MVO_2 implies that the delivery of oxygen to the tissues is inadequate for the patient's needs. In one study, all those who survived ARDS had either an initial MVO_2 greater than 30 mmHg or responded to therapy by increasing MVO_2 above 30 mmHg.[66] All those who did not survive had an MVO_2 less than 30 mmHg in spite of therapy. While some authors have suggested that MVO_2 is a good indicator of overall tissue oxygenation, this point is controversial.[14] The conclusion to be reached from these considerations, however, is that a low MVO_2 (less than 30 mmHg) may signify a poor prognosis and impaired tissue oxygenation. A normal MVO_2 does not eliminate the possibility of inadequate tissue delivery of oxygen, because in the face of severe illness the body may be unable to adequately extract oxygen from the blood and reduce MVO_2.[14]

While shunt is certainly the major factor in causing impaired arterial oxygenation in ARDS, other abnormalities may also be important. Dantzker has demonstrated that in addition to shunt (with a $\dot{V}/\dot{Q}$ ratio of zero), as many as 40 percent of patients with ARDS also have lung units with some ventilation but with perfusion far in excess of this ventilation.[15] These lung units have a low $\dot{V}/\dot{Q}$ ratio but it is not zero. Such lung units also contribute to hypoxemia in much the same way that shunt does. However, the existence of these low ventilation/perfusion ratio lung units is important to recognize because, unlike pure shunt alveoli, these units can accommodate gas during some phase of the respiratory cycle. This becomes clinically relevant because as inspired oxygen tension increases, low-$\dot{V}/\dot{Q}$ alveoli can accept oxygen and can then lead to an increase in PaO_2. This increase in PaO_2 with increases in inspired oxygen fraction (F_{IO_2}), which has been observed in some ARDS patients,[39] would not occur if only shunt was present.

Alveolar units with low $\dot{V}/\dot{Q}$ ratios may result from the reduced compliance of the ARDS lung.[9] The lung volume at the end of expiration, functional residual capacity (FRC), is normally larger than the volume at which alveoli begin to collapse, closing volume (CV). During pregnancy, especially in the supine position, the diaphragmatic elevation caused by the gravid uterus may reduce FRC below CV.[26] In ARDS, the reduced compliance of the lung also leads to a reduction in FRC below CV, and pregnancy may further accentuate this abnormality. Thus, at the end of any expiratory maneuver, the lungs are at a volume less than CV, and alveoli collapse. However, during inspiration, if these alveoli are not flooded, they may open and allow some gas exchange to occur. Such alveoli are not shunt units, but rather are low $\dot{V}/\dot{Q}$ units. In experimental models[8] airway resistance may increase in ARDS, and this may further contribute to $\dot{V}/\dot{Q}$ mismatching and hypoxemia. Some authors[34] have also suggested the possibility that gas exchange abnormalities result from interstitial edema blocking gas diffusion into the blood, but this view is not widely accepted.

Thus, because of altered elastic properties of the ARDS lung and because of alveolar flooding, $\dot{V}/\dot{Q}$ mismatching and shunt can occur and lead to inadequate arterial oxygenation. When oxygenation is considered along with cardiac output and hemoglobin concentration, tissue oxygen delivery can be calculated and the potential effect of lung injury on other organs considered. While an MVO_2 less than 30 mmHg suggests impaired oxygen delivery to tissues and a poor prognosis, the value of serial studies of MVO_2 is at present unknown.

DIAGNOSIS

The clinical features of ARDS have been summarized in Table 2-1 and provide the framework for disease definition and diagnosis. In the proper clinical setting in the absence of left ventricular failure or prior pulmonary disease, the diagnosis can be made in a patient with respiratory distress and refractory hypoxemia. Refractory hypoxemia is defined by Petty as an arterial oxygen tension less than 50 mmHg measured with the patient inhaling at least 60 percent oxygen.[50] The compliance of the lung and chest wall combined is calculated by dividing the tidal volume by the change in ventilator airway pressure required to deliver this volume (peak airway

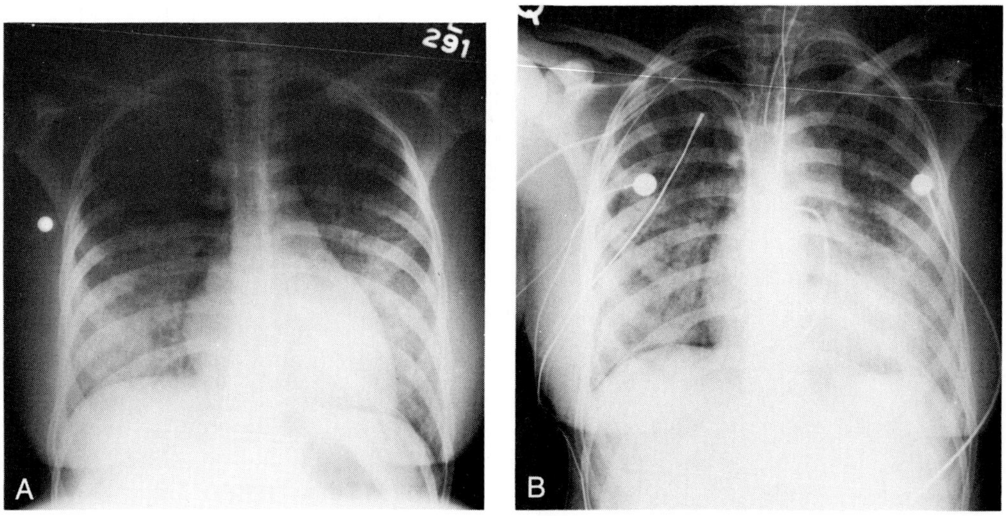

Fig. 2-4 Chest radiographs of an 18-year old female who developed adult respiratory distress syndrome in the immediate postpartum period. Figure 2-4*a* shows bilateral patchy and interstitial densities. Several days later (Fig. 2-4*b*), the infiltrates are more marked in spite of therapy with PEEP. Also visible in Fig. 2-4*b* is an endotracheal tube, a right-sided chest tube, and a pulmonary artery (Swan-Ganz) catheter. A persistent right pneumothorax is also evident and the patient required multiple simultaneous chest tubes. After a protracted course the patient recovered from this illness.

pressure minus PEEP). In ARDS, this value is reduced to less than 30 cc/cmH_2O. When calculated, $\dot{Q}s/\dot{Q}t$ usually exceeds 20 percent.

Chest radiography (Fig. 2-4) can support the clinical diagnosis of ARDS but the radiograph may be normal when the insult occurs. Then a fine reticular or interstitial pattern may appear, followed in 12 to 24 h by patchy, ill-defined nodular densities and then a patchy confluent consolidation.[49] Later, as the disease persists for days or weeks, a diffuse interstitial fibrotic pattern may develop. When therapeutic PEEP is instituted, the radiograph can remain unchanged or may appear to improve.[2] However, when PEEP is discontinued, the infiltrates again become more evident.

THERAPY

Mechanical Ventilation and PEEP

Hypoxemia that is unresponsive to oxygen supplementation is the primary manifestation of ARDS and can be improved by mechanical ventilation. The conventional ventilator delivers intermittent positive-pressure ventilation (IPPV) with large tidal volumes (10 to 15 cc/kg) and can expand collapsed areas of the lungs during inspiration, allowing gas exchange to occur. During expiration, airway pressure falls to atmospheric level and airway and alveolar collapse occurs. Expiratory collapse is a particular problem in ARDS but can be ameliorated by the application of PEEP.

Application of PEEP is the cornerstone of therapy in ARDS and can be accomplished with a conventional ventilator by adding a resistance to expiratory air flow. It can open collapsed alveoli and thus improve ventilation-perfusion relationships. By recruiting alveoli, PEEP makes the lung easier to expand, and this increase in compliance allows FRC to increase above CV. The sum of these effects is an improvement in oxygenation and a decrease in $\dot{Q}s/\dot{Q}t$.[25] However, high levels of PEEP can overdistend the lung and reduce compliance.[69]

Most patients who have ARDS and increases in $\dot{Q}s/\dot{Q}t$ will respond to incremental levels of PEEP with increases in PaO_2.[25] However, there is a limit to this beneficial effect. As the level of PEEP increases, mean intrathoracic pressure also increases, and this may impede venous return and cause a decrease in cardiac index. Depending on the patient's preexisting intravascular volume status and ventricular function, a situation may arise in which the increase in PaO_2 is offset by a decrease in cardiac index sufficient to decrease oxygen delivery to the tissues. Suter et al.[68] have proposed that the optimal or "best" PEEP is that level associated with maximal oxygen delivery (arterial oxygen content × cardiac index). Therefore, some essential cardiovascular and respiratory variables must be known in order to determine optimum ventilator management. These investigators have also shown that when measurements of cardiac output or of mixed venous oxygen tension are not available, compliance may be used to help select the end-expiratory pressure most likely to result in optimal cardiopulmonary function. As levels of PEEP were changed, the best PEEP was associated with maximal compliance of the respiratory system. To utilize this principle at the bedside, the tidal volume is maintained at a constant level and PEEP is increased by increments of 5 cmH_2O. Compliance is then calculated as tidal volume divided by the effective peak airway pressure (peak airway pressure minus PEEP).

In selected patients, PEEP may actually improve ventricular function. This is achieved by multiple effects on the cardiovascular system, most notably a reduction in pulmonary and systemic vascular resistances (right and left ventricular afterload).[28] However, a reduction in cardic index is a more common outcome and is largely due to the decrease in venous return. This is easily corrected by volume expansion, but any increase in fluid loading may be accompanied by adverse effects on pulmonary function. This is a particular problem in ARDS, where the capillary leak predisposes to lung edema. As an alternative to fluid loading, cardiac index may be increased by pharmacologic interventions (alterations in cardiac rate, rhythm and contractility, and vascular resistance) after PEEP is applied, and this may be preferable in individual cases.

The circulatory effects of the gravid uterus compressing the inferior vena cava and abdominal aorta must be considered when hemodynamic changes do occur. In order to minimize this problem, pregnant women on ventilators who are lying supine should have their hips elevated or be positioned on their sides. The normal increase in total blood volume and cardiac index of the pregnant patient should be maintained in the face of any ventilatory maneuver. A decrease in cardiac index to levels that would be considered normal in nonpregnant women indicates a low output state, which requires correction by the appropriate circulatory strategy. Moreover, PEEP can cause a reduction of blood flow in the splanchnic and other circulatory beds, and while there is little data available, it is likely that the uteroplacental circulation may be similarly affected.[46] Such a reduction of uteroplacental blood flow would be expected to magnify the effect of any decrease in cardiac index on fetal well-being, and electronic fetal heart rate monitoring should be a helpful guide in determining optimal respiratory and circulatory interventions.

The pulmonary hypertension in ARDS can be further increased by PEEP and may cause right ventricular failure, as evidenced by an inverse relationship between cardiac index and pulmonary vascular resistance in such patients.[29,77] As a consequence, a specific form of left ventricular dysfunction can occur.[36] As the right ventricle fails, its end-diastolic volume increases. Eventually, a point is reached at which further enlargement can only occur at the expense of the left ventricle because the edematous ARDS lung occupies a considerable volume in the closed chest. The intraventricular septum bulges into the left ventricular cavity and causes a diminution in its volume. Left ventricular contractility increases in an attempt to maintain cardiac index, but ultimately the patient may experience a decreasing cardiac index and an increasing pulmonary capillary wedge pressure (PCWP) in the presence of a small hypercontractile left ventricle.[36] The clinician is usually only in a position to measure the cardiac index and the PCWP and thus may be deceived into diagnosing a loss of left ventricular contractility rather than the primary right heart failure.

Indications for Mechanical Ventilation. Ventilator therapy should be instituted when refractory hypoxemia is present. However, to assure fetal well-being, in the pregnant patient it should also be strongly considered at the earliest recognition of ARDS. With correction of hypoxemia and respiratory alkalosis, fetal oxygen delivery can be maintained at an adequate level, as described in Chapter 12. Other commonly accepted indications for mechanical ventilation are retention of carbon dioxide, impaired consciousness, and inability to clear secretions.[21] However, dangerous hypoxemia is often already present when these situations become manifest.

Ventilatory Parameters. There are three basic types of ventilators: volume-cycled, time-cycled, and pressure-cycled. Volume- and time-cycled ventilators deliver a preset tidal volume, which will remain constant in the face of a changing respiratory compliance. In contrast, pressure-cycled ventilators deliver a variable tidal volume depending on a preset airway pressure. The latter should be avoided in ARDS because the delivered tidal volume can fall to inadequate levels when compliance increases.

The initial setting of a volume- or time-cycled ventilator requires selection of an FIO_2, respiratory rate, tidal volume, and level of PEEP. An FIO_2 of 1.0 (100 percent oxygen) is a safe, conservative initial setting, with subsequent values being dictated by the results of arterial blood gas determinations. Although under normobaric conditions the administration of an FIO_2 of 1.0 for up to 24 h has not been associated with the development of pulmonary oxygen toxicity, an attempt should be made to reduce the FIO_2 as soon as possible.[74] An FIO_2 of 0.5 can be administered indefinitely without adverse sequelae.

The respiratory rate is a major determinant of carbon dioxide elimination, and we recommend rates in the order of 10 to 12 per minute. In conjunction with tidal volume manipulations, respiratory rate can be adjusted to keep arterial carbon dioxide tension ($PaCO_2$) and pH in the normal range.

Ventilated patients should be given a tidal volume of 10 to 15 cc/kg with a respiratory rate of 10 to 12 breaths per minute. This will provide a minute ventilation (rate × tidal volume) of 7 to 10 L/min, which should be sufficient to adequately eliminate carbon dioxide. In selecting a minute volume, hyperventilation should be avoided. The normal $PaCO_2$ of the pregnant patient is 30 to 32 mmHg, and decreases below this level can cause marked reductions in placental perfusion.[42] Mechanical ventilation with low tidal volumes should be avoided because of an increase in the alveolar-to-arterial diffusion gradient for oxygen which can thereby ensue.

Application of PEEP is accomplished by titrating upwards from levels of 5 cmH_2O. By improving ventilation-perfusion relationships, the oxygen concentration required to maintain an arterial saturation above 90 percent can be reduced.[25] By following serial arterial blood samples, PEEP can be increased until either the required FIO_2 is below 0.6 or cardiac output declines. Generally, levels above 15 cmH_2O are not required, but values as high as 20 cmH_2O may occasionally be necessary to provide an appreciable increase in arterial oxygen. Applying PEEP at high levels may lead to retention of excess lung water.[29] If PEEP is then decreased, this lung water can flood alveoli and lead to a deterioration in gas exchange, which is not easily reversed by simply raising levels of PEEP.[45] To avoid this problem, we apply PEEP at low levels (5 cmH_2O) and then gradually increase it as needed.

Intermittent Mandatory Ventilation. Traditional IPPV allows for the delivery of a preset tidal volume at a preset rate and can be adjusted to a control or an assist mode. In the control mode, the ventilator cycles only at the preset rate. In the assist mode, the negative airway pressure associated with initiation of a spontaneous breath by the patient triggers a ventilator-delivered tidal volume. With intermittent mandatory ventilation (IMV), the ventilator is set on the control mode and can deliver a preset tidal volume at a preset rate. However, a system of one-way valves in the inspiratory tubing allows the patient to continue spontaneous breathing efforts via the ventilatory circuit between ventilator-delivered, preset tidal volumes, which are given at intervals varying from 5 seconds to several minutes.[19] As against other techniques of mechanical ventilation, IMV has several potential advantages. Spontaneous respiratory muscle activity is maintained, in contrast to controlled ventilation, in which such activity is largely abolished. With the latter, disuse of respiratory muscles may contribute to discoordination between chest wall and diaphragmatic function. The presence of spontaneous respiratory activity may also be beneficial when considering both cardiovascular function and distribution of inspired gas in the presence of acute lung injury. The ability to maintain adequate circulatory function with IMV and high PEEP, as reported by Kirby et al.,[25,35] is probably due to lower mean airway and pleural pressures during IMV as compared with controlled mechanical ventilation at similar PEEP. Thus, higher levels of PEEP are possible with this method. A further advantage is continued diaphragmatic activity and its theoretical benefit on the distribution of inspired gas. During spontaneous breathing, inspired gas is preferentially distributed to dependent lung regions, in contrast to positive-pressure ventilation, with which distribution favors nondependent regions. Thus, the presence of both spontaneous and passive ventilation during IMV may provide more uniform gas distribution to all regions of the lung.[19]

High-Frequency Ventilation. High-frequency ventilation (HFV) is a relatively new ventilatory technique characterized by ventilatory frequencies ranging from 120 to 1,800 cycles/min delivering tidal volumes at or below the volume of the anatomic dead space.[24,64] It is unclear why ventilation with such low tidal volumes is consistent with effective gas mixing in the lungs. However, the efficacy of the technique has been documented in experimental animals and in humans.[10] Indeed, there are a number of clinical circumstances in which HFV may be more appropriate than conventional ventilation. This mode of gas exchange is associated with a decrease in mean airway pressure; it thus may diminish the potential for ventilator-induced pulmonary barotrauma and could also theoretically reduce the harmful hemodynamic consequences of conventional ventilation. Other potential benefits include its use in patients with head injuries, in whom it can minimize the increase in mean intrathoracic pressure that may result in elevation of intracranial pressure. It also is preferable to conventional ventilation for treating patients with bronchopleural fistula.[10] Although HFV provides a low level of continuous positive airway pressure, this may not be adequate to increase FRC above CV in the ARDS patient. In these patients, an additional positive airway pressure, similar to PEEP, is still required and used as previously described. However, when this additional pressure is used with HFV, the mean airway pressure is still lower than when PEEP is used with conventional ventilation.[10]

The Use of Neuromuscular Blocking Agents. Rarely, the use of intravenously administered neuromuscular blocking agents may be indicated to maintain mechanical ventilation. This intervention should be considered if patient agitation leads to forced expiration (bucking) which impedes ventilation.[56] These agents may also be useful to paralyze chest and abdominal muscles in order to reduce thoracic compliance in patients who consistently demonstrate peak airway pressures greater than 60 cmH_2O on the ventilator and are thus exposed to an increased risk of barotrauma. This may be a particular problem in the pregnant patient when the gravid uterus impedes diaphragmatic excursion and results in a decrease in thoracic compliance. Since an alert patient may be terrified by being paralyzed, the degree of patient awareness must be taken into account when these medications are employed. Ancillary sedative-hypnotic agents should be routinely administered to any alert paralyzed patient. All neuromuscular blocking agents can cross the placenta, and their use has been associated with fetal musculoskeletal anomalies due to changes in fetal position from muscle relaxation.[56] An increased incidence of intraventricular hemorrhage has been noted in neonates given pancuronium bromide and mechanical ventilation for hyaline membrane disease, but it is unclear whether the drug was responsible for this morbidity.[12] If these agents must be used in an obstetrical patient, pancuronium bromide is an acceptable choice in doses of 0.04 to 0.08 mg/kg.[56] The minimum effective dose should be determined by titration of the agents according to objective indices of the degree of neuromuscular blockade, such as the monitoring of twitch height and response to tetanic stimulation by means of a nerve peripheral stimulator. Neuromuscular blocking agents should be discontinued at least 4 h prior to parturition to avoid delivery of a flaccid, apneic neonate.

Endotracheal Intubation and Tracheostomy. Mechanical ventilation necessitates placement of an artificial airway. Adult endotracheal and tracheostomy tubes achieve an airtight seal by means of an inflatable balloon-cuff. Although these cuffs exert a pressure on the tracheal wall, Jenicek, in a retrospective analysis, has demonstrated that long-term use of high cuff pressures does not routinely lead to tracheal damage.[37] However, these cuffs have been experimentally demonstrated to reduce tracheal mucosal blood supply, an effect which may be minimized by using the recently available high-volume, low-pressure cuff systems.[30]

When it appears that prolonged mechanical ventilation is necessary, consideration should be given to tracheostomy. Prolonged endotracheal intubation has been reported to lead to laryngeal damage and tracheal stenosis. Some investigators believe that these complications can be minimized by early institution of tracheostomy.[53] However, in a recent study by Stauffer,[67] prolonged endotracheal intubation was not associated with a higher incidence of tracheal stenosis than tracheostomy. In addition, other complications of tracheostomy can include infection, granuloma formation, and innominate artery hemorrhage. We recommend that a decision regarding tracheostomy be made after 2 weeks of endotracheal intubation. If at this time it appears likely that the patient will be extubated in the following week, tracheostomy should be deferred. However, if continued prolonged ventilatory support is anticipated, tracheostomy should be performed then.

Monitoring Pitfalls. Data derived from pulmonary artery catheterization can be extremely useful in managing the ARDS patient. It can help guide fluid therapy as well as ventilator management. However, there are potential inaccuracies in some of the derived measurements. In the presence of the pulmonary hypertension associated with ARDS, left atrial pressure may be appreciably lower than pulmonary capillary hydrostatic pressure. Therefore, the wedged pulmonary artery catheter, which measures left atrial pressure, may not accurately reflect the hydrostatic forces contributing to the formation of pulmonary edema.[32] The most accurate measurement of PCWP is achieved when measured at end expiration, where the effect of airway pressures are minimal.[27] With high levels of PEEP, PCWP may be falsely elevated because it reflects both intravascular and elevated alveolar pressures.[71] This effect is maximal when the pulmonary artery catheter tip is above the left atrium and airway pressure exceeds pulmonary venous pressure. Shasby[62] has recommended that a lateral chest roentgenogram be obtained to determine the position of the pulmonary artery catheter and to confirm that the tip is positioned below the left atrium. To minimize the effect of transmitted airway pressures on PCWP measurements, it might seem reasonable to discontinue mechanical ventilation while measurements are being obtained. However, such a maneuver could alter hemodynamics and result in a measurement which does not reflect the patient's clinical status.[16] For this reason, we measure PCWP without discontinuing mechanical ventilation.

When the pulmonary artery catheter is used to obtain mixed venous blood for shunt fraction calculations, care should be taken to avoid rapid aspiration from the distal tip. Only by slow withdrawal can one prevent the sample from being contaminated with "arterialized" pulmonary venous blood.

Weaning from Mechanical Ventilation. After the initiation of therapy for ARDS, the patient may begin to show signs of improvement with less impairment of gas exchange, a reduction in $\dot{Q}s/\dot{Q}T$, and increases in lung compliance and MVO_2. If the FIO_2 can then be reduced to less than 0.5 and PEEP to 5 cmH_2O, consideration should be given to weaning from mechanical ventilation. Weaning can be defined as the progressive discontinuation of mechanical ventilation.

The first step in this process is to decide whether the patient has adequate respiratory reserve to sustain unassisted ventilation. Clinical studies have demonstrated that simple bedside measurements can successfully predict the outcome of the weaning process. Vital capacity must be at least 10- to 12 cc/kg, negative inspiratory force -20 cmH_2O, and resting minute ventilation less than 10 L/min.[58] In addition, the patient should be able to double her resting minute ventilation with maximal effort.

Once bedside measurements demonstrate that weaning can be initiated, the next step is to establish that nonrespiratory major organ function can sustain this process. A general principle to follow is that any unresolved acute cardiovascular, renal, neurologic, infectious, or hemorrhagic illness is an absolute contraindication to weaning.

Patients with impaired cardiac function may have difficulty tolerating the physiological changes that accompany the weaning process. Discontinuation of mechanical ventilation and PEEP can increase venous return and left ventricular afterload, thus precipitating acute left ventricular failure. This in turn will lead to pulmonary vascular congestion, interstitial edema, a reduction in lung compliance, and an increased work of breathing, thus dooming the weaning process to failure. In addition, the weaning process is associated with an increase in sympathoadrenal activity, which can add further stress to the cardiovascular system.[65]

The oliguric phase of acute renal failure (ARF) is a very difficult time to wean a patient. In this phase there is always the possibility of intravascular volume overload, even with meticulous attention to fluid balance. In addition, dialysis may be necessary and this can be associated with marked deterioration in respiratory function.[54] In oliguric patients with threatened ARF, large volumes of fluid may be necessary to maintain urine output at the temporary expense of pulmonary function. In such patients not only may fluid therapy preclude weaning, but the cardiovascular response to weaning may lead to a further decline in renal function.

Consideration of the central nervous system is particularly important in the ARDS patient with preeclampsia-toxemia. Hyperventilation may be indicated in such patients to reduce cerebral edema, in spite of its deleterious effects on placental blood flow. When weaning is initiated, this therapeutic modality can no longer be used.

An integral part of the weaning process is the eventual removal of the artificial airway, but extubation can only be performed if several criteria are met. The patient must have an intact gag reflex and must be alert enough to protect her airway from aspiration and obstruction. In addition, she must be able to mobilize and expectorate secretions so that an artifical airway is not required for pulmonary toilet. If these criteria are not met, extubation can not be safely achieved and the weaning process can not be completed.

To initiate weaning, the endotracheal or tracheostomy tube is fitted with a T-piece adapter and connected to a source of humidified oxygen delivered at high flow rates. The inspired oxygen concentration should be the same as that delivered to the patient during controlled ventilation. End-expiratory pressure can still be applied when the patient is intubated but not receiving mechanical ventilation. By providing air flow resistance to the expiratory limb of the T-piece, airway pressure is always positive and the patient receives continuous positive airway pressure (CPAP) while spontaneously breathing.

Arterial blood gases are obtained after 15 min, and patient toleration, vital signs, and cardiac rhythm are monitored. Some women will tolerate this change clinically and will maintain adequate blood gas values ($PaO_2 > 70$ mmHg, $PaCO_2 <$ 40 mmHg, pH > 7.35). These patients can then be extubated, and the weaning process will have been completed.

In the majority of patients, a more gradual weaning process is necessary before successful extubation can be achieved. Patients who have been maintained on mechanical ventilation for longer than 5 days will fall into this group. Intially, the patient is allowed to breathe spontaneously through the T-piece for 15 min every 2 h. Subsequently, the duration of spontaneous ventilation is increased by 15-min increments as tolerated while clinical status and arterial blood gases are evaluated. Once the patient can maintain spontaneous ventilation for 1 h without signs of clinical instability (rapid respiratory rate, restlessness, hypertension, tachycardia, arrhythmia, or diaphoresis), arterial blood gases are again drawn. If these confirm that the patient no longer requires mechanical ventilation, extubation is performed.

An alternate approach to gradual weaning is to use IMV. When the set ventilatory rate is gradually reduced with the ventilator in the IMV mode, spontaneous respiration assumes a larger share in gas exchange and weaning can also be accomplished. While one recent study has shown that this weaning technique did not reduce the length of time required on the ventilator, it does require less moment-to-moment observation than conventional weaning.[59]

Repeated Failure to Wean. When weaning progresses poorly, several patient parameters should be examined. Nutritional status must be assessed because ARDS may be associated with increased catabolism and a severe negative nitrogen balance.[7] As somatic protein stores become depleted, generalized muscle atrophy results in an insufficient muscle mass to perform the work of breathing. These sequelae can be modified by vigorous parenteral alimentation early in the course of the illness. Respiratory muscle discoordination may also be present and results in a lack of synchrony between diaphragmatic and chest wall movement.[44] Specific electrolyte abnormalities (hypophosphatemia, hypermagnesemia, hypomagnesemia, hypokalemia, and hypocalcemia) can also lead to impaired muscular function and must be excluded.

In some patients, ARDS may begin to resolve but the lungs will remain extremely noncompliant. Until further lung repair occurs, the increased work of breathing will prevent completion of the weaning process.

Complications Associated with ARDS

Therapy of ARDS requires knowledge not only of the disease process and its management, but also of associated complications. Table 2-3 lists complications resulting from intubation and mechanical ventilation and also emphasizes that this severe disease can involve many organ systems in addition to the lungs. Two specific complications, pulmonary barotrauma and infection, merit special mention.

Pulmonary barotrauma may be defined as the development of pneumothorax, pneumomediastinum, or subcutaneous emphysema in patients received positive pressure to the airway, either as sustained end-expiratory pressure or intermittent positive pressure. When positive pressure results in alveolar rupture, gas can dissect into the mediastinum and then travel into the pleural cavity and/or appear as subcutaneous emphysema. In one series of ARDS patients, 38 percent of the group were found to have pneumomediastinum or pneumothorax.[17] Pneumothorax may cause further deterioration in gas exchange, and tension pneumothorax may produce immediate life threatening pulmonary and cardiovascular deterioration. Factors which have been implicated as predisposing to barotrauma include high inflation pressures resulting from poor lung compliance, large tidal volumes, and high levels of PEEP. Methods for decreasing the frequency of barotrauma include patient sedation to decrease inflation pressures, lower tidal volumes (10 to 12 cc/kg), the use of IMV to decrease mean airway pressure, avoidance of excessive levels of PEEP, and use of high-frequency jet ventilation.

Infectious complications can play a major role in the morbidity and mortaility of ARDS patients. Approximately two-thirds of all crticially ill patients become colonized with gram-negative bacteria, and Browdie et al.[9] found concurrent infection in a majority of patients with ARDS. Intravenous catheters, endotracheal tubes,

Table 2-3. Complications Associated with the Adult Respiratory Distress Syndrome

I. Pulmonary
  A. Pulmonary emboli
  B. Pulmonary barotrauma
  C. Pulmonary fibrosis
  D. Pulmonary complications of ventilatory and monitoring procedures
    1. Mechanical ventilation
      a. Right main stem intubation
      b. Alveolar hypoventilation
    2. Swan-Ganz catheter
      a. Pulmonary infarction
      b. Pulmonary hemorrhage
    3. Tracheal intubation
      a. Laryngeal injury
      b. Tracheal stenosis
II. Gastrointestinal
  A. Gastrointestinal hemorrhage
  B. Illeus
  C. Gastric distension
  D. Pneumoperitoneum
III. Renal
  A. Renal failure
  B. Fluid retention
IV. Cardiac
  A. Arrhythmia
  B. Hypotension
  C. Low cardiac output
V. Infection
  A. Sepsis
  B. Nocosomial pneumonia
VI. Hematologic
  A. Anemia
  B. Thrombocytopenia
  C. Disseminated intravascular coagulation
VII. Other
  A. Hepatic
  B. Endocrine
  C. Neurologic
  D. Psychiatric

From Bone, RC (ed): Clinics in Chest Medicine. Vol. 3. Philadelphia, W.B. Saunders, 1982, p. 144.

bladder catheters, and intra-arterial cannulae can all be sources of infection. The equipment attached to these devices has also been implicated.[13] Medical personnel, of course, may be another reservoir of infection.[1] Control of infection depends upon aseptic placement of invasive devices, appropriate disinfection of equipment, and surveillance of personnel for sources of sepsis, along with frequent hand washing.

It has been postulated than an impairment of host defense mechanisms is the major variable in determining the frequency of bacterial colonization. Critically ill patients may become colonized in the oropharynx with gram-negative organisms in the absence of an identifiable environmental source. Once colonized, the likelihood of subsequent gram-negative bacillary pneumonia increases almost 10-fold. Johanson[38] has demonstrated that the majority of patients developing oropharyngeal colonization have increased adherence of gram-negative organisms to buccal epithelial cells in vitro. Factors which increase the likelihood of bacterial adherence to upper respiratory tract mucosa include surgery, renal failure, and malnutrition. An increase in bacterial adherence to mucosal cells may explain the critically ill patient's increased risk of bacterial colonization.

Accurate clinical diagnosis of supermimposed bacterial pneumonia is exceedingly difficult in the ARDS patient. Concurrent medical or surgical illness may independently cause fever and leucocytosis. Pulmonary infiltrates are a feature of the primary disease. Culture of tracheal secretions is misleading because of the ubiquitous colonization of the upper respiratory tract of ventilated patients. The technique of obtaining bronchial brushings with a protected bronchial brush may improve the bacteriologic diagnosis of pneumonia.[72]

In one study, 58 percent of patients with ARDS had histologic evidence of pneumonia.[4] However, 36 percent of these cases were not clinically detected and 20 percent of those without pneumonia were incorrectly given this diagnosis. Since veryifying the clinical impression of pneumonia is so difficult in patients with ARDS, it is not easy to know when to administer antimicrobial therapy. We recommend administering antibiotics if the primary etiologic event which precipitated the ARDS is respiratory infection or aspiration pneumonitis. When ARDS has a noninfectious etiology, we give antibiotics to patients who develop persistent fever, leukocytosis, or worsening infiltrates after pathogenic bacteria have been recovered from the sputum. These criteria are merely rough guidelines and may, in some cases, lead to the treatment of patients who do not actually have pneumonia. We do not recommend the use of prophylactic antibiotics in the absence of suspected pneumonia.

Lung Function in the Acute and Recovery Stages

The acutely injured lungs of the patient with ARDS are characterized as having a restrictive abnormality (see Ch. 10), with a reduced total lung capacity and FRC. Also, with the onset of lung injury, the alveolar-arterial oxygen tension gradient is increased and lung compliance is reduced. In one study, serial observations showed that patients who survived ARDS had improvement in both of these parameters within 1 week of the onset of illness.[63]

When survivors of ARDS are studied on a long-term basis, the other abnormalities also appear to improve. In some studies, 40 to 55 percent of survivors are left with no reductions in total lung capacity or vital capacity.[20,40,57] Other survivors have minor reductions in lung volume, rate of air flow, or diffusing capacity. However, all survivors may have exercise-induced widening of the alveolar-arterial oxygen tension gradient, according to one study.[20]

These data demonstrate that the lung can repair itself to a normal or near normal functional state if it can be supported through a phase of severe injury. Such information should provide the impetus to aggressively treat this potentially curable complication of systemic catastrophic illness.

APPENDIX 1

The shunt as a fraction of cardiac output ($\dot{Q}S/\dot{Q}T$) can be calculated from the following equations:

$$\dot{Q}S/\dot{Q}T = \frac{CcO_2 - CaO_2}{CcO_2 - C_vO_2}$$

where CcO_2 = end-capillary blood oxygen content
CaO_2 = arterial blood oxygen content
C_vO_2 = mixed venous blood oxygen content

The value of CaO_2 is calculated from arterial blood gas data, C_vO_2 from pulmonary artery blood gas data drawn from the distal tip of a Swan-Ganz catheter, and CcO_2 by using the ideal alveolar oxygen tension and assuming equilibrium with end-capillary blood.

Oxygen content is calculated as:

$$O_2 \text{ content} = \text{saturation} \times \text{hemoglobin (g)} \times 1.34 \text{ ml oxygen/g hemoglobin} + (PO_2 \times 0.0031)$$

This equation includes the oxygen dissolved in the blood by using the factor 0.0031 to convert oxygen tension (in millimeters of mercury) to oxygen content.

Some studies have confirmed that the shunt is best calculated by using the fraction of inspired oxygen (FIO_2) that the patient is receiving and not 100 percent oxygen, as had been previously recommended.[61]

These equations can be applied to a patient with ARDS and the following clinical data:

T = 37°C	FIO_2 = 0.60
Hb = 15.0 g	Blood gas: pH = 7.40
Mixed venous O_2 = 30 mmHg	$PaCO_2$ = 40 mmHg
	PaO_2 = 58 mmHg

Alveolar oxygen tension (pAO_2)

$$= (\text{barometric pressure} - \text{water vapor pressure})\, FIO_2 - \frac{PaCO_2}{0.8}$$

$$= (760 - 47)(0.60) - \frac{40}{0.8}$$

$$= 377 \text{ mmHg}$$

From the oxyhemoglobin dissociation curve (Fig. 2-3):

Arterial saturation (PaO_2) = 58 mmHg = 89%
Mixed venous saturation (MVO_2) = 30 mmHg = 59%
Capillary saturation (PAO_2) = 377 mmHg = 100%

Then,

$$\dot{Q}s/\dot{Q}T = \frac{[(1.0)(15)(1.34) + 377(0.0031)] - [(0.89)(15)(1.34) + 58(0.0031)]}{[(1.0)(15)(1.34) + 377(0.0031)] - [(0.59)(15)(1.34) + 30(0.0031)]}$$
$$= 0.34$$

Therefore, this patient has a 34 percent shunt fraction.

REFERENCES

1. Albert, R.K. and Condie, F.: Hand-washing patterns in medial intensive-care units. N. Engl. J. Med., *304:*1465, 1981.
2. Altman, A.R. and Johnson, T.H.: Roentgenographic findings in PEEP therapy: indicators of pulmonary complications. JAMA *242:*727, 1979.
3. Anderson, H.F., Lynch, J.P., and Johnson, T.R.B.: Adult respiratory distress syndrome in obstetrics and gynecology. Obstet. Gynecol., *55:*291, 1980.
4. Andrews, C.P., Coalson, J.J., Smith, J.D., and Johanson, W.G.: Diagnosis of nosocomial bacterial pneumonia in acute diffuse lung injury. Chest, *80:*254, 1981.
5. Ashbaugh, D.G., Bigelow, D.B., Petty, T.L. et al.: Acute respiratory distress in adults. Lancet, *2:*319, 1967.
6. Bachofen, M. and Weibel, E.R.: Structural alterations of lung parenchyma in the adult respiratory distress syndrome. P. 35. In: Bone, Roger C., Ed.: Clinics in Chest Medicine. Vol. 3, W.B. Saunders Co., Philadelphia, 1982.
7. Benotti, P. and Blackburn, G.L.: Protein and caloric or macronutrient metabolic management of the critically ill patient. Crit. Care Med., *7:*520, 1979.
8. Brigham, K.L.: Mechanisms of lung injury. P. 9. In: Bone, Roger C., Ed.: Clinics in Chest Medicine. Vol. 3. W.B. Saunders Co., Philadelphia, 1982.
9. Browdie, D.A., Deane, R., Shinozaki, T. et al.: Adult respiratory distress syndrome, sepsis and extracorporeal membrane oxygenation. J. Trauma *17:*579, 1977.
10. Carlon, G.C., Ray, C., and Pierri, M.K.: High-frequency jet ventilation: theoretical considerations and clinical observations. Chest, *81:*350, 1982.
11. Connors, A.F. Jr., McCaffree, D.R., and Rogers, R.M.: The adult respiratory distress syndrome. D.M. *27:*1, 1981.
12. Crone, R.K. and Favorito, J.: The effects of pancuronium bromide on infants with hyaline membrane disease. J. Pediatr., *97:*991, 1980.
13. Cross, A.S. and Roup, B.: Role of respiratory assistance devices in endemic nosocomial pneumonia. Am. J. Med., *70:*681, 1981.
14. Danek, S.J., Lynch, J.P., Weg, J.G., and Dantzker, D.R.: The dependence of oxygen uptake on oxygen delivery in the adult respiratory distress syndrome. Am. Rev. Respir. Dis., *122:*387, 1980.
15. Dantzker, D.R., Brook, C.H., DeHart, P. et al.: Gas exchange in adult respiratory distress syndrome and the effects of positive end-expiratory pressure. Am. Rev. Respir. Dis., *120:*1039, 1979.
16. Davison, R., Parker, M., and Harrison, R.A.: The validity of determinations of pulmonary wedge pressure during mechanical ventilation. Chest, *73:*352, 1978.
17. de Latorre, F.J., Tomasa, A., Klamburg, J. et al.: Incidence of pneumothorax and pneumomediastinum in patients with aspiration pneumonia requiring ventilatory support. Chest, *72:*141, 1977.

18. Divertie, M.B.: The adult respiratory distress syndrome. Mayo Clin. Proc., *57*:371, 1982.
19. Downs, J.B., Klein, E.F., Desautels, D. et al. Intermittent mandatory ventilation: a new approach to weaning patients from mechanical ventilators. Chest, *64*:331, 1973.
20. Elliot, C.G., Morris, A.H., and Cengiz, M.: Pulmonary function and exercise gas exchange in survivors of adult respiratory distress syndrome. Am. Rev. Respir. Dis., *123*:492, 1981.
21. Feeley, T.W. and Hedley-Whyte, J.: Weaning from controlled ventilation and supplemental oxygen. N. Engl. J. Med., *292*:903, 1975.
22. Fein, A., Grossman, R.F., Jones, J.G. et al.: The value of edema fluid protein measurement in patients with pulmonary edema. Am. J. Med., *67*:32, 1979.
23. Finley, T.N., Lenfant, C., Haab, P. et al.: Venous admixture in the pulmonary circulation of anesthetized dogs. J. Appl. Physiol., *15*:418, 1960.
24. Gallagher, T.J.: High frequency ventilation: a passing fancy? Chest, *80*:659, 1981.
25. Gallagher, T.J., Civetta, J.M., and Kirby, R.R.: Terminology update: optimal PEEP. Crit. Care Med., *6*:323, 1978.
26. Garrard, G.S., Littler, W.A., and Redman, G.W.G.: Closing volume during normal pregnancy. Thorax, *33*:488, 1978.
27. Geer, R.T.: Interpretation of pulmonary artery wedge pressure when PEEP is used. Anesthesiology, *46*:383, 1977.
28. Gong, H.: Positive-pressure ventilation in the adult respiratory distress syndrome. P. 69. In: Bone, Roger C., Ed.: Clinics in Chest Medicine. Vo. 3. W.B. Saunders Co., Philadelphia, 1982.
29. Gong, H. and Tierney, D.F.: Respiratory distress syndrome: use of positive end-expiratory pressure and outcome. P. 103. In: Simmons, D.H., Ed.: Current Pulmonology. Vol. 2. Houghton Mifflin, Boston, 1980.
30. Grillo, H.C., Cooper, J.D., Geffin, B., and Pontoppidan, H.: A low pressure cuff for tracheostomy to minimize tracheal injury. J. Thorac. Cardiovasc. Surg., *62*:898, 1971.
31. Hammerschmidt, D.E., Weaver, L.J., Hudson, L.D. et al.: Association of complement activation and elevated plasma—C5a with adult respiratory distress syndrome. Lancet *1*:947, 1980.
32. Hobelmann, C., Smith, D., Virgilio, R.W. et al.: Hemodynamic alterations with positive end-expiratory pressure: the contribution of the pulmonary vasculature. J. Trauma, *15*:951, 1975.
33. Hudson, L.D.: Causes of the adult respiratory distress syndrome—clinical recognition. P. 195. In: Bone, Roger C., Ed.: Clinics in Chest Medicine. Vol. 3. W.B. Saunders Co., Philadelphia, 1982.
34. King, T.K.C., Weber, B., Okinaka, A. et al.: Oxygen transfer in catastrophic respiratory failure. Chest, *65*:40S, 1974.
35. Kirby, R.R., Downs, J.B., Civetta, J.M. et al.: High level positive end-expiratory pressure (PEEP) in acute respiratory insufficiency. Chest, *67*:156, 1975.
36. Jardin, F., Farcot, J.C., Boisante, L. et al.: Influence of positive end-expiratory pressure on left ventricular performance. N. Engl. J. Med., *304*:387, 1981.
37. Jenicek, J., Danner, C., and Allen, C.: Continuous cuff inflation during long term intubation and ventilation: evaluation of technic. Anesth. Analg. (Cleve), *52*:252, 1973.
38. Johanson, W.G., Higuchi, J.H., Chaudhuri, T.R., and Woods, D.E.: Bacterial adherence to epithelial cells in bacillary colonization of the respiratory tract. Am. Rev. Respir. Dis., *121*:55, 1980.
39. Lamy, M., Fallat, R.J., Koeniger, E. et al.: Pathologic features and mechanisms of hypoxemia in adult respiratory distress syndrome. Am. Rev. Respir. Dis., *114*:267, 1976.
40. Lakshminarayan, S., Stanford, R.E., and Petty, T.L.: Prognosis after recovery from adult respiratory distress syndrome. Am. Rev. Respir. Dis., *113*:7, 1976.

41. Lee, C.T., Fein, A.M., Lippman, M. et al.: Elastolytic activity in pulmonary lavage fluid from patients with adult respiratory distress syndrome. N. Engl. J. Med., *304:*192, 1981.
42. Levinson, G., Shnider, S.M., de Lorimier, A.A., and Seffenson, J.L.: Effects of maternal hyperventilation on uterine blood flow and fetal oxygenation and acid-base status. Anesthesiology, *40:*340, 1974.
43. Luce, J.M. and Culver, B.H.: Respiratory muscle function in health and disease. Chest, *81:*82, 1982.
44. Luterman, A., Horovitz, J.H., Carrico, C.J. et al.: Withdrawal from positive end-expiratory pressure. Surgery, *83:*328, 1978.
45. Lynch, J.P., Mhyre, J.G., and Dantzker, D.R.: Influence of cardiac output on intrapulmonary shunt. J. Appl. Physiol., *46:*315, 1979.
46. Manny, J., Justice, R., and Hechtman, H.B.: Abnormalities in organ blood flow and its distribution during positive end-expiratory pressure. Surgery, *85:*425, 1979.
47. Newman, J.H., McMurty, I.F., and Reeves, J.T.: Oxygen toxicity blunts hypoxic vasoconstriction in rat lungs: possible role of prostaglandins. Am. Rev. Respir. Dis., *121:*383 S, 1980.
48. Noble, W.H., Kay, J.C., and Obdrzalek, J.: Lung mechanics in hypervolemic pulmonary edema. J. Appl. Physiol., *38:*681, 1975.
49. Ovenfors, C.O. and Hedgcock, M.W.: Intensive care unit radiology: problems of interpretation. Radiol. Clin. N. Am. *16:*407, 1978.
50. Petty, T.L.: Adult respiratory distress syndrome: definition and historical perspective. P. 3. In: Bone, Roger C., Ed.: Clinics in Chest Medicine. Vol. 3. W.B. Saunders Co., Philadelphia, 1982.
51. Petty, T.L. and Ashbaugh, D.G.: The adult respiratory distress syndrome: clinical features, factors influencing prognosis and principles of management. Chest, *60:*233, 1971.
52. Petty, T.L., Silvers, G.W., Paul, G.W., and Stanford, R.E.: Abnormalities in lung elastic properties and surfactant function in adult respiratory distress syndrome. Chest, *75:*571, 1979.
53. Prolonged endotracheal intubation. Br. Med. J., *1:*321, 1967.
54. Rafferty, T.: Weaning from mechanical ventilation: the adult surgical patient. Curr. Rev. Respir. Ther., *12:*91, 1980.
55. Rinaldo, J.E. and Rogers, R.M.: Adult respiratory distress syndrome: changing concepts of lung injury and repair. N. Engl. J. Med., *306:*900, 1982.
56. Roizen, M.F. and Feeley, T.W.: Pancuronium bromide. Ann. Intern. Med., *88:*64, 1978.
57. Rotman, H.H., Lavelle, T.F., Dimcheff, D.G. et al.: Long-term physiologic consequences of the adult respiratory distress syndrome. Chest, *72:*190, 1977.
58. Sahn, S.A., Lakshminarayan, S., and Petty, T.L.: Weaning from mechanical ventilation. JAMA *235:*2208, 1976.
59. Schachter, E.N., Tucker, D., and Beck, G.J.: Does intermittent mandatory ventilation accelerate weaning? JAMA, *246:*1210, 1981.
60. Schumer, W.: Steroids in the treatment of clinical septic shock. Ann. Surg., *184:*333, 1976.
61. Shapiro, B.A., Cone, R.D., Harrison, R.A., and Steiner, M.C.: Changes in intrapulmonary shunting with administration of 100 percent oxygen. Chest, *77:*138, 1980.
62. Shasby, D.M., Dauber, I.N., Pfister, S. et al.: Swan-Ganz catheter location and left atrial pressure determine the accuracy of the wedge pressure when positive end-expiratory pressure is used. Chest, *80:*666, 1981.
63. Shimada, Y., Yoshiya, I., Tanaka, K. et al.: Evaluation of the progress and prognosis of adult respiratory distress syndrome: simple respiratory physiologic measurement. Chest, *76:*180, 1979.
64. Sjostrand, U.: High frequency positive-pressure ventilation (HFPPV): a review. Crit. Care Med., *8:*345, 1980.

65. Skillman, J.J., Malhotra, I.V., Pallotta, J.A., and Bushnell, L.S.: Determinants of weaning from controlled ventilation. Surg. Forum, *22:*198, 1971.
66. Springer, R.R. and Stevens, P.M.: The influence of PEEP on survival of patients in respiratory failure: a retrospective analysis. Am. J. Med., *66:*196, 1979.
67. Stauffer, J.L., Olson, D.E., and Petty, T.L.: Complications and consequences of endotracheal intubation and tracheotomy: a prospective study of 150 critically ill adult patients. Am. J. Med., *70:*65, 1981.
68. Suter, P.M., Fairley, H.B., and Isenberg, M.D.: Optimum end-expiratory airway pressure in patients with acute pulmonary failure. N. Engl. J. Med., *292:*284, 1975.
69. Suter, P.M., Fairley, H.B., and Isenberg, M.D.: Effect of tidal volume and positive end-expiratory pressure on compliance during mechanical ventilation. Chest, *73:*158, 1978.
70. Tenney, S.M. and Mithoeffer, J.C.: The relationship of mixed venous oxygenation to oxygen transport: with special reference to adaptations to high altitude and pulmonary disease. Am. Rev. Respir. Dis., *125:*474, 1982.
71. Tooker, J., Huseby, J., and Butler, J.: The effect of Swan-Ganz catheter height on the wedge pressure—left atrial pressure relationship in edema during positive-pressure ventilation. Am. Rev. Respir. Dis., *117:*721, 1978.
72. Wallace, R.J.: [Another] new technique for an old disease: the protected brush catheter and bacterial pneumonia. Chest, *81:*532, 1982.
73. Weir, E.K., Mlczoch, J., Reeves, J.T. et al.: Endotoxin and prevention of hypoxic pulmonary vasoconstriction. J. Lab. Clin. Med. *88:*975, 1976.
74. Winter, P.M. and Smith, G.: The toxicity of oxygen. Anesthesiology, *37:*210, 1972.
75. Wynne, J.W. and Modell, J.H.: Respiratory aspiration of stomach contents. Ann. Intern. Med. *87:*466, 1977.
76. Wyszogrodski, I., Kyei-Aboagye, K., Taeusch, H.W., and Avery, M.E.: Surfactant inactivation by hyperventilation: conservation by end-expiratory pressure. J. Appl. Physiol., *38:*461, 1974.
77. Zapol, W.M. and Snider, M.T.: Pulmonary hypertension in severe acute respiratory failure. N. Engl. J. Med., *296:*476, 1977.

3

Fluid Management in the Massively Bleeding Obstetric Patient

Terence D. Rafferty, M.D.
J. Robert Keefer, M.D.
Paul G. Barash, M.D.

INTRODUCTION

Massive maternal hemorrhage can occur at any time during pregnancy and when it does, it threatens the life of the mother and her fetus. Significant blood loss can result in uteroplacental insufficiency, renal failure, cerebral anoxia, adult respiratory distress syndrome, myocardial ischemia and insufficiency, and ultimately death.

The classic responses to acute blood loss are: (1) reduced total blood volume, venous return, and cardiac output; (2) decreasing systemic arterial pressure; (3) reduced baroreceptor activity; (4) vagal inhibition, resulting in tachycardia; and (5) stimulation of the vasomotor center with resultant vasoconstriction and increased systemic vascular resistance. Because of these compensatory responses, a healthy woman can lose 20 percent of her blood volume acutely before hypotension develops, and the loss of 10 percent is usually without clinically obvious consequences. Cerebral and cardiac blood flows are initially maintained at the expense of the renal, muscular, cutaneous, and most importantly, uteroplacental circulations. However, under the conditions of hypoxia and acidosis, which commonly accompany shock states, myocardial contractility becomes impaired and poorly responsive to endogenous catecholamines. This inhibits the compensatory responses to intravascular depletion and exacerbates the low-flow state, which leads to the lethal sequelae of this condition. In order to prevent these complications and adequately replace the blood loss, it is incumbent upon the practitioner to be familiar with the use of fluids for volume expansion and the principles of blood transfusion.

INFUSION OF FLUIDS FOR VOLUME REPLETION

In many instances the availability of blood and blood products does not match immediate needs, and it becomes necessary to administer other fluids in an effort to achieve or maintain hemodynamic stability. Solutions which contain substances with molecular weights in excess of 40,000 (5 percent albumin, salt-poor albumin, Plasmanate, Hespan, Macrodex, and Rheomacrodex) exert a significant oncotic pressure and are termed colloids. Solutions which do not contain such macromolecules (saline, dextrose and water, Ringer's lactate) are called crystalloids. These two types of solution have different effects on respiratory and renal function, and their relative roles in intravascular volume resuscitation are controversial.

Resuscitative Fluid Regimen and Respiratory Function

With rare exceptions, we do not recommend the use of colloidal solutions in resuscitation of the massively bleeding patient. These solutions are expensive, are of little proven benefit, and can have marked disadvantages under specific circumstances. Some authors have argued that colloidal solutions might decrease the potential for pulmonary edema by retaining fluid within the intravascular space. However, severe shock is commonly associated with actual or potential damage to the pulmonary capillary endothelium. This sets the stage for adult respiratory distress syndrome (described in detail in Ch. 2). In this disease, colloidal solutions will simply cross the disordered pulmonary capillary wall with ease and exert an oncotic effect within the interstitium. Resolution of the capillary wall destruction will result in prolongation of pulmonary edema by trapping the oncotically active fluid in the interstitium. While crystalloid solutions will redistribute rapidly throughout the extracellular fluid space irrespective of capillary wall permeability, they have the advantage that they can be readily excreted under all circumstances by diuresis. An examination of the issues involved in the crystalloid versus colloid controversy requires consideration of the forces involved in fluid exchange in the lung and a knowledge of relevant experimental and clinical studies.

Oncotic Pressure and Respiratory Function. The forces involved in fluid exchange in any tissue consist of oncotic and hydrostatic pressures. The extravascular pressures in the lung are difficult to measure. However, in the normal state these pressures are not dominant variables and most experimental studies deal only with the intravascular pressures, i.e., the plasma colloid oncotic pressure and the intravascular hydrostatic pressure. The first precise study describing fluid exchange at the capillary level in the lungs was reported by Guyton and Lindsey in 1959.[21] These investigators used the ratio of wet to dry weight of the lungs as a measure of pulmonary edema, left atrial pressure (LAP) as their measure of the intravascular hydrostatic pressure, and the plasma protein concentration as a measure of plasma colloid oncotic pressure (PCOP). They found that in healthy dogs with a normal plasma protein concentration, fluid began to transude into the lungs when the LAP increased above 24 mmHg. When the plasma protein concentration was halved, fluid began to transude into the lungs at a LAP in excess of 11 mmHg. If the LAP was subtracted from the pressure exerted by the plasma proteins, i.e., the net intravascular force for fluid filtration was derived, this value was directly related to the amount of lung water created. Levine et al.[29] repeated these same experiments measuring the PCOP directly and confirmed the findings of Guyton and Lindsey. Thus, experimentally, in healthy animals with normal lungs the PCOP is an important variable in lung fluid exchange, and the PCOP minus the intravascular hydrostatic pressure is directly proportional to the amount of pulmonary edema.

One cannot necessarily conclude from these experiments that the infusion of solutions such as albumin which possess a high oncotic pressure will preserve respiratory function when treating hemorrhagic shock. Investigations of this issue have produced conflicting results. In a study of hemorrhagic shock performed in rhesus monkeys, in which either Ringer's lactate solution or 5 percent albumin was infused at a rate sufficient to maintain a constant central venous pressure (CVP), pulmonary ultrastructural changes consistent with pulmonary edema occurred only in those animals treated with Ringer's lactate.[17] It is difficult to draw conclusions from this report, however, since the only published evidence that both groups were given comparable amounts of intravascular volume repletion was the constancy of the CVP. In similar studies on baboons, two other groups of investigators have demonstrated resolution of pulmonary edema with saline resuscitation, whereas colloid infusion resulted in distortion of alveolar collagen and the development of interstitial edema.[40,53] Finally, recent experimental evidence suggests that increasing PCOP may actually worsen and prolong pulmonary edema, probably by increasing interstitial oncotic pressure in situations in which increased capillary permeability allows the osmotically active substance to leave the intravascular compartment.[64]

Repeating these studies in a clinical setting presents major methodological problems. The validity of using LAP and, more particularly, mean pulmonary capillary wedge pressure (PCWP) as a measure of pulmonary capillary pressure is questionable when pulmonary artery pressure is elevated.[23,65] In addition, although capillary permeability may be taken to be a constant in experimental models, this is not necessarily valid in the clinical situation.[1,8,12,28] Another factor to be considered is that the contribution of extravascular forces may not be negligible in disease states. Finally, the speed with which changes occur in the forces responsible for fluid movement is crucial because of limitations in the ability of the pulmonary lymphatics to increase drainage of the transudate.[66] With these points in mind, it is hardly surprising that controversy exists as to the clinical importance of net intravascular pressure (PCOP minus PCWP) in the genesis of pulmonary edema.

da Luz, Shubin, Weil et al. have investigated this issue using chest roentgenographic evidence of pulmonary edema as their measure of lung edema and PCWP as their measure of pulmonary capillary pressure.[14] Their study population consisted of coronary care unit admissions, but was nonhomogeneous in that one-third were mechanically ventilated. They reported that although the PCOP alone did not correlate with the presence or degree of pulmonary edema, the net intravascular force for fluid filtration (i.e., PCOP minus PCWP) did. In this series, a rise in PCWP with a constant PCOP, a fall in PCOP with a constant PCWP, or a combination of these effects was associated with pulmonary edema. The normal PCOP in nonpregnant patients is 25 mmHg in the erect position and 22 mmHg in the supine position. The normal range of PCWP is 7 to 15 mmHg. Subtracting 15 mmHg from 22 mmHg gives 7 mmHg as the net intravascular filtration pressure for fluid movement. In this study by Weil's group no patient with a value in excess of 5 mmHg developed pulmonary edema. Rackow et al.[46] using the same study methods, subsequently reported similar findings. Although their study population is not clearly categorized, it consisted of consecutive admissions to a medical intensive care unit, and the majority of their patients seemed to have cardiac disorders. In contrast, Virgilio et al.[62] could not demonstrate an interdependence between the net intravascular filtration pressure and pulmonary edema in mechanically ventilated aortic surgery patients. These authors quantified pulmonary edema by means of shunt fraction ($\dot{Q}s/\dot{Q}_T$). In this series, low and even negative PCOP-PCWP gradients were unattended by adverse sequelae. In a similar study of surgical intensive care unit patients, most of whom had undergone major cardiothoracic operative procedures, Rafferty et al. found the PCOP-PCWP gradient to be a poor predictor of pulmonary edema determined roentgenographically and in terms of $\dot{Q}s/\dot{Q}_T$.[47] These authors speculated that this resulted from the inherent insensitivity of the PCOP-PCWP gradient as an indicator of the intravascular filtration pressure and of $\dot{Q}s/\dot{Q}_T$ and roentgenograms as measurements of lung edema, as well as from the multiplicity of variables involved in the genesis of pulmonary edema in the clinical situation.

Normal pregnancy is associated with a decreased plasma protein concentration and PCOP.[5,55–57] Preeclampsia-toxemia (PET) causes a further lowering of these variables. The mean PCOP of a series of normal pregnant patients in our institution was 20 mm Hg, and that of a matched group of PET patients was 2 mmHg lower (unpublished data). Accordingly, it might be argued that pregnant patients are at particular risk for noncardiogenic pulmonary edema. However, the decreases in PCOP which occur in pregnancy are gradual in onset and are undoubtedly accompanied by reciprocal protective changes in interstitial oncotic pressure. Furthermore, in contrast to Benedetti and Carlson,[5] we have observed low and even negative PCOP-PCWP gradients in term and postpartum patients with normal chest roentgenograms, low $\dot{Q}s/\dot{Q}_T$, and no clinical evidence of respiratory distress.

While the concept of the net intravascular force for fluid filtration in the lung, expressed as the PCOP-PCWP gradient, may be a satisfying academic exercise, we have not found the use of absolute numerical values to define an acceptable range for this variable to be clinically useful. Furthermore, it must be reiterated that the use of colloidal solutions to increase the PCOP-PCWP gradient can be harmful when capillary permeability is abnormal.

Resuscitative Fluid Regimen and Renal Function

Most experimental data indicate that resuscitation with colloidal solutions is less effective in preserving and restoring renal function than treatment with saline. Siegel et al. have studied the renal tubular function of baboons subjected to hemorrhagic shock for several hours and resuscitated with either Ringer's lactate solution alone or Ringer's lactate solution and 5 percent albumin.[52] Those animals treated with Ringer's lactate demonstrated a rapid return of renal tubular function and urine output to control values. In contrast, animals resuscitated with 5 percent albumin and Ringer's lactate solution manifested prolonged depression of tubular absorption of Na^+ and K^+, an inappropriate increase in free water clearance, a reduction in para-aminohippuric acid (PAH) extraction ratio, and a slow return to basal urine output.

Other studies have demonstrated a protective effect of saline loading on experimentally induced acute renal failure (ARF). In several experimental models of ARF, prior salt depletion has been shown to markedly accentuate the acute renal injury.[58] Salt-loaded animals experience better preservation of both glomerular and tubular function. In contrast to salt-depleted animals, which manifested little change in renal morphology and function with time, the appearance and function of the kidneys of salt-loaded animals improved more rapidly with dramatic increases in blood flow and glomerular filtration.

Clinical data also suggest that renal function is less effectively restored by colloidal solutions than by saline. In a pilot study carried out in Vietnam, Carey[11] found that casualties treated with 5 percent albumin did not fare as well clinically, required twice as much blood, and manifested a marked diminution in urine output as compared with a similar group resuscitated with Ringer's lactate solution. A subsequent prospective study, utilizing more sophisticated indices of renal function (glomerular filtration rate (GFR), sodium clearance, and water excretion), confirmed the association between the use of albumin and prolongation of renal dysfunction following resuscitation from shock.[30] Albumin-treated patients also manifested a marked increase in the incidence of ARF.[30]

Most authorities believe that the protective effect of crystalloid solutions is related to induction of a solute diuresis. This is more readily achieved by crystalloid than by colloid solutions. While colloidal solutions increase renal blood flow, they do not necessarily promote a solute diuresis.[31] However, if a severely hypoproteinemic patient experiences massive bleeding, it is wise to administer some colloid so that the fluid being infused can be more effectively maintained in the intravascular space.

BLOOD TRANSFUSION

Restoration of the oxygen-carrying capacity of the blood is as major a therapeutic priority as repletion of intravascular volume. At the present time this can only be accomplished by blood transfusion.

Minimum Hematocrit

A previously healthy nonpregnant patient with massive bleeding can tolerate a hematocrit as low as 20 percent with relative impunity when the deficit in oxygen-carrying capacity is combined with superadequate hydration with saline infusion.[15] The extra fluid and salt are eliminated over the next 1 to 4 days via diuresis, following which erythrocyte concentrations are increased. However, fetal oxygenation is a priority in the pregnant patient, and we recommend maintaining a hematocrit of at least 30 percent as a goal in acutely hemorrhaging pregnant women. It is important to realize that the hematocrit may remain unchanged for several hours following an acute hemorrhage. The decrease, maximal after 4 to 5 h, is due to compensatory fluid transfer from the extravascular compartment into the intravascular space.[2]

Red Cell Concentrates versus Whole Blood

Transfusion of whole blood has been the traditional method of replacing blood lost by massive hemorrhage. Indeed, until a decade ago, whole blood and plasma were the only blood products available clinically. The advent of plastic containers with multiple satellite pouches has made it possible to split freshly donated units of blood into its components without the hazard of bacterial contamination. The densities of red cells, plasma, platelets, and white cells differ sufficiently to make separation by centrifugation feasible. Blood and blood products are scarce resources. Fractionation of donated blood makes it possible to treat a number of people with a single unit of blood. Accordingly, it is the recommendation of the National Research Council's Division of Medical Sciences and the Committee on Transfusion of the American Medical Association that component therapy be practiced whenever possible.[20]

It is estimated that as many as 70 to 80 percent of all bleeding patients can be managed with packed red blood cells (hematocrit 60 to 80 percent) combined with supplemental crystalloid solutions rather than with whole blood.[41] It is certainly irrational to administer whole blood (hematocrit 30 percent) merely to replace red cells. The main objection to administering packed red blood cells (PRBC) to bleeding patients is the slow flow rate during infusion. This problem can be circumvented by diluting PRBC with normal saline prior to administration. Whole blood should be reserved for those patients with truly massive hemorrhage and even then should be combined 1:1 with PRBC.

Storage Lesions

Cold. Acid-citrate-dextrose (ACD) and citrate-phosphate-dextrose (CPD) blood are stored between 1 and 6°C. Transfusion of cold blood causes a lowering of body temperature, which can have a number of adverse effects. Peripheral vasoconstriction and a leftward shift of the oxyhemoglobin dissociation curve can reduce delivery of oxygen to the tissues. Shivering is associated with an increase in metabolic rate. Ventricular irritability increases as body temperature decreases, and core temperatures below 30°C can be associated with spontaneous ventricular fibrillation. These complications can be eliminated entirely by warming blood prior to transfusion. This can be accomplished by the use of a commercially available blood warmer or of coiled tubing submerged in warm water. The heating temperature should not exceed 110°F lest hemolysis occur.[27] Most electric blood warmers are set to shut off at 100°F but must be tested regularly for malfunction.

Depletion of 2,3-Diphosphoglycerate. The oxygen dissociation curve of blood is obtained by plotting percent saturation of hemoglobin against partial pressure of oxygen (PO_2) (Fig. 3-1). The characteristic sigmoidal shape of the curve is beneficial in that the plateau at the upper end ensures that a decrease in the partial pressure of alveolar O_2 (PAO_2) to values as low as 60 mmHg does not appreciably alter the adequacy of the arterial oxygen content. Conversely, the shape of the lower end of the curve ensures that even a small decrease in tissue PO_2 makes considerably more oxygen available to the tissues. A leftward shift in the oxygen dissociation curve decreases the level of PAO_2 above which appreciable saturation of hemoglobin occurs and thus, in this sense, is protective as far as uptake from the lung is concerned. However, the hemoglobin cannot now release oxygen to the same extent that it could previously until the tissue PO_2 has decreased by a similar margin. With a marked leftward shift it is conceivable that oxygen release might not occur even with tissue oxygen tensions within hypoxic ranges.

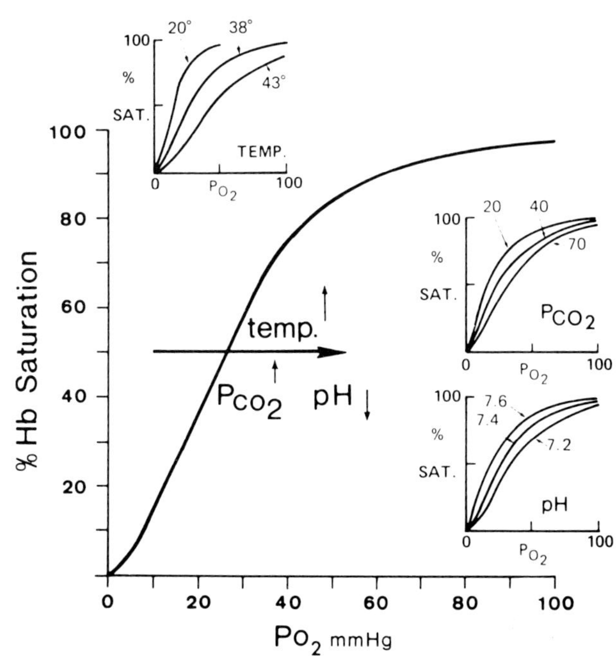

Fig. 3-1 Oxygen dissociation curve with alterations that can shift the curve to the right or left. A leftward shift indicates an increased affinity of hemoglobin for oxygen. (Reprinted with permission from West, J.B., Respiratory Physiology—the Essentials, © 1974, The Williams & Wilkins Co., Baltimore.)

In 1954, Valtis and Kennedy[61] reported that blood stored in ACD solution had a leftward shift in the oxygen dissociation curve, the magnitude of which was related to the duration of storage. This leftward shift is due to depletion of 2,3-diphosphoglycerate (2,3-DPG), an organic phosphate present in the red cell.[10] Other preservatives have been investigated as possible alternatives to ACD solution. The use of CPD solution results in better maintenance of 2,3-DPG levels and CPD is currently the only such preservative licensed in the state of Connecticut. The decrease in 2,3-DPG may be clinically significant. Hechtman,[22] in reviewing his own and other work, has shown that a rightward shift of the oxygen dissociation curve is associated with improved myocardial performance in cases of sepsis and after coronary artery surgery and may improve survival after aortic aneurysm surgery. In addition, Oski[45] has demonstrated improved survival in neonates with severe respiratory distress syndrome when fetal hemoglobin was replaced by adult hemoglobin via exchange transfusion. Accordingly, a decrease in parturient 2,3-DPG levels and a consequent change in the delicate balance between the relative positions of the maternal and fetal oxygen dissociation curves may well cause fetal hypoxia. The effect of reduced 2,3-DPG can be minimized by using the freshest blood possible. Blood should always be warmed before administration because hypothermia causes a leftward shift of the oxygen dissociation curve. Alkalosis also shifts the oxygen dissociation curve to the left, and excessive bicarbonate administration should be avoided. By the same token, acidosis should be avoided as, paradoxically, alkalinization facilitates 2,3-DPG repletion.[32]

The wider use of frozen red blood cells instead of ACD or CPD blood is receiving support from many sources. Frozen red blood cells have a high 2,3-DPG level. In essence, they are a specific form of PRBC. The red blood cells, virtually free of plasma, are suspended in glycerol, frozen in liquid nitrogen, and stored at −85 to 196°C. Additional advantages of this type of PRBC include a shelf life of years, which can be particularly useful with rare blood types; virtual elimination of transfusion hepatitis and megalovirus infections; a minimal chance of immunization to white cells or plasma proteins; and the absence of white cell and platelet debris.[60] However, this blood product has limited availability, and improvements are necessary in the time-consuming washing (removal of the cryoprotective glycerol prior to use) and thawing processes.

Acid-Base Balance. The pH of CPD solution is 5.6. In addition, stored blood accumulates by-products of continued erythrocyte metabolism, including lactic acid, pyruvic acid, and carbon dioxide. The net result is that a unit of stored blood has a pH of 6.6 to 6.8. Accordingly, it is reasonable to assume that the administration of large volumes of blood would create a metabolic acidosis. However, acid-base status remains relatively unchanged after massive blood replacement unless severe shock adds an endogenous source of lactic acid to the exogenous hydrogen ions supplied by the bank blood.[13,35] This is because the excess carbon dioxide is readily blown off in the lungs and the lactate and pyruvate are incorporated in the Krebs cycle. The empirical prophylactic administration of bicarbonate without objective indices of acidosis is never indicated except in cases of prolonged life-threatening shock. We recommend that analysis of arterial blood for pH and arterial carbon dioxide tension

($PaCO_2$) be performed after each 5 units of blood administered. Of course, severe metabolic acidosis thus determined does require bicarbonate therapy.

Paradoxically, metabolic alkalosis may be a delayed complication of massive transfusion. This is partly due to the metabolism of citrate (ACD and CPD solutions) and lactate (Ringer's lactate solution), often compounded by nasogastric suction and the use of diuretics. This acid-base derangement usually requires no specific therapy.

Hyperkalemia. Storage of blood at low temperatures inactivates the Na^+ pump in the red cell membrane. This results in an accumulation of Na^+ within the cell and a loss of intracellular K^+ into the plasma. While fresh blood contains a serum K^+ level of 3.9 mEq/L, 1-week-old blood has a level of 12 mEq/L, 2-week-old blood 17 mEq/L, and 3-week-old blood 21 mEq/L. Accordingly, patients suffering massive hemorrhage might receive significant amounts of K^+ over a short period of time. Despite this, blood must be administered at a rate of more than 1 unit every 3 min for consistent increases in recipient serum K^+ to occur, and the K^+ load will rarely result in serious hyperkalemia if renal function is intact.[9,24,50]

The earliest and most specific electrocardiogram (EKG) abnormalities in hyperkalemia are T wave changes. Tall, peaked, and narrow T waves become apparent with serum K^+ levels of 6.7 to 7.5 mEq/L. With a serum K^+ level in the range of 7.5 to 8 mEq/L, the QRS complex widens, the P-R interval lengthens, and P wave amplitude decreases. As serum K^+ levels increase above 8 to 9 mEq/L, intraventricular conduction time becomes more prolonged, with the QRS complex becoming biphasic. The QRS complex may merge with the elevated T wave, producing a sine wave pattern. Calcium may be given to counteract the membrane effects of hyperkalemia although this will not decrease the serum K^+ level. The serum K^+ level may be lowered acutely without excreting the excess K^+ by moving it intracellularly and establishing a more normal intra- to extracellular K^+ ratio. This can be accomplished with insulin, which augments K^+ uptake by cells. Insulin secretion is stimulated by the intravenous administration of 50 percent glucose. Usually 10 to 20 units of regular insulin are also given to ensure maximal K^+ uptake. Rapid alkalinization of plasma will also cause a shift of K^+ to the intracellular fluid. This can be achieved by hyperventilation and/or administration of sodium bicarbonate.

In contrast to the rare occurrence of hyperkalemia, hypokalemia commonly follows blood transfusion. Metabolism of the citrate in ACD and CPD blood can result in increased serum bicarbonate levels. Renal compensation for this abnormality involves alkalinization of the urine and is associated with a decrease in activity of the renal tubular H^+-K^+ exchange pump mechanism. The resultant urinary loss of K^+ may cause hypokalemia, which requires correction by K^+ supplementation.

Hypocalcemia ("Citrate Intoxication"). The citrate of ACD and CPD solution prevents coagulation by binding calcium. Therefore, transfusion of bank blood could theoretically cause hypocalcemia, but this is exceedingly rare. One unit of ACD blood must be administered every 3 min to a 70-kg patient in order to raise the circulating citrate to levels which may result in significant hypocalcemia. Usually, the citrate is readily metabolized in the liver, and endogenous Ca^{2+} stores are mobilized to replenish depleted serum Ca^{2+}. Therefore, routine Ca^{2+} administration is not indicated, but it should be given in response to EKG changes consistent with hypocalcemia (prolonged QT interval) or laboratory evidence of abnormally low serum levels.[26] Improvement in hemodynamics when Ca^{2+} is given empirically during massive transfusion of blood does not necessarily demonstrate the existence of hypocalcemia, because exogenously administered Ca^{2+} is a nonspecific, inotropic agent even when serum levels are in the normal range.[25,33]

Formation of Microaggregates. As storage time increases, the serum of bank blood accumulates increasing amounts of partculate matter. These microaggregates are composed of cellular debris, platelets, leukocytes, and fibrin. Routine blood administration sets have 170-μm filters. Microaggregates of smaller diameter are transfused directly into the circulation and become trapped in the pulmonary vasculature. This has generated concern not only regarding vascular occlusive phenomena but also that the microaggregates might combine in vivo with platelets and white cells to release vasoactive substances.[6,39] Accordingly, newer blood filters of 25- to 40-μm pore diameter have been used to supplement or replace larger pore filters. While there is little doubt about their effectiveness in removing microaggregates from transfused blood, the necessity of doing thus remains uncertain. Several groups have reported a lower incidence of pulmonary dysfunction in patients transfused through micropore filters.[4,48] However, numerous other reports have failed to validate these findings.[16,54] At the present time, it remains to be proved that microaggregates have a significant adverse effect on pulmonary function. At the very least, one should not delay administering vitally needed blood until a micropore filter can be found and set up.

Dilutional Coagulopathy

Dilution of the normal circulating clotting factors and platelets occurs when intravascular volume repletion is accomplished by the infusion of fluids deficient in these elements. When the degree of dilution is sufficient to cause abnormal bleeding, the condition is termed a dilutional coagulopathy.

Obviously, crystalloid solutions do not contain platelets, and bank blood becomes devoid of viable platelets after 24 h of storage. Acute dilutional thrombocytopenia becomes a clinically significant problem in healthy nonpregnant patients after transfusion of 15 to 30 units of blood.[34] A platelet count of approximately 50,000/mm^3 is a level necessary for surgery to proceed without continuous oozing from cut surfaces.[3] These same numerical values can probably be applied to the obstetrical patient. Although platelet counts in healthy pregnant women have been variously reported to be elevated,[38] subnormal,[51] and normal,[7] the differences in absolute values in reported series are small, and platelet function is normal during pregnancy. Thus, when the tenth unit of blood is transfused and it appears probable that many more will be needed, a platelet count should be performed, and platelet concentrates should be ordered when the count is 100,000/mm^3. Hopefully, the platelet concentrate will be available by the time 20 to 25 units of blood have been administered. One unit of platelets can raise the platelet count approximately 10,000/mm^3 in a 70-

kg adult.[42] Not less than 5 units should be administered to allow a reasonable reserve margin. Although normal circulating platelets have a life-span of 9 to 11 days in pregnancy, the effect of platelet transfusion is limited to a few days.[19] Seventy percent of administered platelets rapidly become sequestered in the spleen and 50 percent of the remainder have only a 1-day survival time.[19] Accordingly, we recommend that the platelet count be followed serially for several days.

Bank blood is deficient in factors V and VIII. Factor VIII is the most unstable of the clotting proteins, with the level in CPD blood falling below 50 percent after less than 24 h of storage at 4°C.[19] Factor V is less labile, the mean level in CPD blood remaining at about 50 percent for more than 2 weeks.[19] Only 30 percent of factor VIII and 5 to 20 percent of factor V are necessary for normal hemostasis to occur. Many authorities believe that a dilutional coagulopathy resulting from deficiencies in these two factors is unlikely in situations where less than 30 units of whole blood have been transfused.[19] However, a PRBC-crystalloid fluid regimen contains almost no clotting factors whatsoever and causes a greater degree of dilution than whole blood. The prothrombin time (PT) and partial thromboplastin time (PTT) are the primary screening tests for abnormalities in clotting proteins. These tests should be performed when 10 units of blood have been transfused. Fresh frozen plasma (FFP) contains all the coagulation factors, and administration of 1 unit of FFP for each 5 units of blood transfused above 10 units should be sufficient to maintain the PT and PTT within normal limits irrespective of the resuscitative fluid regimen.

The use of fibrinogen concentrates is associated with an incidence of hepatitis in excess of 50 percent, and these blood products have no place in the therapy of massive bleeding. Likewise, concentrates containing factors II, VII, IX, and X (Koyne and Proplex) are not recommended. These preparations are associated with a similar incidence of hepatitis and may also cause anaphylaxis.

When any coagulopathy occurs, a differential diagnosis of dilutional coagulopathy, disseminated intravascular coagulation, and primary fibrinolysis must be entertained. Differentiation of these disorders requires further laboratory analysis, including the measurement of fibrinogen levels, thrombin time, and fibrin split products (FSP). It is vital that a hematologist be closely involved in decision making when these diagnoses are seriously considered. The reader is referred to Chapter 9 for an in-depth review of this topic.

Major Immediate Transfusion Reactions

Reactions Involving Red Blood Cells. When the antigen-antibody reaction involves the red blood cells, the cell membrane ruptures. This hemolysis usually involves the donor red blood cells, with the patient furnishing the involved antibody. The reverse phenomenon, i.e., lysis of patient red blood cells by donor plasma antibody, is rare but can occur when O negative (universal donor) blood is administered in an extreme emergency without crossmatching.

Hemolytic reactions usually begin with chills, fever, chest or flank pain, and nausea. When the patient is under general anesthesia, the most common signs are unexplained hypotension, pink- or red-stained urine (hemoglobinuria), and the onset of oozing from surgical wounds and venipuncture sites (disseminated intravascular coagulation, DIC). Hemoglobinemia and hemoglobinuria occur when the release of free hemoglobin following rupture of the red cell membrane exceeds the binding capacity of serum haptoglobin. The DIC may result from activation of the intrinsic coagulation system by elements of the hemolyzed red blood cell membrane.[37]

Investigation of a suspected transfusion reaction involves the following steps: (1) Discontinue the transfusion. (2) Draw a fresh specimen of the patient's blood for blood grouping, serological testing, and crossmatching. (3) Send any unused blood, including the unit being transfused, the infusion set in use, and any "empty" blood containers to the blood bank. (4) Perform a careful check to confirm the identity of the patient and the accuracy of clerical records (40 percent of the 80 transfusion reaction associated fatalities which occurred in the United States between 1976 and 1979 resulted from clerical errors). (5) Obtain specimens of blood and urine for estimation of plasma and urinary hemoglobin levels, respectively. (6) Draw specimens of blood for estimation of PT, PTT, fibrinogen level, thrombin time, and FSP.

A major focus of the treatment of a hemolytic transfusion reaction is the maintenance of renal function. Renal impairment may occur as a result of damage mediated by antigen-antibody-complement complexes.[49] Vigorous hydration and diuresis with mannitol and/or furosemide to maintain the urine output at 1.5 to 2.0 cc/kg/h are recommended. In addition, alkalinization of the urine reduces precipitation of hemoglobin in the renal tubules and can be accomplished by administration of sodium bicarbonate and carbonic anhydrase inhibitors.[43] Finally, if pharmacological agents are required to maintain the patient's circulatory status, alpha-adrenergic vasopressors should be avoided because the ensuing vasoconstriction may contribute to renal damage.[42]

Reactions Involving White Cells, Platelets, and Plasma Proteins. Major immediate reactions to these blood elements take the form of noncardiogenic (increased capillary permeability) pulmonary edema (PE) or anaphylaxis (noncardiogenic PE and cardiovascular collapse). These reactions occur mainly in patients who have received multiple prior transfusions (particularly platelet transfusions), in multiparous women,[37] and in patients with a congenital absence of IgA.[63] Treatment is supportive and involves the use of the antihistamines, epinephrine, corticosteroids, and ventilatory support. The sheer multiplicity of potential antigens precludes elimination of these reactions by crossmatching techniques. They are usually avoided in patients who give a history of untoward responses to blood transfusion by using frozen red blood cells, in which the serum elements are removed in the deglycerolation process, and PRBC prepared by centrifugation and sedimentation.

SYNTHETIC OXYGEN-TRANSPORT FLUIDS

For many years, a search has been underway for oxygen-transporting materials that can be used as a substitute for blood replacement. Hemoglobin preparations have been extensively investigated without a major breakthrough in terms of clinical applicability. An alternate to such oxygen-binding agents is the use of liquids with the capability of dissolving large amounts of oxygen.[18] Recently, several investigators have reported the successful clinical use of perfluorochemicals, which are hydrophobic nonpolar liquids with a high oxygen solubility, as effective oxygen-transport fluids.[36,44,59] These fluids afford biologically useful concentrations of dissolved oxygen at high partial pressures of oxygen, and elimination of the need for blood typing means that emergency situations could be met without delay. These fluids are still in the early stages of evaluation, but in the future they may allow less dependence on blood products for the management of massively bleeding patients.

REFERENCES

1. Achaner, B., Allyn, P., Furnas, D., and Bartlett, R.H.: Pulmonary complications of burns: the major threat to the burn patient. Ann. Surg., *177*:311, 1973.
2. Adamson, J. and Hillman, R.: Blood volume and plasma protein replacement following acute blood loss in normal man. JAMA, *205*:609, 1968.
3. Barrer, M. and Ellison, N.: Platelet function. Anesthesiology, *42*:202, 1977.
4. Barrett, J., Tahir, A.H., and Litwin, M.S.: Increased pulmonary arteriovenous shunting in humans following blood transfusion. Arch. Surg., *113*:947, 1978.
5. Benedetti, T. and Carlson, R.: Studies of colloid osmotic pressure in pregnancy-induced hypertension. Am. J. Obstet. Gynecol., *135*:308, 1979.
6. Bennett, S.H., Geelhoed, G.W., Aaron, R.K. et al.: Pulmonary injury resulting from perfusion with stored bank blood in the baboon and dog. J. Surg. Res., *13*:295, 1972.
7. Bonnar, J., McNicol, G., and Douglas, A.: Fibrinolytic enzyme system and pregnancy. Br. Med. J, *3*:387, 1969.
8. Brigham, K., Woolverton, W., Blake, L., and Staub, N.: Increased lung vascular permeability caused by Pseudomonas bacteremia. J. Clin. Invest., *45*:792, 1975.
9. Bunker, J.: Metabolic effects of blood transfusion. Anesthesiology, *27*:446, 1966.
10. Bunn, H. and Jandl, J.: Control of hemoglobin function within the red cell. N. Engl. J. Med, *282*:1414, 1970.
11. Carey, L., Lowery, B., and Cloutier, C.: Hemorrhagic shock. In: Current Problems in Surgery, Year Book Medical Publishers, Chicago, 1971.
12. Chien, S., Sinclair, D., Dellenback, R. et al.: Effect of endotoxin on capillary permeability to macromolecules. Am. J. Physiol., *207*:518, 1965.
13. Collins, J., Simmons, R., James, P. et al.: The acid-base status of seriously wounded combat casualties: II. Resuscitation with stored blood. Ann. Surg., *173*:6, 1971.
14. da Luz, P., Shubin, H., Weil, M. H. et al.: Pulmonary edema related to changes in colloid osmotic and pulmonary artery wedge pressure in patients after acute myocardial infarction. Circulation, *51*:350, 1975.
15. Dillon, J., Lynch, L., Myers, R., and Butcher, H.: The treatment of hemorrhagic shock. Surg. Gynecol. Obstet., *122*:967, 1966.
16. Durtschi, M. B., Haisch, C. E., Reynolds, L. et al.: Effect of micropore filtration in pulmonary function after massive transfusion. Am. J. Surg, *138*:8, 1979.
17. Gaisford, W., Pandey, N., and Jansen, C.: Pulmonary changes in treated hemorrhagic shock. Am. J. Surg., *124*:738, 1972.
18. Geyer, R.: Oxygen transport in-vivo by means of perfluorochemical preparations. N. Engl. J. Med., *307*:304, 1982.

19. Greenwalt, T. and Perry, S.: Preservation and utilization of the components of human blood. p. 148. In Brown, E. and Moore, C. Eds.: Progress in Hematology. Vol. 6. Grune and Stratton, New York and London, 1969.
20. Greenwalt, T.J., Ed.: General Principles of Blood Transfusion, American Medical Association, Chicago, 1973.
21. Guyton, A. and Lindsey, A.: Effect of elevated left atrial pressure and decreased plasma protein concentration on the development of pulmonary edema. Circ. Res., *7*:649, 1959.
22. Hechtman, H., Grindlinger, G., Vegas, A. et al.: Importance of oxygen transport in clinical medicine. Crit. Care Med., *7*:419, 1979.
23. Hellems, H., Haynes, F., Dexter, L., and Kinney, T.: Pulmonary capillary pressure in animals estimated by venous and arterial catheterization. Am. J. Physiol., *155*:98, 1948.
24. Howland, W., Bellville, J., Zucker, M., and Cliffton, E.: Massive blood replacement. V. Failure to observe citrate intoxication. Surg. Gynecol. Obstet., *105*:529, 1957.
25. Howland, W., Jacobs, R., and Goulet, A.: An evaluation of calcium administration during rapid blood replacement. Anesth. Analg. (Cleve), 39:557, 1960.
26. Howland, W. and Schweizer, O.: Physiologic compensation for storage lesion of blood. Anesth. Analg. (Cleve), *44*:8, 1965.
27. Howland, W. and Schweizer, O.: Blood warming and hemolysis. Anesthesiology, *26*:223, 1965.
28. Katz, S., Aberman, A., Frand, U. et al.: Heroin pulmonary edema—evidence for increased capillary permeability. Am. Rev. Respir. Dis., *106*:472, 1972.
29. Levine, O., Mellins, R., Senior, R., and Fishman, A.: The application of Starling's Law of capillary exchange to the lungs. J. Clin. Invest., *49*:923, 1967.
30. Lucas, C., Ledgerwood, A., and Higgins, R.: Impaired salt and water excretion after albumin resuscitation for hypovolemic shock. Surgery, *86*:544, 1979.
31. Lucas, C., Weaver, D., Higgins, R. et al.: Effects of albumin versus non-albumin resuscitation on plasma volume and renal excretory function. J. Trauma, *18*:564, 1978.
32. Miller, R.: The oxygen dissociation curve and multiple transfusions of ACD blood. p. 43. In Howland, W. and Schweizer, O., Eds.: Management of the patient for radical cancer surgery: Clinical Anesthesia, F. A. Davis, Philadelphia, 1972.
33. Miller, R.: Complications of massive transfusion. Anesthesiology, 39:82, 1973.
34. Miller, R., Robbins, T., and Tong, M.: Coagulation defects associated with massive blood transfusions. Ann. Surg., *174*:794, 1971.
35. Miller, R., Tong, M., and Robbins, T.: Effects of massive transfusion of blood on acid-base balance. JAMA, *216*:1762, 1971.
36. Mitsuno, T., Ohyanagi, H., and Naito, R.: Clinical studies of a perfluorochemical blood substitute (Fluosol-DA). Ann. Surg., *195*:60, 1982.
37. Mollison, P.: Blood Transfusions in Clinical Medicine. 4th Ed. F. A. Davis Co., Philadelphia, 1972.
38. Mor, A., Yang, W., Schwarz, A., and Jones, W.: Platelet counts in pregnancy and labor. Obstet. Gynecol., *16*:338, 1960.
39. Mosely, R. and Doty, D.: Changes in the filtration characteristics of stored blood. Ann. Surg., *171*:329, 1970.
40. Moss, G., Das Gupta, T., Newson, B., and Nyhus, L.: The effect of saline resuscitation on pulmonary sodium and water distribution. Surg. Gynecol. Obstet., *136*:934, 1973.
41. Moss, G., Valeri, C., and Brodine, C.: Clinical experience with the use of frozen blood in combat casualties. N. Engl. J. Med., *278*:747, 1968.
42. Myhre, B., Ed.: Blood Component Therapy: A Physician's Handbook. 2nd Ed. American Association of Blood Banks, Washington, 1975.
43. Nalbandian, R., Mader, I., Margulis, R., and Camp, F.: Preventing death from incompatible transfusions. Postgrad. Med., *45*:84, 1969.

44. Ohyanagi, H., Toshima, K., Sekita, M., and Naito, R.: Clinical studies of perfluorochemical whole blood substitutes: safety of Fluosol-DA (20%) in normal human volunteers. Clin. Ther. 2:306, 1979.
45. Oski, F.: Clinical implications of the oxyhemoglobin dissociation curve in the neonatal period. Crit. Care Med., *7*:412, 1979.
46. Rackow, E., Fein, A., and Leppo, J.: Colloid osmotic pressure as a prognostic indicator of pulmonary edema and mortality in the critically ill. Chest, *72*:709, 1977.
47. Rafferty, T., Ljungquist, R., Firestone, L. et al.: The plasma colloid oncotic pressure—pulmonary artery occlusion pressure gradient. A poor predictor of pulmonary edema in surgical intensive care unit patients. Arch. Surg. (in press).
48. Ruel, G.J., Greenberg, S.D., Lefrak, E.A. et al.: Prevention of post-traumatic pulmonary insufficiency: fine screen filtration of blood. Arch. Surg., *106*:386, 1973.
49. Schmidt, P. and Holland, P.: Pathogenesis of the acute renal failure associated with incompatible transfusion. Lancet, *2*:1169, 1967.
50. Schweizer, O. and Howland, W.: Potassium levels, acid-base balance and massive blood replacement. Anesthesiology, *23*:735, 1962.
51. Shaper, A., Kear, J., Macintosh, D. et al.: The platelet count, platelet adhesiveness and aggregation and the mechanism of fibrinolytic inhibition in pregnancy and the puerperium. J. Obstet. Gynecol. Br. Commonw., *75*:433, 1968.
52. Siegel, D., Cochin, M., Geocaris, T., and Moss, G.: Effects of saline and colloid resuscitation on renal function. Ann. Surg., *177*:51, 1973.
53. Siegel, D., Moss, G., Cochin, A., and Das Gupta, T.: Pulmonary changes following treatment for hemorrhagic shock: saline versus colloid infusion. Surg. Forum, *2*:17, 1980.
54. Snyder, E.L., Barash, P., Hezzey, A., and Palermo, G.: Microaggregate blood filtration in patients with compromised pulmonary function. Transfusion, *22*:21, 1982.
55. Studd, J., Blainey, J., and Bailey, D.: A study of serum protein changes in late pregnancy and identification of the pregnancy zone protein using antigen antibody crossed immunoelectrophoresis. J. Obstet. Gynecol., *77*:42, 1970.
56. Studd, J., Blainey, J., and Bailey, D.: Serum protein changes in the pre-eclampsia eclampsia syndrome. J. Obstet. Gynecol. Br. Commonw., *77*:796, 1970.
57. Studd, J., Shaw, R., and Bailey, D.: Maternal and fetal serum protein concentrations in normal pregnancy and pregnancy complicated by proteinuric pre-eclampsia. Am. J. Obstet. Gynecol., *114*:582, 1972.
58. Thiel, G., McDonald, F., and Oken, D.: Micropuncture studies of the basis for protection of renin depleted rats from glycerol induced acute renal failure. Nephron, *8*:67, 1970.
59. Tremper, K., Friedman, A., Levine, E. et al.: The preoperative treatment of severely anemic patients with a perfluorochemical oxygen-transport fluid, Fluosol-DA. N. Engl. J. Med., *307*:277, 1982.
60. Valeri, C.: Frozen blood. N. Engl. J. Med. *275*:365, 1966.
61. Valtis, D. and Kennedy, A.: Defective gas-transport function of stored red blood cells. Lancet, *1*:119, 1954.
62. Virgilio, R., Rice, C., Smith, D. et al.: Crystalloid versus colloid resuscitation: Is one better? Surgery, *85*:129, 1979.
63. Vyas, G., Perkins, H., and Fudenl : Immunological study of human IgA globulin. I. Anaphylactoid transfusion reactions sociated with anti-IgA. Lancet, *2*:312, 1968.
64. Weaver, D., Lederwood, A., Lucas, C. et al.: Pulmonary effects of albumin resuscitation for severe hypovolemic shock. Arch. Surg., *113*:387, 1978.
65. Zapol, W. and Snider, M.: Pulmonary hypertension in severe acute respiratory failure. N. Engl. J. Med., *296*:476, 1977.
66. Zarins, C., Rice, C., Smith, D. et al.: Role of lymphatics in preventing hypo-oncotic pulmonary edema. Surg. Forum, *27*:257, 1976.

4

Cardiac Surgery in Pregnant Women

Ronald M. Becker, M.D.

Since the advent of human cardiac surgery in the late 1940s and early 1950s, hundreds of cardiac operations have been performed in pregnant patients, and the vast majority have apparently been successful for both mother and fetus.

Most of these operations have been performed for the relief of mitral stenosis, but in recent years virtually the entire spectrum of cardiac pathology has been treated surgically in pregnant patients.

In addition to searching the medical literature, the author has conducted a survey among members of the Society of Thoracic Surgeons (STS). This society contains virtually all the practicing cardiothoracic surgeons in North America and also many prominent surgeons from abroad. A detailed questionnaire was mailed to each member of the society, requesting information on the surgeon's experience with cardiac surgery in pregnant patients. Nearly 2,000 of these questionnaires were mailed out and the response was excellent. Over 500 surgeons replied that they had no experience with cardiac procedures in pregnant patients, while 119 positive responses were returned. Some of these surgeons had already described their experiences in the medical literature but most had not and the responses have been extremely helpful in providing a clear picture of current attitudes, practices, and results regarding cardiac operations in pregnant patients.

It is important to understand the distinction between those procedures requiring use of the heart-lung machine, i.e., cardiopulmonary bypass (CPB) and those which can be performed without resort to cardiopulmonary bypass. The former are referred to as open-heart operations while the latter are called closed procedures. Although coronary bypass surgery is not strictly speaking open-heart surgery, since the chambers of the heart or great vessels are not opened, it is generally performed with the aid of CPB and therefore can be classified with the open-heart procedures.

The distinction between open and closed procedures is important because CPB produces profound alterations in physiology, while closed procedures avoid the effects of CPB and should be no more hazardous to the fetus than any other major procedure requiring general anesthesia. Although it is apparent that the surgeon should feel obligated to select a closed operation whenever possible, mitral stenosis is the only pathologic condition for which a true option between open and closed operations exists.

CARDIOPULMONARY BYPASS AND ITS POTENTIAL EFFECTS ON THE FETUS

Cardiopulmonary bypass (CPB) produces significant physiologic changes but these are surprisingly well tolerated when bypass time is less than 3 to 4 h.

Patients undergoing CPB are heparinized to the point that clotting is virtually absent. In addition, the oxygenators used in CPB traumatize plasma proteins and platelets so that even after CPB is discontinued and heparin reversed, hemostasis is not normal. Nevertheless, spontaneous bleeding at sites remote from the operative field is exceedingly rare, and it is unlikely that bleeding into the placenta, uterus, or fetus itself is a significant hazard.

In CPB the function of the lungs is performed by the oxygenator. The level of oxygenation and the removal of CO_2 must be constantly monitored by frequent blood gas determinations. In most centers, these are performed by the bypass team in the operating room. Normal pH, pCO_2, and O_2 saturation levels are easily and routinely maintained during CPB, and there is no reason why a pregnant woman or her fetus should be unduly at risk for hypoxia, acidosis, or alkalosis. Whether hyperoxia (pO_2 during CPB is usually >200 mmHg) is potentially harmful to the fetus is unknown.

The aspect of CPB which is probably of greatest concern with regard to the fetus is the perfusion of blood. This is generally performed by a roller pump, which produces continuous (i.e., nonpulsatile) return of arterialized blood from the oxygenator to the patient's arterial circulation via a cannula in the aorta or femoral artery. Venous blood returns to the oxygenator via cannulas in the right atrium or cavae by simple gravity drainage. Although nonpulsatile blood flow has theoretical disadvantages and potentially damaging renal effects, in practice it does not produce harmful short- or long-term sequelae when perfusion and oxygenation are otherwise adequate. While some centers have produced pulsatile CPB by use of various devices, there is little evidence to suggest that this has any practical advantage over nonpulsatile CPB.[6] Although I am unaware of any studies of the response of the uteroplacental circulation to nonpulsatile flow, there is no a priori reason to suspect that it should respond differently than flow to other organs.

Most centers strive to maintain a total CPB blood flow which approaches a normal resting cardiac output. This flow is in the range of 2.4 to 2.6 L/min/m^2 for nonpregnant patients and is achieved simply by manipulating the speed of the roller pump. Depending on gestational age, the "normal" cardiac index for pregnant women may be considerably higher. Since it is likely that higher flow rates would maximize perfusion of all maternal and fetal organs, CPB should probably be administered at a rate of 2.8 to $3 L/min/m^2$ during pregnancy. Optimal flow during CPB depends on adequate venous return, and patients operated upon late in pregnancy should be positioned with the right flank elevated to displace the uterus off the inferior vena cava.

The pressure in the arterial circulation during CPB is related to total CPB flow and systemic vascular resistance (SVR). Although SVR tends to rise during CPB, the more important determinant of pressure will be the flow rate. Mean perfusion pressure ≥ 80 mmHg should be the goal and pressures <50 mmHg are unacceptable. If increasing flow rate does not produce adequate pressures, then pharmacologic means should be considered to increase SVR, although the potential harmful effects of vasoconstrictors on uterine or placental vessels must be borne in mind. Organs vary in their responses to changes in pressure (e.g., coronary circulation is quite pressure-dependent while cerebral circulation is more flow-dependent) but as is true of total perfusion flow, it seems wisest to aim for a mean perfusion pressure approaching the normal.

Hypothermia is commonly employed in conjunction with CPB. The perfusate is usually cooled to 20 to 30°C as it is pumped back into the arterial circulation. Hypothermia helps reduce local metabolic activity during the period of cardiac arrest when surgery in or around the heart is being performed. The consequences for the fetus of hypothermia, with its attendant reduction in metabolic rate, are unknown. Of particular concern is the potential for ventricular fibrillation, with cooling to levels below 30°C. Total body hypothermia in conjunction with CPB is not a necessity, since other means are available to achieve local myocardial cooling. Therefore I believe that one should avoid or minimize the use of hypothermia during CPB in the pregnant patient.

There is currently no detailed published data regarding the effects of CPB on the fetus. Therefore it seems appropriate to suggest that what is safest for the mother is likely to also be safest for her fetus. High-flow, high-pressure CPB at normothermia should be the optimal technique. One should recognize that short periods of deviations from the ideal may be well tolerated by the mother but be disastrous for the fetus. The usual monitoring of pressure, flow, blood gases, etc. must be extremely strict, and an extra margin of safety can be gained by electronic fetal heart rate and uterine monitoring.

Fetal Heart and Uterine Monitoring During CPB

Several authors have now reported their results with electronic fetal heart rate monitoring during CPB for various procedures. A consistent finding has been fetal bradycardia occurring with the onset of CPB and persisting throughout the period of its use, despite high flow rates at adequate pressures and satisfactory acid-base balance. The bradycardia may be a response to the moderate hypothermia (30 to 32°C) generally employed or to alterations in placental perfusion patterns in response to nonpulsatile flow. Although the cause of fetal bradycardia during CPB is unknown, it does not portend an adverse outcome. In each of the cases cited, fetal heart rate returned to baseline levels shortly after CPB was discontinued, and healthy infants were eventually delivered at term.

An increased frequency of uterine contractions has also been reported during CPB.[1,5,14] In some cases the contractions disappeared without specific therapeutic measures shortly after the surgery was completed and therefore increased uterine activity does not necessarily indicate the onset of premature labor. However, in all the cases cited the patients were in their third trimester of pregnancy, which reinforces the concept that surgery late in pregnancy does increase the risk of premature labor.

MITRAL STENOSIS

Closed Commissurotomy

Mitral stenosis is the commonest significant sequel to rheumatic heart disease. Reduction in the mitral valvular orifice leads to elevation of the left atrial pressure. With demand for increased cardiac output or with significant increase in circulating blood volume, as occurs during the second trimester of pregnancy, severe elevations in left atrial pressure (LAP) may occur. Elevated LAP will cause pulmonary congestion and dyspnea and eventually frank pulmonary edema. Thus the alterations in cardiovascular physiology which occur during pregnancy may convert a minimally symptomatic patient into a cardiac cripple.

Prior to the availability of cardiac surgery, cardiac disease was said to be the leading cause of maternal mortality during pregnancy, with mitral stenosis by far the most common cardiac lesion.[18,21] In severely compromised patients maternal mortality was as high as 40 percent. Closed mitral commissurotomy during pregnancy was first reported in 1952, and by the late 1950s several large series had been reported.[10,18,20]

Reid[18] described the accumulated experience with 133 procedures done in pregnant women. There were five maternal and nine fetal deaths in this series. Although maternal mortality was higher than expected for a similar group of nonpregnant patients, this was not due to effects of pregnancy per se but rather to the tendency to procrastinate in pregnant patients beyond the point of salvage. Thus it was clear that surgery early in pregnancy would avoid the necessity for urgent, high-risk operations in the face of severe circulatory compromise.

Although results of closed mitral commissurotomy in pregnant patients in the 1950s were excellent, they were nevertheless compromised by: (1) unavailability of open-heart surgery, which forced surgeons to perform closed commissurotomy in less than ideal cases (the optimal valve for closed commissurotomy being one with no calcium, pliable leaflets, no regurgitation, and no thrombus); (2) unsophisticated diagnostic methods, resulting in an occasional operation in patients without significant stenosis; and (3) crude monitoring and anesthesia techniques. With the current widespread availability of echocardiography, confirmation of the diagnosis and identification of appropriate cases should be easier, and the availability of open-heart surgery should eliminate the performance of closed commissurotomy in inappropriate cases. Current results are in fact excellent. In the STS survey, over 100 cases were reported by more than 50 surgeons. There were no maternal deaths and only 3 perinatal losses, one of which occurred after emergency caesarean section and simultaneous commissurotomy in a woman who had respiratory arrest during labor.

On the basis of these results, I believe one can confidently recommend closed mitral commissurotomy in the pregnant patient who progresses beyond early class II symptoms. The operation should ideally be performed at 15 to 20 weeks gestation. Procrastination will increase the risk both for the mother (since increases in blood volume and cardiac output will more severely compromise her circulatory status) and for the fetus (since premature labor is more likely to occur in association with surgery later in pregnancy). Women who have experienced serious difficulties in previous pregnancies should also be considered candidates for elective operation at 15 weeks gestation, although preferably this should be done prior to conception.

Open Mitral Commissurotomy

As increasing experience confirmed the safety of cardiopulmonary bypass, most surgeons in North America abandoned closed mitral commissurotomy in favor of the open approach. With direct vision of the valve the surgeon can achieve a more accurate commissurotomy and also attend to subvalvular fusion if necessary. This results in more predictable outcomes. In addition, thrombus, if present, can be removed and valve replacement can be performed if the valve appears to be unsuitable for simple commissurotomy. The mortality rate for open mitral commissurotomy is under 2 percent[8,19] with excellent long-term results. Since closed commissurotomy is now virtually obsolete in North America, increasingly fewer surgeons are familiar or comfortable with this technique. In the future one can therefore expect that pregnant women will be subjected to the open approach, despite the argument that a closed procedure, without CPB, would be far safer for their fetuses.

The earliest successful open mitral commissurotomies during pregnancy were reported by Zuhdi and Kozam[13] in the mid-1960s. The survey of STS members revealed 19 instances of open mitral commissurotomy during pregnancy with no maternal deaths. In 16 cases the pregnancy continued to term with delivery of a normal infant. In one case, in which surgery was performed at 32 weeks gestation, spontaneous delivery of a healthy baby, weighing slightly less than 4 lb occurred 6 h postoperatively. In another, spontaneous vaginal delivery of a healthy premature neonate occurred at 32 weeks, 3 weeks after cardiac surgery. In this case the premature delivery was felt to be unrelated to the open mitral commissurotomy.

A fetus died in only one case. This occurred at 28 weeks in the immediate postoperative period. Electronic fetal monitoring was used in this instance, and fetal heart tones were lost shortly after the mother was returned to the intensive care unit (ICU). Spontaneous labor with the vaginal delivery of a stillborn occurred approximately 2 h after return to the ICU. Although no specific cause of death was identified, hypothermia (32°F) during CPB had been used.

The overall results (19 of 19 maternal and 18 of 19 fetal survivors) indicate the safety of this operation during pregnancy. It can be performed generally with short CPB time, and normothermic perfusion is certainly compatible with excellent results.

VALVE REPLACEMENT SURGERY

Choice of Prosthesis

When cardiac valve replacement is necessary, the surgeon and patient may choose among several mechanical (i.e., plastic or metal) or biologic (i.e., natural animal tissue) prostheses. In each group valves with acceptable hemodynamic properties are available so that hemodynamic performance is not an important determinant in selection of the appropriate type of valve. The major issues are thrombogenicity versus durability. Currently available mechanical valves (e.g., Bjork-Shiley or Starr-Edwards) have excellent records of durability. However every mechanical valve currently available requires continuous full anticoagulation in order to minimize the risk of thromboembolic complications which may produce systemic emboli or impede the proper functioning of the valve.

On the other hand, porcine or bovine pericardial prostheses produce minimal thromboembolic complications even in the absence of systemic anticoagulation.[2] This is especially true for aortic valve replacements but catastrophic emboli from biologic mitral prostheses are also quite uncommon. The major limitation in the use of these valves is their uncertain durability. The cumulative experience with porcine prostheses suggests that more than 90 percent will function for at least 5 years. However, gradual stiffening and calcification produces an increasing incidence of valve failure so that by 10 years approximately 30 percent of patients require reoperation.[15,17] The risk of valve failure is increased and accelerated in younger patients, especially those less than 35 years old.[15] Experience with bovine pericardial valves is too limited at this time to determine long-term durability. We are hopeful that they will fare better than porcine valves, and Ionescu's experience is quite promising.[11] Recent reports of early failure in children,[7] however, suggest that bovine pericardial valves may behave similarly to porcine valves in young patients.

The options are clear: One may choose a mechanical valve with excellent durability but obligatory anticoagulation and the potential for catastrophic thromboembolism, or one may choose a tissue valve of limited durability which will almost certainly require replacement within a few years but does not require anticoagulation. The difficulties related to adequate anticoagulation in the pregnant woman are so overwhelming that I believe one is forced to choose a tissue valve and accept the need for eventual replacement.

Because coumarin derivatives cross the placental barrier and because the fetal liver is immature, properly controlled anticoagulation in the mother may result in gross hyperanticoagulation of the fetus at any time during the pregnancy.[3] Therefore, coumarin anticoagulants may produce fatal hemorrhagic complications throughout pregnancy in addition to their direct teratogenic effects in the first trimester. Although heparin does not cross the placental barrier, the problems associated with several months of full anticoagulation with heparin are so great that this is an alternative fraught with difficulties. The relatively large number of reports of thrombosed prostheses in pregnant and peripartum patients, to be discussed further below, emphasizes the difficulties of proper anticoagulation in the pregnant patient.

I therefore feel that when valve replacement is necessary in the pregnant woman, a tissue valve should be inserted. Recognizing the probable need for eventual replacement, the patient should be counseled to have any additional children in close succession, so that potential pregnancy will not be a factor in the choice of a valve substitute when re-replacement becomes necessary.

Results of Aortic Valve Replacement

In the survey of STS members 6 isolated aortic valve replacements during pregnancy were reported, and only a handful of others have been published in the literature, so that 11 cases are available for analysis.

Seven patients were operated upon for symptoms related to either congenital or acquired aortic stenosis. All the mothers survived the surgery but only three of the pregnancies were successfully completed. In the other four cases spontaneous abortion occurred within 3 days of operation; three of these operations were during the second trimester and one at 6 weeks.

Three patients were operated upon for complications of endocarditis, two during the second trimester and the third at 32 weeks. In each case the pregnancy was continued to term and an apparently healthy infant was born. In a fourth patient with endocarditis, the infant was delivered by cesarean section just prior to aortic valve replacement. These results suggest that the fetus is not necessarily adversely affected by maternal endocarditis if it is treated aggressively.

Results of Mitral Valve Replacement

Since the first published case by Harthorne et al. in 1967, only 19 women have been reported to have had mitral valve replacements during pregnancy. Fourteen operations were performed for symptoms related to rheumatic mitral valve disease. The mother survived surgery in each instance, although one (and her fetus) died of hepatitis 7 weeks postoperatively. Ten pregnancies were completed successfully. In the other cases, one spontaneous abortion occurred 3 days postoperatively at 20 weeks, one infant born at term had cerebral palsy thought to be related to heparin mismanagement, and one premature infant was born 1 day postoperatively to a patient operated upon at 30 weeks.

One procedure was performed for complications of endocarditis. The mother survived the operation but spontaneous abortion occurred 1 day postoperatively at 15 weeks.

Four patients had emergency replacement of thrombosed mechanical valves. In all four cases the mother survived. Three of these pregnancies were successfully completed although one infant was born with mild hydrocephalus. In the fourth case a stillbirth occurred 3 days postoperatively at 31 weeks. Considering that all four women were in cardiogenic shock at the time of surgery, these results must be considered excellent. In a fifth patient with a thrombosed mitral prosthesis, emergency caesarean section, followed by mitral valve replacement, was performed at 35 weeks, with successful outcome for both mother and fetus. A sixth patient had successful emergency caesarean section followed by mitral valve replacement while on CPB at 36 weeks.[16]

Considering aortic and mitral valve replacement together, it appears that valve replacement is generally successful for both mother and fetus. The incidence of fetal loss is higher than for simple open commissurotomy, no doubt because patients requiring valve replacement are sicker and the period of greatest risk, i.e., the duration of CPB, is longer.

MISCELLANEOUS PROCEDURES

Not surprisingly, very few cases of coronary bypass surgery in pregnant women have been reported. Two of the three reported cases were performed in patients who were not known to be pregnant. All three cases had successful outcomes for both mother and fetus.

Septal defects (seven atrial, one ventricular) were repaired during pregnancy in eight patients, four of whom were not known to be pregnant. Results were successful in all cases except for one spontaneous abortion 4 days postoperatively in a patient who had severe congestive failure and pulmonary hypertension.

Pulmonary embolectomy for cardiogenic shock has been performed in three pregnant patients. All three mothers and two of their fetuses survived. Spontaneous abortion 5 days postoperatively occurred in the third case at 10 weeks.

Attempted repair of dissecting aneurysm was performed in two patients at 30 and 33 weeks of gestation. Both women died but little can be learned from these cases, since surgical repair of dissecting aneurysm is not often successful in the best of circumstances.

Removal of an atrial myxoma has been reported in two cases[4,22] at 23 and 22 weeks of gestation. Both pregnancies were successfully completed.

SUMMARY AND CONCLUSIONS

Cardiac surgery can be performed in pregnant patients with excellent results. The risk for the mother is probably no greater than for the nonpregnant patient. The risk for the fetus can be minimized with proper attention to various factors:

(1) Whenever possible, operations should be performed semielectively early in the second trimester when organogenesis is completed. It should be noted, however, that to date there is no evidence to suggest that operations with CPB are teratogenic. In the second trimester the hemodynamic burden of pregnancy and the risk of induction of labor is less than in the third trimester. (2) When feasible, closed mitral commissurotomy is the procedure of choice in patients with mitral stenosis. (3) When CPB is necessary, high-flow, high-pressure, normothermic perfusion should be employed. (4) Tissue valve prostheses should be used whenever valve replacement is necessary to avoid the necessity for anticoagulation; (5) Electronic fetal heart rate and uterine monitoring should be performed during the perioperative period. Fetal bradycardia and increased uterine contractions are common during and shortly after CPB but are perfectly compatible with a successful outcome. If, however, postoperative premature labor ensues, carefully monitored tocolytic therapy is indicated.

ACKNOWLEDGMENTS

The author is indebted to those members of the Society of Thoracic Surgeons who responded so kindly to the questionnaires. The enormous burden of secretarial work associated with this project was superbly handled by Marie Galella and Frances Cappello.

REFERENCES

1. Bahery, C.M., Ninio, A., Gorodesky, I.G., and Neri, A.: Tococardiography in pregnancy during extracorporeal bypass for mitral valve replacement. Isr. J. Med. Sci., *16*: 395, 1980.
2. Becker, R.M., Sandor, L., Tindel, M., and Frater, R.W.M.: Medium-term follow-up of the Ionescu-Shiley heterograft valve. Ann. Thorac. Surg., 32: 20, 1981.
3. Ben-Ismail, M., Fekih, M., Taktak, M., and Chelli, M.: Prostheses valvulaires cardiaques et grossesse. Arch mal. Coeur 72(2): 192, 1979.
4. Casarotto, D., Bortolotti, V., Russo, R. et al.: Surgical removal of a left atrial myxoma during pregnancy. Chest, 75: 390, 1979.
5. Eilen, B., Kaiser, I.H., Becker, R.M., and Cohen, M.N.: Aortic valve replacement in the third trimester of pregnancy: case report and review of the literature. Obstet. Gynecol., 57: 119, 1981.
6. Frater, R.W.M., Wakayama, S., Oka, Y. et al.: Pulsatile cardiopulmonary bypass: Failure to influence hemodynamics or hormones. Circulation, *62*: I-19, 1980.
7. Galioto, F.M., Midgley, F.M., Kapur, S. et al.: Early failures of Ionescu-Shiley bioprosthesis after mitral valve replacement in children. J. Thorac. Cardiovasc. Surg. *83*: 306, 1982.
8. Halseth, W.L., Elliot, D.P., Walker, E.L., and Smith, E.A.: Open mitral commissurotomy. J. Thorac. Cardiovasc. Surg., *80*: 842, 1980.
9. Harthorne, J.W., Buckley, M.J., Grover, J.W., and Austen, W.G.: Valve replacement during pregnancy. Ann Int Med, *67*: 1032, 1967.
10. Igna, E.J., Detrick, M.F., Lam, C.R., et al.: Pregnancy and cardiac operations. Am. J. Obstet. Gynecol. *71*: 1024, 1956.
11. Ionescu, M.I., Hasan, S.S., Chidambaram, M., and Tandon, A.P.: Clinical durability of

the pericardial xenograft valve: Ten years' experience with mitral valve replacement. Presented at 18th Annual Meeting, Society of Thoracic Surgeons, New Orleans, Jan. 1982.

12. Koh, K.S., Friesen, R.M., Livingstone, R.A., and Peddle, L.J.: Fetal monitoring during maternal cardiac surgery with cardiopulmonary bypass. Can. Med. Assoc. J., *112*:1102, 1975.
13. Kozam, R.L., Conklin, E.F., Giannelli, S. et al.: Open-heart surgery for mitral stenosis during pregnancy. J. Thorac. Cardiovasc. Surg., *53*:587, 1967.
14. Lamb, M.P., Rass, K., Johnstone, A.M., and Manners, J.M.: Fetal heart monitoring during open heart surgery. Br. J. Obstet. Gynecol. *88*:669, 1981.
15. Magilligan, D.J., Lewis, J.W., Jara, F.M., et al.: Spontaneous degeneration of porcine bioprosthetic valves. Ann. Thorac. Surg., *30*:259, 1980.
16. Martin, M.C., Pernoll, M.L., Boruszak, A.N. et al.: Cesarean section while on cardiac bypass: report of a case. Obstet. Gynecol. *57*:415, 1981.
17. Oyer, P.E., Miller, D.C., Stinson, E.B. et al.: Clinical durability of the Hancock porcine bioprosthetic valve. J. Thorac. Cardiovasc. Surg., *80*:824, 1980.
18. Reid, J.M., Berger, R.L., and Stevenson, J.G.: Transventricular mitral valvotomy during pregnancy. Br. Med. J., 1197, 1960.
19. Roe, B.B., Edmunds, L.H., Fishman, N.H., and Hutchinson, J.C.: Open mitral valvulotomy. Ann. Thorac. Surg. *12*:483, 1971.
20. Taylor, W.J., Black, H., Trower, W.B., and Harken D.E.: Valvuloplasty for mitral stenosis during pregnancy. JAMA, *166*:1013, 1958.
21. Tocker, A.M., Crow, E.W., and Evans, G.E.: Pregnancy and heart disease. J Kansas Med Soc, p. 269, 1956.
22. Trimakas, A.P., Maxwell, K.D., Berkay, S. et al.: Fetal monitoring during cardiopulmonary bypass for removal of a left atrial myxoma during pregnancy. Johns Hopkins Med. J., *144*:156, 1979.

5

Anesthesia for the Critical-Care Obstetric Patient

Glen Z. Brooks, M.D.

Even uncomplicated pregnancy cannot be considered a "normal" physiological state. As a consequence, the safe anesthetic management of the healthy obstetric patient is predicated on an understanding of and an appreciation for the physiological changes that evolve during normal gestation. For many critically ill obstetric patients, these changes will have precipitated pregnancy-related decompensation of preexisting disease. For all critically ill obstetric patients, the physiology of pregnancy will have important anesthetic implications. Therefore, a discussion of the anesthetic approach to the critically ill parturient should begin with a brief but relevant review of the physiological profile of the uncomplicated obstetric patient.

HEMODYNAMICS OF PREGNANCY

Early in the first trimester, with uteroplacental circulation still in its "infancy," plasma volume begins to expand[131] (Fig. 5-1). By the middle of the third trimester total blood volume will have increased by 25 to 40 percent.[127,131,157,214] The increase in plasma volume correlates better with fetal size than maternal size.[91] Multigravid patients have greater increases in plasma volume than do primagravidas,[3] and patients with multiple pregnancies have been shown to have greater circulating blood volumes than those with singleton pregnancies.[177]

Plasma volume begins to increase earlier and to a greater extent than does red blood cell volume (Fig. 5-1). Therefore a relative, but not absolute, anemia may occur. While a fall in hematocrit is common during pregnancy, a hemoglobin below 11 mg/dl or a hematocrit less than 35 percent may be abnormal and represent a true anemia.[87]

The hypervolemic state experienced by the normal parturient at term provides a buffer for the blood loss which occurs at the time of delivery. The vaginal delivery of a singleton fetus is usually associated with a maternal blood loss of less than 500 ml.[159] Vaginal delivery of twins or cesarean section for the delivery of a singleton or multiple fetuses may result in blood losses of 1,000 ml or more.[6,159] These losses should be well tolerated by the normal parturient. While bleeding decreases circulating blood volume during delivery and in the early puerperium, the contracting uterus actually "transfuses" an excess of 500 ml of blood back into the circulation following expulsion of the fetus and placenta. At the same time, the contracting uterus decreases the vascular bed requiring perfusion.[82]

The hypervolemic and vasodilated state that accompanies normal pregnancy also provides the gravida with a cushion against precipitous blood pressure falls following regional anesthesia and sympathetic nervous system blockade. In contrast, the chronic or gestational hypertensive patient may have a contracted blood volume

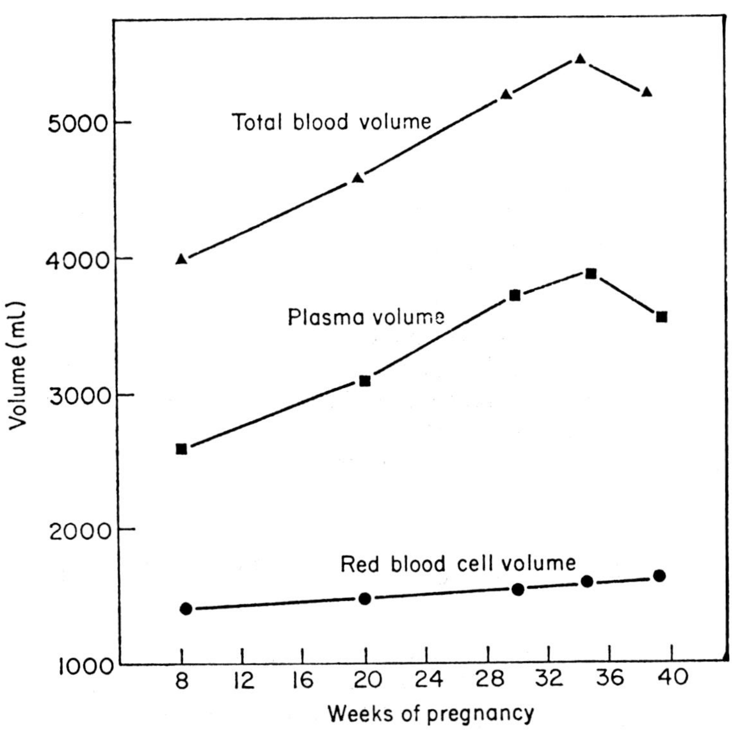

Fig. 5-1 Plasma volume, red blood cell volume, and total blood volume changes in pregnancy. (From Moir, D.D. and Carty, M.J.: Obstetric Anesthesia and Analgesia. Baillière Tindall, London, 1977.)

secondary to diffuse vasoconstriction. These patients are more susceptible to severe hypotension following sympathetic blockade.

Most authors agree that there is a dramatic rise in maternal cardiac output during the first trimester.[112,131,225] (Fig. 5-2). The rise continues into the second trimester, with a peak increase of 30 to 40 percent above nonpregnant values occurring about the 24th week.[218] The increase in cardiac output that occurs during pregnancy parallels the observed increase in blood volume. During early pregnancy, an increase in stroke volume is most responsible for the observed rise in cardiac output. As pregnancy progresses, stroke volume decreases and an increase in heart rate becomes the prime factor responsible for maintaining the increased cardiac output.[218]

Early work led to the belief that cardiac output fell toward preterm levels during the last weeks of pregnancy.[3] While a fall in cardiac output may occur near term, maternal positioning is extremely important in determining to what degree cardiac output will decline.[44,104,112,131,163,218] An early report by Howard et al.[88] noted hypotension associated with tachycardia and pallor occurring in 10 percent of term parturients when kept supine. Pyörälä[163] failed to demonstrate any fall in cardiac output in term patients who were studied in the lateral position, while significant decreases in cardiac output were seen in patients studied when supine. More recent investigators[44,112,218] have also demonstrated the dramatic effect supine positioning has on

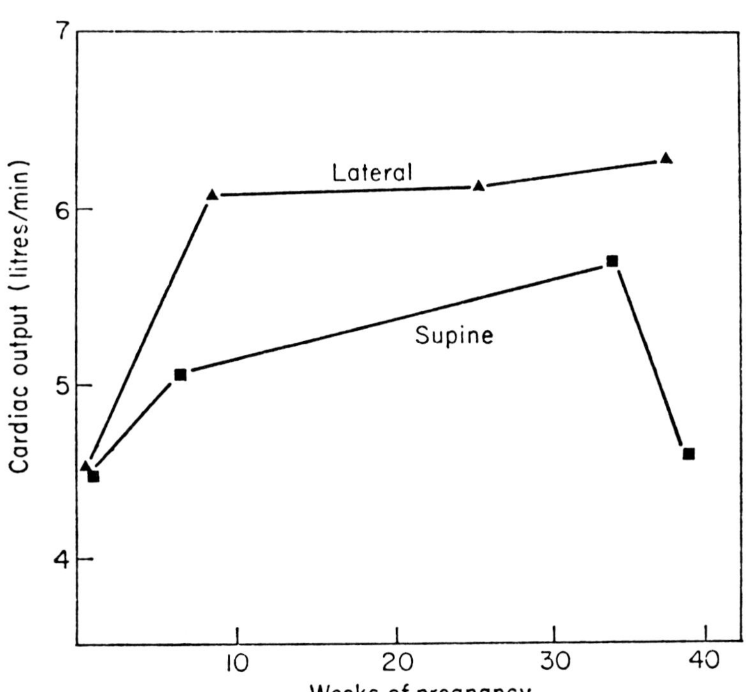

Fig. 5-2 Cardiac output in pregnancy in the supine and lateral positions. (From Moir, D.D. and Carty, M.J.: Obstetric Anesthesia and Analgesia. Baillièr Tindall, London, 1977.)

blood pressure and cardiac output during the later stages of pregnancy and have attributed the phenomenon to compression of the vena cava by the gravid uterus. If significant compression of the vena cava occurs, and blood shunted to the right heart through the azygos and epidural venous plexuses is not sufficient, a fall in stroke volume, cardiac output, and blood pressure will follow.

The aorta and iliac arteries are also susceptible to obstruction by the gravid uterus, resulting in a decrease in uterine blood flow. Bienarz et al.[23] have demonstrated the phenomenon radiographically. However, if cardiac output is shunted to vessels above the obstruction, hemodynamic instability may be masked, i.e., brachial artery pressures may appear normal while arterial pressures distal to the obstruction are markedly decreased.[23,58,118] As a result, even the apparently normotensive and asymptomatic gravida may be hypoperfusing her uterus while supine.[102]

Maintaining the parturient in a lateral position will avoid vena caval and aortic compression.[78] Likewise, elevating the right hip 15° with a wedge will produce left uterine displacement of the gravid uterus off the vena cava.[58] It is imperative that anesthesiologists and obstetricians appreciate the importance of proper positioning during labor and vaginal or abdominal delivery. The sympathetic blockade that accompanies major conduction-block anesthesia decreases vascular tone in the lower extremities. This ablates reflex vasoconstriction in response to decreased perfusion pressure and allows pooling of blood in the capacitance vessels. The result is a more profound decrease in blood pressure and cardiac output when patients are not positioned to avoid aortocaval compression.[122] Obese patients, patients with "tight" abdomens secondary to relatively large uteri (twins, polyhydramnios), and patients of short stature are at even greater risk for supine hypotension. In addition to proper positioning, volume loading before induction of regional anesthesia will also decrease the incidence of supine hypotension.[230]

Few investigators have studied the hemodynamics of labor. Pain and anxiety can increase serum catecholamines, resulting in tachycardia and an increase in cardiac contractility and peripheral vascular resistance. Uterine contractions augment cardiac output by transfusing blood into the venous circulation, and, if painful, by increasing serum catecholamines as well. If the increase in cardiac output is accompanied by an increase in arterial blood pressure, a reflex decrease in heart rate may be seen. Maternal positioning is again important. During early labor, Ueland and Hansen[217] noted that during contractions supine patients increased their cardiac outputs 24 percent above values obtained between contractions. However, when kept in the lateral position, patients had higher baseline cardiac outputs and stroke volumes between contractions, and the hemodynamic changes with contractions were less dramatic. The greatest increases in cardiac output occurred immediately postpartum (Fig. 5-3). In the supine patient receiving only local anesthesia, Ueland and Hansen[217] observed an 80 percent increase in cardiac output over prelabor values. The increase is best explained by a sudden increase in blood volume that accompanies uterine tetany following delivery. Peaks in cardiac output then fell 40 to 50 percent within the first postpartum hour. Within 1 week, cardiac output returns to near prepregnant values.[3] The effects of various anesthetic techniques on the hemodynamics of labor and delivery will be discussed in relation to specific disease states later in the chapter.

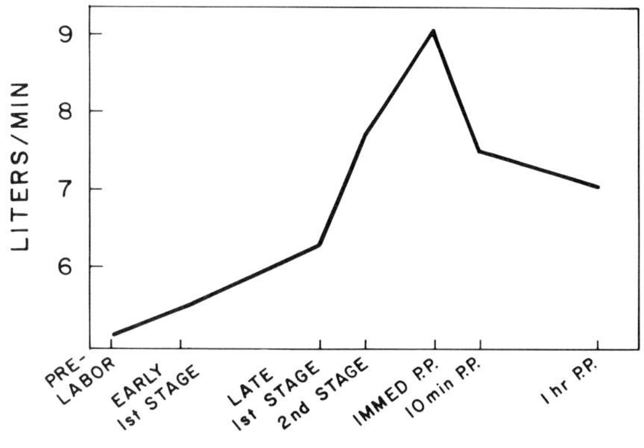

Fig. 5-3 Changes in cardiac output which occur during labor and the early postpartum period. (Modified with permission from Ueland, K. and Hansen, J.M.: Maternal cardiovascular dynamics. Part III: Labor and delivery under local and cardiac analgesia. Am. J. Obstet. Gynecol., *103*:8, 1969.)

Gastrointestinal Changes Associated with Pregnancy

Parturients should always be considered "full stomach" patients regardless of how long they have fasted.[169] Gastric displacement by the gravid uterus results in a change in the angle of the gastroesophageal junction, relaxing the sphincter and its ability to prevent regurgitation. Progesterone also has a relaxing effect on the gastroesophageal sphincter. Pyloric displacement impedes gastric emptying, which is also delayed by a pregnancy-related decrease in gastric motility. Anxiety, labor, and narcotics further delay gastric emptying. Dehydration and ketosis associated with prolonged labor increase gastric acid secretion, which may be already abnormally increased during pregnancy by a placental gastrin.[12] The gravida may also experience raised intragastric pressures resulting from an increase in gastric liquid secretions and swallowed air, intestinal distension, and externally applied fundal pressures at the time of delivery. The combination of a relaxed gastroesophageal sphincter, increased gastric volume, and raised intragastric pressure predisposes the parturient to regurgitation of gastric contents. The sedated, unconscious, or anesthetized patient may be unable to protect her airway, allowing pulmonary aspiration of regurgitated liquid and particulate material. While aspiration of solids is always potentially hazardous, aspiration of liquid contents with a pH less than 2.5[170,212] and a volume greater than 0.4 ml/kg[170] is required to produce symptoms.

The routine administration of oral antacids, 15 to 30 ml every 3 to 4 h[169] will help neutralize gastric acidity and decrease the chemical burn associated with the aspiration of highly acidic material. Repeated antacid therapy, however, may actually increase gastric volume and the risk of aspiration. Taylor[211] reported pneumonitis following aspiration of a large volume of liquid gastric contents with a pH greater than 2.5 following antacid therapy. Furthermore, magnesium and aluminium hydroxides, antacids commonly used in the United States, contain particular matter which also may cause pulmonary damage if aspirated.[74] Sodium citrate, a clear antacid, is an effective and attractive alternative to the particulate preparations,[65,110] but it is not yet commercially available. Cimetidine, a histamine-2 receptor antagonist, has been shown to effectively decrease gastric acid secretion in patients scheduled for elective surgery.[53,56,65,153] However, neither fetal safety nor the efficacy of cimetidine in emergency situations has been established. At the time of this publication, cimetidine has not received FDA approval for routine obstetric use.

While neutralization of gastric contents will decrease the risk of developing pneumonitis if aspiration should occur, it will not protect the patient from aspiration per se or decrease the risk associated with aspiration of solid materials. An awake patient is the best prophylaxis against aspiration. The inspired concentrations of the inhalational anesthetic agents required to produce an anesthetic state decreases during pregnancy.[148] Therefore, even the unmedicated parturient is more likely to become anesthetized at lower anesthetic concentrations than the nonpregnant patient. For the patient who has been receiving narcotics, barbiturates, or tranquilizers, the concentration of inhalational agents required to produce anesthesia can be expected to be even lower, further increasing the risk of losing consciousness and aspirating.

Anesthesiologists and obstetricians must appreciate the fact that pulmonary aspiration is the leading cause of anesthesia-related maternal morbidity and mortality. The increased risk of maternal aspiration associated with general anesthesia must be considered when choosing the most appropriate anesthetic technique for either the uncomplicated or the critically ill obstetric patient.

Respiratory Changes Associated with Pregnancy

Anatomically, the greatest changes in the respiratory system occur during the second half of pregnancy. The gravid uterus displaces the diaphragm cephalad, and there is a flaring of the ribs and an increase in thoracic cage circumference. These compensatory changes maintain, or even increase, vital capacity and total lung capacity (Fig. 5-4). However, important pulmonary reserves are decreased. An increase in tidal volume decreases expiratory reserve volume, while functional residual capacity is diminished by diaphragmatic elevation. The decrease in functional residual capacity is more dramatic while lying than sitting.[178] Although recent evidence[178] indicates that there is no significant change in closing capacity or closing volume during pregnancy, the decrease in functional residual capacity is sufficient to allow airway closure during tidal breathing in at least 50 percent of term parturients while lying.

Pregnancy-related changes in ventilation begin to evolve during the first trimester, with maximal changes occurring by the beginning of the second trimester (Fig. 5-5). The ventilatory state can only be described as hyperventilation, with a marked increase in alveolar ventilation. Progesterone has long been known to be a potent respiratory stimulant and is probably the cause of the increase in respiratory rate and tidal volume. Hyperventilation results in hypocarbia (pCO_2 about 32 mmHg), which persists throughout pregnancy.[28] The gravida compensates for this respiratory alkalosis with a reduction in serum bicarbonate to approximately 22 mEq/L (normal, 26 mEq/L). This maintains pH within normal limits. Increased alveolar ventilation and

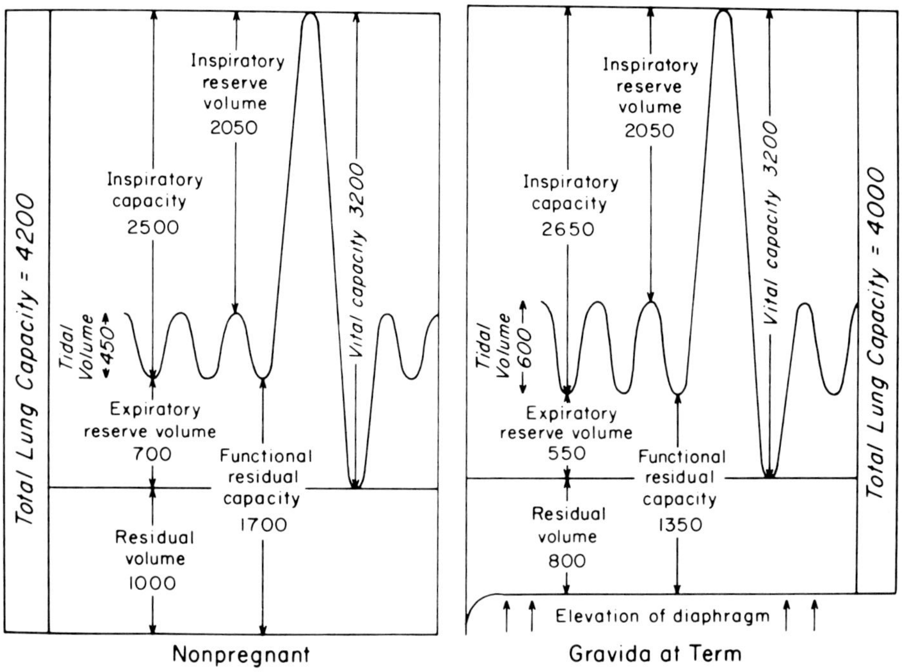

Fig. 5-4 Pulmonary volumes and capacities in the nonpregnant state and those of the pregnant patient at term. (From Bonica, J.J.: Principles and Practice of Obstetric Analgesia and Anesthesia. F.A. Davis, Philadelphia, 1967.)

decreased end-tidal CO_2 are responsible for the hyperoxemia (pO_2 105 mmHg) normally seen during pregnancy.

During labor, pain and anxiety may contribute to further increases in ventilation. Without proper coaching or analgesia, minute ventilation may increase 300 percent or more.[6] This results in a concomitant marked hypocapnia. The expected secondary respiratory alkalosis may be balanced by lactic acidosis caused by the increased work of breathing. Therefore, maternal pH values can range from alkalotic[132] to acidotic.[117]

Fig. 5-5 Changes in ventilatory parameters during pregnancy. Note that almost maximum hyperventilation occurs as early as the second or third month of gestation. (From Bonica J.J.: Obstetric Analgesia and Anesthesia. World Federation of Societies of Anaesthesiologists, Amsterdam, 1980.)

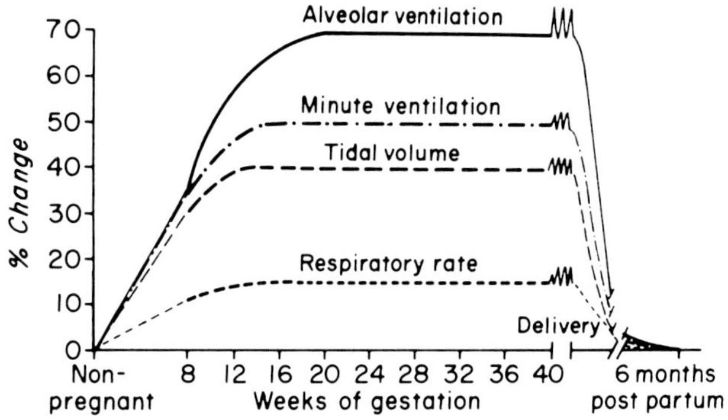

The cost of hyperventilation during labor is an increase in oxygen consumption by as much as 100 percent.[6] A well-conducted regional anesthetic can decrease oxygen consumption[179] and return pCO_2 and acid-base status toward normal.[151]

Functional changes in ventilatory parameters during pregnancy are of considerable significance to the anesthesiologist. The combination of a decrease in functional residual capacity plus an increase in oxygen consumption predisposes the parturient to dramatic falls in venous and arterial oxygenation during periods of apnea.[9] This is especially true when she is horizontal. Any decrease in cardiac output will further decrease blood oxygen levels.[103] Therefore, to avoid hypoxemia during intubation for general anesthesia, obstetric patients should be preoxygenated, and the uterus should be adequately displaced off the vena cava. Intubation should be performed as rapidly as possible following succinylcholine-induced apnea.

The decreased functional residual capacity and increased minute ventilation work together to effect a more rapid rise in alveolar, and thus blood and brain, concentrations of inhalational anesthetic agents. This, combined with the fact that the concentration of inhalational agents required to produce anesthesia in the parturient is decreased,[148] results in a more rapid induction of an anesthetic state. As a result, there is potential danger that during the administration of mask analgesia, the gravida may experience an unwanted loss of consciousness, predisposing her to aspiration of gastric contents through an unprotected airway.

Renal Physiology

Concomitant with increases in cardiac output and plasma volume during early pregnancy are rises in renal plasma flow and glomerular filtration rate. These values increase by as much as 50 percent by the second trimester.[55,191] As a result, in normal pregnancy blood urea nitrogen (BUN) and serum creatinine fall to about half of their prepregnant values. Although these values may begin to rise again during the third trimester, they still remain below nonpregnant values. Chesley and Sloan[39] feel that positioning may play an important role in these third trimester changes, as aortic compression by the gravid uterus decreases renal blood flow. Renograms by Baird et al.[13] support this theory.

GENERAL PRINCIPLES OF ANESTHESIA FOR THE CRITICALLY ILL PARTURIENT

As a result of their extensive involvement with the intraoperative and intensive care unit management of critically ill patients, anesthesiologists of the past two decades have been in a unique position to gain valuable experience in their management. Obstetric anesthesiologists should be considered peripartum consultants, and their involvement should not be limited to providing intraoperative analgesia and anesthesia. They should be consulted early and not called upon at the last minute to provide anesthesia for patients they have not had the opportunity to evaluate.

Preanesthetic evaluation of the critically ill parturient should always begin with a careful history, which includes concurrent, nonpregnancy-related medical problems and medications, drug allergies, and past anesthetic experiences. The patient's family members should also be asked about a history of familial problems related to anesthesia. If regional anesthesia is contemplated, any history of neurological disease or deficit should be elicited. All patients should be examined for oral prostheses and for possible difficulty with airway management or tracheal intubation should these become necessary. Since the critically ill obstetric patient will often present with multiorgan dysfunction, all major organ systems will require thorough evaluation before initiating anesthesia.

Any anesthetic evaluation of the critically ill obstetric patient would be incomplete without a review of all medications the parturient is receiving or has received recently. This information is valuable for two reasons: first, current assessment of the patient's cardiovascular, respiratory, neurological, and psychological status can only be made after considering possible drug effects on these physiological parameters; and second, many drugs used by the anesthesiologist may interact with medications the parturient is receiving. Therefore, appropriate anesthetic techniques, and choices and doses of drugs required for the anesthetic management of these patients will depend upon existing drug therapy.

Intravenous Therapy

For purposes of rapid fluid therapy and drug administration, all critically ill obstetric patients must have at least one large-bore intravenous line prior to the induction of regional or general anesthesia. The anesthesiologist should be aware of all functioning peripheral and central intravenous lines, as well as all fluids and medications being administered intravenously.

SEVERE PREECLAMPSIA

The American College of Obstetrics and Gynecology has recognized that all hypertensive pregnant patients are not experiencing the same disease but merely sharing a common symptom, i.e., abnormally elevated blood pressure. It is important to distinguish between hypertensive patients who become pregnant and patients who develop pregnancy-related hypertension. The patient in the latter group, specifically the preeclamptic-eclamptic patient, is suffering from a complex disorder whose pathophysiology involves nearly every organ system. These patients are at greater risk of becoming critically ill during pregnancy than women with uncomplicated chronic hypertension.

Mean arterial blood pressure tends to decrease during the second trimester of normal pregnancy as a result of a fall in peripheral vascular resistance. The third trimester patients who develop a blood pressure of 140/90 mmHg or greater or who experience a rise in systolic blood pressure of 30 mmHg or in diastolic blood pressure of 15 mmHg above prepregnant values, combined with urine protein loss of 2 g or more per day, are considered to be preeclamptic. Generalized edema and hyperreflexia help support the diagnosis but need not be present. Gestational hypertension greater than 160/110 mmHg combined with proteinuria in excess of 5 g/day is considered severe preeclampsia. Headache, epigastric pain, and visual disturbances are the red flags of impending eclamptic grand mal convulsions. When the severe preeclamptic patient shows evidence of major organ system decompensation, i.e., pulmonary edema with or without congestive heart failure, oliguria less than 400 ml/24 h, eclamptic seizures, or clinically evident disseminated intravascular coagulation, the gravida must then be considered critically ill.

Whether cause or effect, widespread arteriolar vasospasm is a basic pathological component of preeclampsia. This is manifested by an increase in peripheral vascular resistance,[11,197] which leads to hypertension, microangiopathy, and a relative decrease in circulating blood volume when compared with normotensive gravidas.[38,195] The combination of hypovolemia plus a constricted vasculature with increased sensitivity to angiotensin and norepinephrine[210] results in labile blood pressure. Severe hypertension may become "malignant" in response to stressful stimuli, while profound hypotension may occur following sympathetic blockade associated with regional anesthesia. To closely monitor changes in arterial blood pressure in critically ill patients, an intra-arterial line is both indicated and recommended. The severity of the patient's hypertension should also be seen as an indication of the magnitude of other organ system involvement.

The electrocardiogram is a valuable monitor of cardiac arrhythmias, myocardial ischemia, and electrolyte imbalances. All these may occur in the preeclamptic patient secondary to hypertension, hypoxemia, or drug therapy. Preeclamptic patients have been reported to have electrocardiographic changes consisting of T wave inversion without Q wave development, probably caused by focal myocardial lesions.[208]

Volume Status. Severely preeclamptic patients should be considered volume-restricted even in the presence of misleading generalized edema. Both total blood and plasma volumes are significantly lower in the preeclamptic patient when compared with the normotensive parturient.[195] The greater the hypertension, the more restricted the circulating volume. Hemoconcentration is reflected in a higher than normal hematocrit.

In spite of her intense vasospasm and hypovolemia, the severe preeclamptic generally has a cardiac output which equals[11] or exceeds that of the nonpreeclamptic gravida.[20] The increase appears to be secondary to an increase in both heart rate and stroke volume,[20] which implies that preeclampsia is associated with a hyperdynamic left ventricular state.[20,164] Several investigators[20,164,173,204] have now invasively studied the hemodynamics of severe preeclampsia. Pulmonary vascular resistance appears to be unaffected by generalized vasospasm.[20,164] However, both Strauss et al.[204] and

Benedetti et al.[20] found an inconsistent relationship between central venous pressure and pulmonary capillary wedge pressure, especially in patients with pulmonary edema.[204]

The safe anesthetic management of the severe preeclamptic patient is predicated partly on a knowledge of her current volume status. The presence of oliguria may reflect hypovolemia, renal decompensation secondary to preeclampsia, or preexisting renal pathology. Severe preeclampsia complicated by oliguria and unresponsive to intravenous hydration justifies the placement of a central venous catheter to determine volume status and to monitor the response to further rehydration.

The preeclamptic patient who presents with or develops pulmonary edema represents another diagnostic problem. Increased lung water in the face of severe preeclampsia may have several etiologies. Pulmonary edema may be secondary to left ventricular dysfunction and consequent high pulmonary capillary pressures or it may be the result of a low-pressure pulmonary capillary leak syndrome secondary to localized intravascular coagulation.[24] Pneumonitis resulting from silent aspiration in overly sedated patients is another possibility. For diagnosis and management of these critically ill patients, a pulmonary artery (Swan-Ganz) catheter is valuable in establishing the patient's left ventricular function and her intravascular volume.

Knowledge of the critically ill patient's volume status is especially important to the anesthesiologist who is consulted concerning the administration of major conduction-block anesthetic, such as a lumbar epidural block for either labor and delivery or cesarean section. In the presence of an uncorrected hypovolemic state, a sympathetic block associated with epidural anesthesia, superimposed on varying degrees of vena caval compression, may result in profound maternal hypotension. This will endanger not only the parturient but also her fetal-placental unit, which must be assumed to be already compromised.[54]

Pulmonary Status. In spite of the fact that pulmonary vascular resistance appears to be normal even in severe preeclampsia,[20,164] the pulmonary microvasculature may still be pathologically involved. As noted previously, an increase in lung water, secondary to either left ventricular decompensation or low-pressure passive diffusion through an injured capillary endothelium, may be sufficient to interfere with normal gas exchange. The resulting hypoxia will jeopardize both the mother and her compromised fetus. Even before pulmonary edema is evident through auscultation or on chest x-ray, an increase in pulmonary capillary wedge pressure may predict a failing left ventricle or circulatory overload and the potential for the development of frank pulmonary edema. Serial determination of arterial blood gases, preferably through an indwelling intra-arterial line, is a means of accurately monitoring the status of pulmonary gas exchange and its response to therapy.

Patients sedated with narcotics, barbiturates, or tranquilizers and those receiving magnesium sulfate may experience pulmonary complications of their therapy. Oversedation can lead to direct respiratory depression. Likewise, magnesium levels of 15 mEq/L can be expected to cause respiratory arrest.[83] The oversedated patient may also experience silent regurgitation of stomach contents and sustain a life-threatening pulmonary aspiration.

In summary, perioperative evaluation of the pulmonary status of the critically ill preeclamptic-eclamptic patient should include careful assessment of the following: (1) the patient's state of consciousness; (2) the adequacy of her pulmonary mechanics, including respiratory rate; (3) the adequacy of her gas exchange as determined by arterial blood gas values; (4) hemodynamic data, particularly pulmonary capillary wedge pressure; and (5) review of the chest x-rays.

Coagulation Status. A hypercoagulable state exists during normal pregnancy. There is an increase in several clotting factors and fibrinogen, while fibrinolytic activity decreases.[122,208] This imbalance may progress to a serious coagulopathy during severe preeclampsia-eclampsia.

The intravascular coagulation that occurs to varying degrees in preeclamptic patients may be localized to specific vascular beds, such as the kidneys, placenta, and lungs.[29,160] Page[147] feels that an increased release of placental thromboplastin during preeclampsia is responsible for the observed intravascular coagulation. However, Pritchard et al.[160] hypothesize that the marked vasospasm of preeclampsia leads to vascular endothelial damage. This then results in diffuse platelet adherence and a consumptive coagulopathy.

When suspected, a consumption coagulopathy should be diagnosed with a combination of laboratory tests. A decrease in platelet count and fibrinogen level in the presence of an increase in fibrin split products and prothrombin and partial thromboplastin times indicates consumption of procoagulants. The anesthetic implications of coagulation defects are serious enough to warrant a thorough laboratory analysis of clotting parameters before performing any regional anesthetic technique on the severe preeclamptic. The major concern is the possibility of producing an epidural hematoma as a result of trauma to an epidural vein by either spinal or epidural needles or an epidural catheter. When there is evidence of coagulopathy, regional anesthesia is contraindicated.

Renal Function. The renal pathophysiological changes of preeclampsia involve both glomeruli and renal tubules. Classical glomerular changes include endothelial cell swelling with subendothelial cell fibrin deposition and narrowing of the capillary lumen. The fibrin which is phagocytized by the glomerular endothelial cells may be the product of a disseminated intravascular coagulation which is initiated by placental thromboplastin.[220] The result is a varying degree of decreased glomerular filtration,[180] with a fall in both sodium and uric acid clearances. Only in cases of moderately advanced renal involvement will BUN and serum creatinine rise to abnormal levels. Therefore, they are not useful indicators of early disease. Histologically, the renal tubules appear plugged by protein and protein casts resulting from reabsorption of protein from glomerular filtrate. The quantity of protein "spilled" into the urine provides a good clinical correlation for the extent of glomerular disease.[122,155]

Knowledge of the preeclamptic's renal function is important for both her obstetric and her anesthetic management. Urinalysis and measurements of serum electrolytes, BUN, serum creatinine, and uric acid should be performed upon admission, and repeat values obtained as necessary to assess both progression of the disease and response to management. Placement of a Foley catheter allows accurate monitoring of urine output during hospitalization. The severe preeclamptic who presents with oliguria or anuria may be suffering from renal decompensation. Decreased urine output may also reflect hypovolemia and volume constriction. In the presence of decreased renal function and oliguria unresponsive to intravenous hydration, monitoring of right (central venous) and/or left (pulmonary capillary wedge) heart pressures will be necessary in order to avoid volume overloading.

Physicians involved with the management of the preeclamptic patient with compromised renal function must also be aware of the altered excretion of many drugs, and their active polar metabolites, which require renal excretion. Included in this group are magnesium sulfate, the narcotics, and the nondepolarizing neuromuscular blockers used during general anesthesia.

Hepatic Function. During normal pregnancy, hepatic enzymes may be slightly elevated although specific histological changes in the liver do not seem to occur. While hepatic blood flow and function remain normal during pregnancy, the activity of pseudocholinesterase, which is produced by the liver, decreases significantly.[61,186] This decrease does not, however, cause a clinically significant prolongation of action of either succinylcholine[26] or ester-type local anesthetic agents which are metabolized by plasma pseudocholinesterase.

Liver involvement is minimal in patients with mild preeclampsia. However, as the severity of disease increases, hepatic blood flow decreases and hepatic function becomes impaired. Fibrin thrombi result in areas of ischemic damage and periportal hemorrhage. In the presence of advanced disease, liver necrosis can result in maternal death.[122,229]

Critically ill preeclamptic patients should have baseline liver function tests upon admission. If these are abnormal, drugs requiring hepatic metabolism for elimination should be used with caution, and agents that are potentially hepatotoxic should be avoided. An increased percentage of drugs that are normally bound to protein will be unbound and in the active state. Since the liver is responsible for the synthesis of a myriad of serum proteins and enzymes necessary to maintain homeostasis, the critically ill patient with severe hepatic dysfunction may be expected to develop ascites, coagulation disorders, and hepatic encephalopathy.

Central Nervous System. The central nervous system of the preeclamptic-eclamptic patient is irritable. This is manifest clinically by hyperactivity of the deep tendon reflexes. Early work has indicated that global cerebral blood flow is not changed during toxemia,[124] although areas of focal ischemia secondary to edema, vasospasm, or hemorrhage may occur. The etiology of the grand mal type seizure that is the hallmark of eclampsia remains unclear.

The first concern in the management of the eclamptic patient is airway maintenance and protection. Turning her into a lateral position will decrease the risk of aspiration. Placement of an oropharyngeal or nasopharyngeal airway will aid in the establishment and maintenance of the airway. I prefer securing the airway with a cuffed endotracheal tube. This significantly decreases the risk of pulmonary aspiration and allows for controlled or assisted ventilation. Endotracheal tube placement can be facilitated with the administration of succinylcholine, 0.75 mg/kg. Succinylcholine also decreases muscular activity and thus lactic acid production as a consequence of seizure activity. During a seizure, apnea rapidly leads to both maternal and fetal hypoxia.[27] Therefore, controlled ventilation with oxygen is recommended until the patient is breathing adequately. Treatment of the seizure itself with an intravenous barbiturate, such as thiopental, 75 to 100 mg, or diazepam, 5 to 10 mg, will decrease cerebral lactate production by decreasing cerebral metabolism. However, both drugs add to postictal depression. To avoid aspiration, hypoxia, and hypercarbia in the postictal period, depressed patients should remain intubated and ventilated. The patient's acid-base status should be monitored with arterial blood gases, and severe metabolic acidosis should be corrected with sodium bicarbonate.

Patients who develop focal neurological signs or who fail to regain a normal level of consciousness following seizure should undergo computerized craniotomography (CT scan) to rule out intracranial hemorrhage or cerebral edema.[18] If recovery is not rapid, intracranial pressure should be monitored. Significant cerebral edema should be treated as discussed in Chapter 13.

To reduce fetal exposure to additional sedatives and to remove the underlying cause of the preeclampsia-eclampsia, delivery should be accomplished as expeditiously as possible as soon as seizure activity and hypertension are controlled. Patients who recover normal mentation following eclamptic convulsions may undergo induction of labor with oxytocin in an attempt to achieve a vaginal delivery. Many of these patients, however, will ultimately require cesarean section for failed induction or fetal distress.

Placental Function and Fetal Well-Being. Nadji and Sommers[137] suggested that a first-trimester placental vasculitis secondary to an antigen-antibody reaction between maternal and fetal tissue may play an important role in the development of the preeclamptic syndrome. Vasculitis leads to placental ischemia, which triggers a release of both placental "thromboplastin" and uterine renin. Subsequent fibrin deposition[105] and diffuse vasoconstriction cause the placenta to become a target organ as well as an initiator of the disease. The end result is an infarcted and degenerated placenta with compromised function and blood flow.[68] Placental perfusion is further impaired by a reduction in uterine blood flow,[35] perhaps initiated by a decrease in the synthesis of placental prostaglandins necessary to maintain normal uteroplacental blood flow and to antagonize the action of vasopressors.[221] The preeclamptic patient's dysfunctional placenta is also at greater risk for abruption.[182] Ultimately, the fetus suffers both nutritional and oxygen deficiencies[121] and is at significant risk for death in utero. The fetus who has only marginal reserves may be further compromised by any additional insult to uteroplacental perfusion resulting from uterine contractions, vasopressor administration, the release of endogenous maternal catecholamines associated with pain and stress, or maternal hypotension secondary to aortocaval compression, sympathetic blockade, or hemorrhage. The fetus, often premature as well as growth-retarded, is also at greater risk for depression from drugs used in the management of preeclampsia.

For the reasons cited, it is imperative that the fetus be monitored throughout labor for abnormal fetal heart rate patterns, which may indicate fetal distress. These abnormal patterns include a decrease in fetal heart rate variability,[150] the presence of bradycardia or tachycardia,[16] late decelerations,[108] and severe variable decelerations.[79] Although the presence of an abnormal fetal heart rate pattern may not necessarily reflect distress in utero,[150] it may indicate the need for fetal scalp pH sampling to establish fetal well-being. If the scalp sampling reveals severe fetal acidosis, either measures that rapidly correct the situation or delivery is indicated.

The anesthesiologist called upon to provide anesthesia either for labor and vaginal delivery or for cesarean section must be aware of abnormal fetal heart rate tracings during labor and the results of any fetal pH samples obtained. The fetal status should be discussed with the obstetrician before anesthetic options are presented to the patient. In the presence of overt fetal distress, anesthetic techniques which may further compromise placental perfusion should be avoided. If a major conduction-block anesthetic is administered, continuous fetal heart rate monitoring must be conducted throughout the remainder of labor.

Maternal Medications. The patient who appears overly sedated, or even obtunded, may either be suffering from true cerebral dysfunction secondary to her disease or be oversedated from the barbiturates, diazepam, or narcotics she has been receiving singly or in combination. The distinction should be made, and if drugs are responsible, they should be restricted or even reversed if possible. Judicious sedation may be necessary to help control further deterioration of the preeclamptic state. However, patients who cannot respond appropriately to verbal commands, whether secondary to drug therapy or to organic disease, should not be considered candidates for major conduction block anesthesia. The poorly responsive patient can neither understand the procedures, give informed consent, nor notify the anesthesiologist of paresthesias occurring during the procedure or aberrant responses to injections of local anesthetic test doses.

Patients with severe hypertension, peripheral edema, or congestive heart failure may be receiving diuretics. The use of these drugs can lead to or exacerbate electrolyte imbalances. Hypokalemia, often associated with diuretic therapy, may lead to cardiac arrhythmias or to a decrease in cardiac inotropy if the imbalance goes uncorrected. The risk of developing serious arrhythmias increases even more during general anesthesia. Therefore, serum electrolytes should be followed in all critically ill preeclamptic patients, especially those receiving diuretic therapy.

Diuretics will also cause an additional reduction of the preeclamptic's already contracted intravascular volume. Although these women are hypertensive in the unanesthetized state, their blood pressures will be extremely volatile during regional or general anesthesia if intravascular volumes are not returned to normal.

Magnesium sulfate is widely used in the management of the preeclamptic-eclamptic patient. While a direct depression of the central nervous system is doubtful,[7,196] there is clinical evidence that magnesium sulfate can control and even prevent eclamptic convulsions.[161] Physicians familiar with the attributes of magnesium sulfate are also aware of its potential for maternal and fetal toxicity. Peripherally, magnesium sulfate acts at the neuromuscular junction to reduce hyperreflexia. It accomplishes this by decreasing acetylcholine release from the prejunctional motor neuron, thus diminishing motor end-plate sensitivity to acetylcholine, and by depressing muscle membrane excitability.[63] Magnesium's activity at the neuromuscular junction also results in an increased sensitivity to depolarizing and nondepolarizing neuromuscular blockers used to provide muscle relaxation during surgery.[72] When magnesium levels exceed the therapeutic range (4 to 6 mEq/L), respiratory paralysis,[233] cardiac conduction defects, and bradycardia[193] can occur (Table 5-1). Magnesium sulfate administration has also been associated with hypotension, possibly secondary to relaxation of skeletal muscle. This effect is most obvious following intravenous bolus administration.[233]

Patients receiving magnesium therapy should be followed clinically for early signs of toxicity. Since loss of deep tendon reflexes precedes either respiratory paralysis or cardiac arrest, monitoring reflexes will help prevent overdose. Patients with impaired renal function are unable to clear rising plasma levels of magnesium, which increases their risk of developing toxicity. Laboratory determinations of magnesium plasma levels are more precise than clinical signs and should be followed when possible.

Since magnesium crosses the placenta, the neonate may also display decreased muscle tone, respiratory depression, or even apnea as toxic manifestations of maternal magnesium therapy.[114] Calcium increases the release of acetylcholine from the prejunctional motor neuron and may be beneficial in reversing both maternal and neonatal magnesium toxicity.

In addition to magnesium sulfate, severe preeclamptic patients whose blood pressures ramain higher than 160/110 mm Hg may be receiving antihypertensive drugs at the time of anesthetic evaluation. The two most popular agents used today are hydralazine, a direct-acting peripheral vasodilator, and alpha-methyldopa, a false neurotransmitter. Hydralazine may be administered orally, intramuscularly, as an I.V. bolus, or as an I.V. drip. Its advantages during hypertensive crisis include a relatively rapid onset of action following I.V. administration (15 to 20 min) and apparent increases in renal[207] and uterine blood flow.[31,168] However, the reduction in peripheral vascular resistance produced by hydralazine also causes an increase in heart rate and cardiac output and thus in oxygen consumption. This may produce chest pain and electrocardiographic changes consistent with anginal attacks. Since the effect of hydralazine can be likened to a chemical sympathectomy, the severely volume-contracted patient may experience profound falls in blood pressure following bolus I.V. injection. Therefore, initial therapy should consist of small doses, 5 to 10

Table 5-1. Effects of Increasing Plasma Magnesium Levels

Observed Condition	mEq/L
Normal plasma level	1.5–2.0
Therapeutic range	4.0–6.0
ECG changes	5.0–10
(P-Q interval prolonged, QRS complex widens)	
Loss of deep tendon reflexes	10
Sinoatrial and atrioventricular block	15
Respiratory paralysis	15
Cardiac arrest	25

From Gutsche, B.B.: Anesthetic considerations for eclampsia-preeclampsia. p. 224. In Shnider, S.M. and Levinson, G. (eds): Anesthesia for Obstetrics. © 1979, The Williams & Wilkins Co., Baltimore.

mg, titrated to desired effect. Hydralazine's vasodilating properties may be potentiated by coincident narcotic administration or sympathetic blockade associated with major conduction-block anesthesia. Common side effects associated with hydralazine include paresthesias and nasal congestion. Patients experiencing paresthesias present the anesthesiologist with a dilemma concerning the use of conduction-block techniques. I suggest avoiding conduction blockade in women with paresthesias when other alternatives exist. Nasal congestion necessitates oral breathing during mask administration of oxygen or inhalational analgesics. During general anesthesia, the passing of nasal airways or suction catheters is likely to initiate bleeding.

Alpha-methyldopa's hypotensive action is due in part to the accumulation of a false neurotransmitter, alpha-methylnorepinephrine, at nerve endings. In addition norepinephrine production is decreased. Since alpha-methyldopa effectively depletes terminal nerve endings of norepinephrine, vasopressors such as ephedrine, which act indirectly by releasing endogenous norepinephrine, will have an unpredictable effect. Therefore, profound hypotension following conduction-block anesthesia may be more difficult to correct.

Following alpha methyldopa therapy, heart rate and cardiac output are reduced and renal blood flow is slightly curtailed. Alpha-methyldopa also has a CNS depressant effect which may be beneficial in the management of preeclamptic patients. Because of its central effect, patients on methyldopa therapy will require a lower alveolar concentration of an inhalational anesthetic agent to produce anesthesia.[129] Therefore, as is also true of narcotics or sedatives, alpha-methyldopa-treated patients receiving inhalational analgesia by mask are more likely to enter an anesthetic state at lower inspired concentrations. To reduce the risk of aspiration, the patient's state of consciousness should be continuously assessed.

Anesthesia for the Severe Preeclamptic

Anesthesia for Labor and Vaginal Delivery. Anesthetic options for the critically ill parturient must be individualized and will depend upon several factors. During the first stage of labor, effective analgesia will decrease the maternal stress associated with painful uterine contractions. By reducing maternal catecholamine release during contractions, the severe preeclamptic will be able to maintain a more stable blood pressure with less risk of cerebrovascular damage or myocardial decompensation. Concomitantly, there will be less oxygen consumption, lactate production, and hypocarbia secondary to hyperventilation and increased muscle tension in response to pain.

During early labor, narcotics and sedatives may be used to decrease maternal pain and anxiety. Narcotics must be respected for their potential to cause maternal respiratory depression. Likewise, they may exacerbate the respiratory depression caused by other drugs the preeclamptic patient is receiving, such as tranquilizers and magnesium sulfate. Because of their vasodilating properties, narcotics may also potentiate the action of hypotensive agents used to control blood pressure. Narcotics may also cause nausea and vomiting, and delay gastric emptying, increasing the risk of aspiration.

Narcotics rapidly cross the placenta and may be associated with alterations in fetal heart rate and neonatal respiratory depression.[33] Altered neonatal neurobehavior following maternal narcotic administration can be detected for more than 2 days following delivery.[84] The premature or already compromised fetus and neonate is even more sensitive to narcotic depression. To minimize narcotic side effects in the mother and her fetus-neonate, both dosages and drug administration to delivery intervals should be carefully considered. By limiting narcotic doses to 50 mg of meperidine or its equivalent and by avoiding narcotics if delivery is expected to take place more than 1 or less than 4 h following I.M. administration, neonatal depression will be minimized.[30,189] Fortunately, narcotic depression of the mother or neonate can be effectively reversed with the narcotic antagonist naloxone. However, since the duration of action of naloxone is short (1.5 to 2 h), both mother and neonate must be observed postpartum for late signs of depression caused by narcotic which has not been metabolized or eliminated.[84] When administering narcotics, it should also be remembered that severe preeclamptics with significant hepatic and/or renal dysfunction may have a decreased ability to metabolize or excrete the parent drugs and their active metabolites.

Because of diazepam's sedative and anticonvulsive properties and minimal hemodynamic effects, it would appear to be a useful agent in the management of the severe preeclamptic. However, diazepam will interact with narcotics, barbiturates, magnesium sulfate, and the inhalational anesthetic agents, increasing their potential for respiratory depression. There has also been controversy concerning the use of diazepam during labor because of its effects on the fetus and neonate. Diazepam rapidly crosses the placenta[45,52] and may attain fetal blood levels that exceed those in the mother. Limited neonatal metabolism results in detectable infant blood levels of diazepam for days after delivery.[45] Following the maternal administration of small doses of diazepam during labor, investigators were unable to demonstrate significant acid-base changes in either the mother, the fetus[181] or the neonate.[232] Rolbin et al.[174] demonstrated that small doses (2.5 to 10 mg) of I. V. diazepam given to nonpreeclamptic mothers did not adversely affect Apgar scores or acid-base status, although the Scanlon neurobehavioral examination, a more sensitive indicator of neonatal drug effects, did reveal decreased muscle tone at 4 h of age. Larger doses of diazepam (20 mg or greater) have been shown to be associated with an increased incidence of lower Apgar scores and hypotonia.[62] McCarthy et al.[125] reported neonatal hypotonia and areflexia lasting 4 days in two babies following the administration of 180 to 200 mg of diazepam to their severely preeclamptic mothers during labor. The significance of early hypotonia is unknown. Neonatal hypothermia has also been reported following maternal diazepam administration.[45,146] Since the fetus of the preeclamptic patient is often premature and already compromised, it seems prudent to avoid any medications which may augment fetal depression unless there are sound maternal indications for their usage.

Paracervical Block. During the first stage of labor, pain results from uterine contractions and cervical dilatation. This pain is mediated by sympathetic fibers which leave the uterus and pass through the paracervical tissues. These fibers then enter the lumbar sympathetic chain at the level of L_2 to L_5 and terminate in the dorsal horn of the spinal cord at T_{10} to L_1. This pathway lends itself to conduction blockade by local anesthetic agents placed in several different locations. The afferent fibers can be blocked as they course paracervically, as they travel in the lumbar sympathetic chain, or by local anesthetic which has been placed in the lumbar epidural space in quantities sufficient to reach lower thoracic levels.

The advantages of performing a paracervical block include its ease of administration and the rapid onset of effective analgesia. However, the block is not without potential fetal and maternal side effects. Paracervical block has been associated with fetal bradycardia and acidosis[135,152,228] and fetal mortality.[223] Possible etiologies of fetal distress following paracervical block include: (1) high levels of local anesthetic reaching the fetus, perhaps by direct uptake of drug through uterine vessels in the paracervical area[10,17]; (2) uterine vasoconstriction from local anesthetic placed in close proximity to uterine arteries[76,166]; and (3) an increase in uterine tone caused by high concentrations of local anesthetic perfusing the uterus.[219]

Since the fetal placental unit of the severe preeclamptic must be considered compromised even in the absence of overt fetal distress, I believe that any technique such as paracervical block, which may further depress the fetus, should be avoided when possible.

Lumbar Sympathetic Block. Lumbar sympathetic block is an alternative to paracervical block for the management of first-stage labor pain. Since sympathetic fibers are blocked exclusively, only visceral pain arising from uterine contractions will be ablated. The block cannot be extended to include somatic nerves during the second stage of labor. Although lumbar sympathetic block can provide effective analgesia while avoiding the problems of fetal bradycardia associated with the deposition of local anesthetic in the paracervical area, it has two disadvantages. First, it is technically difficult to administer during labor, especially with the patient moving during painful contractions. Second, lumbar sympathetic block does not selectively affect only afferent sympathetic fibers arising from the uterus but also blocks efferent sympathetic fibers responsible for vascular tone in the lower extremities. Therefore, serious hypotension can be expected following lumbar sympathetic blockade in the severe preeclamptic if her blood volume is not acutely expanded before performing the procedure.

Inhalational Analgesia and Ketamine. Inhalational analgesia may be used as an alternative or supplement to regional anesthesia during the second stage of labor. While the analgesia provided by inhalational agents will not be as profound as that obtained with a well-conducted regional anesthetic technique, inhalational analgesia will be preferred by some patients and adequate for their needs. Advantages of the technique include ease of administration by well-trained personnel, little to no effect on the progress of labor, and limited fetal and neonatal depression when used in low concentrations and for short periods of time. Inhalational agents will be rapidly eliminated by the breathing neonate while fixed drugs, such as the narcotics, will require slower hepatic metabolism and renal excretion for elimination.

The major disadvantage of inhalational analgesia is the increased risk of pulmonary aspiration of gastric contents associated with any altered state of consciousness. Therefore, it is imperative that inhalational analgesia not become inhalational anesthesia unless the airway is protected with a cuffed endotracheal tube. To ensure that the parturient is able to maintain and protect her airway while receiving inhalational analgesia, the anesthesiologist or nurse-anesthetist in attendance must continually assess the patient's level of consciousness. If she becomes nonresponsive to verbal commands, confused, or disoriented, the technique should be discontinued until normal mentation is reestablished. Eclamptic patients who are postictal and preeclamptic patients who are heavily sedated and poorly responsive are not candidates for inhalational analgesia by mask.

For patients who are alert and cooperative, the potent inhalational agents (methoxyflurane, enflurane, and isoflurane) may be administered with oxygen. I prefer the continuous or intermittent administration of 30 to 40 percent nitrous oxide in oxygen, with the addition of a low concentration (0.25 to 0.5 percent) of one of the more potent inhalational agents as required. Stefani et al.[201] have shown that nitrous oxide and enflurane analgesia do not adversely affect neonatal neurobehavior. However, both methoxyflurane and enflurane undergo hepatic biotransformation. Inorganic fluoride, an important metabolite of both halogenated ethers, has been associated with renal toxicity.[42] Clark et al.[40] and Wikstrom[227] have measured serum fluoride ion concentrations in pregnant patients receiving methoxyflurane[40] or enflurane[227] and found levels to be well below the 80 to 100 μmol/L felt to be necessary to produce clinical nephrotoxicity. Although toxicity following a short exposure to either agent is unlikely, some authors feel that the administration of any potentially nephrotoxic agent should be avoided in the preeclamptic patient.

Ketamine is a parenteral anesthetic agent which can be used alone to produce analgesia for labor and delivery or as a supplement to incomplete regional anesthesia. By using a "low-dose" technique, 10 to 15 mg I.V. every 5 to 10 min with a maximum of 100 mg over a 30-min period,[5] the parturient can experience analgesia without loss of consciousness or the ability to maintain and protect her airway. If high doses of ketamine are avoided, the incidence of hallucinations will be minimal. The addition of nitrous oxide, 40%, with oxygen will enhance the analgesia produced by low-dose ketamine and reduce the dose required to produce effective analgesia.[226] When ketamine doses are kept below 1 mg/kg, only minimal increases in uterine tone are observed.[67,119] Janeczko et al.[95] were also unable to demonstrate neonatal depression as determined by Apgar scores with ketamine doses of less than 1 mg/kg. Hodgkinson and his group[86] compared the effects of thiopental (less than 4 mg/kg), ketamine (0.7 mg/kg), and epidural anesthesia with 2-chloroprocaine on neonatal neurobehavior following vaginal delivery. Neurobehavior was less depressed following maternal ketamine administration than following thiopental, while babies born to mothers who had received epidural anesthesia with 2-chloroprocaine scored best overall. In doses greater than 1 mg/kg ketamine causes significant uterine hypertonus[67] and a higher incidence of neonatal depression.[66,95,115] Because of its sympathomimetic effects, ketamine is associated with an increase in blood pressure and heart rate.[113] This cardiovascular support might be beneficial during the anesthetic management of the hypovolemic patient. However, most authors agree that ketamine should be used cautiously or avoided completely in the severe preeclamptic.

Pudendal Block. A combination of pudendal block and local anesthetic infiltration of the perineum has been a popular method for providing pelvic and perineal somatic analgesia during the second stage of labor and vaginal delivery. It avoids the potential problem of hypotension associated with sympathetic blockade following an epidural or a subarachnoid block and maintains the patient's ability to push effectively. It also allows the parturient to remain awake and limits her exposure to parenteral or inhalational agents and the risk of aspiration.

While the technique is generally considered safe, it must be remembered that the fetus can acquire detectable blood levels of amide-type local anesthetics following the block.[19,235] Zador et al.,[235] comparing lidocaine with epinephrine to plain lidocaine, have shown that peak maternal and fetal blood levels are achieved within 10 to 20 min of administering a pudendal block. By limiting the dose of lidocaine to 200 mg, the highest fetal blood lidocaine level recorded in the lidocaine only group was 0.82 g/ml. While this is well below the 5 μg/ml plasma level considered to be toxic in the adult, it may represent a significant drug level in the already depressed or premature infant. With the addition of epinephrine, 1:200,000, to lidocaine, both maternal and fetal drug levels were reduced. However, since the effects of epinephrine on uterine tone and blood flow remain uncertain and since this agent may exacerbate the preeclamptic's hypertension, I feel that the use of epinephrine should be avoided. By using the rapidly metabolized ester local anesthetic, 2-chloroprocaine, high fetal drug levels and toxicity can be avoided.

Spinal Anesthesia. For the normotensive parturient, a low-level subarachnoid block, e.g., at the S_1 to S_5 sensory level (saddle block), will generally provide safe and effective anesthesia for vaginal delivery and episiotomy repair. By increasing the dose of local anesthetic injected or by altering maternal position so that the hyperbaric local anesthetic solution extends more cephalad, a level of anesthesia extending to the lower thoracic segments can be attained. This level will also block uterine sympathetic fibers, thereby eliminating the pain associated with contractions and the application of forceps at the time of delivery. There are two major advantages of a subarachnoid block: first, there is a rapid onset of complete analgesia, and second, it requires a much smaller dose of local anesthetic than is necessary for a pudendal block or lumbar or caudal epidural anesthesia. By limiting drug dosage, maternal and fetal exposure to high concentrations of potentially toxic local anesthetic agents can be avoided. However, segmental spread of the local anesthetic during spinal anesthesia can be more difficult to control, and severe hypotension may result from unintentional cephalad extension of the block. When sensory levels of anesthesia are kept below T_4, compensatory vasoconstriction of the upper torso and extremities can help limit declines in central venous and systemic blood pressures. As subarachnoid block extends to include upper thoracic sympathetic efferent fibers, however, less compensation is possible, and hypotension may become more profound.[230] When the anesthetic spread extends to involve T_1 and T_2 fibers, a blockade of the cardioacceleratory fibers occurs, limiting the heart's ability to correct hypotension by responding with an increase in heart rate.

As noted previously, vena caval compression associated with pregnancy augements the hypotensive effects of sympathetic blockade. Partial vena caval occlusion shunts blood through the azygous system and epidural venous plexus. Increased epidural venous flow decreases the volume of the subarachnoid space and enhances the spread of drug injected into the cerebrospinal fluid. If the uterus is contracting or the patient bears down during injection, anesthetic spread becomes even more difficult to predict or control. This, of course, increases the likelihood of an exaggerated spread of the anesthetic agent and subsequent hypotension.

The vasospastic and volume-constricted severe preeclamptic is even more likely to become severely hypotensive secondary to abrupt vasodilatation from a chemical sympathectomy than the normotensive and normovolemic parturient. Any significant decrease in uterine perfusion pressure will be poorly tolerated by the fetus of a woman with severe preeclampsia. Therefore, because it is difficult to control and may cause hemodynamic instability, subarachnoid block is generally considered to be a poor anesthetic choice for vaginal delivery or cesarean section in the severe preeclamptic.

Epidural Anesthesia. Most clinicians now agree that when properly administered, lumbar epidural anesthesia can be an important adjunct in the successful management of the severe preeclamptic. Lumbar epidural analgesia provides the parturient with effective pain relief during the first and second stages of labor and can be extended to provide anesthesia for abdominal delivery when indicated. However, the value of epidural anesthesia in the care of a woman with toxemia goes beyond its flexibility and capacity to relieve pain per se. Severe preeclampsia represents a hyperdynamic state [20,164] as evidenced by an increase in left ventricular stroke work index. This hyperdynamic state is associated with an increase in myocardial oxygen consumption and in some cases may lead to cardiac decompensation. The pain associated with labor and delivery can place additional demands on the myocardium. Pain and stress have been shown to cause an elevation in maternal catecholamines,[190] which further increases myocardial inotropy, chronotropy, cardiac output[217] and oxygen consumption.

Since the preeclamptic has a vasculature which is more sensitive to catecholamines than that of a nontoxemic patient,[210] she is also more likely to develop an exaggerated hypertensive response to pain-induced catecholamine secretion. This increases both cardiac work and the risk of intracranial hemorrhage. Shnider et al.[187] have demonstrated that lumbar epidural anesthesia will effectively decrease the release of maternal endogenous catecholamines during labor. A well-conducted regional anesthetic will also decrease maternal requirements for narcotics and tranquilizers, decreasing the likelihood of unwanted oversedation.

Most parturients hyperventilate in response to pain and isometrically contract various muscle groups. This leads to a further increase in peripheral oxygen consumption and cardiac output. Curtis noted wide fluctuations in the transcutaneous measurement of blood oxygen levels associated with hyperventilation.[46] Hyperventilation can contribute to lactic acidosis if anaerobic metabolism occurs.[98,117] Following the administration of effective regional analgesia during the first stage of labor, decreases in tidal volume,[179] oxygen consumption, and lactic acid production have been observed.[98,117,151]

While epidural anesthesia should not be administered for the purpose of controlling maternal blood pressure, an attentuation of preeclampsia-related vasospastic hypertension is generally observed once the block is established. There are two reasons for this: first, as has been mentioned, pain relief results in a decrease in maternal catecholamines; and second, lumbar epidural anesthesia causes a blockade of the lumbar sympathetic nervous system. This results in a dilatation of resistance and capacitance vessels, decreasing peripheral vascular resistance and causing a pooling of blood in the veins of the pelvis and lower extremities.

The fetus should also benefit from a well-conducted lumbar epidural anesthetic. Primate[136] and sheep[190] studies have shown that maternal stress can reduce uterine blood flow and even produce fetal asphyxia,[136] most likely as a result of increasing maternal catecholamine secretion. Elevated maternal catecholamines not only jeopardize already compromised placental perfusion but also decrease uterine activity and the progress of labor.[111] Jouppila and his group,[99] using radioactive xenon-133, have shown that placental blood flow tends to increase in preeclamptics following epidural anesthesia as long as systemic hypotension is avoided. James and Davies[93] have also shown that gestational hypertensive patients whose labor management included lumbar epidural anesthesia delivered newborns with acid-base and blood gas values comparable with those of normotensive controls. By providing adequate maternal analgesia, epidural anesthesia will eliminate further maternal narcotic and sedative requirements, thereby decreasing fetal exposure to these drugs and secondary fetal and neonatal depression.

Because the untreated severe preeclamptic is volume-depleted, she is more susceptible to serious hypotension following a lumbar sympathetic block than is the normotensive parturient. Fear of producing maternal hypotension and a dramatic decrease in placental perfusion has been the basis of much opposition to major conduction-block anesthesia in the management of the severe preeclamptic.[161] However, by using continuous epidural anesthesia as an adjunct to existing and careful medical management, i.e., as a means of providing pain relief and not as antihypertensive therapy, profound and dangerous hypotension can be avoided. Severe and volatile maternal hypertension should be brought into good medical control with appropriate antihypertensive agents before epidural anesthesia is administered. Intravascular volume depletion should be corrected with intravenous infusions and urine output should exceed 30 ml/h. Failure to rapidly correct oliguria with intravenous hydration necessitates assessment of the parturient's volume status with invasive monitoring (central venous or pulmonary capillary wedge pressure). Prior to the induction of epidural anesthesia in this setting, the central venous pressure should be raised to 6 to 8 cm H_2O. This can accomplished by infusing balanced salt solution, colloid, or a combination of both. There is recent evidence that volume expansion with 25 percent albumin may actually decrease diastolic blood pressure while raising central venous pressure and increasing urine output.[101]

If after administering an epidural anesthetic, significant relative hypotension (systolic blood pressure less than 100 mm Hg) occurs in spite of prophylactic volume expansion and adequate left uterine displacement, initial treatment to prevent a further decline in blood pressure should include head-down positioning and further crystalloid or colloid administration. Since the preeclamptic is very sensitive to adrenergic drugs, vasopressors should be titrated in smaller doses than normally used. Of the cardiotropic agents and vasopressors currently available, ephedrine and mephentermine have been shown to most consistently return uterine blood flow toward normal while correcting spinal hypotension.[94] I prefer ephedrine. To avoid a hypertensive response to ephedrine, the initial dose should be limited to 5 mg and repeated if necessary.

Most often, the severe preeclamptic will be receiving supplemental oxygen therapy when seen. If not, oxygen should be administered via a clear plastic face mask or nasal prongs once epidural anesthesia has been administered. Not only will oxygen therapy increase fetal oxygen tension,[8,69,167,234] but it also increases the margin of maternal safety in the event that hypoventilation or a fall in cardiac output occurs following the establishment of the block.

Since the management of pain associated with the first stage of labor requires only blockade of sympathetic afferent fibers entering the cord at T_{10} to L_1 (segmental block), the initial volume of local anesthetic required for lumbar epidural analgesia is only 6 to 8 ml. While this small volume will ablate labor pain, the chance of fetal malpresentation will be limited by avoiding the premature blockade of sacral nerves and relaxation of pelvic floor muscles that occur with higher doses. Other benefits of using small doses of local anesthetic include: (1) a block with limited cephalad spread, which decreases the incidence and severity of subsequent hypotension; (2) limited paralysis of the lower extremities; and (3) limited maternal and fetal exposure to potentially depressive local anesthetic agents.

The development of neonatal neurobehavioral assessment techniques during the past 25 years has allowed the objective evaluation of subtle effects caused by drugs used during labor. Although early studies were hampered by a lack of "pure" control groups and their study designs, more recent work has shown that well-conducted epidural anesthesia using bupivacaine,[1,41,48] etidocaine,[48] lidocaine,[1] or 2-chloroprocaine[1,48] will not adversely affect neurobehavior in the newborn.

The most important difference between the amide-type local anesthetics (bupivacaine, etidocaine, and lidocaine) and the esters (2-chloroprocaine, procaine, and tetracaine) is their routes of metabolism. The amides require hepatic degradation by the mixed-function oxidase system whereas the esters are rapidly metabolized in the blood. In full-term neonates, the half-lives of the amides are measured in hours.[144] The fetus of the severe preeclamptic is often premature and even more limited in its ability to metabolize local anesthetics than a fetus at term. It may therefore be extremely susceptible to the potential CNS and myocardial depressive effects associated with these agents. The already acidotic fetus is more likely to ionize and trap local anesthetic molecules within its circulation,[22,34] increasing the risk of further depression. Of all the amides, bupivacaine appears to be associated with the lowest fetal/maternal drug ratios. This has been attributed to a greater limitation in transplacental transfer of bupivacaine. Bupivacaine's high pKa (8.05) results in an increased ionization and trapping of drug in the maternal circulation.[32] In addition, bupivacaine is highly bound to maternal proteins.[213] Etidocaine also has pharmacokinetic properties which limit its placental transfer. However, when it is used in doses and concentrations suitable for the obstetric patient, a prolonged motor block of the lower extremities with only a patchy and incomplete sensory block of the abdomen has been observed.[48]

Unlike the amides, the ester, 2-chloroprocaine, undergoes rapid metabolic degradation in both maternal and fetal blood by plasma pseudocholinesterase. O'Brien et al.[140] found the half-life of 2-chloroprocaine to be 21 s in maternal blood and 43 s in umbilical cord blood. As a result of this rapid metabolism, Kuhnert et al.[109] found trace levels of 2-chloroprocaine in only half of the neonates whose mothers had received epidural anesthesia with 2-chloroprocaine. Therefore, because of rapid maternal and fetal metabolism and the lack of neonatal depression associated with 2-chloroprocaine, it would seem to be the most acceptable local anesthetic for obstetric use and is my choice for epidural anesthesia in the severe preeclamptic.

If a lumbar epidural catheter is in place during the second stage of labor, the patient need only be reinforced in a semisitting position with a dose of local anesthetic slightly larger than that required for segmental block during the first stage. This will result in good vaginal and perineal analgesia for episiotomy, forceps-assisted delivery, and any necessary repairs of the birth canal. Although complete perineal analgesia will ablate the parturient's reflex urge to bear down, she should nevertheless be able to push effectively with proper coaching.

General Anesthesia for Vaginal Delivery. On rare occasions, the severe preeclamptic will require general anesthesia for vaginal delivery. Fetal distress occurring during the second stage of labor may be managed best by vaginal delivery under general anesthesia because of the rapid induction time and the complete operative anesthesia provided. Munson and Embro[134] have shown that potent inhalational agents (halothane, enflurane, and isoflurane) have a dose-related effect on uterine contractility and are equally depressant at equipotent concentrations. In concentrations equal to or greater than 1 MAC (minimum alveolar concentration), these potent agents will rapidly relax a tetanic uterus to allow intrauterine manipulation and extraction of a malpositioned fetus or retained placenta. General anesthesia also may be indicated when regional techniques are contraindicated or refused by the patient. The induction and maintenance of general anesthesia for the critically ill preeclamptic will be discussed in the section dealing with general anesthesia for cesarean section.

Anesthesia for Cesarean Section. The same parameters considered during the anesthetic evaluation of a severe preeclamptic patient during labor and vaginal delivery should be studied before selecting the most appropriate anesthetic technique for cesarean section. In the absence of overt fetal distress, consideration can and should be given to administering regional anesthesia. Obvious advantages include an awake patient, who can protect her airway from aspiration, and avoidance of the interactions between drugs used during medical management of preeclampsia and those required for general anesthesia. Hodgkinson and his associates[85] found epidural anesthesia to be hemodynamically superior to general anesthesia for cesarean section in volume-corrected severely preeclamptic women (Fig. 5-6A and B). Laryngoscopy and tracheal intubation during general anesthesia resulted in a rise in mean arterial pressure of 45 mm Hg, and rises in mean pulmonary artery and pulmonary capillary wedge pressures of 20 mm Hg (Fig. 5-6A). Increases in pressures of this magnitude place the patient at greater risk for cerebrovascular accident and cardiac decompensation with pulmonary edema. In contrast, except for a slight fall in mean arterial pressure, patients who received epidural anesthesia displayed laudable cardiovascular stability, with no significant changes in pulmonary artery or pulmonary capillary wedge pressures (Fig. 5-6B).

Most investigators would agree that the potential risk of secondary hypotension following epidural anesthesia in the severe preeclamptic is a major disadvantage of

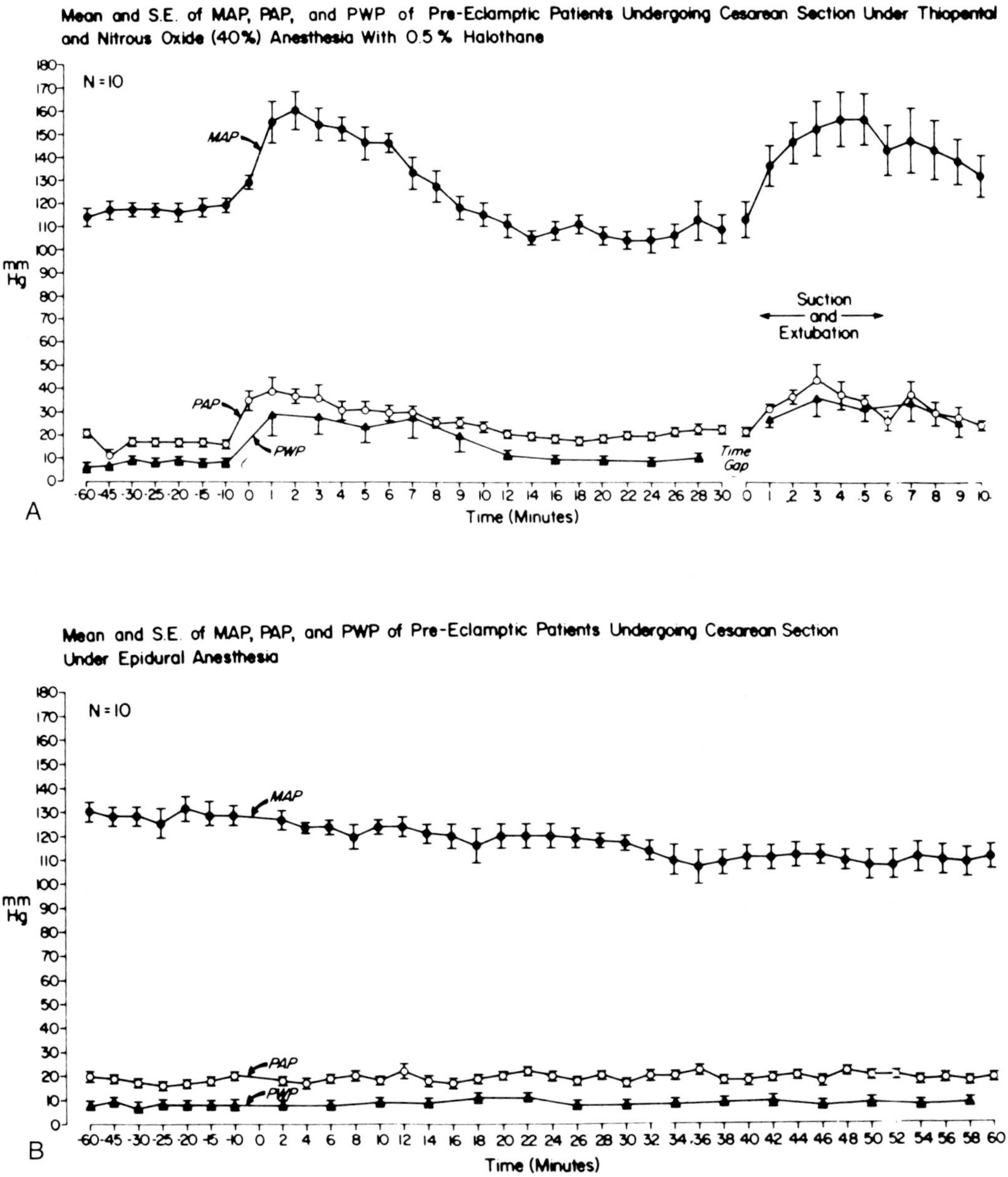

Fig. 5-6 (A) Values before induction of anesthesia are indicated as −60 to −10 min. The start of induction is indicated by the first 0. The second 0 refers to the start of suction and extubation. (B) Values before the administration of the epidural injection of bupivacaine at 0 min are indicated as −60 to −10 min. and values during epidural anaesthesia as 2 to 60 min. (From Hodgkinson, R., Husain, F.J., and Hayashi, R.H.: Systemic and pulmonary blood pressure during caesarean section in parturients with gestational hypertension. Can. Anaesth. Soc. J., *27*:389, 1980.)

the technique. However, with adequate rehydration, careful invasive monitoring when indicated, and avoidance of aortocaval compression, epidural anesthesia may be used safely in these women without creating additional hemodynamic instability.[80,85,100] Because the preeclamptic patient is more sensitive to vasopressors, prophylactic use of ephedrine is not recommended. An uncorrected volume deficit, laboratory evidence of coagulopathy, a confused or disoriented patient, and patient refusal of regional anesthesia should all be considered contraindications to the administration of epidural anesthesia for cesarean section.

Spinal anesthesia might seem to be an attractive alternative to epidural anesthesia for cesarean section in severe preeclamptics because of its rapid onset of action and minimal maternal and fetal drug exposure. However, the combination of a rapid onset of sympathetic block, difficulty in controlling the cephalad spread of the blockade, and varying degrees of vena caval compression by the gravid uterus all may result in greater hemodynamic instability[47,216] than that seen with epidural anesthesia. The severe preeclamptic with an uncorrected and constricted intravascular volume is at great risk for developing hypotension following chemical sympathectomy. Because hypotension represents a serious threat to both mother and the already compromised fetal-placental unit, I do not recommend spinal anesthesia for cesarean section in these women.

General anesthesia is indicated for cesarean section in the critically ill preeclamptic patient under the following circumstances: (1) overt fetal distress, where the possibility of developing hypotension following regional anesthesia is not acceptable; (2) uncorrected hypovolemia secondary to preeclampsia-related vasospasm or hemorrhage (abruptio placentae); (3) a hypocoagulable state, which may lead to an intraspinal hematoma following inadvertent vascular trauma secondary to needle or epidural catheter placement; (4) a patient who is unresponsive or confused secondary to preeclampsia-related cerebral involvement or oversedation from drug therapy; and (5) patient refusal of regional anesthesia.

There are several advantages to using general anesthesia for cesarean section in the critically ill preeclamptic woman: (1) it is a reliable and effective technique; (2) the time from the induction of anesthesia to delivery of the fetus is rapid, limiting the distressed fetus's time in utero; (3) the hypotension which may follow spinal or epidural anesthesia can be avoided; and (4) intubation with a cuffed endotracheal tube secures and protects the patient's airway. Intubation also enables high concentrations of oxygen to be administered to the mother, improving both maternal and fetal oxygen tensions.[71,171]

The major disadvantages of general anesthesia for cesarean section in the severe preeclamptic include: (1) an increased risk of maternal aspiration when compared with regional techniques; (2) an exacerbation of the patient's hypertensive state during laryngoscopy and tracheal intubation and during light anesthesia (Fig. 5-6A); and (3) the interaction of drugs used for perioperative management of preeclampsia with those required for induction and maintenance of general anesthesia.

As discussed in an earlier section, all parturients are considered to be full-stomach patients and at risk for lethal aspiration. In addition to oral antacid therapy, which has been advocated by other investigators,[36,169] I also recommend a rapid-sequence induction and endotracheal intubation with a cuffed endotracheal tube. During induction and intubation, manual cricoid pressure (Sellick maneuver)[184] collapses the esophagus and further decreases the risk of aspiration. Another technique to prevent aspiration is that of awake intubation under topical anesthesia. This is recommended especially if there is any doubt concerning the ability to intubate following paralysis with succinylcholine. Intraoperatively, an orogastric tube can be used to partially empty the stomach of liquid and solid contents. Postoperatively, the patient should be awake and able to protect her airway before she is extubated. The best way to prevent aspiration, however, is to avoid general anesthesia and administer regional anesthesia whenever possible.

Nonpregnant hypertensive patients display an exaggerated circulatory response to laryngoscopy and tracheal intubation, manifested by tachycardia and increases in mean arterial blood pressure.[162] In addition, preeclamptic patients have been observed to develop increases in pulmonary artery and pulmonary capillary wedge pressures during intubation.[85] Shnider et al.[188] have shown that plasma norepinephrine levels rise significantly in preeclamptics following endotracheal intubation. Since preeclamptic women are known to be more responsive to both endogenous and exogenous vasopressors than normal pregnant patients,[210] the cardiovascular responses noted during laryngoscopy and intubation might be predicted. The preeclamptic's hemodynamic lability in response to the induction of general anesthesia and maintenance of a light anesthetic state places her at great risk for cardiovascular complications during those periods. The cardiovascular responses during induction of general anesthesia should be less dramatic, however, if blood pressure has been under good control during labor.

For a detailed discussion of the antihypertensive agents used to treat the preeclamptic patient during labor, the reader is referred to Chapter 11. For rapid control of hypertension prior to emergency surgery, I prefer hydralazine (Apresoline), a direct-acting vasodilator. Concomitant with a fall in blood pressure following the administration of this drug, reflex increases in heart rate and cardiac output can be expected. In pregnant ewe models, hydralazine has been shown to increase uterine blood flow while reducing blood pressure.[31,168]

Two potent hypotensive agents are currently being investigated for use during pregnancy. Sodium nitroprusside is widely used in nonobstetric patients to control hypertension. However, concern about the transplacental passage of nitroprusside's toxic metabolite, cyanide, has limited its use in controlling preeclampsia-related hypertension.[138] Ellis et al.,[60] studying norepinephrine-induced hypertension in sheep, did not find toxic levels of cyanide in mother or fetus following short-term administration of sodium nitroprusside in amounts that might be infused prior to the induction of anesthesia. However, nitroprusside itself rapidly crosses the placenta.[138] There is also evidence that in the phenylephrine-induced hypertensive pregnant ewe model, nitroprusside does not significantly improve uterine blood flow while correcting hypertension.[168] Therefore, at this time the use of nitroprusside prior to operative delivery in severely hypertensive obstetric patients should probably be restricted to those rare cases which have not responded to intravenous hydralazine.

Snyder and his associates[194] have investigated the use of nitroglycerin for the management of severe pregnancy-related hypertension in humans during general anesthesia for cesarean section. They found nitroglycerin to be an effective antihypertensive agent with a rapid onset but short duration of action, allowing flexible blood pressure control. More recently, nitroglycerin therapy for phenylephrine-induced hypertension in pregnant ewes has been investigated by Craft et al.[43] They found nitroglycerin to rapidly return maternal mean arterial blood pressure to control values while increasing uterine blood flow from 50 percent below control values to 30 percent below control values. Fetal arterial pH increased significantly from 7.30 to 7.35. Nitroglycerin crosses the placenta, but not as freely as does sodium nitroprusside.[51] In animal models, nitroglycerin has been shown to disturb the autoregulation of cerebral blood flow, resulting in an increase in intracranial pressure despite a reduction in mean arterial pressure.[92,172,231] Since little is known about intracranial hemodynamics during severe preeclampsia, and since the effects of nitroglycerin on human uterine blood flow and the fetus are unknown, further investigation of nitroglycerin is indicated before its widespread use for the management of hypertension during general anesthesia for the severe preeclamptic patient can be recommended.

Ideally, a patient with severe preeclampsia will have her blood pressure monitored with an intra-arterial line. This will also allow access to arterial blood for blood gas determinations. If, upon arrival to the operating room, the diastolic blood pressure is above 100 mm Hg, I administer hydralazine as a bolus, 10 to 15 mg. During the time required for preparing the patient for surgery, hydralazine begins to lower the blood pressure and will ablate the subsequent and otherwise severe hypertensive response often observed following laryngoscopy and tracheal intubation. In the nonpregnant patient this hypertensive response can also be blunted by administering I.V. lidocaine, 1.5 mg/kg, prior to induction.[2,202] When lidocaine was given as an I.V. bolus in this dose, however, Abou-Madi et al.[2] measured serum lidocaine levels of 1.86 μg/ml within 2 to 3 min. Therefore, since lidocaine rapidly crosses the placenta and can depress the fetal myocardium and brain, it is preferable that this technique be avoided in severely preeclamptic women.

The common practice of administering a small dose of *d*-tubocurarine or pancuronium before induction to limit succinylcholine-induced fasciculations is probably unnecessary in preeclamptic patients receiving magnesium sulfate, since the later drug will accomplish the same effect. Following several minutes of preoxygenation to decrease the risk of hypoxemia during apnea, anesthesia is induced with thiopental, 4 mg/kg. Ketamine should be avoided as an induction agent in hypertensive patients because of its sympathiomimetic effects. Succinylcholine, 0.75 to 1.5 mg/kg, will provide neuromuscular blockade to facilitate intubation. Cricoid pressure should be maintained during induction and intubation to prevent aspiration. Following intubation, anesthesia can be maintained with oxygen and nitrous oxide, 50 percent. This combination may be supplemented with halothane, 0.5 percent, prior to delivery to decrease the level of maternal awareness during otherwise light anesthesia.[188] In spite of reduced awareness, Shnider et al.[188] were unable to show any significant decreases in norepinephrine levels or blood pressure in preeclamptic patients who were supplemented with 0.5% halothane, as compared with those receiving oxygen and nitrous oxide alone. Halothane, 0.5 percent, does not appear to worsen acid-base values in the already distressed fetus[49] or to adversely affect neonatal neurobehavior.[188] While oxygen and nitrous oxide supplementation with enflurane or methoxyflurane will also decrease the level of maternal awareness, it has been recommended that these agents be avoided in the preeclamptic because of the release of nephrotoxic inorganic fluoride during their biotransformation.[83]

Magnesium potentiates the neuromuscular blockade produced by both depolarizing (*d*-tubocurarine, pancuronium) and nondepolarizing (succinylcholine) skeletal muscle relaxants,[72,75] (Fig. 5-7). Because the preeclamptic patient receiving magnesium sulfate will have greater sensitivity to these agents, initial doses should be smaller than those usually administered. The magnitude of the effect of magnesium on a given patient's neuromuscular function is difficult to predict. Therefore, these women should be monitored throughout surgery with a blockade monitor. Additional drug can then be titrated to individual needs and prolonged paralysis avoided.

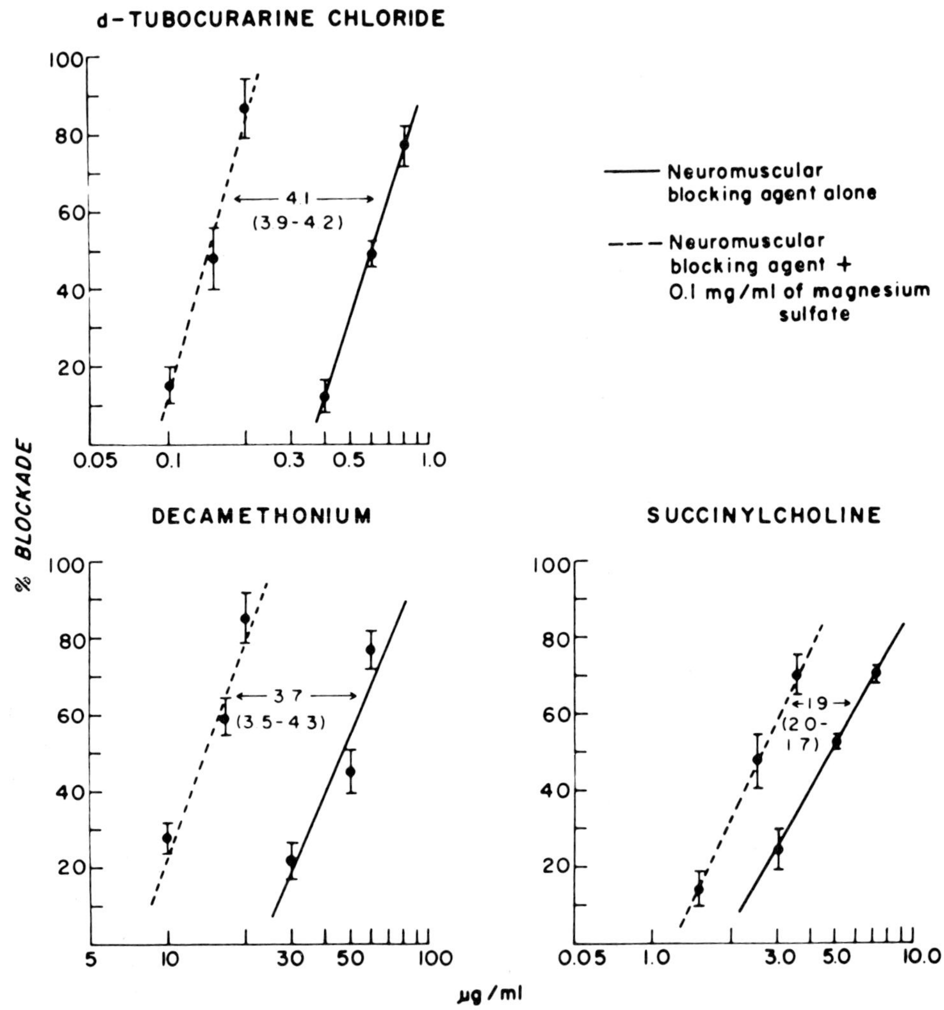

Fig. 5-7 Dose response curves of *d*-tubocurarine, decamethonium, and succinylcholine, using the rat phrenic nerve–diaphragm preparation. Each point represents the mean of five observations; vertical bars indicate standard error. 0.1 mg/ml of magnesium sulfate is a subliminal dose. The magnitude of potentiation is shown in between the curves, with their fiducial limits. (From Ghoneim, M.M. and Long, J.P.: Interaction between magnesium and other neuromuscular blocking agents. Anesthesiology, 32:23, 1970.)

Following delivery of the fetus, anesthetic depth can be deepened by increasing the inspired concentration of the chosen inhalational anesthetic agent or by supplementing oxygen and nitrous oxide with a combination of narcotics and diazepam. The choice and doses of the agents selected will be in part based on the patient's cardiovascular response to surgery as reflected by heart rate, blood pressure, and, if monitored, pulmonary capillary wedge pressure.

Since the neonate of the severe preeclamptic is often premature, growth-retarded, and depressed,[133] personnel familiar with newborn resuscitation should be present at the time of delivery. Any neonate displaying flaccidity and respiratory depression may be suffering from neonatal hypermagnesemia.[114] If severe, the infant may require mechanical ventilation and intravenous calcium to antagonize the effect of magnesium.

Involvement of the anesthesiologist in the management of the critically ill preeclamptic patient should not end with delivery of fetus. Because the preeclamptic's hemodynamic instability may continue for several days, the anesthesiologist remains a valuable consultant during the critical postpartum period.

SEVERE HEPATIC DYSFUNCTION

The liver is responsible for a myriad of important physiological and biochemical functions. Since it is the site of both glycogen breakdown and glucose synthesis, severe parenchymal disease will limit the liver's ability to maintain metabolic homeostasis. For example, glucose can be synthesized from either amino acids, glycerol, or lactic acid produced by skeletal muscle during the anaerobic metabolism of carbohydrates. During labor, the unanesthetized parturient is often in a state of mild lactic acidosis[117] secondary to the intense skeletal muscle activity associated with hyperventilation and isometric muscle tension in response to pain. Laboring patients with concomitant liver dysfunction will have difficulty metabolizing lactate and may experience severe metabolic acidosis.

The liver produces many of the clotting factors necessary for the adequate coagulation of blood. Although severe liver impairment is usually required before production of these proteins is critically reduced, laboratory studies to evaluate the adequacy of coagulation (fibrinogen levels, and prothrombin and partial thromboplastin times) are indicated during the preanesthetic evaluation of patients with hepatic dysfunction. Since the gastrointestinal absorption of vitamin K may also be impaired, patients with severe hepatic disease often require parenteral vitamin K supplementation.

If hepatic disease is severe enough to limit albumin production, drug binding will be seriously affected. While protein-bound, drugs are inactive. With serum albumin levels below 3.5 g/dl, the reduction in protein-binding sites becomes significant. When this occurs, the number of unbound drug molecules will increase and their biological activity will be greater than expected. A further increase in activity may become apparent during the administration of more than one drug as they compete for available protein-binding sites. Drug groups that can be expected to show increased activity in this setting include the barbiturates,[73] benzodiazepines,[81] narcotics, and amide-type local anesthetics.

In addition to alterations in protein binding, decreased hepatic uptake, and impaired intrahepatic metabolism of drugs secondary to reduced microsomal enzyme activity delays their biotransformation to inactive compounds and polar molecules which the kidney can excrete. Delayed biotransformation of a drug results in a prolongation of its plasma half-life and biological activity.[89,106,185] Since protein binding and metabolism are important in limiting the transplacental passage of maternally administered drugs,[32] the risk of fetal toxicity increases as the maternal blood levels of unbound active drugs rise.

Pseudocholinesterase activity is decreased in the presence of severe hepatic dysfunction. This enzyme is responsible for the biotransformation of succinylcholine and the ester-type local anesthetics. While the rate of hydrolysis of succinylcholine is limited in patients with severe liver disease, critical prolongation of biological activity (apnea) was not observed by Foldes[63] following the I.V. administration of 0.6 mg/kg of this drug. Toxicity resulting from high blood levels of the ester 2-chloroprocaine following regional anesthetic techniques in patients with decreased pseudocholinesterase activity is also unlikely.

In addition to coagulation studies and the measurement of serum albumin, the preanesthetic laboratory evaluation of patients with significant hepatic disease should include a complete liver function profile. These tests will serve as an indication of the site of hepatic involvement (prehepatic, intrahepatic, or posthepatic), the severity of the disease, and the patient's operative risk.[205] Specific tests should include serum bilirubin, direct and indirect, serum alkaline phosphatase, serum glutamic oxylacetic transaminase (SGOT), serum glutamic pyruvic transaminase (SGPT), and lactic dehydrogenase (LDH). Since patients with severe hepatic disease also may develop renal failure (hepatorenal syndrome), renal function should also be assessed. The presence of hepatic encephalopathy and the status of the fetus are also important factors in determining anesthetic options in these critically ill patients.

There is no universal approach to the anesthetic management of the obstetric patient with severe liver disease. The selection of anesthetic techniques and of drugs and their dosages should be made only after careful preanesthetic evaluation of the patient and her fetus. Laboring patients should receive supplemental oxygen to discourage anaerobic metabolism. Lactate production will be decreased during labor by providing adequate analgesia and avoiding maternal hyperventilation.[98,151] All parenteral drugs should be administered in small doses and titrated to patient needs and tolerances. Regional anesthesia may be considered if blood coagulation is adequate and the patient is not obtunded. Segmental lumbar epidural anesthesia can be administered early in labor and the level of anesthesia extended caudad to include sacral roots for vaginal delivery or cephalad for abdominal delivery. Effective regional anesthesia will decrease the amounts of potentially toxic parenteral drugs that may otherwise be required. Local anesthetic agents should be administered in the smallest doses that will provide effective analgesia. Because of 2-chloroprocaine's rapid metabolism and low fetal and maternal toxicity, it is a safer agent than the amide-type local anesthetics, which depend upon protein binding and hepatic microsomal enzyme metabolism to limit their maternal toxicity and transplacental passage.

In order to avoid any decrease in hepatic perfusion, which may add hypoxic insult to the already injured hepatocytes, adequate intravascular volume and cardiac output should be maintained. Displacement of the gravid uterus from the vena cava will help to ensure hemodynamic stability following sympathetic blockade. If regional analgesia is contraindicated, inhalational analgesia offers the advantage of rapid elimination of inspired agents following delivery. Parenteral drugs which require hepatic biotransformation will be eliminated slowly. General precautions concerning inhalational analgesia outlined earlier in this chapter should be observed. The choice of inhalational agents for patients with hepatic disease will be discussed below.

There is no one preferred method of anesthesia for cesarean section in the presence of hepatic dysfunction. The advantages of and contraindications to regional anesthesia discussed above for labor and delivery also apply for cesarean section. Because of the small dose of local anesthetic required for spinal anesthesia, it would appear to be an attractive alternative to epidural anesthesia. As a disadvantage, spinal anesthesia for cesarean section is associated with a high incidence of hypotension, partly due to vena caval compression. If hepatic disease is complicated by significant ascites, raised intra-abdominal pressure will further compromise blood return through the vena cava, making it difficult to maintain adequate cardiac output following sympathetic blockade. Blood shunted from the vena cava through the vertebral canal will cause epidural venous distension, decreasing the size of the subarachnoid space and making doses of local anesthetic required for spinal anesthesia difficult to predict.

General anesthesia avoids the problems associated with coagulation defects and is less likely to cause hypotension. It further enables the anesthesiologist to safely control the patient's airway and deliver high concentrations of oxygen during surgery. However, potential problems exist with this technique. During induction, dosages of thiopental and succinylcholine can be difficult to predict. To avoid prolonged apnea or sleep, normal doses should be adjusted. Oxygen and nitrous oxide, 50%, may be used for maintenance of anesthesia. To avoid maternal awareness, low concentrations of a more potent inhalational agent may be added prior to delivery of the fetus. True halothane hepatotoxicity is rare and occurs unpredictably, but there is animal evidence to suggest that hypoxia and prior microsomal enzyme induction can cause increased metabolism of this agent via reductive pathways. Since general and regional anesthetic techniques all appear to decrease hepatic blood flow by 20 to 40 percent, parenchymal hypoxia may occur during anesthesia. Halothane's reductive metabolites, binding covalently to hepatic proteins, lipoproteins, and lipids, may then cause further hepatic parenchymal cell damage.[126] If reductive metabolites of halothane are potentially hepatotoxic, it would seem prudent to avoid this agent and the risk of further injury to the liver. Alternatives to halothane include enflurane and isoflurane, two halogenated ethers which are metabolized to a lesser extent and are thus, theoretically, less hepatotoxic.

Because of changes in the volume of distribution and the protein binding of the nondepolarizing neuromuscular blockers in the presence of severe liver disease, dose requirements of these drugs are difficult to predict.[57,203] By using a blockade monitor, the doses of *d*-tubocurarine and pancuronium can be titrated to each patient's needs without fear of a prolonged effect.

Following the delivery of the fetus, anesthesia may be deepened by increasing the concentration of the inhalational agent administered or by supplementing oxygen and nitrous oxide with narcotics and diazepam. Large doses of fixed I.V. drugs should be avoided to prevent prolonged postoperative CNS or respiratory depression.

RENAL FAILURE

Compromised renal function, regardless of the etiology, has important implications in the anesthetic management of the pregnant patient. In these women, intravascular volume status must be assessed prior to anesthetic induction. Hypervolemia with secondary peripheral and pulmonary edema and hypertension may be seen in association with renal failure. Occasionally, on the other hand, hypovolemia and hypotension occur immediately following dialysis. Central monitoring may therefore be necessary as a guide to fluid therapy.

The kidney is also vitally important in electrolyte balance and acid-base homeostasis. The undialyzed patient in renal failure may be hyperkalemic, hypocalcemic, hypermagnesemic, and metabolically acidotic. Ideally, serial determinations of serum electrolytes will be obtained throughout labor and abnormalities corrected prior to elective or semiurgent surgery. Hyperkalemia predisposes the patient to the development of serious ventricular arrhythmias in the perioperative period. Proceeding with elective surgery in patients with a serum potassium value greater than 5.5 mEq/L is not advised, since succinylcholine, intraoperative hypoxia or hypercarbia, and the administration of bank blood can all cause further increases in potassium to occur. If necessary, elective surgery should be delayed and the patient medically treated or dialyzed immediately prior to the operation. Dialysis will improve acid-base and water balance as well as restore electrolyte balance.

For the patient with renal disease undergoing elective cesarean section, both regional and general anesthesia may be considered. The advantages of spinal or epidural anesthesia in this group include the avoidance of drugs and intraoperative events which can alter biochemical homeostasis and of anesthetic agents which require renal excretion following surgery. Contraindications to regional anesthesia include coagulopathy secondary to uremia-related platelet dysfunction[59] or systemic heparinization, labile blood pressure, and fetal distress.

If general anesthesia is chosen, induction should be a rapid-sequence technique with cricoid pressure as prophylaxis against aspiration. A short-acting barbiturate (thiopental) may be used safely in sleep doses. Although increases in serum potassium have been reported following the administration of succinylcholine for intubation,[156,176] serious hyperkalemia should not occur if serum potassium levels have been normalized prior to surgery.[130]

Following intubation, anesthesia may be maintained with a combination of oxygen and nitrous oxide, 50 percent, and low concentrations of an inhalational agent to prevent maternal awareness. The recently dialyzed patient, if hypovolemic, may be very sensitive to the cardiovascular effects of the potent inhalational agents. Adequate preoperative fluid replacement will help prevent a decrease in cardiac output and subsequent fall in uterine perfusion. Halothane, 0.5 percent, or isoflurane, 0.5 percent, are the inhalational agents I prefer. Enflurane, 0.75 percent, may be used in the anephric patient, but the biotransformation of this agent results in the release of inorganic fluoride,[42] which is nephrotoxic. While Wikstrom[227] has shown that the levels of this metabolite thought to be nephrotoxic are not reached following a brief anesthetic exposure to enflurane, it should probably be avoided in women with functioning kidneys unless there is a specific indication for its use. Following delivery of the fetus, anesthesia may be deepened by increasing the concentration of the chosen inhalational agent. Although I.V. narcotics can be used for supplementation during this period, many anesthesiologists would avoid administering agents which require renal elimination. Since many patients with significant renal dysfunction are anemic, high concentrations of oxygen should be administered throughout the surgery.

The nondepolarizing neuromuscular blockers are all excreted to some extent by the kidney. Gallamine, the agent most dependent upon renal excretion, should be avoided in patients with renal failure. *d*-Tubocurarine and pancuronium, though largely excreted by the kidney, can also undergo hepatic biotransformation and biliary excretion. However, since the elimination half-lives of these drugs are prolonged, doses administered should be modified and titrated to patient needs.

Although successful pregnancies have been reported in patients undergoing chronic hemodialysis,[107] fetal growth retardation is common. Anesthesia and pediatric personnel should be prepared to resuscitate a depressed and uremia-poisoned newborn.

PERIPARTUM HEMORRHAGE

Antepartum shock represents a serious pathophysiological crisis which threatens both maternal and fetal well-being. There are two major causes of third-trimester antepartum hemorrhage: (1) encroachment of the placenta upon the internal cervical os (placenta previa) and (2) premature separation of the placenta from the wall of the uterus (abruptio placentae).

In general, placenta previa presents as painless, bright red vaginal bleeding without uterine hyperactivity or tenderness. In contrast, bleeding from an abruptio is often associated with contractions and may appear per vagina or remain concealed. The clinical presentation is a function of the location of the separation and its severity. Since concealed blood loss in patients with abruptions may exceed 5 L,[158] it is difficult to estimate the amount of hemorrhage by visual inspection alone. Furthermore, since normal pregnancy is characterized by a state of hypervolemia, tachycardia and hypotension may not become apparent in the recumbent patient until blood loss exceeds 2 L.

Placenta Previa

Patients who present with vaginal bleeding are assumed to have placenta previa until proved otherwise. They should not be examined vaginally unless this condition has been ruled out. Occasionally, however, the diagnosis cannot be excluded by ultrasound, and the degree of cervical dilatation and position of the placental margin relative to the internal os must be known to optimize obstetric management. In this setting, a "double setup" examination can be peformed in the operating room with the patient's abdomen prepped and draped for surgery. Both the obstetrician and the anesthesiologist must be prepared to proceed with immediate cesarean section and the management of sudden hemorrhage should it occur.

A double setup should be performed only after the patient's cardiovascular status has been stabilized and she has been prepared for general anesthesia and possible sudden massive blood loss. The severity of hemorrhage prior to the procedure can be estimated by the observed blood loss, the patient's blood pressure and heart rate in response to postural changes, and her hematocrit. Urine output is an indication of adequate vital organ perfusion. Monitoring central venous pressure provides more direct insight into intravascular volume status[70] and serves as a guide to fluid resuscitation. Uterine blood flow is a function of maternal blood pressure and blood volume.[175] Likewise, placental oxygenation is a function of maternal cardiac output and the concentration of inspired oxygen. Therefore, to avoid maternal and fetal hypoxia and acidosis during hemorrhage, fluid resuscitation should be rapid and adequate, and supplemental oxygen should be administered throughout the resuscitative period.

The initial fluid replacement of massive blood loss can be accomplished with crystalloid (lactated Ringer's solution) or 5 percent albumin solution (Plasmanate). While the use of albumin solution helps to maintain colloid osmotic pressure, there does not appear to be any deleterious cardiopulmonary effect from the administration of large volumes of crystalloid without albumin during resuscitation.[37,192,222] Since severe hemorrhagic shock may result in pulmonary capillary endothelial damage, albumin solutions administered to these patients may translocate across pulmonary capillary beds to extravascular spaces and actually contribute to the development of pulmonary insufficiency. These issues are further discussed in Chapter 3. Following initial resuscitation with fluids which do not contain red blood cells, the patient should be transfused with whole blood or packed red blood cells to a hematocrit of at least 30 percent. Central venous pressure should be restored to a level of 8 to 10 cmH_2O prior to proceeding with vaginal examination in the delivery room.

In preparation for anesthesia, the patient should receive 30 ml of an oral antacid. Two large-bore intravenous lines are indicated as well. Blood pumps and warmers should be available for the rapid administration of blood and balanced salt solutions. Two, and preferably four, units of whole blood should be in the delivery room or immediately available. After the patient has been placed in the lithotomy position with left uterine displacement, a small dose of *d*-tubocurarine, 3.0 mg, or pancuronium, 0.5 to 1.0 mg, may be injected to block succinylcholine-induced fasciculations which raise intragastric pressure and encourage regurgitation. Pure (100%) oxygen is administered during aseptic preparation of the abdomen and perineum. Only when the obstetric, anesthesia, and pediatric teams are ready should the cervical os be examined.

If the diagnosis of placenta previa is confirmed without inducing bleeding and immediate delivery of a premature fetus is not indicated, the patient may return to her room and be placed at bed rest. Once mature, the fetus can be delivered by elective cesarean section under general or regional anesthesia. If a complete placenta previa is confirmed and the fetus is mature, cesarean section is usually performed immediately following the double setup examination. For the patient with complete previa who is not actively bleeding and hemodynamically stable, cesarean section may be performed under general anesthesia or a regional anesthetic technique if preferred by the patient and her anesthesiologist.[21]

If examination initiates hemorrhage, immediate cesarean section is performed under general anesthesia. Adequate volume replacement may be difficult, or even impossible, until the placenta is removed. If the patient becomes hypotensive with a falling central venous pressure, induction with ketamine, 1 mg/kg, is recommended. Because of its sympathomimetic properties, ketamine will support the maternal cardiovascular system better than will thiopental. In a dose of 1 mg/kg, ketamine will not cause any direct adverse effects on uterine blood flow or the neonate. Induction of anesthesia in the presence of severe hypotension (systolic pressure less than 70 mm Hg) and obtundation should be accomplished with succinylcholine alone, 1.0 to 1.5 mg/kg, to facilitate endotracheal intubation. In this situation, the use of ketamine may cause cardiovascular collapse. If vasopressors are required prior to delivery of the fetus, ephedrine, 10 to 15 mg I.V., is recommended. Potent alpha-adrenergic agonists (phenylephrine or norepinephrine) may be used to treat life-threatening maternal hypotension until intravascular volume can be restored. Possible adverse effects on uterine blood flow following the use of alpha-adrenergic agonists must be disregarded when maternal safety is jeopardized.

Prior to delivery of the fetus, agents used for the maintenance of anesthesia will depend upon the status of the mother. If tolerated, nitrous oxide may be added to oxygen in concentrations not exceeding 50 percent. Halothane, 0.5 percent, or enflurane, 0.75 percent, may be added to prevent maternal awareness if blood pressure and central venous pressure are stable. Neuromuscular blockade may be provided with a succinylcholine infusion, 0.1 to 0.2 percent, or incremental doses of pancuronium. Once the fetus and placenta are delivered, blood loss can be controlled and hemodynamic stability restored. Anesthesia may then be maintained with a combination of inhalational and intravenous agents as preferred by the anesthesiologist.

Since maternal hypotension will result in altered uterine blood flow, the neonate may be severely asphyxiated at birth. In the presence of a velamentous cord insertion, vaginal hemorrhage may reflect fetal blood loss and in that situation, a delay in delivery can result in fetal exsanguination. Pediatric and anesthesia personnel must be prepared to treat neonatal asphyxia with immediate tracheal intubation and ventilation with 100 percent oxygen. The hypovolemic neonate will require rapid volume replacement with crystalloid, plasma, or preferably, fresh whole blood via an umbilical artery catheter.

Abruptio Placentae

The anesthetic management of the patient with abruptio placentae will depend upon several factors: (1) the severity of the abruption, and as a direct corollary, the presence or absence of maternal shock; (2) the status of the fetus; and (3) the presence of an associated maternal coagulopathy.

The magnitude of vaginal bleeding may or may not indicate the severity of the separation. In the case of a concealed abruption, the severity of hemorrhage may only be appreciated by the presence of maternal shock, or evidence of fetal distress or demise. Because of the compensatory capabilities of the cardiovascular system of the young and otherwise healthy gravida, blood pressure and heart rate may appear stable initially, even in the presence of a massive concealed hemorrhage. The intravascular volume status of a patient suspected of having a significant abruption can be better assessed and corrected by monitoring her central venous pressure[141] or pulmonary capillary wedge pressure. Using central venous pressure as a guide to blood volume replacement, O'Driscoll[141] reported that his patients with severe abruption required an average of 7 units of blood to replace hemorrhagic losses. The potential threat to mother and fetus is apparent.

The patient with a small abruption may deliver vaginally without complications and remain undiagnosed until the placenta is inspected, whereas mild uterine hyperactivity and localized tenderness, in the absence of maternal hypotension or evidence of fetal distress, usually indicate a mild to moderate abruption. Maternal blood pressure, heart rate, central venous pressure, urine output, serial hematocrits, and fetal heart rate tracings can all be used to assess the progression of a suspected abruption and the adequacy of fluid replacement. If there is no immediate threat to mother or fetus, these patients may be considered candidates for lumbar epidural analgesia during labor. Because abruptio placentae and preeclampsia (which often accompanies abruptio) are both associated with coagulopathies, the patient who is suspected of having an abruption should have a coagulation profile performed before epidural analgesia is administered. Maternal hypovolemia, fetal distress, and abnormal clotting studies should all be considered contraindications to regional analgesia.

Severe abruptio may occur precipitously. The sudden onset of fetal distress and uterine tetany, with or without maternal shock, indicates a rapid extension of the abruption. Again, vaginal bleeding may not be indicative of the magnitude of intrauterine hemorrhage. Immediate cesarean section may be necessary to save the life of the fetus. If a lumbar epidural catheter is in place and anesthesia is adequate for surgery, cesarean section may be performed under the existing block. However, an existing epidural block, if inadequate for surgery, should not be extended because of the risk of worsening hypotension following extension of the sympathectomy.

Induction and maintenance of general anesthesia prior to delivery of the fetus is aimed at supporting maternal hemodynamic stability and optimizing maternal and fetal oxygenation. Suggested techniques and agents are the same as those discussed above for the bleeding patient with placenta previa. Following delivery of the fetus and placenta, hemorrhage may persist due to uterine atony or the presence of disseminated intravascular coagulation. In addition to replacing acute blood losses with balanced salt solutions and whole blood, fresh frozen plasma, platelets, and cryoprecipitate may be required to replace consumed clotting factors. The potent inhalational anesthetic agents may contribute to maternal hypotension and uterine atony and should be avoided. The goals of therapy include restoration of blood volume and cardiac output, reversal of the coagulopathy, maintenance of acid-base balance, and prevention of end organ failure. In addition to monitoring urine output, arterial blood gases, and central venous pressure, monitoring of pulmonary capillary wedge pressure may provide important additional information regarding left ventricular function and the etiology of pulmonary edema should it develop.

Severe abruptio placentae is associated with a high incidence of perinatal mortality. Blair,[25] in his series of 189 cases, reported 85 stillbirths and 21 neonatal deaths for a perinatal mortality of 55 percent. The neonate who survives a severe abruption can be expected to be asphyxiated and hypovolemic and to require extensive resuscitative efforts followed by intensive neonatal care.

Postpartum Hemorrhage

Blood loss in excess of 500 ml following vaginal delivery is considered to be a postpartum hemorrhage (PPH). The most common causes of postpartum hemorrhage are uterine atony, retained placental fragments, and traumatic injuries to the perineum, vagina, cervix, or uterine fundus. Disseminated intravascular coagulation associated with abruptio placentae or preeclampsia may also contribute to excessive postpartum bleeding. For a comprehensive discussion of the causes of PPH and their medical and surgical management, the reader is referred to Chapters 9 and 10.

If uterine atony, regardless of its etiology, does not respond to medical management, emergency ligation of the hypogastric arteries or abdominal hysterectomy may be necessary to control hemorrhage and save the mother's life. Because the decision to proceed with the surgery usually follows unsuccessful attempts to control the bleeding, these patients may be severely hypovolemic and acidotic. Transport to the operating room should be in the head-down position with supplemental oxygen administered en route. The principles of the anesthetic management of these patients, including invasive monitoring, fluid therapy, and anesthetic techniques are similar to those discussed above in the sections dealing with hemorrhage secondary to placenta previa and abruptio placentae. Besides its sympathomimetic effects, an additional advantage of using ketamine rather than thiopental for induction in patients with uterine atony is that ketamine actually increases uterine tone.[67] Again, in the presence of severe hypotension and obtundation, neither ketamine or thiopental should be used. Because the fetus has been delivered and its welfare is no longer a consideration, vasopressors normally avoided during the antepartum period may be used as needed to support maternal hemodynamics until the hemorrhage is controlled and blood volume replaced. Halothane and other potent inhalation agents should be avoided in the presence of uterine atony and hemorrhage. These agents will antagonize uterine contractility, depress the myocardium, and decrease reflex vasomotor tone.

The definitive treatment of active bleeding secondary to retained placental fragments is manual uterine exploration and curettage. The manual exploration should always be done first to rule out a uterine rupture as the cause of the bleeding. Patients who do not already have an adequate epidural or subarachnoid block should not be administered a regional technique at this time because of the risk of serious hypotension following chemical sympathectomy in a hypovolemic patient. Often mask analgesia will be sufficient for intrauterine exploration and placental extraction. Oxygen and nitrous oxide, 40 to 50 percent, plus a low concentration, 0.25 to 0.5 percent, of one of the halogenated ethers (enflurane, isoflurane, or methoxyflurane) will provide adequate analgesia for most patients without loss of consciousness and risk of aspiration. If either analgesia or uterine relaxation is not sufficient to allow intrauterine manipulation, general anesthesia with a cuffed endotracheal tube is recommended. Higher concentrations of the potent inhalational agents mentioned above will provide rapid uterine relaxation and allow manual removal of retained placental fragments. Caution must be exercised in the use of these agents in the hypovolemic patient to avoid profound hypotension and prolonged uterine relaxation. The inhalational agents should be discontinued immediately following placental removal. Continued bleeding secondary to anesthetic-related tocolysis may be controlled with uterine massage and an oxytocin infusion.

When the retained placenta has an abnormal adherence to the uterine wall with villi in direct contact with the myometrium (placenta accreta), manual removal may be very difficult and can result in profound hemorrhage. If ligation of the hypogastric arteries or hysterectomy is required to control hemorrhage, the anesthetic considerations in management of these patients are similar to those discussed in previous sections dealing with acute peripartum hemorrhage and shock.

Lacerations to the birth canal may arise during spontaneous descent and expulsion of the fetus or iatrogenically secondary to forceps-assisted vaginal delivery. Bleeding will not be controlled in these patients until the lacerations are located and sutured. During inspection and repair of the birth canal, blood loss must be rapidly replaced with available fluids. Placing the patient in a head-down lithotomy position will augment venous return to the heart. Supplemental oxygen should be administered continuously. As with other causes of peripartum hemorrhage and shock, anesthetic techniques and agents which may further threaten maternal hemodynamic stability should be avoided.

CARDIAC DISEASE

The anesthetic management of the obstetric patient with hemodynamically significant heart disease is determined by individual disease processes and guided by appropriate monitoring of peripartum physiological changes and the effects of therapeutic intervention. There is no anesthetic protocol which will be universally applicable to all cardiac patients, even those who share a common cardiopulmonary lesion. Recommendations made in this section will be based on current understanding of the pathophysiology of each disease discussed and the known physiologic effects of anesthetic techniques and agents. Though all cardiac disorders will not be specifically addressed, the principles discussed should be of value as the reader formulates an anesthetic approach to any pregnant woman with cardiac disease. This section is intended to complement the more thorough discussion of serious cardiac disorders in pregnancy found in Chapter 19.

For the obstetric patient without heart disease, the cardiovascular changes that occur during pregnancy, though significant, pose no threat to maternal well-being. Whether pregnancy is well tolerated in a patient with cardiac disease depends upon the nature of her lesion and the functional classification of her disability. For example, patients with noncyanotic congenital lesions, or acquired aortic stenosis or mitral insufficiency who have no limitation of physical activity (New York Heart Association Class I) generally tolerate pregnancy and labor well. However, all patients with primary pulmonary hypertension or Eisenmenger's syndrome and those with mitral stenosis who display marked limitation of physical activity (Class III or IV) are at greater risk for pregnancy-related cardiopulmonary decompensation.[165] Approximately 85 percent of maternal cardiac deaths have been reported to occur in patients in Class III or IV.[145]

Ideally, the anesthesiologist should be informed of any obstetric patient with significant heart disease during her second trimester. This will allow sufficient time for a personal interview and a preanesthetic evaluation of the gravida's cardiac disease and medications. Working with the patient's perinatologist and cardiologist, the anesthesiologist can then contribute to the formulation of plans for her peripartum management.

For the critically ill cardiac patient, regardless of the nature of her lesion, invasive hemodynamic monitoring is both valuable and appropriate. An intra-arterial line not only provides continuous assessment of changes in blood pressure but also allows access to arterial blood for serial determination of arterial blood gases. This is especially important in patients with cyanotic heart disease. Placement of a balloon-tipped, thermodilution, pulmonary artery catheter enables the measurement of central venous, pulmonary artery, and pulmonary capillary wedge pressures and determination of pulmonary and peripheral vascular resistances and cardiac output. In patients without mitral valve disease, pulmonary capillary wedge pressure correlates with changes in left ventricular end diastolic pressure and therefore reflects the inotropic state of the left ventricle as well as the patient's intravascular volume status. Invasive hemodynamic monitoring not only helps in detecting pathologic events as they occur but also serves as a measurement of the effectiveness of therapy.

Mitral Stenosis

Szekley and Snaith[209] found mitral stenosis to be the most common acquired valvular heart disease associated with pregnancy. Unfortunately, significant mitral stenosis is also one of the most dangerous cardiovascular lesions complicating pregnancy.

To appreciate the potential insult that pregnancy and parturition represent for the patient with mitral stenosis, an understanding of the pathophysiology of the disease is essential. The stenotic mitral valve limits the rate of blood flow from the left atrium to the left ventricle. Transvalvular blood flow, and thus cardiac output, becomes a function of the cross-sectional area of the valve, left atrial pressure, and duration of diastole. During normal pregnancy, both heart rate and cardiac output increase. In order to maintain an increase in cardiac output in the presence of a stenotic mitral valve and a decrease in diastolic filling time, left atrial pressure must increase. Patients with mitral stenosis who are asymptomatic or mildly symptomatic prior to conception may experience cardiac decompensation during pregnancy. This will occur if the demands for increased cardiac output and transvalvular flow cannot be met or if left atrial pressure and, as a result, pulmonary capillary hydrostatic pressure increase until a transudation of fluid into the interstitial and alveolar spaces occurs. Pregnant women with significant stenosis have been shown to have a higher pulmonary capillary blood volume than normal gravidas.[71] Patients with increased left atrial pressures also have an increased incidence of atrial fibrillation and paroxysmal atrial tachycardia.[209] Therefore, during labor and vaginal delivery or during cesarean section, the patient with severe mitral stenosis will benefit from careful hemodynamic monitoring. A radial artery line and pulmonary artery catheter are recommended.

Pain associated with labor will cause an increase in heart rate, which in turn further limits the diastolic filling time of the left ventricle. This results in a decrease in cardiac output, an increase in left atrial pressure, and an increased risk of developing pulmonary edema. By administering adequate analgesia throughout labor tachycardia can be avoided. I recommend that a segmental lumbar epidural block be placed early to ablate any discomfort caused by uterine contractions. The block may be extended during the second stage of labor to provide sacral root analgesia. A forceps-assisted delivery or vacuum extraction is recommended to avoid the hemodynamic consequences of the Valsalva maneuver during pushing.

Hypotension following sympathetic blockade may cause a compensatory increase in heart rate and should be avoided. Crystalloid solutions should be infused in volumes sufficient to maintain pulmonary capillary wedge pressure in a range consistent with optimal cardiac output. Cardiac output can be serially determined throughout parturition by using a thermodilution tip pulmonary artery catheter. Adequate left uterine displacement will help maintain central venous volume. If vasopressors are required to increase peripheral vascular resistance and correct hypotension, the alpha-adrenergic agonist phenylephrine, 10 mg in 500 ml saline, or metaraminol,[116] 10 mg in 250 ml saline, may be administered by slow infusion until hypotension is corrected. By using commercially available pumps to control infusion rates, wide fluxes in blood pressure can be avoided. Hypotension must be treated very cautiously in these women because significant increases in afterload secondary to iatrogenic hypertension may precipitate pulmonary edema. It should also be remembered that alpha-adrenergic agonists will increase pulmonary vascular resistance as well as peripheral vascular resistance. Patients who already have significant pulmonary hypertension may decompensate during alpha-agonist therapy and will benefit from close monitoring of pulmonary artery and central venous pressures. Although ephedrine will correct spinal hypotension and improve uterine blood flow in normal obstetric patients,[94] it also causes tachycardia and therefore may worsen the situation in patients with severe mitral stenosis.

Because pulmonary edema and impaired gas exchange may develop during the peripartum period, continuous supplemental oxygen via a face mask or nasal prongs is recommended.

While either regional or general anesthesia may be used for cesarean section, well-conducted epidural anesthesia offers some advantages. The awake patient has less risk of aspiration. A regional anesthetic technique, when properly performed, also avoids the dramatic hemodynamic fluctuations often associated with general anesthesia. Following the placement of a lumbar epidural catheter, the level of anesthesia can be slowly raised. This will allow time for compensatory vasoconstriction above the level of the block and for gentle hydration to maintain pulmonary capillary wedge pressure and cardiac output within the range of control values. When the procedure is properly performed, tachycardia and large fluctuations in blood pressure can be avoided. Prophylactic ephedrine is not recommended because of the possibility of inducing tachycardia. In normal pregnancy, cardiac output increases dramatically following delivery owing to increases in heart rate and stroke volume secondary to the autotransfusion of uterine blood. For the patient with severe mitral stenosis, marked increases in central blood volume and tachycardia may lead to dramatic increases in pulmonary capillary wedge pressure and pulmonary edema. With an indwelling epidural catheter, the level of sympathetic blockade can be extended at this time to encourage the peripheral pooling of blood in capacitance vessels and avoid cardiac decompensation. Concurrent diuretic therapy will further decrease preload and help restore normal central volume and intracardiac pressures. I do not recommend spinal block for cesarean section in patients with severe mitral stenosis because of the rapid and extreme hemodynamic changes associated with subarachnoid anesthesia during pregnancy.

When cutaneous lumbar epidural anesthesia is contraindicated or refused, general anesthesia may be administered for cesarean section. Drugs which produce tachycardia, such as atropine, ketamine, and pancuronium, should be avoided when possible. Stress associated with light general anesthesia will also cause an unwanted tachycardia and catecholamine release. Increases in left atrial pressure, pulmonary capillary wedge pressure, and pulmonary vascular resistance may result and lead to a fall in cardiac output. In the absence of left or right ventricular dysfunction, thiopental induction, 4 mg/kg, is usually indicated. Intravenous fentanyl (in doses to 50 μg/kg I.V.) may be used in patients with mitral valve disease to decrease the tachycardia and hypertension associated with induction.[200] In patients with left or right heart dysfunction, fentanyl also decreases the requirements for thiopental, a myocardial depressant. For maintenance, oxygen and nitrous oxide, 50 percent, can be used. If tachycardia develops following induction, it can be managed by deepening anesthesia with additional narcotic or inhalational agent or by administering incremental doses of intravenous propranolol. The appropriate depth of anesthesia and/or dosage of propranolol should be determined by closely monitoring subsequent cardiovascular responses.

Hypoxia and acidosis are known pulmonary vasoconstrictors and should be avoided. If increased pulmonary vascular resistance leads to right ventricular compromise, low-dose isoproterenol, nitroprusside, or nitroglycerin may be necessary to treat pulmonary hypertension and right ventricular failure. Many of these drugs may have adverse effects on uterine blood flow or the fetus. However, when they are required to support or improve maternal hemodynamics, I feel that their potential benefits outweigh possible fetal risks.

Many patients with severe mitral stenosis will be digitalized prior to admission either because of a history of atrial fibrillation with a rapid ventricular response or as prophylaxis in the event that atrial fibrillation or paroxysmal atrial tachycardia should develop during pregnancy. Serum potassium levels should be closely followed in these patients, with supplemental potassium administered when necessary.

Peripartum Cardiomyopathy

Peripartum cardiomyopathy (PPCM) is a disease of cardiac muscle which develops during the last month of pregnancy (7 percent) or during the first 5 postpartum months (93 percent).[50] The diagnosis of PPCM precludes myocardial disease due to any other demonstrable cause. Hormonal changes, autoimmune mechanisms, poor nutrition, drug therapy, and viral infection have all been cited as possible etiological factors in the development of this condition. Whether pregnancy is causally associated or predisposes obstetric patients with asymptomatic preexisting myocardial disease to cardiac decompensation is unclear.

While the etiology of PPCM remains uncertain, the clinical significance of the disease is not. Patients present with signs and symptoms of left and/or right heart failure,[50,208] including shortness of breath, peripheral edema, anginal-type chest pain, and arrhythmias.[208] Cardiomegaly and pulmonary venous congestion are apparent on chest x-ray. In addition to arrhythmias, electrocardiographic changes frequently noted are ST segment depression and T wave inversion. A decrease in cardiac output with an increase in venous oxygen desaturation can be expected.[90] Invasive hemodynamic investigations have supported the diagnosis of biventricular involvement in some patients, with raised pulmonary capillary wedge pressures and right ventricular end diastolic pressures both being observed.[96]

The hemodynamic changes occurring during the third trimester and the peripartum period place antepartum patients with PPCM at great risk for further myocardial decompensation if treatment is not aggressive. Bed rest, salt restriction, diuretics, and digitalization form the cornerstones of therapy. Because of the hypercoagulable state of pregnancy and the high incidence of mural thrombosis and thromboembolism associated with PPCM,[206] prophylactic anticoagulant therapy has been advocated.[208]

During the preanesthetic evaluation, information concerning current drug therapy must be elicited. Patients who are receiving diuretics may have serum potassium levels less than 3.5 mg/dl. It is important that serum potassium levels be kept within normal limits, especially when digitalis is being given. For women who are fully anticoagulated, regional anesthesia is contraindicated. The anesthetic management of patients receiving minidose heparin and having normal partial thromboplastin times remains controversial. In the absence of studies to support or refute the safety of intraspinal techniques in these patients, I prefer to avoid regional anesthesia unless the probable maternal benefits greatly outweigh the risks of developing an intraspinal hematoma.

When not contraindicated, continuous lumbar epidural anesthesia is recommended for labor and vaginal delivery. The stress and catecholamine release normally associated with painful uterine contractions can be avoided. As a result, tachycardia and increases in the left and right heart afterload secondary to raised peripheral and pulmonary vascular resistances will be ablated. Patients with left ventricular compromise will also benefit from the decreases in both preload and afterload resulting from sympathectomy. As with other serious cardiac diseases, patients with significant PPCM should be followed with continuous intracardiac monitoring of left and right heart function during labor and delivery. A fall in cardiac output secondary to decreases in preload can be corrected with slow rehydration. Following delivery, on the other hand, the marked increases in preload normally experienced can be blunted by maintaining or extending the level of sympathetic blockade until diuresis corrects the intravascular volume overload. A fall in cardiac output resulting from left or right ventricular failure can be improved with the administration of the inotrope dopamine, 200 mg in 500 ml of saline, or epinephrine, 2 mg in 500 ml of saline. Oxygen should be administered during labor and in the postpartum period until the patient's cardiovascular status is stable.

Either regional or general anesthesia may be used for cesarean section. If a regional technique is chosen, I prefer the slow administration of a continuous lumbar epidural anesthetic to the administration of a spinal anesthetic which can be more difficult to control. Suggested hemodynamic monitoring and the management of complications during epidural anesthesia for cesarean section are similar to those discussed above for vaginal delivery.

For the induction of general anesthesia, ketamine, 1 mg/kg, is recommended rather than thiopental because of thiopental's negative inotropic potential. Anesthesia maintenance can be achieved with oxygen and nitrous oxide, 50%, and supplemented with narcotic (fentanyl), diazepam, and a neuromuscular blocker as tolerated. The potent inhalational agents are myocardial depressants and should be avoided in the presence of cardiac failure. Inotropic support and afterload reduction with nitroprusside may be required. Following surgery, the anesthesiologist remains a valuable consultant as the patient with PPCM progresses through the hemodynamically unstable early postpartum period.

Pulmonary Arterial Hypertension and Eisenmenger's Syndrome

For patients with primary pulmonary arterial hypertension, pregnancy represents a serious threat with a reported maternal mortality rate of over 50 percent.[123] When pulmonary arterial hypertension is associated with a right-to-left or bidirectional shunt at the aortopulmonary, atrial, or ventricular level (Eisenmenger's syndrome), maternal mortality rates of 27 to 70 percent have been observed.[97,139,154] Maternal and fetal risk and prognosis depend upon the level of pulmonary hypertension[116,215] and the pulmonary artery's reponsiveness to vasodilators. Spinnato et al.[198] have suggested that fixed pulmonary hypertension, unresponsive to oxygen therapy, may represent an absolute indication for termination of pregnancy.

In pregnant patients with Eisenmenger's syndrome, any increase in pulmonary vascular resistance secondary to hypoxia, acidosis, or catecholamine release in response to pain will result in an increase in right to left shunting and the delivery of desaturated venous blood to the systemic circulation. Decreases in preload or afterload, whether secondary to blood loss or a decrease in peripheral vascular resistance associated with sympathectomy, will decrease systemic blood pressure and consequently increase right-to-left shunting in patients with pulmonary hypertension. Regardless of the cause, shunting of desaturated blood from the pulmonary to the systemic circulation will decrease peripheral and central oxygen delivery, placing both mother and fetus at risk for hypoxia, acidosis, and death.

For labor and vaginal delivery or for cesarean section, patients with Eisenmenger's syndrome require continuous hemodynamic and acid-base evaluation. Therefore, a balloon-flotation, thermodilution pulmonary-artery catheter and a radial arterial line are both recommended. Supplemental oxygen will improve hemoglobin oxygen saturation and decrease pulmonary vascular resistance. Adequate left uterine displacement will help maintain central volume and preload. Systemic analgesics and paracervical block are acceptable modes of analgesia for first-stage labor pain. Because a decrease in peripheral vascular resistance might lead to an increase in right-to-left shunting, some authors have recommended that lumbar epidural and spinal anesthesia be used with caution or avoided completely in patients with Eisenmenger's syndrome.[6,116] However, Midwall et al.[128] noted no significant effect on shunt flow in laboring patients who received epidural anesthesia. During the second stage of labor, pudendal block supplemented with low-dose intravenous ketamine or inhalational agents will provide effective analgesia for forceps-assisted delivery without significantly decreasing preload or afterload. Blood loss should be kept at a minimum, and intravascular volume should be expanded as necessary. Because of the lack of sympathetic nervous system blockade associated with the administration of intraspinal narcotics, this technique may prove to be valuable in providing analgesia for obstetric patients who will not tolerate significant hemodynamic changes.[4] Further investigation of intraspinal narcotics for this purpose is warranted.

For cesarean section, general anesthesia with a ketamine induction will maintain peripheral vascular resistance and discourage right-to-left shunting. Oxygen and nitrous oxide, 40% or less, can be used for maintenance of anesthesia with narcotic and diazepam supplementation following delivery. A succinylcholine infusion or pancuronium is recommended for neuromuscular blockade. By monitoring intracardiac pressures, determining pulmonary and systemic vascular resistances, and measuring arterial and mixed venous oxygen saturations, hemodynamic changes can be followed and treated. If not fixed, pulmonary hypertension and shunt can be improved with high oxygen concentrations and correction of any hypercarbia and acidosis. A failing right ventricle (increasing central venous pressure) may be supported with an inotrope such as dopamine, and high concentrations of oxygen to decrease right ventricular afterload. Hypovolemia (low central venous pressure, falling blood pressure) can be corrected with fluid therapy. Patients with fixed pulmonary vascular resistance may only improve their right-to-left shunts and systemic oxygenation by maintaining high peripheral vascular resistance. Their prognosis is guarded.

As noted above, a theoretical objection to using lumbar epidural anesthesia for vaginal delivery or cesarean section in patients with Eisenmenger's syndrome exists because of the risk of decreasing peripheral vascular resistance and increasing right-to-left shunting following sympathectomy. However, Spinnato et al.[198] reported remarkable hemodynamic stability during epidural anesthesia for cesarean section in a patient with Eisenmenger's syndrome. Although cardiac output in the supine position decreased by 24 percent following epidural block, arterial pressure and oxygen saturations were well maintained. Pulmonary vascular resistance increased slightly.

It therefore appears that a carefully conducted lumbar epidural anesthetic, combined with continuous hemodynamic and serial blood gas monitoring, can be a safe and effective technique for cesarean section in patients with Eisenmenger's syndrome.

Because of their unstable hemodynamic status and high rate of mortality during the early postpartum period,[152,208] patients with Eisenmenger's syndrome will be more safely managed following delivery by admission to an intensive care unit, where invasive monitoring can be continued and treatment rapidly instituted.

Recent Myocardial Infarction

Ginz[77] has estimated the incidence of myocardial infarction during pregnancy and the puerperium to be 1 in 10,000 deliveries. The maternal and fetal mortality rates in a retrospective study of 39 cases exceeded 28 percent. Of those patients studied, 62 percent were over the age of 30. It has been suggested that the incidence of coronary artery disease in young women is increasing.[143,149] The cause(s) responsible for the increased incidence are unclear. In patients who have other risk factors, the use of oral contraceptives may be contributory.[142,143] Since a greater number of women are delaying pregnancy until their fourth decade, it is increasingly more likely that many perinatologists and anesthesiologists will become involved in the care of patients who have suffered a myocardial infarction during pregnancy.

In order to minimize the risk of myocardial ischemia and reinfarction during the peripartum period, it is essential that myocardial oxygen supply be adequate to meet myocardial oxygen demands. To maximize oxygen delivery, any anemia should be corrected. Supplemental oxygen, via face mask or nasal prongs, will improve arterial oxygen saturation and should be administered continuously during labor. Furthermore, tachycardia, which decreases coronary artery perfusion time, should be avoided. Arterial disastolic pressure is also an important factor in coronary artery perfusion. Sustained hypotension will seriously jeopardize myocardial blood flow and should be corrected if it occurs.

The major determinants of myocardial oxygen demand are heart rate, myocardial contractility, and myocardial wall tension. Peripartum events can have significant effects on each of these variables. Stress associated with painful uterine contractions and anxiety results in the release of serum catecholamines. Catecholamines, in turn, produce tachycardia, an increase in the myocardial contractile state, and a rise in myocardial wall tension secondary to increased peripheral vascular resistance. The tachycardia and increased stroke volume that are responsible for the dramatic increase in cardiac output noted immediately postpartum create serious additional demands for myocardial oxygen availability.

Postinfarct patients with angina who are already receiving nitrates to decrease wall tension and/or propranolol to decrease heart rate and myocardial contractility should have these medications continued throughout pregnancy and parturition.

While not all postinfarct patients will require invasive monitoring during labor and delivery or for cesarean section, a radial arterial line and pulmonary-artery catheter are highly recommended in those women with recent infarcts, unstable angina, or uncompensated congestive heart failure. The electrocardiogram is also useful as a monitor of myocardial ischemia. By alternate monitoring of leads V_5 and II, anterolateral and inferior wall ischemia, respectively, can be diagnosed throughout the peripartum period.

For labor and vaginal delivery, lumbar epidural anesthesia placed early during the first stage offers several advantages. By eliminating the pain and stress associated with uterine contractions, myocardial ischemia secondary to catecholamine-induced tachycardia and hypertension can be minimized. The block can be extended caudad to provide sacral-root analgesia during the second stage. This will allow an early application of forceps and avoidance of the hemodynamic effects of the Valsalva maneuver, which accompanies pushing. Sympathetic blockade produced by epidural anesthesia will cause peripheral pooling of blood in capacitance vessels (decreased preload) and blunt the hypervolemic state occurring immediately postpartum. By decreasing preload, intracardiac volume and thus myocardial wall tension will be decreased as well. However, epidural anesthesia and sympathetic blockade are not without possible hemodynamic complications. By utilizing invasive monitoring, excessive decreases in central volume following sympathectomy can be diagnosed and corrected with positioning and administration of crystalloid solutions. If sympathectomy produces a severe decrease in afterload (diastolic blood pressure less than 50 mm Hg), metaraminol or a pure alpha-agonist such as phenylephrine can be used to increase peripheral vascular resistance and restore coronary artery perfusion pressure. Following the correction of central venous volume and/or peripheral vascular resistance, the tachycardia associated with chemical sympathectomy will most often resolve. When tachycardia does not improve and is associated with myocardial ischemia, propranolol may be used to restore normal heart rate and coronary artery diastolic filling time.

It is not possible to recommend a single anesthetic technique for cesarean section which would be appropriate for all patients who have suffered a recent myocardial infarction. If regional anesthesia is chosen, I recommend continuous lumbar epidural anesthesia rather than subarachnoid anesthesia because of the poor controllability and rapid hemodynamic changes that can occur with spinal block. By using a continuous epidural anesthetic technique, the level of anesthesia can be raised slowly and cardiovascular responses to sympathectomy can be corrected gradually, as discussed in previous sections. As noted above, the ability to produce a chemical sympathectomy can also be of therapeutic value in managing the rapid hemodynamic changes during the postpartum period.

A major problem with general anesthesia in patients with coronary artery disease is the stress-related tachycardia and hypertension that occur during induction and surgery. The narcotic anesthetic techniques can blunt these hemodynamic responses and can be valuable in managing patients with coronary insufficiency.[15,199] However, unless large doses of narcotic are employed, hypertension and tachycardia will probably still occur.[224] Two disadvantages of using large doses of narcotic for induction and maintenance of anesthesia for cesarean section are increased risk of aspiration during induction and fetal exposure to maternally administered opiates. Inhalational agents, alone or in combination with smaller doses of narcotic, will minimize tachycardia and hypertension, thus decreasing myocardial oxygen consumption. For patients without evidence of myocardial failure, a thiopental induction, 4 mg/kg, followed by oxygen and nitrous oxide, 50 percent, and an inhalational agent such as halothane, 0.5 percent, for maintenance is recommended. Significant increases in heart rate (above 100 beats per minute) or blood pressure (systolic pressure greater than 150 mm Hg) occurring before or after delivery should be treated by deepening anesthesia with narcotic and/or higher concentrations of an inhalational agent. If required, sodium nitroprusside and propranolol may be used to lower peripheral vascular resistance and heart rate, respectively.

For patients with failing ventricular function, the major problems encountered during anesthesia are poor cardiac output and rising ventricular volumes and pressures, which result in both pulmonary congestion and further myocardial ischemia. The medical management of these patients requires measures which will improve myocardial contractility (inotropes) and/or decrease peripheral vascular resistance (vasodilators). In concert, they will improve cardiac output and decrease cardiomegaly and myocardial oxygen demands. Because lumbar epidural anesthesia will decrease peripheral vascular resistance while avoiding myocardial depression, it may be considered the preferred technique for cesarean section in patients with congestive heart failure.

When regional anesthesia is contraindicated or refused for cesarean section in patients with congestive heart failure, general anesthesia may be used. The potent inhalational agents are myocardial depressants and should be avoided in the presence of ventricular dysfunction. Large-dose narcotic techniques are alleged to preserve myocardial function.[14,15] While a narcotic induction may increase the risk of maternal aspiration and fetal opiate depression, its probable benefits in avoiding myocardial decompensation in these critically ill patients outweigh possible maternal and fetal risks. Transfer to an intensive care unit following surgery will be necessary to maintain controlled ventilation and continue hemodynamic monitoring during the volatile postpartum period. If preload becomes excessive following delivery, it can be corrected with diuretics and/or venodilators.

REFERENCES

1. Abboud, T.K., Williams, V., Miller, F. et al.: Comparative fetal, maternal, and neonatal responses following epidural analgesia with bupivacaine, chloroprocaine, and lidocaine. Anesthesiology, 55:A315, 1981.
2. Abou-Madi, M.N., Keszler, H., and Yacoub, J.M.: Cardiovascular reactions to laryngoscopy and tracheal intubation following small and large intravenous doses of lidocaine. Can. Anaesth. Soc. J., 24:12, 1977.
3. Adams, J.Q.: Cardiovascular physiology in normal pregnancy: Studies with the dye dilution technique. Am. J. Obstet. Gynecol., 67:741, 1954.
4. Ahmad, S., Hawes, D., Dooley, S. et al.: Intrathecal morphine in a parturient with a single ventricle. Anesthesiology, 54:515, 1981.
5. Akamatsu, T.J., Bonica, J.J., Rehmet, R. et al.: Experiences with the use of ketamine for parturition: 1. Primary anesthesia for vaginal delivery. Anesth. Analg. (Cleve), 53:284, 1974.
6. Albright, G.A.: Anesthesia in obstetrics. Maternal, fetal, and neonatal aspects. Addison-Wesley Publishing Co., Reading, Mass., 1978.
7. Aldrete, J.A., Barnes, D.R., and Aikawa, J.K.: Does magnesium produce anesthesia? Evaluation of its effects on the cardiovascular and neurologic systems. Anesth. Analg. (Cleve), 47:428, 1968.

8. Althabe, O., Jr., Schwarcz, R.L., Pose, S.V. et al.: Effects on fetal heart rate and fetal pO_2 of oxygen administration to the mother. Am. J. Obstet. Gynecol., *98:*858, 1967.
9. Archer, G.W. and Marx, G.F.: Arterial oxygen tension during apnoea in parturient women. Br. J. Anaesth., *46:*358, 1974.
10. Asling, J.H., Shnider, S.M., Margolis, A.J. et al.: Paracervical block anesthesia in obstetrics. II. Etiology of fetal bradycardia following paracervical block anesthesia. Am. J. Obstet. Gynecol., *107:*626, 1970.
11. Assali, N.S., Holm, L.W., and Parker, H.R.: Systemic and regional hemodynamic alterations in toxemia. Circulation, suppl. II, *29,30:*11, 1964.
12. Attia, R.R., Ebeid, A.M., and Fischer, J.E.: Gastrin: Placental, maternal and plasma cord levels, its possible role in maternal residual gastric acidity. p. 547. In: Abstracts of Scientific Papers, Annual Meeting, American Society of Anesthesiologists, San Francisco, 1976.
13. Baird, D.T., Gasson, P.W., and Doig, A.: The renogram in pregnancy. Am. J. Obstet. Gynecol., *95:*597, 1966.
14. Barash, P.G. and Kopriva, C.J.: Narcotics and the circulation. p. 91. In Kitahata, L.M. and Collins, J.G., Eds.: narcotic Analgesics in Anesthesiology. Williams & Wilkins, Baltimore, 1982.
15. Barash, P., Kopriva, C., Giles, R. et al.: Global ventricular function and intubation: radionuclear profiles. Anesthesiology, *53:*S109, 1980.
16. Beard, R.W., Knight, C.A., and Roberts, G.M.: The significance of the changes in the continuous fetal heart rate in the first stage of labour. J. Obstet. Gynaecol. Br. Commonw., *78:*865, 1971.
17. Beazley, J.M., Taylor, G., and Reynolds, F.: Placental transfer of bupivacaine after paracervical block. Obstet. Gynecol., *39:*2, 1972.
18. Beck, D.W. and Menezes, A.H.: Intracerebral hemorrhage in a patient with eclampsia. JAMA, *246:*1442, 1981.
19. Belfrage, P., Berlin, A., Lindstedt, M. et al.: Plasma levels of bupivacaine following pudendal block in labour. Br. J. Anaesth., *45:*1067, 1973.
20. Benedetti, T.J., Cotton, D.B., Read, J.G. et al.: Hemodynamic observations in severe pre-eclampsia with a flow-directed pulmonary artery catheter. Am. J. Obstet. Gynecol., *136:*465, 1980.
21. Biehl, D.R.: Antepartum and postpartum hemorrhage. p. 243. In: Shnider, S.M. and Levinson, G., Eds.: Anesthesia for Obstetrics. Williams & Wilkins Co., Baltimore, 1979.
22. Biehl, D., Shnider, S.M., Levinson, G. et al.: Placental transfer of lidocaine: effects of fetal acidosis. Anesthesiology, *48:*409, 1978.
23. Bieniarz, J., Crottogini, J.J., Curuchet, E., et al.: Aortocaval compression by the uterus in late human pregnancy. II. An arteriographic study. Am. J. Obstet. Gynecol., *100:*203, 1968.
24. Birmingham Eclampsia Study Group: Intravascular coagulation and abnormal lung scans in pre-eclampsia and eclampsia. Lancet, *2:*889, 1971.
25. Blair, R.G.: Abruption of the placenta. A review of 189 cases occurring between 1965 and 1969. J. Obstet. Gynaecol. Br. Commonw. *80:*242, 1973.
26. Blitt, C.D., Petty, W.C., and Alberternst, E.E.: Correlation of plasma cholinesterase activity and duration of action of succinylcholine during pregnancy. Anesth. Analg. (Cleve) *56:*78, 1977.
27. Boehm, F.H. and Growdon, J.H.: The effect of eclamptic convulsions on the fetal heart rate. Am. J. Obstet. Gynecol., *120:*851, 1974.
28. Bonica, J.J.: Obstetric Analgesia and Anesthesia. World Federation of Societies of Anaesthesiologists, Amsterdam, 1980.
29. Bonnar, J., Menicol, G.P., and Douglas, A.S.: Coagulation and fibrinolytic systems in pre-eclampsia and eclampsia. Br. Med. J., *2:*12, 1971.

30. Brice, J.E.H., Moreland, T.A., and Walker, C.H.M.: Effects of pethidine and its antagonists on the newborn. Arch. Dis. Child., *54:*356, 1979.
31. Brinkman, C.R. III and Assali, N.S.: Uteroplacental hemodynamic response to antihypertensive drugs in hypertensive pregnant sheep. p. 363. In Lindheimer, M.D., Katz, A.I., and Zuspan, F.P., Eds.: Hypertension in Pregnancy. John Wiley & Sons, New York, 1976.
32. Bromage, P.R.: Choice of local anesthetics in obstetrics. p. 109. In Shnider, S.M. and Levinson, G., Eds.: Anesthesia for Obstetrics. Williams & Wilkins, Baltimore, 1979.
33. Brooks, G.Z. and Ngeow, Y.F.: Narcotics, mother, fetus, and neonate. p. 157. In Kitahata, L.M. and Collins, J.G., Eds.: Narcotic Analgesics in Anesthesiology. Williams & Wilkins, Baltimore, 1982.
34. Brown, W.U., Bell, G.C., and Alper, M.H.: Acidosis, local anesthetics and the newborn. Obstet. Gynecol., *48:*27, 1976.
35. Browne, J.C.M. and Veall, N.: The maternal placental blood flow in normotensive and hypertensive women. J. Obstet. Gynaecol. Br. Commonw., *60:*141, 1953.
36. Burgess, G.E. III: Antacids for obstetric patients. Am. J. Obstet. Gynecol., *123:*577, 1975.
37. Carrico, C.J., Canizaro, P.C., and Shires, T.S.: Fluid resuscitation following injury. Rationale for the use of balanced salt solutions. Crit. Care Med., *4:*46, 1976.
38. Chesley, L.C.: Plasma and red cell volumes during pregnancy. Am. J. Obstet. Gynecol., *112:*440, 1972.
39. Chesley, L.C. and Sloan, D.M.: The effect of posture on renal function in late pregnancy. Am. J. Obstet. Gynecol., *89:*754, 1964.
40. Clark, R.B., Beard, A.G., Thompson, D.S. et al.: Maternal and neonatal plasma inorganic fluoride levels after methoxyflurane analgesia for labor and delivery. Anesthesiology, *45:*88, 1976.
41. Corke, B.C.: Neurobehavioural responses of the newborn. The effect of different forms of maternal analgesia. Anaesthesia, *32:*539, 1977.
42. Cousins, M.J., Greenstein, L.R., Hitt, B.A. et al.: Metabolism and renal effects of enflurane in man. Anesthesiology, *44:*44, 1976.
43. Craft, J.B., Jr., Co., E.G., Yonekura, M.L. et al.: Nitroglycerin therapy for phenylephrine-induced hypertension in pregnant ewes. Anesth. Analg. (Cleve), *59:*494, 1980.
44. Crawford, J.S., Burton, M., and Davies, P.: Time and lateral tilt at caesarean section. Br. J. Anaesth., *44:*477, 1972.
45. Cree, J.E., Meyer, J., and Hailey, D.M.: Diazepam in labour: its metabolism and effect on the clinical condition and thermogenesis of the newborn. Br. Med. J., *4:*251, 1973.
46. Curtis, J., Shnider, S.M., Saito, C. et al.: The effects of painful uterine contraction, position, and epidural anesthesia on maternal transcutaneous oxygen tension. Anesthesiology, *53:*S315, 1980.
47. Datta, S. and Alper, M.H.: Anesthesia for cesarean section. Anesthesiology, *53:*142, 1980.
48. Datta, S., Corke, B.C., Alper, M.H. et al.: Epidural anesthesia for cesarean section: A comparison of bupivacaine, chloroprocaine and etidocaine. Anesthesiology, *52:*48, 1980.
49. Datta, S., Ostheimer, G.W., Naulty, J.S. et al.: General anesthesia for cesarean section: effects of halothane on maternal and fetal acid-base and lactic acid concentration. Anesthesiology, *55:*A309, 1981.
50. Demakis, J.G. and Rahimtoola, S.H.: Peripartum cardiomyopathy. Circulation, *44:*964, 1971.
51. deRosayro, M., Nahnwold, M.L., Hill, A.B. et al.: Plasma levels and cardiovascular effects of nitroglycerin in pregnant sheep. Can. Anaesth. Soc. J., *27:*560, 1980.
52. DeSilva, J.A.F., D'Arconte, L., and Kaplan, J.: The determination of blood levels and the placental transfer of diazepam in humans. Curr. Ther. Res., *6:*115, 1964.
53. Detmer, M.D., Pandit, S.K., and Cohen, P.J.: Prophylactic single-dose oral antacid therapy in the preoperative period—comparison of cimetidine and Maalox. Anesthesiology, *51:*270, 1979.

54. DeWolf, F., Robertson, W.B., and Brosens, T.: The ultrastructure of acute atherosis in hypertensive pregnancy. Am. J. Obstet. Gynecol., *123*:164, 1975.
55. Dignam, W.J., Titus, P., and Assali, N.S.: Renal function in human pregnancy. I. Changes in glomerular filtration rate and renal plasma flow. Soc. Exp. Biol. Med., *97*:512, 1958.
56. Dobb, G., Jordan, M.J., and Williams, J.G.: Cimetidine in the prevention of the pulmonary acid aspiration (Mendelson's) syndrome. Br. J. Anaesth., *51*:967, 1979.
57. Duvaldestin, P., Agoston, S., Henzel, D. et al.: Pancuronium pharmacokinetics in patients with liver cirrhosis. Br. J. Anaesth., *50*:1131, 1978.
58. Eckstein, K. and Marx, G.F.: Aortocaval compression and uterine displacement. Anesthesiology, *40*:92, 1974.
59. Eknoyan, G., Wacksman, S.J., Glueck, H.I. et al.: Platelet function in renal failure. N. Engl. J. Med., *280*:677, 1969.
60. Ellis, S.C., Wheeler, A.S., James, F.M. III et al.: Sodium nitroprusside for hypertension in gravid ewes. Anesthesiology, *55*:A302, 1981.
61. Evans, R.T. and Wroe, J.M.: Plasma cholinesterase changes during pregnancy. Their interpretation as a cause of suxamethonium-induced apnoea. Anaesthesia, *35*:651, 1980.
62. Flowers, C.E., Rudolph, A.J., and Desmond, M.M.: Diazepam (Valium) as an adjunct in obstetric analgesia. Obstet. Gynecol., *34*:68, 1969.
63. Foldes, F.F.: Factors which alter the effects of muscle relaxants. Anesthesiology, *20*:464, 1959.
64. Foldes, F.F., Swerdlow, M., Lipschitz, E. et al.: Comparison of the respiratory effects of suxamethonium and suxethonium in man. Anesthesiology, *17*:559, 1956.
65. Foulkes, E. and Jenkins, L.C.: A comparative evaluation of cimetidine and sodium citrate to decrease gastric acidity: effectiveness at the time of induction of anaesthesia. Can. Anaesth. Soc. J., *28*:29, 1981.
66. Galbert, M.W. and Gardner, A.E.: Ketamine for obstetrical anesthesia. Anesth. Analg. (Cleve), *52*:926, 1973.
67. Galloon, S.: Ketamine for obstetric delivery. Anesthesiology, *44*:522, 1976.
68. Gant, N.F., Hutchinson, H.T., Siiteri, P.K. et al.: Study of the metabolic clearance rate of dehydroisoandrosterone sulfate in pregnancy. Am. J. Obstet. Gynecol., *111*:555, 1971.
69. Gare, D.J., Shime, J., Paul, W.M. et al.: Oxygen administration during labor. Am. J. Obstet. Gynecol., *105*:954, 1969.
70. Gauer, O.H., Henry, J.P., and Sieker, H.O.: Changes in central venous pressure after moderate hemorrhage and transfusion in man. Circ. Res., *4*:79, 1956.
71. Gazioglu, K., Kaltreider, N.L., Rosen, M. et al.: Pulmonary function during pregnancy in normal women and in patients with cardiopulmonary disease. Thorax, *25*:445, 1970.
72. Ghoneim, M.M. and Long, J.P.: The interaction between magnesium and other neuromuscular blocking agents. Anesthesiology, *32*:23, 1970.
73. Ghoneim, M.M. and Pandya, H.: Plasma protein binding of thiopental in patients with impaired renal or hepatic function. Anesthesiology, *42*:545, 1975.
74. Gibbs, C.P., Schwartz, D.J., Wynne, J.W. et al.: Antacid pulmonary aspiration. p. 26. In Abstracts of Scientific Papers, Annual Meeting, Society for Obstetric Anesthesia and Perinatology, Memphis, 1978.
75. Giesecke, A.H., Morris, R.E., Dalton, M.D. et al.: Of magnesium, muscle relaxants, toxemic parturients, and cats. Anesth. Analg. (Cleve), *47*:689, 1968.
76. Gintautas, J. and Kraynack, B.: Action of local anesthetics on human uterine arteries. Anesthesiology, *55*:A324, 1981.
77. Ginz, B.: Myocardial infarction in pregnancy. J. Obstet. Gynaecol. Br. Commonw., *77*:610, 1970.
78. Goodlin, R.C.: Importance of the lateral position during labor. Obstet. Gynecol., *37*:698, 1971.

79. Goodlin, R.C.: Inappropriate fetal bradycardia. Obstet. Gynecol., *48*:117, 1976.
80. Graham, C. and Goldstein, A.: Epidural analgesia and cardiac output in severe pre-eclamptics. Anaesthesia, 35:709, 1980.
81. Greenblatt, D.J. and Koch-Weser, J.: Clinical toxicity of chlordiazepoxide and diazepam in relationship to serum albumin concentration: A report from the Boston Collaborative Drug Surveillance Program. Eur. J. Clin. Pharmacol., *7*:259, 1974.
82. Gutsche, B.B.: Anesthetic considerations for pre-eclampsia–eclampsia. p. 224. In: Shnider, S.M. and Levinson, G.: Anesthesia for Obstetrics. Williams & Wilkins, Baltimore, 1979.
83. Gutsche, B.B.: Maternal physiologic alterations during pregnancy. p. 3. In: Shnider, S.M., Levinson, G.: Anesthesia for Obstetrics. Williams & Wilkins, Baltimore, 1979.
84. Hodgkinson, R., Bhatt, M., Grewal, G. et al.: Neonatal neurobehavior in the first 48 hours of life: effect of the administration of meperidine with and without naloxone in the mother. Pediatrics, *62*:294, 1978.
85. Hodgkinson, R., Husain, F.J., and Hayashi, R.H.: Systemic and pulmonary blood pressure during caesarean section in parturients with gestational hypertension. Can. Anaesth. Soc. J. *27*:389, 1980.
86. Hodgkinson, R., Marx, G.F., Kim, S.S. et al.: Neonatal neurobehavioral tests following vaginal delivery under ketamine, thiopental, and extradural anesthesia. Anesth. Analg. (Cleve), *56*:548, 1977.
87. Holly, R.G.: Anemia in pregnancy. Obstet. Gynecol., *5*:562, 1955.
88. Howard, B.K., Goodson, J.H., and Mengert, W.F.: Supine hypotensive syndrome in late pregnancy. Obstet. Gynecol., *1*:371, 1953.
89. Hug, C.C., Murphy, M.R., Sampson, J.F. et al.: Biotransformation of morphine and fentanyl in anhepatic dogs. Anesthesiology, *55*:A261, 1981.
90. Hughes, R.A.C., Kapur, P., Sutton, G.C. et al.: A case of fatal peripartum cardiomyopathy. Br. Heart J. *32*:272, 1970.
91. Hytten, F.E. and Paintin, D.B.: Increase in plasma volume during normal pregnancy. J. Obstet. Gynecol. Br. Commonw., *70*:402, 1963.
92. Ivankovich, A.D., Sheth, D.J., Shulman, M. et al.: Autoregulation of cerebral blood flow during infusion of trimethaphan or nitroglycerin in the goat. p. 77. In: Abstracts of Scientific Papers, Annual Meeting, American Society of Anesthesiologists, Chicago, 1978.
93. James, F.M. III and Davies, P.: Maternal and fetal effects of lumbar epidural analgesia for labor and delivery in patients with gestational hypertension. Am. J. Obstet. Gynecol., *126*:195, 1976.
94. James, F.M. III, Greiss, F.C., Jr., and Kemp, R.A.: An evaluation of vasopressor therapy for maternal hypotension during spinal anesthesia. Anesthesiology, *33*:25, 1970.
95. Janeczko, G.F., El-Etr, A.A., and Younes, S.: Low-dose ketamine anesthesia for obstetrical delivery. Anesth. Analg. (Cleve), *53*:828, 1974.
96. Johnson, J.B., Mir, G.H., Flores, P. et al.: Idiopathic heart disease associated with pregnancy and the puerperium. Am. Heart J., *72*:809, 1966.
97. Jones, A.M. and Howitt, G.: Eisenmenger syndrome in pregnancy. Br. Med. J., *1*:627, 1965.
98. Jouppila, R. and Hollmen, A.: The effect of segmental epidural analgesia on maternal and foetal acid-base balance, lactate, serum potassium and creatine phosphokinase during labor. Acta Anaesthesiol. Scand. *20*:259, 1976.
99. Jouppila, R., Jouppila, P., Hollmen, A. et al.: Epidural analgesia and placental blood flow during labor in pregnancies complicated by hypertension. Br. J. Obstet. Gynaecol., *86*:969, 1979.
100. Joyce, T.H. III, Debnath, K.S., and Baker, E.A.: Pre-eclampsia—relationship of CVP and epidural analgesia. Anesthesiology *51*:S297, 1979.

101. Joyce, T.H. III and Loon, M.: Pre-eclampsia: Effect of albumin 25% infusion. Anesthesiology, *55:*A313, 1981.
102. Kauppila, A., Koskinen, M., Puolokka, J. et al.: Decreased intervillous and unchanged myometrial blood flow in supine recumbency. Obstet. Gynecol., *55:*203, 1980.
103. Kelman, G.R., Nunn, J.F., Prys-Roberts, C. et al.: The influence of cardiac output on arterial oxygenation: A theoretical study. Br. J. Anaesth., *39:*450, 1967.
104. Kerr, M.G., Scott, D.B., and Samuel, E.: Studies of the inferior vena cava in late pregnancy. Br. Med. J., *1:*532, 1964.
105. Kitzmiller, J.L. and Benirschke, K.: Immunofluorescent study of placental bed vessels in pre-eclampsia of pregnancy. Am. J. Obstet. Gynecol., *115:*248, 1973.
106. Klotz, U., Avant, G.R., Hoyumpa, A. et al.: The effects of age and liver disease on the disposition and elimination of diazepam in adult man. J. Clin. Invest., *55:*347, 1975.
107. Kobayashi, H., Matsumoto, Y., Otsubo, O. et al.: Successful pregnancy in a patient undergoing chronic hemodynamics. Obstet. Gynecol., *57:*382, 1981.
108. Kubli, F.W., Hon, E.H., Khazin, A.F. et al.: Observations on heart rate and pH in the human fetus during labor. Am. J. Obstet. Gynecol., *104:*1190, 1969.
109. Kuhnert, B.R., Kuhnert, P.M., Prochaska, A.L. et al.: Plasma levels of 2-chloroprocaine in obstetric patients and their neonates after epidural anesthesia. Anesthesiology, *53:*21, 1980.
110. Lahiri, S.K., Thomas, T.A., and Hodgson, R.M.H.: Single-dose antacid therapy for prevention of Mendelson's syndrome. Br. J. Anaesth., *45:*1143, 1973.
111. Lederman, R.P., Lederman, E., Work, B.A. et al.: The relationship of maternal anxiety, plasma catecholamines, and plasma cortisol to progress in labor. Am. J. Obstet. Gynecol., *132:*495, 1978.
112. Lees, M.M., Scott, D.B., Kerr, M.G. et al.: The circulatory effects of recumbent postural change in late pregnancy. Clin. Sci. Mol. Med., *32:*453, 1967.
113. Levinson, G., Shnider, S.M., and Gildea, J.E.: Maternal and foetal cardiovascular and acid-base changes during ketamine anesthesia in pregnant ewes. Br. J. Anaesth., *45:*1111, 1973.
114. Lipsitz, P.J.: The clinical and biochemical effects of excess magnesium in the newborn. Pediatrics, *47:*501, 1971.
115. Little, B., Chang, T., and Chucot, L.: Study of ketamine as an obstetric anesthetic agent. Am. J. Obstet. Gynecol., *113:*247, 1972.
116. Mangano, D.T.: Anesthesia for the pregnant cardiac patient. p. 180. In Shnider, S.M. and Levinson, G., Eds.: Anesthesia for Obstetrics. Williams & Wilkins, Baltimore, 1979.
117. Marx, G.F. and Green, N.M.: Maternal lactate, pyruvate and excess lactate production during labor and delivery. Am. J. Obstet. Gynecol., *90:*786, 1964.
118. Marx, G.F., Husain, F.S., and Shiav, H.F.: Brachial and femoral blood pressures during the prenatal period. Am. J. Obstet. Gynecol., *136:*11, 1980.
119. Marx, G.F., Hwang, H.S., and Chandra, P.: Postpartum uterine pressures with different doses of ketamine. p. 301. In: Abstracts of Scientific Papers, Annual Meeting, American Society of Anesthesiologists, New Orleans, 1977.
120. Marx, G.F. and Mateo, C.V.: The effects of different oxygen concentrations during general anesthesia for elective caesarean section. Can. Anaesth. Soc. J., *18:*587, 1971.
121. Marx, G.F., Smith, B.E., and Greene, N.M.: Umbilical vein blood biochemical data and neonatal condition. Pediatrics *66:*989, 1965.
122. Marx, G.F. and Wang, C.N.: Anesthetic considerations in hypertensive disorders of pregnancy. Curr. Probl. Anesth. Crit. Care Med., *1*(8):1, 1978.
123. McCaffrey, R.M. and Dunn, L.J.: Primary pulmonary hypertension in pregnancy. Obstet. Gynecol. Surv., *19:*567, 1964.
124. McCall, M.L.: Cerebral circulation and metabolism in toxemia of pregnancy. Observa-

tions on the effects of veratrum viride and apresoline (1-hydrazinophthalazine). Am. J. Obstet. Gynecol., *66:*1015, 1953.

125. McCarthy, G.T., O'Connell, B., and Robinson, A.E.: Blood levels of diazepam in infants of two mothers given large doses of diazepam during labour. J. Obstet. Gynaecol. Br. Commonw., *80:*349, 1973.
126. McLain, G.E., Sipes, I.G., and Brown, B.R.: An animal model of halothane hepatotoxicity: roles of enzyme induction and hypoxia. Anesthesiology, *51:*321, 1979.
127. McLennan, C.E. and Thovin, L.G.: Blood volume in pregnancy. Am. J. Obstet. Gynecol., *55:*189, 1948.
128. Midwall, J., Jaffin, H., Herman, M.V. et al.: Shunt flow and pulmonary hemodynamics during labor and delivery in the Eisenmenger syndrome. Am. J. Cardiol., *42:*299, 1978.
129. Miller, R.D. and Way, W.L.: The effect of alpha-methyldopa on the alveolar concentration of halothane required for anesthesia. Anesthesiology, *29:*204, 1968.
130. Miller, R.D., Way, W.L., Hamilton, W.K. et al.: Succinylcholine-induced hyperkalemia in patients with renal failure? Anesthesiology, *36:*138, 1972.
131. Moir, D.D. and Carty, M.J.: Obstetrical Anesthesia and Analgesia. Baillière Tindall, London, 1977.
132. Moya, F.: Considerations in maternal and placental physiology. Anesth. Analg. (Cleve), *42:*661, 1963.
133. Muller, G., Philippe, E., Lefakis, P. et al.: Les lesions placentaires de la gestose: étude anatomo-clinique. Gynecol. Obstet. (Paris) *70:*309, 1971.
134. Munson, E.S. and Embro, W.J.: Enflurane, isoflurane, and halothane and isolated human uterine muscle. Anesthesiology, *46:*11, 1977.
135. Murphy, P.J., Wright, J.D., and Fitzgerald, T.B.: Assessment of paracervical nerve block anaesthesia during labour. Br. Med. J., *1:*526, 1970.
136. Myers, R.E.: Maternal physiological stress and fetal asphyxia: a study in the monkey. Am. J. Obstet. Gynecol., *122:*47, 1975.
137. Nadji, P. and Sommers, S.C.: Lesions of toxemia in first trimester pregnancies. Am. J. Clin. Pathol., *59:*344, 1973.
138. Naulty, J., Cefalo, R.C., and Lewis, P.E.: Fetal toxicity of nitroprusside in the pregnant ewe. Am. J. Obstet. Gynecol., *139:*708, 1981.
139. Neilson, G., Galea, E.G., and Blunt, A.: Eisenmenger's syndrome and pregnancy. Med. J. Aust., *1:*431, 1971.
140. O'Brien, J.E., Abbey, V., Hinsvark, O. et al.: Metabolism and measurement of 2-chloroprocaine, an ester-type anesthetic. J. Pharm. Sci., *68:*75, 1979.
141. O'Driscoll, K. and McCarthy, J.R.: Abruptio placentae and central venous pressures. J. Obstet. Gynaecol. Br. Commonw., *73:*923, 1966.
142. Oliver, M.F.: Oral contraceptives and myocardial infarction. Br. Med. J., *1:*210, 1970.
143. Oliver, M.F.: Ischaemic heart disease in young women. Br. Med. J., *2:*253, 1974.
144. Ostheimer, G.W.: Neurobehavioral effects of local anesthesia and fetal resuscitation. Reg. Anesth., *6:*136, 1981.
145. Ostheimer, G.W. and Alper, M.H.: Intrapartum anesthetic management of the pregnant patient with heart disease. Clin. Obstet. Gynecol., *18:*81, 1975.
146. Owen, J.R., Irani, S.F., and Blair, A.W.: Effect of diazepam administered to mothers during labour on temperature regulation of neonate. Arch. Dis. Child., *47:*107, 1972.
147. Page, E.W.: On the pathogenesis of pre-eclampsia and eclampsia. J. Obstet. Gynaecol. Br. Commonw., *79:*883, 1972.
148. Palahniuk, R.J., Shnider, S.M., and Eger, E.I. II: Pregnancy decreases the requirement for inhaled anesthetic agents. Anesthesiology, *41:*82, 1974.
149. Parrish, H.M., Carr, C.A., Silberg, S.L. et al.: Increasing autopsy incidence of coronary heart disease in women. Arch. Intern. Med., *118:*436, 1966.

150. Paul, R.H., Sudan, A.K., Yeh, S. et al.: Clinical fetal monitoring. VII. The evaluation and significance of intrapartum baseline FHR variability. Am. J. Obstet. Gynecol., *123:*206, 1975.
151. Pearson, J.F. and Davies, P.: The effect of continuous lumbar epidural analgesia on maternal acid-base balance and arterial lactate concentration during the second stage of labour. J. Obstet. Gynaecol. Br. Commonw., *80:*225, 1973.
152. Petrie, R.H., Paul, W.L., and Miller, F.C.: Placental transfer of lidocaine following paracervical block. Am. J. Obstet. Gynecol., *120:*791, 1974.
153. Pickering, B.G., Palahniuk, R.J., and Cumming, M.: Cimetidine premedication in elective caesarean section. Can. Anaesth. Soc. J., *27:*33, 1980.
154. Pitts, J.A., Crosby, W.M., and Basta, L.L.: Eisenmenger's syndrome in pregnancy. Does heparin prophylaxis improve the maternal mortality rate? Am. Heart J., *93:*321, 1977.
155. Pollak, V.E. and Nettles, J.B.: The kidney in toxemia of pregnancy: A clinical and pathologic study based on renal biopsies. Medicine (Baltimore), *39:*469, 1960.
156. Powell, J.N.: Suxamethonium-induced hyperkalemia in a uraemic patient. Br. J. Anaesth., *42:*806, 1970.
157. Pritchard, J.A.: Changes in the blood volume during pregnancy and delivery. Anesthesiology, *26:*393, 1965.
158. Pritchard, J.A.: Haematological problems associated with delivery, placental abruption, retained dead fetus and amniotic fluid embolism. Clin. Haematol. *2:*563, 1973.
159. Pritchard, J.A., Baldwin, R.M., Dickey, J.C. et al.: Blood volume changes in pregnancy and the puerperium. II. Red blood cell loss and changes in apparent blood volume during and following vaginal delivery, cesarean section, and cesarean section plus total hysterectomy. Am. J. Obstet. Gynecol., *84:*1271, 1962.
160. Pritchard, J.A., Cunningham, F.G., and Mason, R.A.: Coagulation changes in eclampsia: their frequency and pathogenesis. Am. J. Obstet. Gynecol., *124:*855, 1976.
161. Pritchard, J.A. and Pritchard, S.A.: Standardized treatment of 154 consecutive cases of eclampsia. Am. J. Obstet. Gynecol. *123:*543, 1975.
162. Prys-Roberts, C., Greene, L.T., Meloche, R. et al.: Studies of anaesthesia in relation to hypertension. II. Haemodynamic consequences of induction and endotracheal intubation. Br. J. Anaesth. *43:*531, 1971.
163. Pyörälä, T.A.: Cardiovascular response to the upright position during pregnancy. Acta Obstet. Gynecol. Scand., *45:*suppl. 5, 1–117, 1976.
164. Rafferty, T.D. and Berkowitz, R.L.: Hemodynamics in patients with severe toxemia during labor and delivery. Am. J. Obstet. Gynecol., *138:*263, 1980.
165. Rafferty, T.D. and Berkowitz, R.L., Brooks, G.Z.: A prospective analysis of prophylactic pulmonary artery (PA) catheterization for labor and delivery of cardiac parturients—New York Heart Association (NYHA) Class I versus Class III. p. 76. In Abstracts of Scientific Papers, Annual Meeting, Society for Obstetric Anesthesia and Perinatology, Boston, 1980.
166. Ralston, D.H. and Shnider, S.M.: The fetal and neonatal effects of regional anesthesia in obstetrics. Anesthesiology, *48:*34, 1978.
167. Ramanathan, S., Gandhi, S., Arismendy, J. et al.: Oxygen transfer from mother to fetus during cesarean section under epidural anesthesia. Anesth. Analg. (Cleve), *61:*596, 1982.
168. Ring, G., Krames, E., Shnider, S.M. et al.: Comparison of nitroprusside and hydralazine in hypertensive pregnant ewes. Obstet. Gynecol., *50:*598, 1977.
169. Roberts, R.B. and Shirley, M.A.: Reducing the risk of acid aspiration during cesarean section. Anesth. Analg. (Cleve), *53:*859, 1974.
170. Roberts, R.B. and Shirley, M.A.: The obstetrician's role in reducing the risk of aspiration pneumonitis with particular reference ot the use of oral antacids. Am. J. Obstet. Gynecol., *124:*611, 1976.

171. Robertson, A., Fothergill, R.J., Hall, R.A. et al.: Effects of anaesthesia with a high oxygen concentration on the acid-base state of babies delivered at elective caesarean section. S. Afr. Med. J., *48*:2309, 1974.
172. Rogers, M.C., Hamburger, C., Owen, K. et al.: Intracranial pressure in the cat during nitroglycerin-induced hypotension. Anesthesiology, *51*:227, 1979.
173. Rolbin, S.H., Cole, A.F.D., and Hew, E.M.: Haemodynamic monitoring in the management of severe pre-eclampsia and eclampsia. Can. Anaesth. Soc. J., *28*:363, 1981.
174. Rolbin, S.H., Wright, R.G., Shnider, S.M. et al.: Diazepam during cesarean section: Effects of neonatal Apgar scores, acid-base status, neurobehavioral assessment and maternal and fetal plasma norepinephrine levels. p. 449. Abstracts of Scientific Papers, Annual Meeting, American Society of Anesthesiologists, New Orleans, 1977.
175. Romney, S.L., Gabel, P.V., and Takeda, Y.: Experimental hemorrhage in late pregnancy. Effects on maternal and fetal hemodynamics. Am. J. Obstet. Gynecol., *87*:636, 1963.
176. Roth, F. and Wüthrich, H.: The clinical importance of hyperkalemia following suxamethonium administration. Br. J. Anaesth., *41*:311, 1969.
177. Rovinsky, J.J. and Jaffin, H.: Cardiovascular hemodynamics in pregnancy. I. Blood and plasma volumes in multiple pregnancy. Am. J. Obstet. Gynecol., *93*:1, 1965.
178. Russell, I.F. and Chambers, W.A.: Closing volume in normal pregnancy. Br. J. Anaesth., *53*:1043, 1981.
179. Sangoul, F., Fox, G.S., and Houle, G.L.: Effect of regional analgesia on maternal oxygen consumption during the first stage of labor. Am. J. Obstet. Gynecol., *121*:1080, 1975.
180. Sarles, H.E., Hill, S.S., LeBlanc, A.L. et al.: Sodium excretion patterns during and following intravenous sodium chloride loads in normal and hypertensive pregnancies. Am. J. Obstet. Gynecol., *102*:1, 1968.
181. Scher, J., Hailey, D.M., and Beard, R.W.: The effects of diazepam on the fetus. J. Obstet. Gynaecol. Br. Commonw., *79*:635, 1972.
182. Schulte, F.J., Schrempf, G., and Hinze, G.: Maternal toxemia, fetal malnutrition, and motor behavior of the newborn. Pediatrics, *48*:871, 1971.
183. Scott, D.B. and Kerr, M.G.: Inferior vena caval pressure in late pregnancy. J. Obstet. Gynaecol. Br. Commonw., *70*:1044, 1964.
184. Sellick, B.A.: Cricoid pressure to control regurgitation of stomach contents during induction of anesthesia. Lancet, *2*:404, 1961.
185. Shideman, F.E., Kelly, A.R., Lee, L.E. et al.: The role of the liver in the detoxification of thiopental (Pentothal) by man. Anesthesiology, *10*:421, 1949.
186. Shnider, S.M.: Serum cholinesterase activity during pregnancy, labor and the puerperium. Anesthesiology, *26*:335, 1965.
187. Shnider, S.M., Abboud, T., Artal, R. et al.: Maternal endogenous catecholamines decrease during labor after lumbar epidural anesthesia. Anesthesiology, *53*:S299, 1980.
188. Shnider, S.M., Abboud, T., Levinson, G. et al.: General anesthesia for cesarean section: Maternal and fetal norepinephrine levels and neonatal neurobehavioral status. Anesthesiology, *53*:S302, 1980.
189. Shnider, S.M. and Moya, F.: Effects of meperidine on the newborn infant. Am. J. Obstet. Gynecol., *89*:1009, 1964.
190. Shnider, S. M., Wright, R. G., and Levinson, G.: Uterine blood flow and plasma norepinephrine changes during maternal stress in the pregnant ewe. Anesthesiology, *50*:524, 1979.
191. Sims, E.A.H. and Krantz, K.E.: Serial studies of renal function during pregnancy and the puerperium in normal women. J. Clin. Invest., *37*:1764, 1958.
192. Skillman, J.J., Restall, D.S., and Salzman, E.W.: Randomized trial of albumin vs. electrolyte solutions during abdominal aortic operations. Surgery, *78*:291, 1975.
193. Smith, P.K., Winkler, A.W., and Hoff, H.E.: Electrocardiographic changes and concen-

tration of magnesium in serum following intravenous injection of magnesium salts. Am. J. Physiol., *126:*720, 1939.

194. Snyder, S.W., Wheeler, A.S., and James, F.M. III: The use of nitroglycerin to control severe hypertension of pregnancy during cesarean section. Anesthesiology, *51:*563, 1979.
195. Soffronoff, E.C., Kaufmann, B.M., and Connaughton, J.F.: Intravascular volume determinations and fetal outcome in hypertensive diseases of pregnancy. Am. J. Obstet. Gynecol., *127:*4, 1977.
196. Somjen, G., Hilmy, M., and Stephen, C.R.: Failure to anesthetize human subjects by intravenous administration of magnesium sulfate. J. Pharmacol. Exp. Ther., *154:*652, 1966.
197. Spetz, S.: Studies on peripheral circulation in normal pregnancy and in pregnancy complicated by toxaemia and diabetes mellitus. Acta Obstet. Gynecol. Scand., *44:*suppl. 1, 1–24, 1965.
198. Spinnato, J.A., Kraynack, B.J., and Cooper, M.W.: Eisenmenger's syndrome in pregnancy: Epidural anesthesia for elective cesarean section. N. Engl. J. Med., *304:*1215, 1981.
199. Stanley, T.H., Philbin, D.M., and Coggins, C.H.: Fentanyl-oxygen anaesthesia for coronary artery surgery: cardiovascular and antidiuretic hormone responses. Can. Anaesth. Soc. J., *26:*168, 1979.
200. Stanley, T.H. and Webster, L.R.: Anesthetic requirements and cardiovascular effects of fentanyl-oxygen and fentanyl-diazepam-oxygen anesthesia in man. Anesth. Analg. (Cleve), *57:*411, 1978.
201. Stefani, S.J., Hughes, S.C., Shnider, S.M. et al.: Neonatal neurobehavioral effects of inhalation analgesia for vaginal delivery. Anesthesiology, *56:*351, 1982.
202. Stoelting, R.K.: Circulatory changes during direct laryngoscopy and tracheal intubation: Influence of duration of laryngoscopy with or without prior lidocaine. Anesthesiology, *47:*381, 1977.
203. Stovner, J., Theodorsen, L., and Bjelke, E.: Sensitivity to tubocurarine and alcuronium with special reference to plasma protein pattern. Br. J. Anaesth., *43:*385, 1971.
204. Strauss, R.G., Keefer, J.R., Burke, T. et al.: Hemodynamic monitoring of cardiogenic pulmonary edema complicating toxemia of pregnancy. Obstet. Gynecol., *55:*170, 1980.
205. Strunin, L.: Preoperative assessment of the patient with liver dysfunction. Br. J. Anaesth., *50:*25, 1978.
206. Stuart, K.L.: Cardiomyopathy of pregnancy and the puerperium. Q. J. Med., *37:*463, 1968.
207. Sullivan, J.M.: Blood pressure elevation in pregnancy. Prog. Cardiovasc. Dis. *16:*375, 1974.
208. Szekely, P. and Julian, D.G.: Cardiovascular physiology of pregnancy. Curr. Probl. Cardiol., *4:*1, 1979.
209. Szekely, P. and Snaith, L.: Heart Disease in Pregnancy. Churchill Livingstone, Edinburgh, 1974.
210. Talledo, O.E., Chesley, L.C., and Zuspan, F.P.: Renin-angiotensin system in normal and toxemic pregnancies. III. Differential sensitivity to angiotensin II and norepinephrine in toxemia of pregnancy. Am. J. Obstet. Gynecol., *100:*218, 1968.
211. Taylor, G.: Acid pulmonary aspiration syndrome after antacids. A case report. Br. J. Anaesth., *47:*615, 1975.
212. Teabeaut, J.R. II: Aspiration of gastric contents. An experimental study. Am. J. Pathol., *28:*51, 1952.
213. Tucker, G.T., Boyes, R.N., and Bridenbaugh, P.G. et al.: Binding of anilide-type local anesthetics in human plasma. II. Implications in vivo, with special reference to transplacental distribution. Anesthesiology, *33:*304, 1970.

214. Ueland, K.: Maternal cardiovascular dynamics. VII. Intrapartum blood volume changes. Am. J. Obstet. Gynecol., *126*:671, 1976.
215. Ueland, K.: Pregnancy and cardiovascular disease. Med. Clin. North Am., *61*:17, 1977.
216. Ueland, K., Gills, R.E., and Hansen, J.M.: Maternal cardiovascular dynamics. I. Cesarean section under subarachnoid block anesthesia. Am. J. Obstet. Gynecol., *100*:42, 1968.
217. Ueland, K. and Hansen, J.M.: Maternal cardiovascular dynamics. III. Labor and delivery under local and caudal analgesia. Am. J. Obstet. Gynecol., *103*:8, 1969.
218. Ueland, K., Novy, M.J., and Peterson, E.N.: Maternal cardiovascular dynamics. IV. The influence of gestational age on the maternal cardiovascular response to posture and exercise. Am. J. Obstet. Gynecol., *104*:856, 1969.
219. Vasicka, A., Robertazzi, R., Raji, M. et al.: Fetal bradycardia after paracervical block. Obstet. Gynecol., *38*:500, 1971.
220. Vassalli, P., Morris, R.H., and McCluskey, R.T.: The pathogenic role of fibrin deposition in the glomerular lesions of toxemia of pregnancy. J. Exp. Med., *118*:467, 1963.
221. Venuto, R.C., O'Doriso, T., Stein, J.H. et al.: Uterine prostaglandin E secretion and uterine blood flow in the pregnant rabbit. J. Clin. Invest., *55*:193, 1975.
222. Virgilio, R.W., Rice, C.L., Smith, D.E. et al.: Crystalloid vs. colloid resuscitation: is one better? Surgery, *85*:129, 1979.
223. Vroman, S. and Thiery, M.: Fetal Mortality after Paracervical Block Analgesia in Labor. Proceedings of the 1st National Congress of the Belgian Royal Society of Gynecology and Obstetrics. Editions Ortho Pharmaceutica, Turnhout, Belgium, 1972.
224. Waller, J.L., Hugg, C.C., Jr., Nagle, D.M. et al.: Fentanyl/oxygen "anesthesia" and coronary bypass surgery. Anesth. Analg. (Cleve), *59*:562, 1980.
225. Walters, W.A.W., MacGregory, W.G., and Hills, M.: Cardiac output at rest during pregnancy and the puerperium. Clin. Sci. Mol. Med., *30*:1, 1966.
226. Wessels, J.V. Allen, G.W., and Slogoff, S.: The effect of nitrous oxide on ketamine anesthesia. Anesthesiology, *39*:382, 1973.
227. Wickström, I., Kjellmer, I., Kristianson, B. et al.: Anesthesia for cesarean section. VII. Early effects on neonatal renal function of enflurane anesthesia for cesarean section. Acta Anaesthesiol. Scand., *24*:190, 1980.
228. Williamson, J.G.: The use of paracervical nerve block anaesthesia in labour. Ir. J. Med. Sci., *3*:581, 1970.
229. Wilson, R.J., Beecham, C.T., and Carrington, E.R.: Obstetrics and Gynecology, 4th ed., The C.V. Mosby Co., St. Louis, 1971.
230. Wollman, S.B. and Marx, G.F.: Acute hydration for prevention of hypotension of spinal anesthesia in parturients. Anesthesiology, *29*:374, 1968.
231. Writer, W.D.R., James, F.M. III, Stullken, E.H., Jr. et al.: Intracranial effects of nitroglycerin—an obstetrical hazard? Anesthesiology, *53*:S309, 1980.
232. Yeh, S.Y., Paul, R.H., Cordero, L. et al.: A study of diazepam during labor. Obstet. Gynecol., *43*:363, 1974.
233. Young, B.K. and Weinstein, H.M.: Effects of magnesium sulfate on toxemic patients in labor. Obstet. Gynecol., *49*:681, 1977.
234. Young, D.C., Popat, R., Luther, E.R. et al.: Influence of maternal oxygen administration on term fetus before labor. Am. J. Obstet. Gynecol., *136*:321, 1980.
235. Zador, G., Lindmark, G., and Nilsson, B.A.: Pudendal block in normal vaginal deliveries. Acta Obstet. Gynecol. Scand. [Suppl.] *34*:51, 1974.

6

Hyperalimentation during Pregnancy

Ramón Martin, M.D.
George L. Blackburn, M.D., Ph.D.

INTRODUCTION

Nutritional status is a prime concern of the obstetrician in following a woman throughout pregnancy. In general, maternal weight gain correlates well with both fetal weight gain and outcome. Maternal malnutrition is related directly or indirectly to several complications of pregnancy, including some cases of intrauterine growth retardation (IUGR) and preeclampsia.

There are three major questions regarding maternal protein-calorie malnutrition (PCM): (1) What constitutes inadequate maternal nutrition? (2) At what point does PCM affect fetal development? (3) What interventions are available to reverse malnutrition? While these issues may be of minor importance in most cases, severe maternal malnutrition unresponsive to conventional oral diet or food supplementation will occasionally necessitate intravenous hyperalimentation to treat maternal PCM and avoid fetal complications. Intravenous hyperalimentation refers to the process of infusing amino acids and hypertonic glucose through a central vein. When calories derived from fat are added, the process is called total parenteral nutrition (TPN).

The maternal and fetal circulations are separated by the placenta, which maintains a concentration gradient between them. Placental growth is important to en-

---

Supported in part by grants GM-22691 and GM-24206, awarded by the National Institute of General Medical Sciences, DHHS. This is article #722 from the Cancer Research Institute of the New England Deaconess Hospital.

sure continued blood flow and nutrient supply for the fetus. This is of particular importance in pregnancies complicated by primary PCM.

The development of TPN has dramatically expanded the therapeutic possibilities in managing maternal malnutrition caused by gut failure. The use of TPN during pregnancy is a recent development. Prevailing opinion has been that illness severe enough to require TPN would either be associated with infertility or lead to early abortion. Consequently, there have only been a few case reports of TPN use during pregnancy. This technique, however, has been demonstrated to be effective in the care of obstetrical patients with inflammatory bowel disease, prolonged postoperative ileus, and severe hyperemesis gravidarum.

This chapter will review the nutritional interrelationship between mother and fetus in normal gestation as well as the adaptive mechanisms which accompany maternal PCM. Techniques of nutritional assessment will be presented in order to provide measures other than maternal weight gain for evaluating PCM. Published reports of TPN in pregnancy will be reviewed, as well as our experience with TPN in pregnancy. Several problems, real and theoretical, in providing hyperalimentation will also be considered, along with its effects on both mother and fetus.

NORMAL NUTRITIONAL REQUIREMENTS IN PREGNANCY

During pregnancy an increase in energy substrates is necessary because of the metabolic demands of the fetus, placenta, and uterus. In addition, maternal metabolic work is increased as a result of the various alterations in physiology necessary to sustain the pregnancy. For pregnancy, the average total extra energy necessary to meet all these functions is 80,000 kcal, or about 300 kcal/day in addition to basal needs.[48] Slightly more calories are needed in the younger age group[56] (Table 6-1). The rate of energy expenditure rises asymptotically, reaching its maximum near the end of the first trimester and remaining at this level until term. Maternal factors such as expanded blood volume, fat accumulation, and growth of the uterus and breasts account for the second-trimester increase in energy expenditure, whereas the third-trimester burden is due mainly to growth of the fetus and placenta.

The increased dietary or energy intake is also reflected in weight gain. At term, the average weight gain in U.S. women is 11 kg, or 24 lb. Weight gain begins at the end of the first trimester and increases linearly (Fig. 6-1). Based on experiments in the rat, the shifts in maternal stores during gestation have been divided into an anabolic and a catabolic phase, which correlate well with human gestation. The former period corresponds to the first two trimesters, during which protein stores are accumulated. Fat stores are also accumulated owing to an increased conversion of glucose to fatty acids (lipogenesis) and a decrease in free fatty acid release from adipose tissue (lipolysis) in response to a relative hyperinsulinemia. Other contributing factors are the increased serum levels of progesterone and a secondary reduction in the secretion of free cortisol.

During the catabolic phase or third trimester, fetal demands increase more

Table 6-1. Mean Height and Weights and Recommended Energy Intake for Women

Age (years)	Weight (kg)	Weight (lb)	Height (cm)	Height (in)	Energy Needs (kcal)
15–18	55	120	163	64	2,100
19–22	55	120	163	64	2,100
23–50	55	120	163	64	2,000
Pregnancy					+300
Lactation					+500

Adapted from Recommended Dietary Allowances, 9th Rev. Ed., National Research Council, National Academy of Sciences, 1980.

rapidly and are met by mobilizing maternal muscle protein stores. Triglyceride formation from fatty acids in adipose tissue declines as maternal lipolysis leads to net mobilization of free fatty acids. This is reflected in decreased tissue responsiveness to insulin as gestation progresses. Levels of estrogen increase, as well as the synthesis of corticosteroids by the maternal adrenal gland, mediated by ACTH secretion. Corticosteroids foster catabolism of maternal muscle protein to maintain amino acid pools for fetal uptake.

The composition of maternal weight gain as either protein or fat has been approximated by indirect means. Total body potassium determinations in pregnant teenage girls demonstrate an accumulation of potassium that is greater than the estimations for lean tissue gain from fetus, placenta, and accessory tissue.[33] A similar study in older pregnant women (24 to 34 years old) also showed excess potassium retention; however, the difference was not as large as in the younger group. These findings support the belief that maternal lean body mass increases during pregnancy.

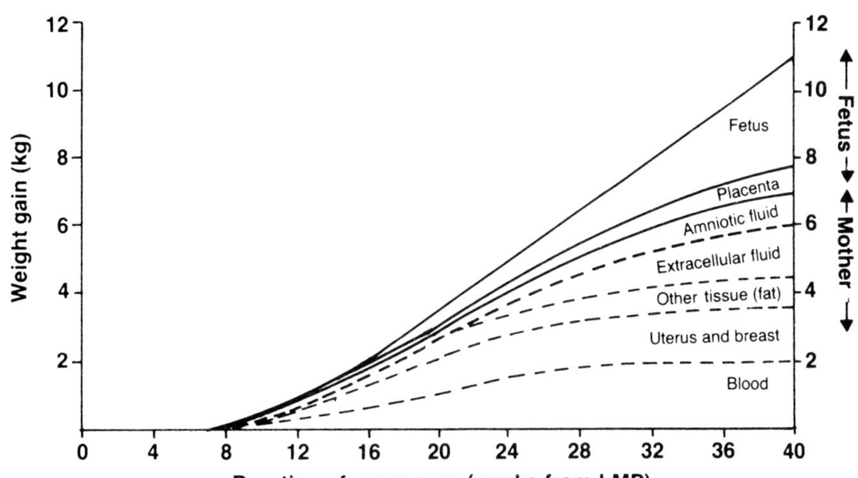

Fig. 6-1 Pattern and components of maternal weight gain during pregnancy. (Adapted from Pitkin, R.M.: Obstetrics and gynecology. In Anderson, C.E., Coursin, D.B., and Schneider, H.A., Eds.: Nutritional Support of Medical Practice. Harper & Row, Hagerstown, Md., 1977.

Results from nitrogen balance studies have led to similar conclusions.[12] An estimate of the protein needs of obstetrical patients has been made by calculating the amounts of nitrogen added during pregnancy in the known sites of protein storage: blood, breast, uterus, fetus, placenta, and amniotic fluid. The result corresponds to approximately 1 kg of protein. Spread over the duration of pregnancy, this means that an accretion of 4 g of protein a day is necessary in order to achieve optimal levels. In order to achieve this positive protein balance an approximate daily intake of 1.3 protein/kg/day is recommended (calculated from the Recommended Dietary Allowance (RDA) for the nonpregnant woman with the addition of 30 g each day for pregnancy). The remainder of maternal weight gain is fat tissue.

Importance of Nutritional Support of the Placenta. The pivotal organ in maternal-fetal nutrient transfer is the placenta. The placenta has a variety of functions, including endocrine support of the pregnancy and transport of nutrients and respiratory gases to the fetus against a concentration gradient. It produces several protein hormones, including human chorionic gonadotropin (HCG), human placental lactogen (HPL), and possibly human chorionic corticotropin (HCC). Both HCG and HPL are secreted primarily into the maternal circulation. HCG reaches its maximum level at day 70 of gestation, then declines gradually[26] but HPL rises slowly throughout gestation and disappears rapidly after delivery. HPL has a diabetogenic, glucose-sparing effect and also stimulates maternal lipolysis, causing an increase in maternal-serum free fatty acid levels.[30] Since the mother can then utilize larger amounts of free fatty acids as fuel, this frees maternal stores of glucose and amino acids for use by the fetus. HCG stimulates the corpus luteum to produce progesterone during the first trimester, may possibly direct steroid production by the fetal gonads,[1] and increases the catabolism of glycogen.[24] This may have a glucose-sparing effect in the placenta and make more glucose available for the fetus.

The progesterone produced by the placenta also has a diabetogenic, glucose-sparing effect in the mother. The primary role of estrogen is in stimulating uterine growth by increasing local DNA and protein synthesis. Another estrogen effect is to increase placental and uterine blood flow, thus increasing the transport of nutrients to the fetus.

Placenta Gradient and Active Transport. Table 6-2 lists substances that cross the placenta as well as currently accepted transport mechanisms. In the case of glucose, both placental metabolism and facilitated diffusion contribute to the differences in concentration between maternal and fetal circulation.[64]

An active transport of amino acids is suggested by the fourfold higher concentrations of amino acids in the fetal as compared with the maternal circulation.[67] In addition, amino acid concentrations in umbilical venous blood exceed those in umbilical arterial blood. Large proteins and polypeptides cross the placenta very slowly, probably by pinocytosis or through breaks in the membranes.[10] Free fatty acids exchange readily, although not as quickly as oxygen and carbon dioxide.[52] The diffusion of cholesterol and steroids is relatively slow and depends upon their molecular configuration.

Water-soluble vitamins are found in higher concentrations in the fetal blood

Table 6-2. Substances That Cross the Placenta and Currently Accepted Mechanisms of Transport

Transport Mechanism	Substances Transported
Passive diffusion	Oxygen
	Carbon dioxide
	Fatty acids
	Steroids
	Nucleosides
	Electrolytes
	Fat-soluble vitamins
Facilitated diffusion	Sugars
Active transport	Amino acids
	Some cations
	Water-soluble vitamins
Solvent drag	Electrolytes
Pinocytosis, breaks in membrane	Proteins

than in the maternal blood.[61] Although they are probably actively transported, their protein binding in the fetal blood is also increased and might account for the large gradient. Fat-soluble vitamins readily cross the placenta by passive diffusion.

The concentration of water in both circulations is affected by both hydrostatic and osmotic pressure differences. Changes in the concentration of any of the above-mentioned substances can affect the osmotic pressure gradient across the placenta and thereby influence water exchange. The osmotic water flux is also influenced by water shifts, due to carbon dioxide exchange, between red cells and plasma, which then can change the plasma concentrations of various solutions.

Fetal and Placental Growth. Fetal growth, as measured by changes in fetal body weight, increases gradually throughout pregnancy. Biochemical analyses of various fetal organs have shown that fetal growth is proliferative up to the 25th week of gestation but becomes both hyperplastic and hypertrophic thereafter.[65] This pattern is similar to the growth pattern of the placenta. In this respect, therefore, the placenta can be considered to be a fetal organ. In early gestation, the placenta is larger than the fetus and probably has greater growth requirements. In later gestation, the rate of fetal growth exceeds that of the placental growth. This is reflected by an increase in the fetal weight/placental weight ratio. Because of this shift, the placenta must increase the amount of substrate per gram of placental tissue which is transferred into the fetal circulation to meet fetal needs.[55] This osmotic gain in turn affects fetal blood volume, venous return, cardiac output, and delivery of nutrients to fetal tissues.

Fetal Growth Factors. There are several recently recognized growth factors that may also play a role in fetal growth. The fetal blood concentration of somatomedin A has been correlated with birth weight. Somatomedin A has binding sites in the placenta and there is indirect evidence that it is synthesized there. Somatomedin C, found in fetal red blood cells, also has placental binding sites. It is found in increasing concentrations in the fetal pig placenta as gestation advances while at the same time insulin binding is decreasing. This suggests a possible role for somatomedins in placental growth.[19] Human placental lactogen has been shown to increase somatomedin production, which suggests that HPL may regulate placental growth through this mechanism.[62] In addition to the somatomedins, there are insulinlike growth factors (IgF_1 and IgF_2) about which little is known.

THE EFFECTS OF MATERNAL NUTRITIONAL DEPRIVATION ON THE FETUS AND PLACENTA

Studies in pregnant rats pair-fed 50 percent of the food normally consumed by nonpregnant controls showed no change in body composition of the mother. However, fetal mean body weights were significantly reduced.[13] When pregnant rats were restricted to 75 percent of their ad libitum intake, the mothers gained 9 g of net body weight while the mean fetal weight remained within control values. With a decrease in the restriction to 50 percent of normal intake, the mothers lost 8 percent of the initial weight, with a decrease in mean fetal weight of 12 percent. At a 25 percent intake restriction, there was a 26 to 32 percent loss of initial body weight, with a 45 to 56 percent decrease in mean fetal weight. This was also associated with a 64 to 92 percent embryonic death rate.[21] These data suggest that there is no apparent effect on fetal growth in food-restricted rats unless the restriction is so severe that the mother cannot gain weight.

If nutrients are available and the mother increases her intake above normal, a portion of the excess goes to the fetus. When food intake is severely limited, however, the fetus is not favored over the mother. The maternal preference for nutrients is continued with refeeding. In pregnant guinea pigs, a low protein diet resulted in (1) a 10 to 12 percent reduction of initial maternal weight; (2) a 50 percent fetal mortality; and (3) a 22 to 38 percent reduction in the fetal birth weight.[68] Pigs fed a low-protein diet during pregnancy lost 17 percent of initial body weight, while the fetuses were 33 percent below control body weights.[46] The same has been found in rhesus monkeys.[50,51] When rats were restricted to 24 percent of normal intake for the first 5 days of pregnancy and then allowed to eat ad libitum for the remainder of the pregnancy, maternal and fetal weights were similar to those of controls. If refeeding was not permitted until the last 12 days of pregnancy, however, maternal net body weight increased 23 percent, with a 7 percent decrease in fetal body weight as compared with controls. When refeeding was begun during the last 10 days of gestation, maternal body weight increased by 21 percent and fetal body weight decreased by 12 percent.[6] This demonstrates that the mother is favored over the fetus when nutrients are available. These results also support the concept that nutrients go preferentially to the mother rather than the fetus during periods of starvation.

The Dutch famine during the winter of 1944–1945 demonstrated the effects of starvation on maternal weight gain. It has been estimated that the average daily intake during this time was approximately 1,200 calories. When this occurred during the second and third trimesters, there was a 250-g decrease in mean fetal body weight (10 percent reduction). Rosso has estimated that the mean loss of weight for the mother was 1.5 kg of initial body weight or less than 3 percent.[57] This is consistent with the experimental animal data described previously and suggests that with semistarvation the mother maintains her own body stores rather than adapting to maintain fetal growth. If there are extra body stores, then she can maintain normal fetal growth even with inadequate food intake. If the stores are small, however, the amount of food intake becomes the critical factor in the maintenance of fetal growth.

The metabolic changes that the mother undergoes during starvation are still largely unknown. In pregnant rats that have been protein-restricted, the rate of urea synthesis and the levels of hepatic enzymes involved in amino acid catabolism are reduced.[4,44] Women on low-protein diets have reduced urea excretion, which suggests a similar mechanism to reduce amino acid catabolism[7] although the reason for this is not clear. In humans as well as in experimental animal models, protein restriction beginning just after conception causes a significant reduction in the expected expansion of plasma volume.[8,11] If blood volume is inadequate, uterine blood flow may be decreased, with subsequent compromise of fetal development. It has been shown that the volume of maternal plasma correlates with infant birth weight.[16]

Effects of Maternal Nutritional Deprivation on the Placenta. The lack of normal plasma volume expansion and its consequent reduction in uterine blood flow may adversely influence nutrient transfer across the placenta. In addition, changes in placental morphology may reduce the size of the effective exchange area and thereby the rate of transfer for substances moved by simple or facilitated diffusion. A reduction in the metabolic activity of the trophoblast would influence active transport. Measurements of maternal cardiac output and regional blood flow have shown less expansion in cardiac output and placental blood flow for malnourished pregnant rats compared with controls, although the percentage of cardiac output distributed to the uterus was the same for both groups.[31] It was the lack of plasma volume expansion that accounted for the decreased placental blood flow and decreased nutrient supply.

Etiology of Lack of Fetal Weight Gain. The primary cause for the lack of weight gain in the nutritionally growth-retarded fetus is decreased placental transport. This is suggested by the frequent occurrence of hypoglycemia seen in nutritionally growth-retarded guinea pig fetuses. Plasma-free fatty acids in these fetuses are also depressed as is the arterial oxygen saturation.[36] In both guinea pig and human fetuses that suffer from nutritional IUGR, venous alanine concentrations are elevated owing to increased protein catabolism. Fetal serum ammonia levels are high because of inadequate clearing by the placenta, as well as a poorly developed fetal urea cycle. Fetal hepatic glycogen is reduced in the rat,[28] but not in the monkey[43] or guinea pig.[36] Triglyceride stores are also reduced with nutritional IUGR. Both glycogen and triglycerides are rapidly mobilizable energy stores for the neonate. Decreased glycogen storage probably accounts for the hypoglycemia that occurs frequently in human newborns who have experienced PCM during gestation.

Organ Effects of Malnutrition. Our understanding of fetal changes in response to maternal malnutrition is largely based on animal studies. A consistent feature seen with nutritional IUGR in both animal models and humans is an asymmetric effect on organ growth.[36] Length is not affected as much as the decrease in body weight. When compared with the reduction in total body weight, the decrease in brain weight is proportionally less and the decrease in lung, heart, and kidney weight is the same (Fig. 6-2).

In addition to a decrease in organ weight, there are also changes in morphology. The liver shows less cytosol, fewer mitochondria, and less endoplasmic reticulum. Hepatic enzyme function is also altered. Low levels of phosphoenolpyruvate carboxykinase suggest impairment of gluconeogenesis. Decreased activity of aminotransferase is consistent with reduced rates of peripheral amino acid metabolism.[36]

In the brain, the decrease in mass is associated with a fall in DNA, RNA, and protein content. In humans, most neurogenesis and some myelination have occurred by 26 weeks of gestation. If growth restriction starts after that time, brain mass at birth is reduced, but if postnatal nutrition is adequate, "catch-up" growth will compensate to produce a normal-size brain.[20] Growth restriction before 26 weeks, however, leads to permanent stunting of brain growth and measurable neurological damage.[23]

The skeletal system is also affected by nutritional IUGR. In guinea pigs, there is delayed ossification, probably secondary to a decrease in factors that cause sulfate to be incorporated into cartilage.[36] These changes are caused primarily by decreased nutrient supply, although secondary changes in the circulating levels of insulin and glucagon have an effect as well.

There is clearly a relationship between maternal weight gain, fetal weight gain, and fetal outcome. A question yet to be answered is whether one can quantitate the relationship between the degree of maternal weight loss and the severity of fetal outcome. It is, of course, important to know what populations are at increased risk for

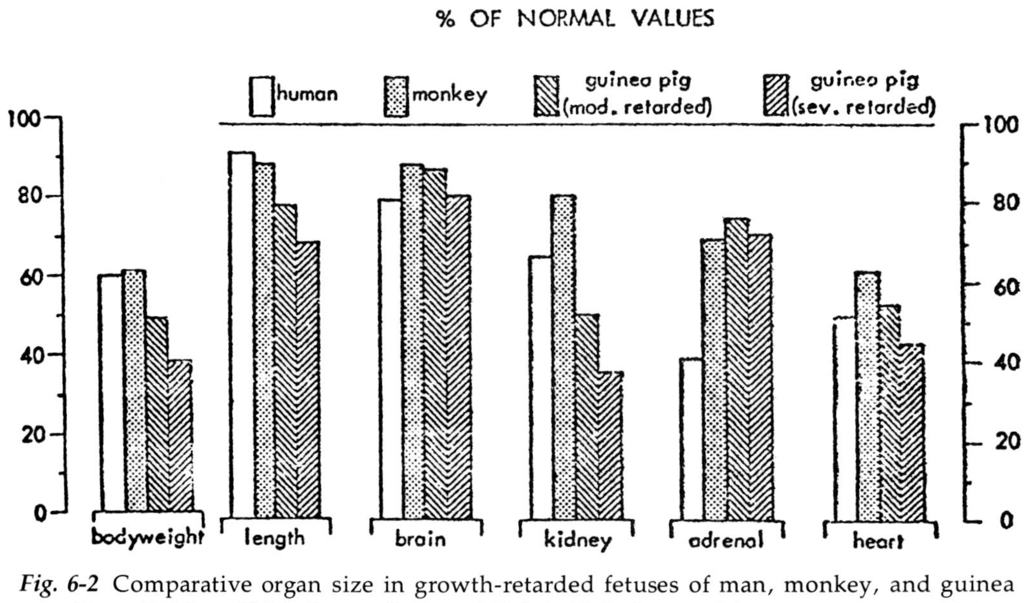

Fig. 6-2 Comparative organ size in growth-retarded fetuses of man, monkey, and guinea pig. (From Lafeber, H.N., Jones, C.T., and Rolph, T.P.: Some of the consequences of intrauterine growth retardation. p. 47. In Visser, H.K.A., Ed.: Nutrition and metabolism of the fetus and infant. Martinus Nijhoff, The Hague, 1979.)

weight loss and to be aware of nutritional assessment techniques other than serial measurements of weight which may be useful in following these patients. A good deal of experience with these techniques has been gained in hospitalized patients with general medical and surgical conditions.

EVALUATION OF THE MALNOURISHED PATIENT

Pitkin has suggested the following definitions to be used as guidelines in the nutritional assessment of obstetrical patients[45]:

1. *Underweight:* prepregnant weight 10 percent or more below standard weight for height and age (i.e., ideal body weight (IBW))
2. *Overweight:* prepregnant weight 20 percent or more above IBW
3. *Inadequate gain:* gain of 1 kg or less per month during the second or third trimester
4. *Excessive gain:* gain of 3 kg or more per month

The first and third categories comprise a group of women who may develop nutritional deficiency.[14] Patients who are at increased risk for this problem include:

1. Adolescents, especially those who are not married
2. Women with low income or for whom food purchase is an economic problem
3. Women with a history of frequent conceptions
4. Women with a history of infants with low birth weight
5. Women with diseases that influence nutritional status: diabetes, tuberculosis, inflammatory bowel disease, anemia, drug addiction, alcoholism, mental depression
6. Women known to be dietary faddists or with frank pica
7. Women who have undergone an operation with a prolonged postoperative ileus

Maternal weight gain has thus far been the only factor mentioned as a reflection of nutritional intake, with fetal outcome being directly related to an appropriate increase in this variable. Other factors may also be important in this regard.

Need for Nutritional Assessment

In evaluating the patient with malnutrition, a nutritional assessment is an important first step in treatment and is relevant to the medical evaluation of an obstetrical patient. Such an assessment can objectively detect the presence of malnutrition and provide guidelines for therapy. Although severe cases of malnutrition can be easily recognized, all cases are best managed by a protocol that includes serial measurements to evaluate the effects of therapy. The following parameters are included in nutritional-metabolic profiles:

1. Height in centimeters
2. Weight in kilograms
3. Basal energy expenditure in kilocalories per day
4. $\frac{\text{Actual weight}}{\text{IBW}} \times 100\%$
5. Actual triceps skinfold thickness as a percentage of the standard value
6. Actual mid-upper arm muscle circumference as a percentage of the standard value
7. Creatinine/height index
8. Serum albumin level
9. Serum transferrin level or total iron-binding capacity
10. Total lymphocyte count
11. Measure of cell-mediate immunity (delayed hypersensitivity reaction)
12. Nitrogen balance
13. Apparent net protein utilization
14. Weight change as percent of usual weight (with time)
15. Caloric intake as a multiple of basal energy expenditure
16. Body surface area in square meters

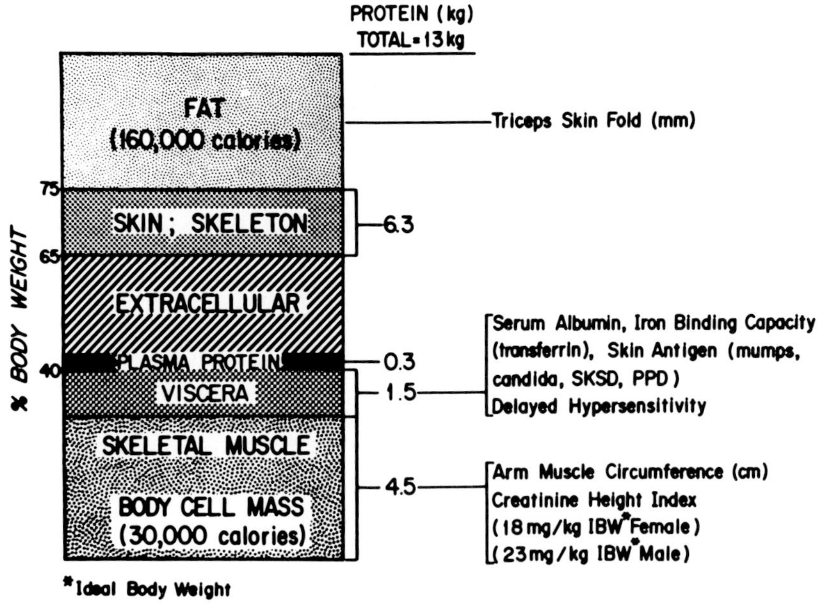

Fig. 6-3 The major parameters for the assessment of nutritional status with corresponding components of body composition. (From Blackburn, G.L., Bistrian, B. R., Maini, B. S. et al. Nutritional and metabolic assessment of the hospitalized patient. J. Parenteral Enteral Nutr *1*:11, 1977.)

Such an assessment effectively identifies any areas of deficit and, more importantly, reflects the status of the components of body cell mass (Fig. 6-3). Knowledge of the patient's weight and height, percentage weight loss, serum albumin, and delayed cutaneous hypersensitivity allows one to classify the type of protein-calorie malnutrition as:

1. *Marasmus:* reduction in body weight and anthropometrics (triceps skinfold and arm muscle circumference), with preservation of serum albumin and immune function (visceral protein)
2. *Adult kwashiorkor-like syndrome:* hypoalbuminemia, low transferrin, and increased likelihood of anergy to skin tests, with preservation of anthropometrics
3. *Hypoalbuminemic malnutrition (mixed kwashiorkor-marasmus):* depression of both visceral protein stores and anthropometrics

Differentiating Starvation From Malnutrition

Decreased nutrient intake and stress determine the type of malnutrition. When energy supply cannot keep up with demands, the deficit is provided from breakdown of skeletal muscle protein, visceral organs, and fat. Fat is the largest store of energy, containing more than 150,000 kcal. Skeletal muscle is a source of amino acids for energy production and protein synthesis. Visceral tissues contain much less protein than skeletal muscle. With semistarvation (marasmus), muscle and fat are utilized preferentially, which accounts for the depressed triceps skinfold (an index of fat stores) and arm muscle circumference (a measure of muscle mass), with normal albumin and immune function (visceral protein), When stress from injury or infection is added, there is an increase in protein mobilization from both skeletal muscle and viscera. This causes hypoalbuminemia as well as anergy and is called kwashiorkor. When a severe stress (such as an extensive burn or prolonged sepsis) occurs in an otherwise healthy individual, hypoalbuminemia and anergy can develop rapidly. This is a variant of hypoalbuminemic malnutrition.

The importance of differentiating the types of malnutrition relates to their effects on mortality rates. In marasmus, there is no increase in mortality until weight loss is 40 percent or greater because of the differential loss of tissue from fat, skeletal muscle, and visceral organs. However, in kwashiorkor (semistarvation plus stress), a weight loss of 25 percent can be lethal.

Visceral protein status is reflected by the serum transferrin concentration. This value may be approximately derived from the total iron-binding capacity (TIBC):

$$\text{Serum transferrin} = 0.8 \times \text{TIBC} - 43 \qquad \text{(normal range: 170–300 mg/dl)}$$

The total lymphocyte count (TLC) is a measure of immune function and may be determined by multiplying the percentage of lymphocytes in a peripheral blood smear by the total white blood cell count (WBC):

$$\text{TLC} = \%\ \text{lymphocytes} \times \text{WBC} \qquad \text{(Normal range: } >1500\text{)}$$

The creatinine/height index (CHI) is a useful measure of muscle mass and allows estimation of lean body mass. It requires a 24-h urine collection.

$$\text{CHI} = \frac{\text{actual urinary creatinine}}{\text{ideal urinary creatinine}} \times 100$$

The ideal value is obtained from a table (see Table 6-3) and is dependent on the patient's weight and height. Urine urea nitrogen (UUN), also obtained from a 24-h urine collection, gives an estimation of nitrogen or protein metabolism. The UUN is also useful in following the effectiveness of nutritional therapy. Nitrogen balance is calculated by:

$$\text{Nitrogen balance} = \frac{\text{protein intake}}{6.25} - (\text{UUN} + 4)$$

Table 6-3. Ideal Urinary Creatinine Values

Height (cm)	Ideal Creatinine (mg)
147.3	830
149.9	851
152.4	875
154.9	900
157.5	925
160.0	949
162.6	977
165.1	1,006
167.6	1,044
170.2	1,076
172.7	1,109
175.3	1,141
177.8	1,174
180.3	1,206
182.9	1,240

Creatinine coefficient = 18 mg/kg of ideal body weight

CONSIDERATIONS IN ADMINISTERING TPN DURING PREGNANCY

The components of TPN (dextrose, amino acids, fat, vitamins, and trace minerals) are the critical nutritional substrates for normal physiologic processes. During pregnancy, as overall requirements increase, the maternal requirements for some of the individual components also increase.

Carbohydrate

The carbohydrate in TPN is dextrose, a monosaccharide chosen because of its physiologic acceptability for parenteral administration. Recent evidence suggests that the optimal rate of parenteral glucose administration during TPN is 4 to 5 mg/kg/min or about 4 to 500 g glucose in a 70-kg person. Additional calories to meet energy requirements are optimally provided by parenteral fat.

During pregnancy, fasting plasma glucose concentrations are somewhat lower than in the nonpregnant state, and they do not change significantly as pregnancy progresses. Fasting plasma insulin concentrations, however, rise slightly during pregnancy. In response to a standard glucose load, there is a rise in serum glucose during the first hour, with a return to fasting levels by 2 to 2½ h. There is, though, a wide range in serum glucose values. In some patients there is only a small rise in serum glucose, whereas in others there is a secondary increase after the first peak. The insulin response for the former is probably rapid, causing an increase in diffusion from plasma to the extracellular space, as well as increased uptake by tissue. For the latter response there is a corresponding secondary rise in plasma insulin. As pregnancy progresses, the time necessary to reach maximum glucose concentration increases. By 38 weeks of gestation, the mean time to peak plasma glucose is 55 min, compared with 34 min in the nonpregnant state. A return to fasting level, however, is still attained in 2 to 2½ h.[17] The insulin response is characterized by a gradually increasing peak value throughout gestation as well as by a delay in reaching this peak. By 2 h, the insulin level is still above the fasting concentration. These factors suggest that glucose homeostasis during TPN in pregnancy may be altered, but studies have not been conducted to confirm this. However, clinically TPN has been well tolerated in the limited number of pregnant subjects treated by this modality.

Glycosuria—What Does It Mean? The glomerular filtration rate (GFR) rises in pregnancy to about 50 percent above the prepregnancy level.[17] With the rise in postprandial glucose levels, this means an increase in the filtered load presented to the renal tubules. It has been shown that with elevated plasma glucose levels tubular reabsorption increases, but with decreasing efficiency, which leads to glycosuria. In a study of urinary glucose excretion in 30 healthy pregnant women, it was found that 10 women excreted glucose in the normal, nonpregnant range of less than 100 mg/24 h.[39] The rest excreted more than 100 mg/24 h on some days. Of the latter group, 10 women excreted as much as 1,000 mg/24 h. All patients had normal oral glucose tolerance tests. Evaluation of possible influencing variables (relationship to meals, time of day, etc.) showed no significant relationship. In addition to the glucose loss from glycosuria during pregnancy, there is also increased excretion of water-soluble vitamins as well as amino acids. In a well-nourished woman during pregnancy, this loss does not affect maternal-fetal nutritional balance. In the presence of PCM, however, intermittent glycosuria could be another potentially significant source of nutritional loss.

Maintenance of Glucose Homeostasis in the Fetus. Intravenous glucose tolerance tests (IGTT) have been used in infants and neonates to calculate the rate of disappearance of glucose (K_G). In healthy full-term infants the mean K_G starts at 1 percent/min and increases to 2 percent/min by 6 months (similar to the adult level). Infants of diabetic mothers have higher K_G values within the first 24 h after birth, as do infants who are small for gestational age (S.G.A.) or those with significant hypoglycemia.[29] The K_G values for premature infants that were appropriate for gestational age (A.G.A.) were less than those of full-term infants for the first 24 h; however, there was a rapid increase in the K_G for the former, so that at 2 months the K_G was the same as that of normal infants at 6 months. In S.G.A. infants, after the elevated K_G during the first 24 h the pattern was similar to the K_G of the A.G.A. infants.[29]

Amino Acids

As mentioned previously, the placenta has an active transport mechanism for amino acids, specifically the L-amino acids. Studies[32] in rhesus monkeys of the ratio of amino acid levels in cord and maternal blood (C/M) showed that the cord levels were greater than those of the mother for all amino acids. For lysine, taurine, and 3-methylhistidine, the elevated C/M is secondary to an increase in free amino acids in the fetus as well as reduced maternal levels. For the other amino acids, the elevated ratio is entirely due to a reduction in maternal serum levels. Taurine, alanine, lysine, and 3-methylhistidine serum levels were elevated in full-term monkey fetuses as compared with 1-year-old animals. The serum levels of the other amino acids were either unchanged or decreased.

Ghadimi and Pecora[25] studied free amino acid levels at delivery in simultaneously drawn cord and maternal serum in humans during the second and third trimester of pregnancy. As in the monkey, cord blood has a higher concentration of amino acids than maternal blood. The fetal/maternal ratios all favored the fetus, most showing a twofold greater concentration in the fetus. When maternal blood was analyzed 6 to 8 weeks postpartum, all amino acid concentrations were found to have increased from maternal levels at delivery. When the fetuses were stratified for gestational age (immature, <30 weeks; premature, 30 to 37 weeks; and full-term, >37 weeks), the differences in the C/M ratios were larger in the immature deliveries. Three diabetic mothers and their full-term infants were also included. Their C/M ratios did not differ from those of nondiabetic women with full-term deliveries. The amino acids in the Krebs-ornithine cycle, i.e., aspartic acid, glutamic acid, and ornithine, have higher ratios in the immature group than in full-term group. This suggests an immaturity of the Krebs-ornithine cycle in early pregnancy, resulting in increased fetal concentrations of these amino acids.

These data indicate that the placenta concentrates amino acids in the fetal circulation. This system is probably best suited for periods of maternal nutritional deprivation.

Fatty Acid and Ketone Metabolism

The fetus needs fatty acids for structure (i.e., phospholipids) and storage. Although the fetus can synthesize some fatty acids, it cannot make essential fatty acids. Linoleic acid accounts for approximately 2.5 percent of fetal adipose tissue stores.[66] This indicates that fatty acids cross the placenta in sizable amounts. Studies in perfused human placenta have demonstrated fatty acid transfer and suggested that the flow to the fetus is determined by the free fatty acid concentration in the maternal serum. Elphick et al. infused 200 ml of a fat emulsion (10 percent Intralipid) over 1 h into six pregnant women about 1 to 2 h prior to delivery.[22] The umbilical vein levels of all triglyceride fatty acids were higher than those in the umbilical artery, indicating placental transfer secondary to the establishment of a large maternal-fetal gradient of oleic and linoleic acids. There was a similar increase for free fatty acids. Maternal phospholipid levels were only slightly affected, with no significant umbilical venous-arterial difference. The profile of the venous-arterial cord levels for both free fatty acids and triglycerides reflects the imprint of the infused Intralipid.

During periods of maternal fasting, there is a reduction in both maternal and fetal serum glucose levels. The resulting maternal lipolysis and free fatty acid mobilization lead to increased ketone body formation. Because the fetus has limited ability to mobilize hepatic glycogen stores, increase gluconeogenesis, or extract free fatty acids from maternal serum, its serum ketone concentration also increases. This is the result of both placental transfer and endogenous production in the fetus. Under normal conditions in the human, measurements of arterial-venous differences show that the fetal brain extracts glucose, ketone bodies, and oxygen. After prolonged fasting, the fetal brain extracts more ketone bodies than glucose. This utilization is particular for the fetus. When one compares fractional extraction rates of ketone bodies by brain among the neonate, infant, and adult, there is a gradual decrease with progressive age. This would explain why neonates are able to tolerate periods of hypoglycemia better than older infants.

Vitamins

The multivitamin solution MVI-12 (see Table 6-4), added daily to TPN solutions, meets and surpasses the RDA values. Vitamin deficiency is of concern during pregnancy and is seen commonly in women with PCM. Baker et al. analyzed vitamin

Table 6-4. Components of Multivitamin Preparation (MVI-12) Added Daily to TPN

Component	Dose
Vitamin C	100 mg
A	3,300 IU
D	200 IU
B_1 (thiamine)	3.0 mg
B_2 (riboflavin)	3.6 mg
B_6 (pyridoxine)	4.0 mg
Niacinamide	40.0 mg
Pantothenic acid	15.0 mg
E	10 IU
Biotin	60 μg
Folic acid	400 mg
B_{12}	5 μg

Table 6-5. Components of Trace Element Solution (2 ml) Added Daily to TPN

Zinc	3.0 mg
Copper	1.0 mg
Manganese	0.4 mg
Iodine	0.056 mg
Chromium	0.01 mg
Magnesium sulfate	8.1 mEq
Calcium gluceptate	9.0 mEq

profiles of 174 women and their newborn infants at term[2]; 133 of these women reported having taken supplemental vitamins during their pregnancies. There was a 1:2 to 1:5 ratio of serum vitamin levels between the mother and the neonate for all the women and infants studied. The exceptions were vitamins A, B_6, and E, and β-carotene. Of the mothers found to be hypovitaminemic, serum levels of folate, thiamine, and vitamins B_{12}, C, and A were the most depressed. In women not taking supplemental vitamins, vitamins B_6 and nicotinate were also depressed. In this latter group, the incidence of low serum folate and thiamine levels was 71 and 53 percent, respectively. The hypovitaminosis was also seen in the neonate. Based on these results, it is evident that most vitamins cross the placenta and accumulate in the fetus against a concentration gradient. The fat-soluble vitamins are the exception.

Baker et al.[3] studied placental transfer in a group of women (hypovitaminemic and normovitaminemic) who took no supplemental vitamins throughout gestation. In the hypovitaminemic group the vitamin depletion in both maternal and fetal serum was the same as in the above-mentioned study; however, the placentas of hypovitaminemic women had depressed levels of only vitamin B_{12} and folate when compared with placentas of normovitaminemic women. This suggests that the placenta not only is selective in the transport of vitamins but as a growing organ has its own vitamin requirements and stores.

When the I.M. and P.O. routes for administration of vitamins were compared, an increase in levels of thiamine, B_{12}, biotin, folate, and B_6 in the mother, placenta, and fetus were noted when either route was employed. Riboflavin, pantothenate, and nicotinate were not increased acutely in the placenta or neonate when either I.M. or P.O. supplements were given shortly before birth. The reason for this is not known. The placental levels for these latter three vitamins were similar to those in unsupplemented mothers, indicating that the placental concentration was probably adequate for fetal demands.

Trace Elements and Minerals

The need for iron supplementation during pregnancy is well established and has been reviewed.[47] The trace elements added daily to TPN solutions are listed in Table 6-5. Deficiency states of minerals and trace elements are rare. Dawson et al. measured maternal levels in 244 pregnant adolescents.[18] These women had not had any mineral supplements. The samples were drawn serially from the tenth week of pregnancy to term. The serum concentrations of calcium, magnesium, iron, and zinc decreased progressively throughout pregnancy. Plasma copper levels rose slightly. All pregnancies in this series were uncomplicated.

In the fetus, copper is stored primarily in the liver, and its concentration at birth is lower than at any other time during life. Ceruloplasmin is a copper-binding protein enzyme that is found only in maternal serum and accounts for the higher maternal concentrations. The non–ceruloplasmin-bound copper concentrations are the same on both sides of the placenta. The role of the placenta in the maternal-fetal exchange of minerals and trace elements is still not clearly defined.

PRINCIPLES OF HYPERALIMENTATION DURING PREGNANCY

Solutions Used for TPN

Commercially available crystalline amino acid (CAA) and fat emulsion solutions for central vein use are listed in Tables 6-6 and 6-7. The appropriate concentration of CAA depends on the total volume of fluid the patient needs or can tolerate, as well as on the relative amounts of dextrose (supplied as a base solution concentration of 70 percent) and protein the patient should receive. The recent advent of premixed solutions can relieve a patient receiving TPN at home from compounding her own solution.

Techniques of TPN

When there is a definite need for nutritional support, the route of administration must be determined. Generally, if the gastrointestinal tract is functioning and can be used safely, the enteral route is chosen. The clinical situations in which enteral feeding is indicated are the same in pregnancy as in general medical-surgical patients and include the following:

- Neurological and psychiatric
  - Central nervous system disorders, cerebrovascular accidents, neoplasms, trauma, inflammation, demyelinating diseases, severe depression, anorexia nervosa
- Oropharyngeal and esophageal
  - Neoplasms, inflammation, trauma
- Gastrointestinal
  - Pancreatitis, inflammatory bowel disease, short bowel syndrome, malabsorption, fistulas
- Burns
- Chemotherapy and radiotherapy

There are several excellent reviews of types of feeding tubes, techniques of tube placement, and dietary formulas, so that these topics will not be reviewed here.[9,54]

When the oral route or gastrointestinal tract is not available for use, then the superior vena cava can be cannulated by a number of approaches: (1) subclavian vein (subclavicular or supraclavicular approach); or (2) internal jugular vein. For short-term use, polyvinylchloride tubing is adequate. To eliminate the needle after inserting the catheter, a catheter change over a wire can be performed.[53]

The Broviac catheter and, more recently, the Hickman catheter have been used for long-term central venous access in home patients receiving chronic TPN. These Silastic catheters are less thrombogenic than the polyvinylchloride catheters,

Table 6-6. Protein Products for Intravenous Use—Crystalline Amino Acid Solutions (CAA)

	Aminosyn (Abbott)			Travasol (Travenol)			Freamine III (McGaw)	Veinamine (Cutter)
Protein concentration	5%	7%*	10%	5%*	8.5%*	10%	8.5%	8%
Nitrogen (g/100 ml)	0.79	1.10	1.57	0.92	1.34	1.68	1.3	1.33
Osmolarity (mOsm/L)	500	700	1,000	520	860	1,000	810	950
Electrolytes (mEq/L)								
Sodium	—	70	—	70	70	3.0	10	40
Potassium	5.4	66	5.4	60	60	—	—	30
Magnesium	—	10	—	10	10	—	—	6
Chloride	—	96	—	70	70	40	2	50
Acetate	60	124	148	100	135	87	74	50

* Also available without electrolytes.

Table 6-7. Fat Emulsions for Intravenous Use

	Liposyn (Abbott)	Intralipid (Cutter)
Concentration	10%	20%
Osmolarity (mOsm/L)	300	300
Component fatty acids:		
Linoleic	77%	50%
Oleic	13%	26%
Palmitic	7%	10%
Stearic	2.5%	
Linolenic	0.1%	9%

generally used for short-term central access. The methods of insertion have been well described and should be accomplished in the operating room with local or general anesthesia (depending on patient tolerance).[40] The care of the catheter, including the technique of dressing changes and infusion, can be learned by the average patient in 1 week to 10 days.

Most patients on home TPN have short bowel syndrome resulting from inflammatory bowel disease or surgical resection of large portions of bowel following a vascular accident (e.g., mesenteric venous thrombosis). These situations are often associated with a low antithrombin III (AT III) level in the plasma, which predisposes to an increased risk of thrombosis. For this reason, women with low AT IIIs on home TPN may benefit from prophylactic anticoagulation to normalize the AT III and therefore decrease the incidence of thrombosis. Since coumadin is a teratogen, its use in pregnancy is relatively contraindicated.

Cyclic Therapy

Cyclic hyperalimentation is a parenteral feeding technique in which the administration of the hypertonic dextrose and amino acids is discontinued during part of the day. This allows for the development of a postabsorptive state facilitating the mobilization and utilization of calories stored as fat during the hypertonic dextrose infusion. The length of the cycle depends on the fluid requirements of the patient and the desired flow rate for the solution.

With cyclic hyperalimentation, the infusion is usually nocturnal, the opposite of the normal daily food intake. In the off stage of the cycle, the placenta obviously modulates glucose transport, and during maternal fasting it transports ketone bodies to the fetus, which is capable of using them for metabolism, particularly by the brain.[35] The cyclic fasting and feeding that occur with TPN probably closely simulate normal variations in maternal serum concentrations of nutrients.

Osteomalacia

Metabolic bone disease is a complication that occurs in patients receiving long-term TPN. This is of concern for both the mother and fetus. Klein et al. reported bone pain as well as patchy osteomalacia developing in patients receiving home TPN for more than 3 months.[34] Serum levels of calcium, phosphorus, and PTH were normal. The symptoms abated within 2 months of stopping the TPN. Deficiencies of copper, zinc, essential fatty acids, and phosphorus were excluded. Shike et al. suggested that the vitamin D in the TPN solution might be causative.[58,59] In a group of 11 patients receiving TPN for 14 to 109 months, serial bone biopsies revealed a picture similar to that of osteomalacia. In three patients, in addition to the histological abnormality there were fractures, hypercalcuria, hypercalcemia, and loss of skeletal calcium. The remainder of the patients had only the histological findings. Withdrawal of the vitamin D from the TPN of the first three patients resulted in reversal of bone pain and cessation of further osteomalacia. Why these three patients developed a more severe form of the bone disease is not known. In fact, there is no known link between vitamin D and/or its metabolites and this osteomalacia-like picture. Although most people receive TPN for a relatively short time (maximum use in pregnancy would be several months), an osteomalacia-like syndrome should be considered a potential complication.

Calculation of Nutritional Requirements

From the basal energy expenditure (BEE) and ideal body weight (IBW), one can calculate the caloric intake as well as protein needed to reverse weight loss. The BEE provides a guideline as to how much caloric intake is desirable. It is calculated from the following equations:

For men: $BEE = 66 + (13.7 \times W) + (5 \times H) - (6.8 \times A)$
For women: $BEE = 655 + (9.6 \times W) + (1.7 \times H) - (4.7 \times A)$

where W is actual weight in kg, H is height in cm, and A is age in years. Calculation of the daily kilocalorie requirement:

Anabolic therapy	
Parenteral	1.75 kcal × BEE
Enteral	1.50 kcal × BEE
Maintenance therapy	1.20 kcal × BEE

As an example, the 22-year-old pregnant woman in case 1 (of the two New England Deaconess Hospital cases described later in this chapter) was 152 cm tall and weighed 60 kg. Her basal energy expenditure was calculated to be:

$$655 + (9.6 \times 60) + (1.7 \times 152) - (4.7 \times 22) = 1386 \text{ kcal}$$

Her maintenance requirements therefore were:

$$1.2 \times BEE = 1.2 \times 1{,}386 \text{ kcal} = 1.663 \text{ kcal}$$

Her parenteral requirements necessary for anabolism were:

$$1.75 \times BEE = 1.75 \times 1{,}386 \text{ kcal} = 2{,}425 \text{ kcal}$$

Determination of Protein Requirements

The amount of protein required is initially based on body weight (in kilograms) but should be adjusted according to serum urea nitrogen levels as well as nitrogen balance. For patients who have undergone semistarvation or mild stress, the intake should be 1.2 to 1.5 times the IBW. With severe stress, it should be 1.7 times the IBW. For the woman in case 1, her protein requirements were:

Parenteral:	$60\text{ kg} \times 1.5 = 90\text{ g/day}$
Enteral:	$60\text{ kg} \times 1.2 = 72\text{ g/day}$

Dividing the grams of protein per day by 6.25 gives the grams of nitrogen per day:

$$\text{Parenteral:} \quad 90\text{ g protein/day} \div 6.25\,\frac{\text{g nitrogen}}{\text{g protein}} = 14\text{ g nitrogen/day}$$

$$\text{Enteral:} \quad 72\text{ g protein/day} \div 6.25\,\frac{\text{g nitrogen}}{\text{g protein}} = 12\text{ g nitrogen/day}$$

During the course of nutritional therapy, serial evaluations should include daily weight measurements, twice weekly nitrogen balance studies, and weekly TLC, anthropometric, and serum transferrin studies. Skin tests should be repeated every 3 weeks. This section has outlined general guidelines for nutritional supplementation. More specific recommendations regarding enteral or parenteral feeding will be made after reviewing the literature on TPN in pregnancy.

THE USE OF TPN DURING PREGNANCY

Total parenteral nutrition is a new form of therapy and its use in high-risk pregnancy is anecdotal at this point. In the Longwood Medical area of Boston, where there are approximately 10,000 deliveries each year, there have been five instances since 1979 of women requiring TPN during pregnancy. Although there have been several recent reports about the use of hyperalimentation in pregnancy, the number of disease states in which it has been employed is still limited. In certain conditions such as inflammatory bowel disease, there may be a place for nutritional intervention early in pregnancy, but most studies to date have been in the third trimester.

Recent case reports describe the use of both enteral and parenteral hyperalimentation in women who would otherwise probably not have been able to continue a pregnancy. Cox et al. followed a 26-year-old woman with acute Crohn's disease whose weight had decreased 1.6 kg from her prepregnancy weight over two trimesters.[15] After an initial unsuccessful trial of elemental diets, she was begun on TPN through a permanently implanted Silastic (Broviac) catheter in the subclavian vein. This began at 32 weeks gestation and continued to term. The patient was followed on a home parenteral nutrition program in which she received in a cyclic manner 3.5 L of 5 percent amino acids with 20 percent dextrose (providing 3,080 calories) over a 20-h infusion period. Intralipid was not used. The only maternal serum abnormalities were transaminase elevations. After a normal spontaneous delivery, the infant did well except for an episode of hypoglycemia 1 h postpartum. This was treated with oral 10 percent dextrose in water and did not recur. The placenta was grossly normal.

Main et al. reported a similar case of a pregnant woman with Crohn's disease.[42] They too initially began with a 5-week course of nasogastric tube feeding with Vivonex (3,600 kcal daily). At 27 weeks gestation, because of a bowel obstruction she was switched to parenteral TPN (2,800 kcal daily, of which 1,000 kcal was supplied by 500 ml of 20 percent Intralipid). With this supplementation, the patient's weight and anthropometric measurements increased. Positive nitrogen balance was achieved. The only abnormality with maternal or fetal serum was an elevation in alkaline phosphatase. The TPN was continued until 36 weeks, when a fall in urinary estriols led to a cesarean section. A 2,400-g female was delivered and subsequently did well. The placenta was small (20th percentile), with ischemic necrosis of the villi.

Smith et al.[60] administered liquid meal replacement (Ensure) through pediatric nasogastric tubes to enterally feed two pregnant, diabetic women with prolonged hyperemesis gradivarum. In one woman, these feedings were begun at 29 weeks gestation when, because of hyperemesis, there was a 2-kg weight loss as well as poor diabetic control. The enteral feedings were continued until 38 weeks (Ensure at 2,200 kcal daily), when labor was induced electively. During the course of the feedings, the mother's blood sugars stabilized as insulin requirements increased from 30 units per day on admission to 78 units per day. No fetal or maternal problems were encountered. The infant's birthweight was 2,567 g and its 1- and 5-min Apgar scores were 8 and 8. The second woman presented with similar problems and was begun on enteral hyperalimentation at 18 weeks gestation. She received 2,600 kcal/day. This was stopped at 24 weeks because of improved P.O. intake. Within 2 weeks, however, recurrent hyperemesis led to reinstitution of the enteral feedings, which were continued until delivery at 38 weeks by cesarean section. The infant weighed 2,620 g and its 1- and 5-min Apgar scores were 7 and 9.

McBurney and Wilmore reported their experience with three pregnant women who required nutritional support (one peripherally, one with central TPN, and one with both). Positive nitrogen balance was achieved only in the woman who received central TPN.[41]

Beischer has attempted to use TPN to treat IUGR based on low 24-h urine estriol excretion.[5] Infusing 25 percent dextrose and/or amino acid and Intralipid into a study group during the third trimester, he found that in comparison with untreated controls (also with low urinary estriols), there was a decreased incidence of SGA infants (19 percent vs. 35 percent) as well as of perinatal mortality (5 percent vs. 16 percent), with no significant difference in the number of congenital anomalies.

Lakoff and Feldman[37] used TPN to reverse weight loss in a 26-year-old woman with a diagnosis of anorexia nervosa. Her prepregnancy weight was 122 lb. Despite psychiatric counseling and oral supplements, her weight had decreased to 95 lb by 32 weeks gestation. She received 3,000 kcal daily of fat, protein, and carbohydrate for 12 days. Her weight increased from 95 to 112 lb. When her oral intake increased, TPN was stopped and she was continued on oral supplements. Her subsequent weight remained approximately 110 lb. There was evidence of IUGR, but urinary estriol levels were normal. At 40 weeks gestation, she delivered a 4 lb 13 oz female with a 5-

min Apgar score of 9. The placenta was histologically normal. Six months postpartum, the infant had no signs of developmental retardation.

Webb[63] used only protein and carbohydrate in providing TPN to a pregnant woman with small bowel obstruction secondary to metastatic embryonal sarcoma of the small bowel. TPN was begun at 28 weeks gestation and continued after delivery at 32 weeks, when premature rupture of membranes occurred. This was followed shortly by vaginal delivery of a 2 lb 14 oz female infant with good Apgar scores. There was no respiratory distress and the infant subsequently developed normally. The mother requested that TPN be stopped 2 weeks postpartum and she died shortly thereafter.

Case Histories

At the New England Deaconess Hospital, two pregnant women have required TPN. Their case histories are given below

Case 1. L.C. was a 22-year-old $G_3P_1Ab_1$ female whose last menstrual period occurred on 4/1/81 and whose EDC was 1/6/82. She had a 12-yr history of juvenile-onset diabetes mellitus and was most recently managed with a split dose of NPH units of insulin (16 units at 8 a.m. and 14 units at 8 p.m.). When she presented on 6/11/81 for her first prenatal visit at 11 weeks gestation, she was 60 in (152 cm) tall and weighed 60 kg (prepregnancy weight 61 kg). When seen again on 6/30/81, there had been no interval weight gain and the patient complained of intermittent anorexia, nausea, and vomiting. An ultrasound to assess fetal growth also demonstrated a 6-cm diameter, solid, hyperechoic left hepatic mass. She was followed as an outpatient until a second ultrasound revealed no change in the hepatic mass. The fetus appeared to have been growing normally. She was admitted to the New England Deaconess Hospital and underwent a left hepatic lobectomy and splenectomy on 8/19/81. The pathology revealed the liver lesion to be focal nodular hyperplasia. From 8-20 to 8-24 she received 2 to 2½ L daily of I.V. solutions containing 3.5 percent amino acids with 5 percent dextrose. The nasogastric tube was removed on 8/21/81, but the patient developed persistent nausea and vomiting. The Nutrition Support Service was consulted on 8/28/81 when the patient was 21 weeks pregnant by dates. At that time, her initial assessment was:

Anthropometrics	
Mid arm circumference (MAC)	28.5 cm (98% of standard)
Triceps skin fold (TSF)	21.5 mm (126% of standard)
Arm muscle circumference (AMC)	21.8 cm (100% of standard)
Ideal body weight	48.6 kg
Actual weight	60.0 kg
Serum total protein	5.0 g/dl
Albumin	2.2 g/dl

BEE	1,386 kcal/day	
Calculated calories required for anabolism	Parenteral	2,425 kcal/day
	Enteral	2,181 kcal/day
Calculated nitrogen (amino acids) required	Parenteral	14 g/day
	Enteral	12 g/day
Calculated protein required	Parenteral	90 g/day
	Enteral	72 g/day

The patient had the adult kwashiorkor-like form of PCM (based on the hypoalbuminemia with normal weight and anthropometrics), and it was felt that she could benefit from TPN to help heal her surgical wound as well as reverse the lack of weight gain with pregnancy. Through a right internal jugular catheter she was given daily infusions of 2 L of 5 percent amino acids and 20 percent dextrose, as well as 500 ml of 10 percent Intralipid. This provided approximately 2,300 kcal/day (100 g protein, 400 g carbohydrate, 50 g fat). Regular insulin was added to the TPN but the patient remained hyperglycemic (see Table 6-8). The TPN was continued until 9/8/81. The patient's P.O. intake gradually improved and she was discharged at 24 weeks gestation. At 29 weeks gestation her renal function began to deteriorate and she was given a course of dexamethasone to accelerate fetal pulmonary maturation. At 30 weeks gestation, she underwent primary cesarean section. A live-born, female infant weighing 1814 g was delivered. Because of respiratory distress syndrome, the infant was initially intubated but subsequently did well. The placenta was grossly unremarkable.

Table 6-8. Blood Sugars for the patient in Case 1

Date	Fasting	3 p.m.	8 p.m.	2 a.m.
8/29	435	371	320	375
8/31	420	370	200	
9/2	132	132	250	
9/4	167	286	199	
9/7	136	97	82	

Case 2. B.P. was a 31-year-old $G_2P_0Ab_1$ woman who noted anorexia, nausea, and vomiting early in gestation. Her prepregnancy weight was 46 kg. When first seen at 9 weeks gestation, she weighed 39 kg. Workup revealed no psychological or organic causes for her symptoms. She was admitted to another hospital and begun on peripheral venous alimentation for two weeks; however, her symptoms persisted. A right subclavian catheter was inserted and she received 3 L of 4.25 percent amino acids and 25 percent dextrose as well as 500 ml 10 percent Intralipid daily. This provided 3,560 kcal. Over a 2-week period, she gained 5.4 kg. Because continued nausea and vomiting meant that the patient would need TPN to assure continued weight gain and fetal growth, she was transferred to the New England Deaconess Hospital at 11 weeks gestation for consideration for home TPN. Her nutritional assessment revealed:

Anthropometrics			
MAC	21.0 cm (76% of standard)		
TSF	11.0 mm (58% of standard)		
AMC	17.6 cm (83% of standard)		
Ideal body weight	46.8 kg		
Actual weight	44.4 kg		
Serum total protein	5.8 g/dl		
Albumin	3.3 g/dl		
BEE	1,249 kcal/day		
Calculated calories required for anabolism		Parenteral	2,198 kcal/day
		Enteral	1,923 kcal/day
Calculated nitrogen (amino acids) required		Parenteral	13 g/day
		Enteral	11 g/day
Calculated protein required		Parenteral	86 g/day
		Enteral	69 g/day

The patient was thought to have the marasmus form of PCM (based on her decreased weight and anthropometrics with normal serum albumin). After her transfer, her formula was decreased to 2 L/day of 5 percent amino acids and 20 percent dextrose, as well as 500 ml 10 percent Intralipid. This provided 2,300 kcal daily (100 g protein, 400 g dextrose, 50 g fat). A Hickman catheter was placed into the right subclavian vein and tunneled under the skin of the anterior chest wall in the operating room under local anesthesia. Prior to the placement of the Hickman catheter and for the week afterward, she was instructed in the care of the catheter and in how to compound, infuse, and disconnect her solution. She was maintained at home on a 12-h nocturnal cycle of 2 L of 5 percent amino acids and 25 percent dextrose. Three times a week she infused 500 ml 10 percent Intralipid.

At 34 weeks gestation, the patient spontaneously went into premature labor and precipitately delivered vaginally a live-born 2640-g male infant. The Apgars were 1 at 1 min and 4 at 5 min. Because of grunting and chest wall retractions, the infant was intubated. A chest x-ray showed an infiltrative process consistent with respiratory distress syndrome. The ventilatory support was gradually weaned and the infant was extubated 6 days after delivery. The infant has subsequently done well. The placenta was grossly normal. Immediately after delivery, the patient's symptoms of nausea and vomiting subsided and she began to eat again. The Hickman catheter was removed on the third postpartum day.

Conclusions from the Reported Cases of TPN in Pregnancy.

These cases help clarify several issues regarding the use of TPN in pregnancy. In addition, lessons may be learned from the use of long-term cyclic TPN in patients with other disease processes.

For most of the reported cases of TPN during pregnancy, caloric intake was 2,700 to 3,000 kcal. Such a large intake surpasses the RDA recommendations and raises two questions about possible fetal sequelae. Whether enteral or parenteral, uninterrupted infusions supplying a continuous flow of nutrients to the placenta might have effects similar to those encountered in the pregnancies of diabetic women. The elevated glucose levels associated with continuous infusions stimulate fetal insulin as well as placental HPL, resulting in increased fetal fat storage. This might result in the clinical stigmata seen in the infants of diabetic mothers (macrosomia, hydramnios, large placentas, intrauterine fetal demise, etc.) Presumably, by meeting the RDA requirements and simply reversing weight loss rather than attempting to achieve absolute weight gain, one might avoid these theoretical problems.

For home patients, cyclic hyperalimentation offers both the mother and the fetus the chance to utilize the fat stored during the infusion period. There have been no body composition studies done in fetuses; however, Reichman et al.[49] compared growth with the cumulative protein, fat, and carbohydrate accretion in low-birth-weight (LBW) premature infants and in term infants. The LBW infants were fed a formula such that their weight gain was similar to that of a fetus of similar age. Of the 150 kcal/kg/day provided, 67.8 kcal/day was stored (almost twice the estimated caloric accumulation of a fetus during the third trimester). Fat deposition was the major component—nearly three times more than that of fetuses of similar postconceptual age. This accounted for 32 percent of weight gain. Protein was accumulated at a rate of 1.92 g/kg/day, which was comparable with that in neonates of similar age and accounted for 11 percent of weight gain. Carbohydrate accretion (1.8 g/kg/day) was also greater than expected.

Another issue raised initially by Heller relates to the possible risks of using parenteral fat emulsions during pregnancy.[27] In pregnant rats he found that when fat comprised 50 percent of caloric intake, there was fatty infiltration of the placenta. This might inhibit triglyceride transport. This fatty infiltration was not seen in pregnant rats when the fat contribution was 20 percent of the total caloric intake. In humans the only reported occurrence of fatty infiltration of the placenta was in a woman with hyperlipidemia. No abnormalities have been seen in the placentas of pregnant women who received fat as a part of TPN.

Heller[27] also noted in rats that when the infusion rate was high and the pregnancy was near term, there was an increase in uterine contractions. This is perhaps a result of synthesis of arachidonic acid from the infused linoleic acid, with subsequent conversion to prostaglandins. Where Intralipid has been used during TPN in pregnancy, there have thus far been no episodes of premature labor or increased uterine irritability. Jeejeebhoy (personal communication) indicated that he has used Intralipid to provide as much as 50 percent of the caloric intake without precipitating premature labor. Since Intralipid structurally resembles chylomicron, theoretically the infusion of this fat emulsion should be similar to ingestion of a fatty meal.

The metabolic complications seen in neonates receiving TPN have also raised questions about the effects of long-term TPN in pregnancy. From the available data about amino acid transport mentioned previously, it is known that placental transport mechanisms maintain a higher blood level in the fetus than in the mother. Thus maternal amino acid concentrations (including excesses) are reflected in fetal levals. Metabolic acidosis has occurred because of the large amino acid load of the solutions; however, the maternal buffering system should generally offset this. Protein hydrolysate solutions contain large amounts of ammonia. This has been linked to neonatal subclinical liver disease. Liver function abnormalities are frequently seen in neonates receiving TPN. Transient hepatic enlargement is usually noted during the first week of therapy in premature infants receiving TPN. This may or may not be associated with intermittent elevations in liver enzymes and bilirubin in the serum. In addition, cholestasis is seen but the etiology is not known. In a number of cases underlying gastrointestinal disorders might contribute to the hepatic abnormality; however one must still consider the possibility of the infused substances being responsible.

Given the present knowledge about TPN during pregnancy, a solution to meet the caloric needs of the mother and infant should contain a mixture of protein, carbohydrate, and fat, as well as a multivitamin preparation and trace elements. After calculating the amount of calories required for anabolism, the required protein should next be calculated. Using the values for the woman in Case 1 as an example, 90 g of protein equals 360 kcal. Of the remaining requirements, 500 kcal daily would be desirable as a fat emulsion, not only to prevent maternal essential fatty acid deficiency, but also to provide linoleic acid for the fetus. These fat calories would decrease the carbohydrate load and hopefully also decrease the diabetogenic effects of continuous hypertonic dextrose solutions. At this point, there have been no adverse effects (e.g., neonatal pulmonary fat infiltration, premature uterine contractions, fat infiltration of the placenta) when fat emulsions have been used as part of TPN in a pregnant woman (500 ml of 10 percent Intralipid equals 500 kcal). The rest of the caloric requirement can be provided with dextrose, as 400 g of dextrose or 2 L of 20 percent dextrose would equal 1,400 kcal. Until further studies are done to determine parenteral need in pregnancy, standard doses (which exceed RDA requirements) of trace elements, minerals, and vitamins should be used.

The questions raised in this discussion are theoretical and can only be answered with more patient experience. Although there are still potential problems with the use of TPN in pregnancy, for the patient in which it is indicated TPN may offer the only chance to continue with the pregnancy and avoid the real problems attendant on poor weight gain or protein-calorie malnutrition.

RECOMMENDATIONS

Certain groups of patients are at high risk of PCM during pregnancy. The following factors should make one alert to the possibility of the need for nutritional intervention:

1. Prepregnancy weight 10 percent less than ideal body weight
2. Excessive weight loss (e.g., 5 to 6 kg during the first trimester)
3. Inadequate weight gain during the second and third trimesters

A nutritional assessment is useful to delineate any deficiencies and to document the effectiveness of nutritional therapy. Once a decision is made to use enteral or parenteral therapy, the goal should be reversal of weight loss. Recommended Daily Allowance requirements should be met (between 2,100 and 2,700 kcal/day), and this will be similar to the anabolic requirements.

When TPN is used, the pregnancy should be monitored closely as follows:

1. Periodic nutritional assessment.
2. Watch for glycosuria.
3. Serial ultrasound examinations to assess fetal growth.
4. Electronic fetal heart rate monitoring to assess fetal well-being.
5. If an amniocentesis is performed for any reason (e.g., to assess fetal lung maturation), an aliquot of amniotic fluid should be sent for an amino acid profile.
6. At delivery, both maternal and cord blood should be checked for amino acid concentrations, fatty acid profile, and vitamin and trace element profiles.
7. After delivery, the neonate should be observed for episodes of hypoglycemia.
8. After 28 weeks gestation, 24-h urine collections for estriol and nitrogen levels should be started.
9. With any persistent febrile episode, catheter infection, either primary (usually by a skin contaminant) or by hematogenous spread from another site, should be ruled out by blood cultures through the line and a line change over a wire to culture the catheter itself.

CONCLUSIONS

A small group of obstetrical patients is at risk for poor fetal outcome because of inflammatory bowel disease, prolonged hyperemesis gravidarium, or postoperative ileus. Total parenteral nutrition can have an impact on this group. Whereas in normal pregnancy all physiological and endocrine changes are directed toward developing a healthy placenta and fetus, an apparent paradox exists in advanced states of PCM. Refeeding studies demonstrate preferential uptake by maternal tissues at the expense of transfer to the fetus. For this reason, efforts should be made as early as possible to identify and treat PCM. At present, the use of TPN in pregnancy should be limited to centers with experience in the utilization of this technique.

REFERENCES

1. Abramovich, R., Baker, T.G., and Neal, P.: Effect of human chorionic gonadotropin on testosterone secretion by the fetal human testis in organ culture. J. Endocrinol., *60:*179, 1974.
2. Baker, H.: Vitamin profile of 174 mothers and newborns at parturition. Am. J. Clin. Nutr., *28:*56, 1975.
3. Baker, H.: Role of placenta in maternal-fetal vitamin transfer in humans. Am. J. Obstet. Gynecol., *141:*792, 1981.

4. Beaton, G.H., Beare, J., Ryu, M.H. et al: Protein metabolism in the pregnant rat. J. Nutr. *54:*291, 1954.
5. Beischer, N.: Treatment of fetal growth retardation. Aust. N.Z. J. Obstet. Gynaecol., *18:*28, 1978.
6. Berg, B.N.: Dietary restriction and reproduction in the rat. J. Nutr., *87:*344, 1965.
7. Beydoun, S.N., Cuenca, V.G., and Evans, L.P.: Maternal nutrition. I. The urinary urea nitrogen/total nitrogen as an index of protein nutrition. Am. J. Obstet. Gynecol., *114:*198, 1972.
8. Blechner, J.N., Stenger, V.G., and Prystowsky, H.: Uterine blood flow in women at term. Am. J. Obstet. Gynecol., *120:*633, 1974.
9. Bothe, A., Wade, J.E., and Blackburn, G.L.: Enteral nutrition—An overview. p. 76. In Hill, G.L., Ed.: Nutrition and the Surgical Patient. Churchill Livingstone, Edinburgh, 1981.
10. Brambell, F.W.R.: Transport of proteins across the fetal membrane. Cold Spring Harbor Symposium. Quant. Biol., *19:*71, 1954.
11. Bruc, N.W.: The distribution of blood flow to the reproductive organs of the rat near term. J. Reprod. Fertil., *45:*359, 1976.
12. Calloway, D.H.: Nitrogen balance during pregnancy. p. 79. In Winick, M., Ed.: Nutrition and Fetal Development. John Wiley & Sons, New York, 1974.
13. Child, C.M.: Some considerations concerning the nature and origin of physiological gradients. Biol. Bull., *39:*147, 1920.
14. Christakis, G.: Maternal Nutritional Assessment. Am. J. Public Health, suppl. *63:*57, 1973.
15. Cox K.: Home TPN during pregnancy: A case report. J.P.E.N., *5:*246, 1981.
16. Croall, J., Sheriff, S., and Matthews, J.: Non-pregnant maternal plasma volume and fetal growth retardation. Br. J. Obstet. Gynaecol., *85:*1978.
17. Davison, J.M.: Changes in renal function and other aspects of homeostasis in early pregnancy. J. Obstet. Gynaecol. Br. Commonw., *81:*1003, 1974.
18. Dawson, E.B.: Plasma vitamins and trace metal changes during teenage pregnancy. Am. J. Obstet. Gynecol., *104:*953, 1969.
19. D'Ercole, A.J., Foushee, D.B., and Underwood, L.E.: Somatomedin-C receptor ontogeny and levels in porcine fetal and human cord serum. J. Clin. Endocrinol. Metab., *43:*1069, 1976.
20. Dobbing, J.: The influence of early nutrition on the development of myelination of the brain. Proc. R. Soc. Lond. [Biol.], *159:*503, 1964.
21. Eastman, N.J. and Jackson, J.: Weight relationships in pregnancy. 1. The bearing of maternal weight gain and pre-pregnancy weight on birth weight in full term pregnancies. Obstet. Gynecol. Surv., *23:*1003, 1968.
22. Elphick, M.C.: The passage of fat emulsion across the human placenta. Br. J. Obstet. Gynaecol., *85:*610, 1978.
23. Fancourt, R., Harvey, D.R., Norman, A.P. et al: Follow-up study of small-for-dates babies. Br. Med. J., *1:*1435, 1976.
24. Gabbe, S.G., Demers, L.M., Greep, R.O. et al: The effects of hypoxia on placental glycogen metabolism. Am. J. Obstet. Gynecol., *114:*540, 1972.
25. Ghadimi, H. and Pecora, P.: Free amino acids of cord plasma as compared with maternal plasma during pregnancy. Pediatrics, *30:*500, 1964.
26. Grumbach, M.M., Kaplan, S.L., Sciarra, J.J. et al: Chorionic growth hormone-prolactin (CGP): Secretion, disposition, biological activity in man and postulated function as "growth hormone" of the second half of pregnancy. Ann. NY Acad. Sci., *148:*501, 1968.
27. Heller, L.: Clinical and experimental studies in complete parenteral nutrition. Scand. J. Gastroenterol., *4:*suppl. 4,7, 1968.

28. Hehenauer, L. and Oh, W.: Body composition in experimental intrauterine growth retardation in the rat. J. Nutr., *99:*23, 1969.
29. Isles, T.E., Dickson, M., and Farquhar, J.W.: Glucose tolerance and plasma insulin in newborn infants of normal and diabetic mothers. Pediatr. Res., *2:*198, 1968.
30. Kalkhoff, R.K., Kisselbah, A.H., and Kim, H.K.: Carbohydrate and lipid metabolism during normal pregnancy: relationship to gestational hormone action. Semin. Perinatol., *2:*291, 1978.
31. Kava, R. and Rosso, P.: Mechanisms for fetal growth retardation in undernourished pregnant rats. Fed. Proc., *38:*871, 1979.
32. Kerr, G.R. and Waisman, H.A.: Transplacental ratios of serum amino acids during pregnancy in the Rhesus monkey. p. 429. In Nyhan, W.L., Ed.: Amino Acids Metabolism and Genetic Variation, McGraw-Hill, New York, 1967.
33. King, J.C., Calloway, D.H., and Margen, S.: Nitrogen retention, total body ^{40}K and weight gain in teenage pregnant girls. J. Nutr., *103:*772, 1973.
34. Klein, G., Ament, M.E., Bluestone, R. et al: Bone disease associated with total parenteral nutrition. Lancet, 1041, November 1980.
35. Kraus, H. and Stumpf, B.: Interrelationship of glucose and ketone body metabolism in brain during early infancy. p. 233. In Soling, H. and Seufert, C., Eds., Biochemical and Clinical Aspects of Ketone Body Formation. George Thieme, Stuttgart, 1978.
36. LaFever, H.N., Jones, C.T., and Rolph, T.P.: Some of the consequences of intrauterine growth retardation. p. 43. In Visser, H.K.A., Ed.: Nutrition and Metabolism of the Fetus and Infant. Martinus Nijhoff, The Hague, 1979.
37. Lakoff, K.: The use of total parenteral nutrition in pregnancy and anorexia nervosa. Obstet. Gynecol., *39:*699, 1972.
38. Lind, T., Billewicz, W.Z., and Brown, G.: A serial study of changes occurring in the oral glucose tolerance test during pregnancy. J. Obstet. Gynaecol. Br. Commonw., *80:*1033, 1973.
39. Lind, T. and Hytten, F.E.: The excretion of glucose during normal pregnancy. J. Obstet. Gynecol. Br. Commonw., *79:*961, 1972.
40. Linos, D.A. and Mucha, P.: A simplified technique for the placement of permanent central venous catheters. Surg. Gynecol. Obstet., *154:*248, 1982.
41. MacBurney, M. and Wilmore, D.: Decision making for i.v. nutritional support during pregnancy. p. 577. 6th Clinical Conference Abstracts, Nov./Dec. 1981.
42. Main, A.H.: Intravenous feeding to sustain pregnancy in a patient with Crohn's disease. Br. Med. J., *283:*1221, 1981.
43. Myers, R.G., Hill, D.E., Holt, A.B. et al: Fetal growth retardation produced by experimental placental insufficiency in the Rhesus monkey II. Chemical composition of the brain, liver, muscle and carcus. Biol. Neonate, *18:*379, 1971.
44. Naismith, D.J.: Adaptations in the metabolism of protein during pregnancy and their nutritional implications. Nutr. Rep. Int., *7:*383, 1973.
45. Pitkin, R.: Nutrition during pregnancy: The clinical approach. p. 27. In Winick, M., Ed.: Current Concepts in Nutrition. John Wiley & Sons, New York, 1977.
46. Pond, W.G., Stracham, D.N., Sinha, Y.N. et al: Effect of protein deprivation of the swine during all or part of gestation on birth weight, postnatal growth rate and nucleic acid content of brain and muscle of progeny. J. Nutr., *99:*61, 1969.
47. Pritchard, J.A.: Anemias complicating pregnancy and the puerperium. In: Maternal Nutrition and the Course of Pregnancy. National Academy of Sciences, Washington, 1970.
48. Recommended Dietary Allowances. p. 26. 9th Rev. Ed. National Academy of Sciences, Washington, 1980.
49. Reichman, B.: Diet, fat accretion and growth in premature infants. N. Engl. J. Med., *305:*1495, 1982.

50. Riopelle, A.J., Hill, C.W., and Li, S.C.: Protein deprivation in primates vs. fetal mortality and neonatal status of infant monkeys born of deprived mothers. Am. J. Clin. Nutr., *28:*989, 1975.
51. Riopelle, A.J.: Weight gain of non-pregnant and pregnant monkeys fed low protein diets. Am. J. Clin. Nutr., *28:*802, 1975.
52. Robertson, A.F. and Sprecher, H.: A review of human placental lipid metabolism and transport. Acta Paediatr. Scand. 57: suppl. 183, 1, 1968.
53. Rodman, G. and Civetta, J.: Bedside pulmonary artery catheterization. Arch. Surg., *109:*840, 1974.
54. Rombeau, J.L. and Barot, L.R.: Enteral nutritional therapy. Surg. Clin. North A., *61:*605, 1981.
55. Rosso, P.: Changes in transfer of nutrients across the placenta during normal gestation in the rat. Am. J. Obstet. Gynecol. *122:*2761, 1975.
56. Rosso, P.: Maternal nutrition, nutrient exchange and fetal growth. p. 3. In Winick, M., Ed.: Nutritional Disorders of American Women. John Wiley & Sons, New York, 1977.
57. Rosso, P.: Nutrition and maternal-fetal exchange. Am. J. Clin. Nutr., *34:*744, 1981.
58. Shike, M., Harrison, J.E., Sturtridge, W.C. et al: Metabolic bone disease in patients receiving long term total parenteral nutrition. Ann. Intern. Med., *92:*343, 1980.
59. Shike, M., Harrison, J.E., Sturtridge, W.C. et al: A possible role of vitamin D in the genesis of TPN-induced metabolic bone disease. Am. J. Intern. Med., *95:*560, 1981.
60. Smith, C.: Long term enteral hyperalimentation in the pregnant woman with insulin-dependent diabetes: a report of two cases. Am. J. Obstet. Gynecol., *141:*180, 1981.
61. Snelling, C.E. and Jackson, S.H.: Blood studies of vitamin C during pregnancy, birth and early infancy. J. Pediatr., *14:*447, 1939.
62. Takano, K.T., Hizuka, N., and Shizuma, N.: The effects of growth hormone and fasting on the serum levels of somatomedin in rats and man determined by radioreceptor assay. Acta. Endocrinol. (Copenh), *85:*189, 1977.
63. Webb, G.: The use of hyperalimentation and chemotherapy in pregnancy. A case report. Am. J. Obstet. Gynecol., *137:*263, 1980.
64. Widdas, W.F.: Inability of diffusion to account for placental glucose transfer in the sheep and consideration of the kinetics of a possible carrier transfer. J. Physiol. (Lond), *118:*23, 1952.
65. Widdowson, E.M., Grabb, D.E., and Milver, R.D.G.: Cellular development of some human organs before birth. Arch. Dis. Child., *47:*652, 1972.
66. Widdowson, E.M., Southgate, D.A.T., and Hey, E.N.: Body composition of the fetus and infant. p. 169. In Visser, H.K.A., Ed.: Nutrition and Metabolism of the Fetus and Infant. Martinus Nijhoff, The Hague, 1979.
67. Young, M. and Prenton, M.A.: Maternal and fetal plasma amino acid concentrations during gestation and in retarded fetal growth. J. Obstet. Gynaecol. Br. Commonw., *76:*333, 1969.
68. Young, M. and Widdowson, E.: The influence of diets deficient in energy or in protein in conceptus weight and the placental transfer of non-metabolizable amino acid in the guinea pig. Biol. Neonate, *27:*184, 1975.

7

Pelvic Artery Embolization

Morton G. Glickman, M.D.

The emergence of arteriography as a well-defined subspecialty of radiology has resulted in rapid development and refinement of catheterization techniques that permit catheter placement in smaller and smaller arteries farther and farther from the aorta. Arteries such as the uterine branches of the internal iliac arteries can be catheterized safely and relatively quickly even in the presence of massive retroperitoneal hematomas which distort and displace pelvic vessels. Radiology teaching programs emphasize arteriography, and radiologists skilled in these new techniques are now widely available.

Arteriography is valuable not only in the diagnosis of vascular disease and parenchymal diseases associated with abnormal vascularity but also in the definitive therapy of otherwise uncontrollable hemorrhage. Therapeutic arteriography is effective in arresting massive hemorrhage from multiple small arterial bleeding sites such as those that result from erosive gastritis and from necrosis in malignant tumors. This is particularly important since surgical compression, packing, ligation, or even resection may not control diffuse hemorrhage from multiple sites.[26,27]

Recent publications of large series have documented the efficacy of arteriographic techniques in controlling hemorrhage in the pelvis from trauma and tumor.[2,14,16] The fact that only a few isolated case reports have appeared describing arteriographic control of postpartum hemorrhage suggests that therapeutic arteriography may be underutilized in obstetrical patients. Our experience at Yale University suggests that arteriography for demonstration of the site and nature of bleeding and for control of hemorrhage should be seriously considered for those postpartum patients with severe vaginal or internal pelvic hemorrhage that cannot be controlled by more conservative measures.[23]

Arteriographic techniques for arresting hemorrhage include infusion of pharmacologic vasoconstrictors directly into bleeding arteries, embolization of peripheral arteries by injection of particulate material, and obstruction of central arteries with expansile devices such as balloon catheters. Although vasoconstrictor infusion is probably safer than embolization, these agents are seldom successful in controlling hemorrhage in the pelvis.[2] While hemorrhage that arises from the internal or external iliac artery may require central arterial obstruction, embolization of peripheral vessels is probably the arteriographic method of choice in most obstetric patients with hemorrhage.

Internal iliac artery ligation and hysterectomy are surgical alternatives to arterial embolization but are associated with greater risk.[5,26] Hysterectomy definitively controls hemorrhage that is confined to the uterus but sacrifices reproductive capability. While pregnancy following embolization of uterine arteries has not been documented, it seems unlikely that prior embolization would influence the ability of a uterus to harbor and nourish a developing fetus. Successful pregnancies have been reported following surgical ligation of both internal iliac arteries.[20,29] Since the ovarian arteries have not required embolization in controlling pelvic hemorrhage in the experience acquired to date, subsequent ovulation should not be affected by embolization in the postpartum period. Thus attempts to control pelvic hemorrhage by arteriography and embolization may be justified prior to hysterectomy for preservation of reproductive potential.[5] If embolization fails to control hemorrhage, the surgical options remain. It is unlikely that prior embolization would increase the risk or technical difficulty of performing either internal iliac artery ligation or hysterectomy.

While the goals and the mechanisms of achieving hemostasis are the same for internal iliac artery ligation and pelvic artery embolization, the latter is probably more often effective, since emboli obstruct peripheral arterial branches whereas the internal iliac arteries are ligated near their origins. In a series of 17 patients with a variety of gynecologic diseases, Burchell[6] found that the rate of blood flow in the internal iliac arteries distal to ligation decreased by only 49 percent after unilateral surgical ligation and 48 percent after bilateral ligation. Although pulse pressure distal to the ligation decreased by 85 percent after a bilateral procedure, the arterial pressure remained higher than systemic venous pressure. The rich network of collaterals in the pelvis may thus sustain hemorrhage distal to the ligation, particularly in obstetrical patients because of the pelvic hypervascularity associated with pregnancy (Fig. 7-1). In two of three cases of postpartum hemorrhage successfully controlled by embolization that have been reported to date, prior internal iliac artery ligation had been unsuccessful. Internal iliac artery ligation may be technically difficult if the hematoma extends beyond the uterus into the retroperitoneal soft tissues[28] and may be dangerous, since incision of the retroperitoneum removes the tamponade effect that restricts venous bleeding.[24]

Particulate emboli injected through an arterial catheter lodge peripheral to major collaterals and induce thrombosis of small arteries at or near the site from which hemorrhage arises. Embolization, in comparison with ligation, increases the likelihood of ischemia in the distribution of the obstructed vessels, but if the size of the particulate emboli is carefully chosen and if absorbable material is used for embolization, small mural collaterals peripheral to the site of obstruction are capable of maintaining viability of critical organs such as the bladder and rectum until the arteries recanalize. Although embolization remains feasible after internal iliac artery ligation, prior surgical interruption of these vessels increases the technical difficulty

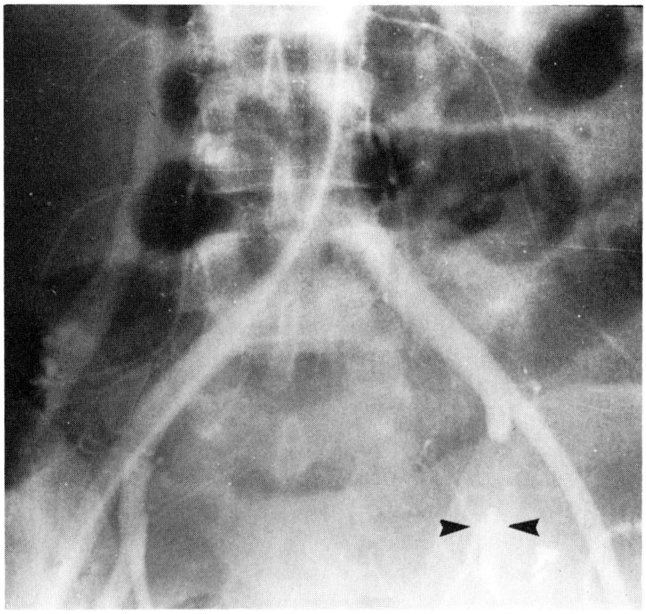

Fig. 7-1 Reconstitution of the internal iliac artery following surgical ligation. The left internal iliac artery was ligated in an attempt to control pelvic hemorrhage that followed cesarean section and hysterectomy (same patient as Fig. 7-4). The Aortogram shows the opacified stump of the internal iliac artery proximal to the site of ligation. Although the lumen is completely occluded, the bifurcation of the internal iliac artery is reconstituted distal to the site of ligation (arrows) via collateral circulation. Since the injection of contrast medium ended 1 s before this film, very little contrast medium remains to opacify the distal aorta. The collateral circulation that reconstitutes the internal iliac artery must have been immediately available, since this aortogram was performed within 2 h of the internal iliac artery ligation.

of the arteriographic procedure by eliminating the most direct route of access to the bleeding sites.[12,23]

DIAGNOSTIC ARTERIOGRAPHY

Embolization must be preceded by diagnostic arteriography in order to demonstrate the arterial anatomy and identify any anatomic variants, and to evaluate the patency of potential collateral circulation. If the site of bleeding can be identified, embolization can be limited to only those arteries from which hemorrhage arises. The arteriographic sign that identifies the site of arterial bleeding is extravasation of contrast medium from the arterial lumen (Fig. 7-2A and B).

Nusbaum and Baum[21] investigated the minimum rate of arterial bleeding that can be demonstrated by arteriography. They surgically transected small arteries in the gastrointestinal tracts of dogs, mechanically controlled the rate of bleeding, and performed aortography and either celiac, superior mesenteric, or inferior mesenteric arteriography. They reported that hemorrhage at the rate of 5 ml/min was necessary for demonstration by aortography, but with selective injections bleeding at rates as low as 0.5 ml/min could be consistently detected. Although subsequent authors citing these data have suggested that selective arteriography in humans is equally sensitive, this has not been documented experimentally and is probably not the case. Because of the size difference between dogs and humans, the differences between controlled

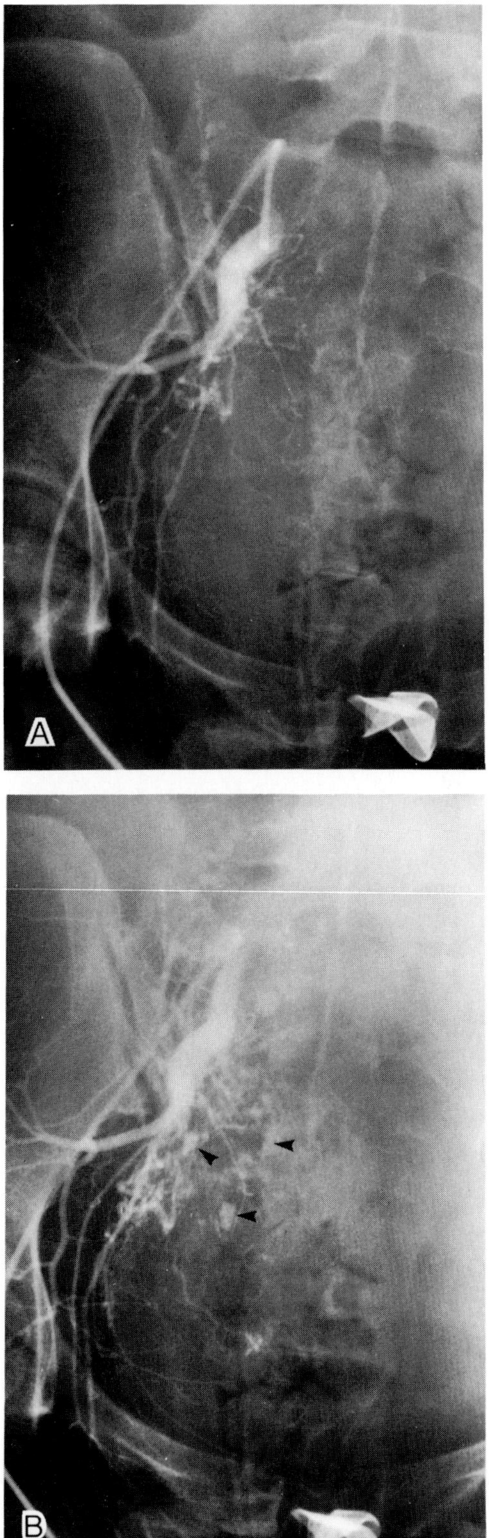

Fig. 7-2 Internal iliac artery embolization for postpartum hemorrhage. A 32-year-old woman with hypofibrinogenemia resulting from liver disease had severe hemorrhage following vaginal delivery of a full-term infant. The hemorrhage did not respond to intravenous and intrauterine oxytocin, Methergine, intrauterine lavage, vaginal packing, dilatation and curettage, intrauterine packing, and repair of surgical and vaginal lacerations. Arteriographic embolization was performed in preference to hysterectomy in an attempt to preserve reproductive capability. (A) Selective injection of the right internal iliac artery shows marked diminution in size of the arteries supplying the pelvis, a result of vasoconstriction due to hemorrhage and vasoconstrictor therapy. (B) Film obtained 3 s later demonstrates extravasation of contrast medium from multiple sites (arrowheads). The fact that extravasation was delayed until the parenchymal phase of the arteriogram suggests that the hemorrhage arises from small peripheral arterial branches. Because of the vasoconstriction the catheter could not be readily manipulated into the anterior division of the internal iliac artery for selective embolization. Consequently, another catheter was inserted through the left femoral artery, and selective catheterization of the anterior division of the right internal iliac artery was achieved. Gelfoam particles were prepared by shaving a Gelfoam pad with a scalpel blade and suspending the shavings in saline. After injection of a total of 1.2 ml of Gelfoam suspension in small increments, no further extravasation was visible at fluoroscopy, and vaginal hemorrhage ceased.

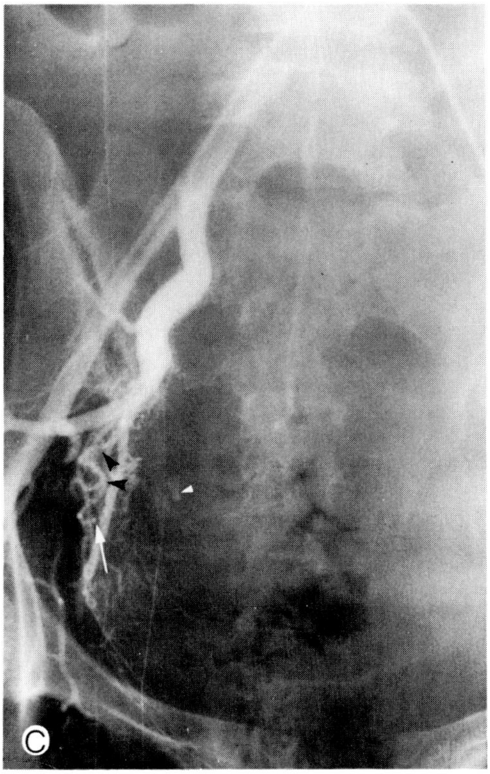

Fig. 7-2 (continued) (C) Subsequent injection of the right internal iliac artery shows that the degree of vasoconstriction has diminished. The main trunk of the uterine artery (black arrowheads) remains patent, but the peripheral portion has been obstructed within the broad ligament (white arrow). Only one small arterial branch (white arrowhead) is opacified by collaterals in the uterine wall. No extravasation is present.

experiments in dogs under general anesthesia and unanesthetized patients, the physiologic differences between hemorrhage from surgically transected vessels and clinical hemorrhage, and a variety of other variables, arteriographic detection of hemorrhage at a rate of 0.5 ml/min in human patients is unlikely.

The sensitivity of arteriography in demonstrating small vessels and extravasation also varies with the location of the catheter (Fig. 7-3). The closer the catheter is to the bleeding site, the more sensitive the arteriogram will be in demonstrating pelvic arterial anatomy and extravasation. Since postpartum hemorrhage most commonly arises from the uterus, the cervix, and the vagina, the diagnostic arteriogram should begin with catheterization of one or both internal iliac arteries. The catheter, whenever possible, should be advanced into the anterior division of the internal iliac artery so that the injection will optimally opacify the uterine, vaginal, and internal pudendal branches of the internal iliac artery.

In most patients with hemorrhage severe enough to warrant arteriography, visible extravasation can be anticipated on the diagnostic arteriogram. Occasionally, however, extravasation may not be visible even in the presence of continued active hemorrhage. Although the absence of visible extravasation does not preclude successful control of hemorrhage by embolization (Fig. 7-3), technical maneuvers to improve sensitivity, such as more selective catheterization, are warranted in order to permit more selective embolization.

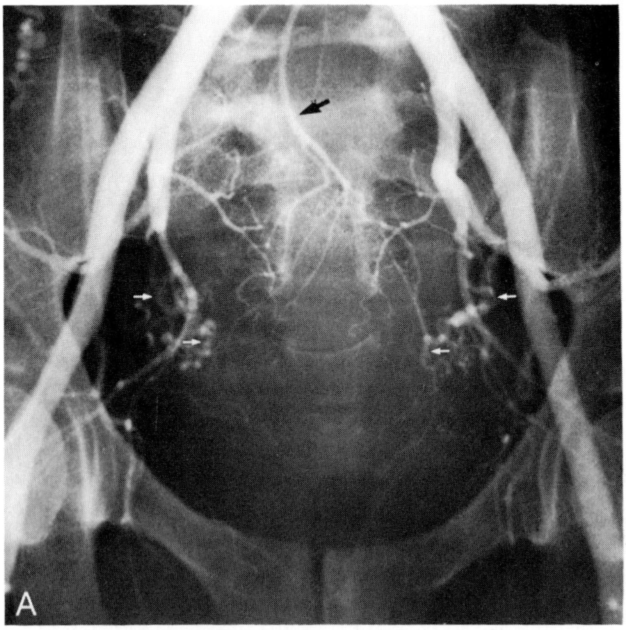

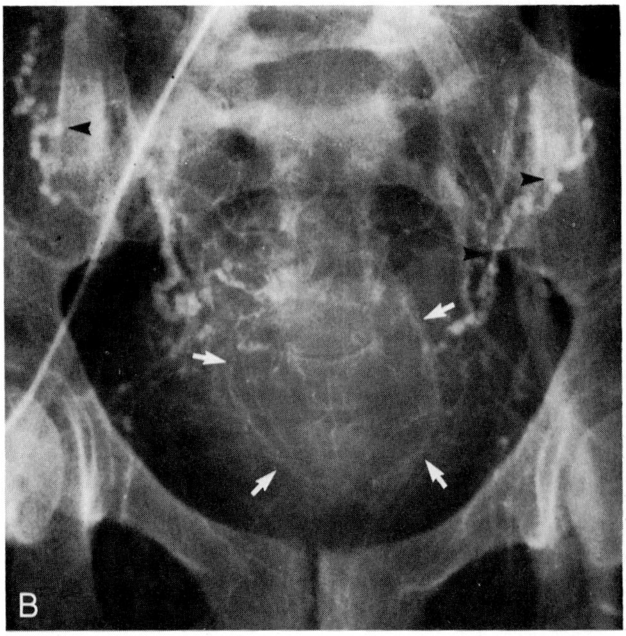

Fig. 7-3 Postpartum hemorrhage 1 week following normal vaginal delivery. Hemorrhage could not be controlled by repeated curettage, intramuscular Methergine, intravenous oxytocin, and sharp dilatation and curettage. After transfusion with 5 units of blood, arteriography was performed. (A) Injection into the abdominal aorta at the level of the renal arteries shows large, tortuous uterine arteries (white arrows) and the rectal branch of the inferior mesenteric artery (black arrow). (B) After 4 s the contrast medium has washed out of the central arterial branches. The distal segments of the dilated ovarian arteries (black arrowheads) are opacified, and rectal artery branches opacify the rectal wall (white arrows). In spite of the hypervascularity of the uterus, however, the uterine artery branches in the corpus were not opacified until the catheter was selectively advanced into the internal iliac artery.

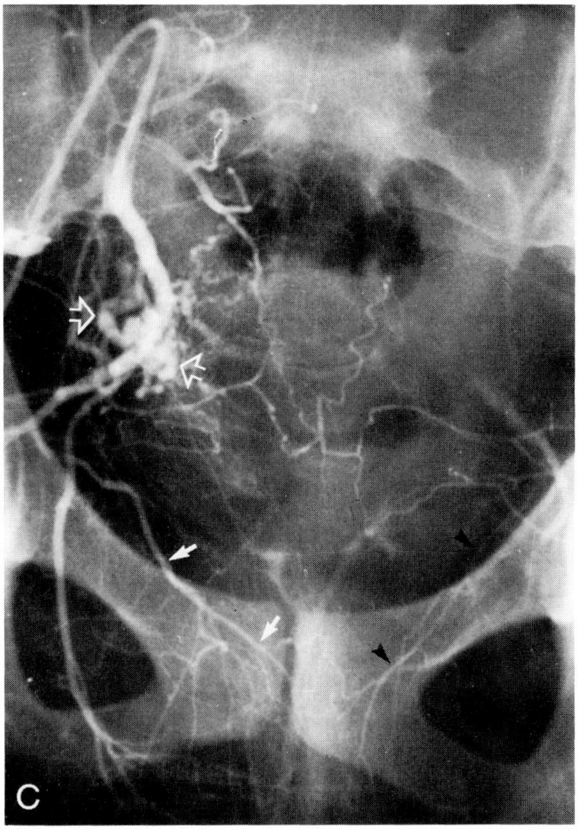

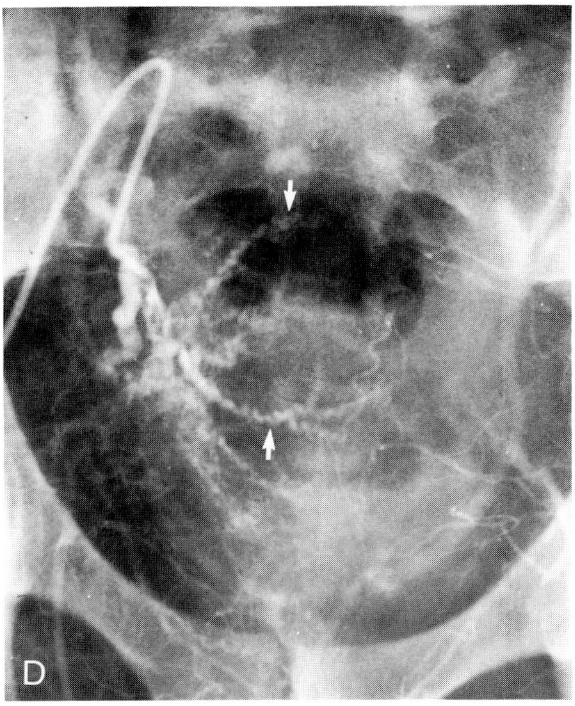

Fig. 7-3 (continued) (C) Selective injection of the right internal iliac artery in the arterial phase shows denser opacification of the uterine artery (open white arrows) and the superior vesical artery (white arrows) than was achieved by aortography. The pressure of injection transmitted to the bladder wall opacifies the left superior vesical artery (black arrowheads) as well. (D) In the parenchymal phase, uterine artery branches are opacified around the circumference of the uterus (arrowheads) as well as within the corpus. Although extravasation of contrast medium could not be identified, brisk vaginal bleeding continued, and Gelfoam emboli were injected selectively into the anterior division of the right internal iliac artery.

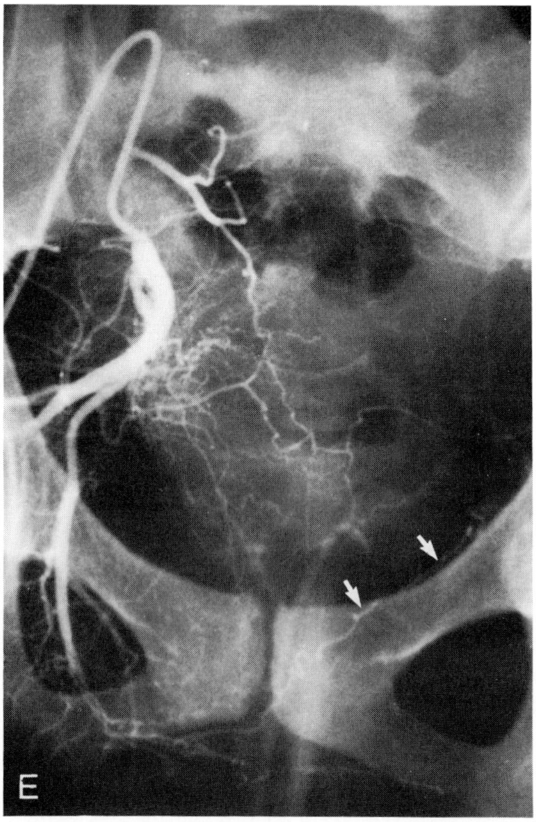

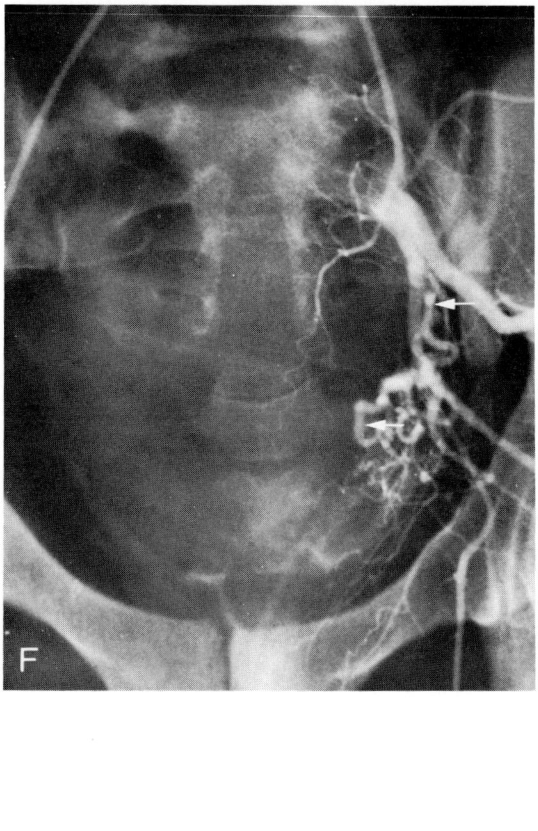

Fig. 7-3 (continued) (E) Following injection of 0.4 ml of suspended Gelfoam shavings, the uterine artery and the right superior vesical artery are no longer opacified. However, collateral flow via pudendal branches opacifies the left superior vesical artery (white arrows). The abundance of collateral circulation minimizes the likelihood of ischemic injury to pelvic organs such as the bladder. (F) The catheter was then advanced over the aortic bifurcation into the left internal iliac artery, and contrast medium injection opacifies the uterine (arrows), vesical, and muscular arteries. The catheter was advanced selectively into the origin of the left uterine artery and Gelfoam emboli were injected. Following embolization vaginal bleeding stopped. (Reprinted from Pais, S.O., Glickman, M.G., Schwartz, P. et al.: Embolization of pelvic arteries for control of postpartum hemorrhage. Obstet. Gynecol., *55,* 754, 1980, by permission of the American College of Obstetricians and Gynecologists.

Technique

Many types of equipment are commercially available which are suitable for arteriography but vary in their levels of sophistication. Since extravasated contrast medium is usually quite dense, diagnostic arteriography and documentation of the degree of obstruction following embolization do not require optimal image resolution. Consequently, any radiographic equipment capable of performing rapid serial filming and of recording images suitable for routine arteriography is suitable for embolization procedures. However, since the diagnostic accuracy, safety, and efficacy of embolization are improved by selective catheter placement in specific arterial branches as close as possible to the bleeding site, the quality of the image-intensifying fluoroscope may be quite important.

Precise catheter manipulation requires optimal resolution of the fluoroscopic image. Cesium iodide phosphors in the image intensifier system convert a higher percentage of the incident x-rays to light than the standard phosphors in older image-intensifying fluoroscopes. Cesium iodide phosphors produce greater image contrast and therefore improve image resolution.

Catheter manipulation is also simplified if the image intensifier is equipped with dual-field sizes. The field size of the standard fluoroscope is 9 in, and recently developed image intensifiers are capable of viewing fields as large as 14 in in diameter. Image intensifiers capable of dual-field imaging permit pushbutton conversion to smaller field sizes, such as 6 in in diameter. In the 6-in mode the fluoroscope views a field only 6 in in diameter, but the smaller field fills the viewing screen of the television monitor, producing a magnified image with improved resolution that permits more precise catheter control.

If the fluoroscope is equipped with a spot-film camera, high-resolution films can be obtained without moving the patient. Spot films instantly document the changes in the catheter position during the various steps in the embolization procedure and the degree of occlusion achieved after each injection of emboli without requiring rapid-sequence filming and multiple radiographs. A spot-film device therefore reduces the time required for the procedure and the radiation exposure of the patient.

Femoral artery puncture is the simplest and safest route of access to the vascular system. All the arteries that supply the pelvis can be selectively catheterized by this route. Although both the ipsilateral and contralateral internal iliac arteries can usually be catheterized from either femoral artery, occasionally bilateral femoral puncture and catheterization may reduce the time required for catheter manipulation and simplify the procedure (Fig. 7-2).

If internal iliac arteriography fails to demonstrate extravasation, aortography should be performed. Injection of the abdominal aorta at, or slightly distal to, the level of the renal arteries, with rapid sequence filming of the pelvis, demonstrates the location and course of all the arteries that supply the pelvis, including the lumbar and gonadal arteries, the inferior mesenteric artery, and the pudendal branches of the femoral arteries, as well as the branches of the internal iliacs. After diagnostic arteriography demonstrates the site of extravasation, the artery from which hemorrhage arises is selectively catheterized and emboli are injected.

Placement of the emboli is fluoroscopically monitored with injections of small volumes of contrast medium. When the target vessel is completely obstructed and extravasation from that artery is no longer visible, the catheter is moved to the contralateral internal iliac artery for injection of contrast medium to opacify the collateral circulation. When the primary artery supplying the bleeding site is obstructed, collateral vessels can immediately dilate and sustain hemorrhage (Figs. 7-1 and 7-4). Additional selective arterial catheterization and embolization should be performed if bleeding from collaterals is detected.

Selective injection of the contralateral internal iliac artery is never sufficient to document the absence of further extravasation without aortography to demonstrate all potential collateral circulation to the pelvis (Fig. 7-4). Even arteries that do not normally supply the pelvis, such as the superior mesenteric artery, may sustain hemorrhage in the pelvis if prior surgery or mesenteric inflammatory disease has established potential collateral arteries through adhesions to pelvic viscera. The arteriographic procedure is terminated only when a final aortogram shows no further extravasation.[27]

Pelvic arteriography and embolization can often be completed in less than 2 h.[27] However, if hemorrhage from collateral circulation requires embolization, as can be anticipated following internal iliac artery ligation, the procedure may be prolonged by several hours. Vital signs, urine output, and continuous electrocardiography should be carefully monitored throughout the procedure. Since contrast medium results in osmotic diuresis, fluid and blood replacement must be carefully attended.

Embolic Materials

A variety of substances have been used for arteriographic embolization with success and documented safety. The embolic material which is probably most appropriate for treating hemorrhage from small vessels of the pelvis, however, is surgical gelatin sponge (Gelfoam). The safety of this substance as an internal foreign body has been established by many years of use as a hemostatic material during surgery.[17] Gelfoam injected into the vascular system mechanically obstructs arteries and induces thrombosis. Although a local inflammatory reaction develops in the arterial wall, the arteritis is mild and self-limited.[3,30] Gelfoam is broken down and removed from the vascular system by phagocytosis within 1 to 3 weeks after injection in humans and in several animal species.[15] Consequently, the risk of migration or late infection of the foreign body is small.

Since pelvic hemorrhage in obstetrical patients results from an acute, self-limited event which is followed by healing, the hemostasis provided by Gelfoam embolization should be sufficient to avoid recurrence of hemorrhage. After Gelfoam is metabolized, the embolized arteries may remain permanently closed if the remaining thrombus organizes, or alternatively the lumen may be reestablished.[3] The possibility of recanalization and restoration of normal blood flow to the affected viscera makes absorbable material preferable to permanent emboli in therapy of benign conditions.

Gelfoam is readily available, inexpensive, and easy to use. A Gelfoam pad is cut with scissors or scalpel blade to prepare particles of the appropriate size. Particle size is determined by reference to the size and appearance of the bleeding arteries on the diagnostic arteriogram. An appropriate number of particles are placed in a 1-ml syringe, suspended in saline or contrast medium, and injected through the arteriographic catheter. Injection of a small volume of contrast medium is then observed fluoroscopically to determine whether extravasation persists. If injection shows continued extravasation, additional emboli are injected.

Autologous blood clot has also been used as an embolic material for pelvic hemorrhage, and some authors consider it preferable to Gelfoam in patients with benign disease.[16] Firm clot can be prepared for embolization even in patients with coagulopathies by heating the blood sample or by adding ϵ-aminocarproic acid or thrombin. Autologous clot usually undergoes lysis earlier than Gelfoam, often within 48 h of injection, and this minimizes the likelihood of ischemic complications.[22] However, blood clot is more difficult to handle than Gelfoam and particle size cannot be as easily controlled. Furthermore, the marked pelvic hypervascularity in obstetrical patients may require a longer-lived embolic material than blood clot for definitive control of hemorrhage.

Maximum size of particulate emboli is limited by the diameter of the lumen of the catheter through which the emboli are injected. If the optimal site of obstruction is located at a point where the lumen of the artery is larger than the lumen of the arteriographic catheter, several embolic materials and mechanical devices are available that enlarge after they leave the catheter.

The most commonly used device for obstructing arteries that are larger than the lumen of the catheter is a stainless steel coil to which Dacron strands are attached (Fig. 7-5).[1,9] The coils are straightened so that they can pass through the catheter. They are pushed through the catheter by a standard arteriographic guidewire. When the embolus emerges from the tip of the catheter, it assumes a coiled shape. These devices are commercially available in different coil diameters so that the appropriate diameter can be selected for the vessel to be obstructed. Careful choice of coil diameter permits localization of the coil at the proper site along the vessel. Once injected, the coil can be advanced farther distally by pushing it with a guidewire. The Dacron fibers attached to the coil are thrombogenic, and shortly after placement the coil is surrounded by thrombus that obstructs the vessel lumen. These are permanent foreign bodies, and are inexpensive and readily available.

Isobutyl cyanoacrylate, a rapidly hardening liquid tissue adhesive, polymerizes on contact with electrolyte solutions such as blood. Since it firmly and permanently adheres to tissue even when it polymerizes in a liquid medium such as blood, cyanoacrylate is an effective embolic agent for vessels larger than the arteriographic catheter.[8,10] The catheter lumen is first filled with a nonelectrolyte solution such as D5W and then liquid cyanoacrylate is injected, followed by another bolus of D5W. Priming the system with D5W prevents polymerization until the adhesive leaves the catheter.

Cyanoacrylate produces a nonmetabolizable, permanent cast of the vessel lumen just distal to the catheter tip. The material can be diluted so that it polymerizes more slowly if the optimal site of obstruction is peripheral to the catheter tip. Because polymerization may occur at a time when a portion of the adhesive remains in contact with the catheter, causing adhesion of the catheter to the embolized artery, cyanoacrylate embolization should be performed with a coaxial catheter system. The catheter through which the adhesive is injected is passed through the lumen of a

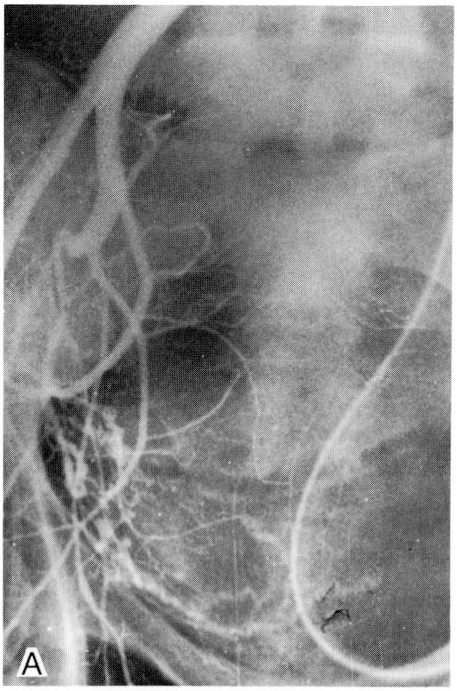

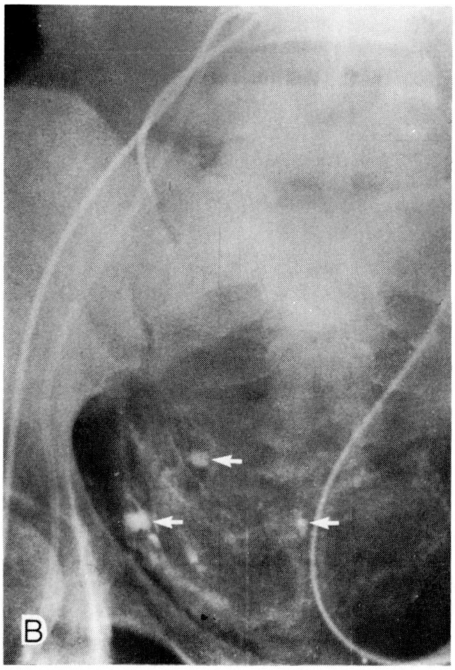

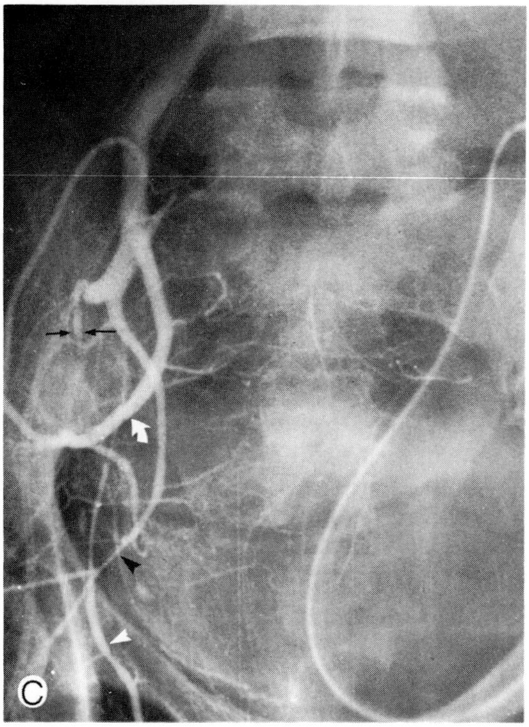

Fig. 7-4 Pelvic hemorrhage following surgical removal of extrauterine fetus. A 38-year-old woman underwent cesarean section because of preeclampsia at 38 weeks of gestation. An unsuspected extrauterine fetus was discovered within the abdominal cavity. The placenta appeared to derive its arterial supply from the left internal iliac artery via the broad ligament. The fetus was removed and hysterectomy was performed but massive hemorrhage arose from placental insertion sites. Multiple individual bleeding sites and then the left internal iliac artery were ligated, but hemorrhage continued following surgery, and arteriography was performed. (A) Right internal iliac artery injection shows generalized vasoconstriction as a result of continued hemorrhage. Tortuous pelvic visceral branches extend across the midline to the left hemipelvis. (B) At 4 s after the end of the arterial injection, several collections of extravasated contrast medium (arrows) indicate active bleeding in the right hemipelvis. The catheter was advanced into the orifice of the internal iliac artery branch from which the extravasation arose and Gelfoam shavings were injected. (C) Postembolization injection shows the stump of the embolized uterine artery (arrows). The obturator artery (white arrowhead), the inferior gluteal artery (black arrowhead), and the superior gluteal artery (curved arrow) remain patent.

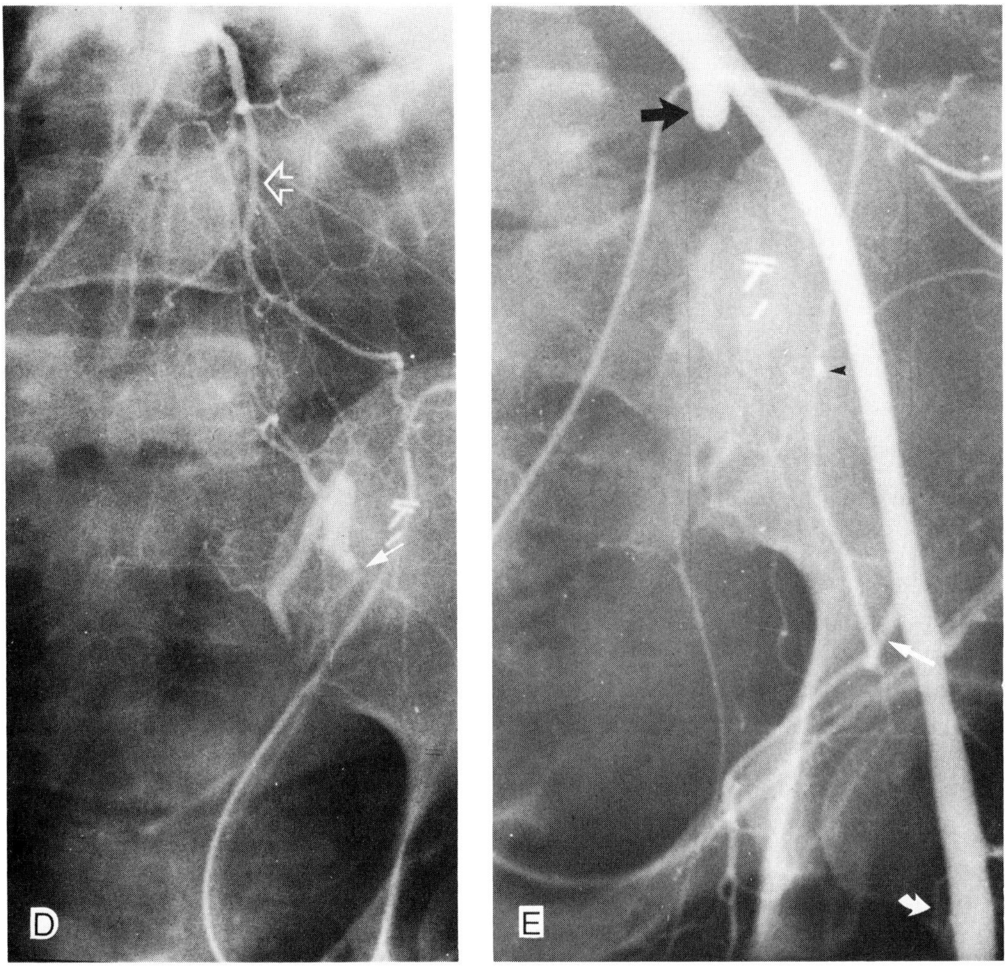

Fig. 7-4 (continued) Aortography showed reconstitution of the left internal iliac artery distal to the ligation site (Fig. 7-1), primarily via the left third lumbar artery. (D) Selective injection of the left third lumbar artery (open white arrow) shows the reconstituted left internal iliac artery branches. The anterior division of the internal iliac artery, which normally supplies the pelvic viscera, abruptly narrows (white arrow), but small pelvic visceral branches remain patent. Extravasation from these branches was identified on late films. The catheter was advanced beyond the origin of the branch that supplies the spinal cord and Gelfoam emboli were injected. (E) Aortogram following lumbar artery embolization shows the ligated stump of the left internal iliac artery (black arrow), the inferior epigastric branch of the external iliac artery (white arrow), and the pudendal branch of the common femoral artery (curved arrow). A small site of contrast medium extravasation (arrowhead) arises from the inferior epigastric artery.

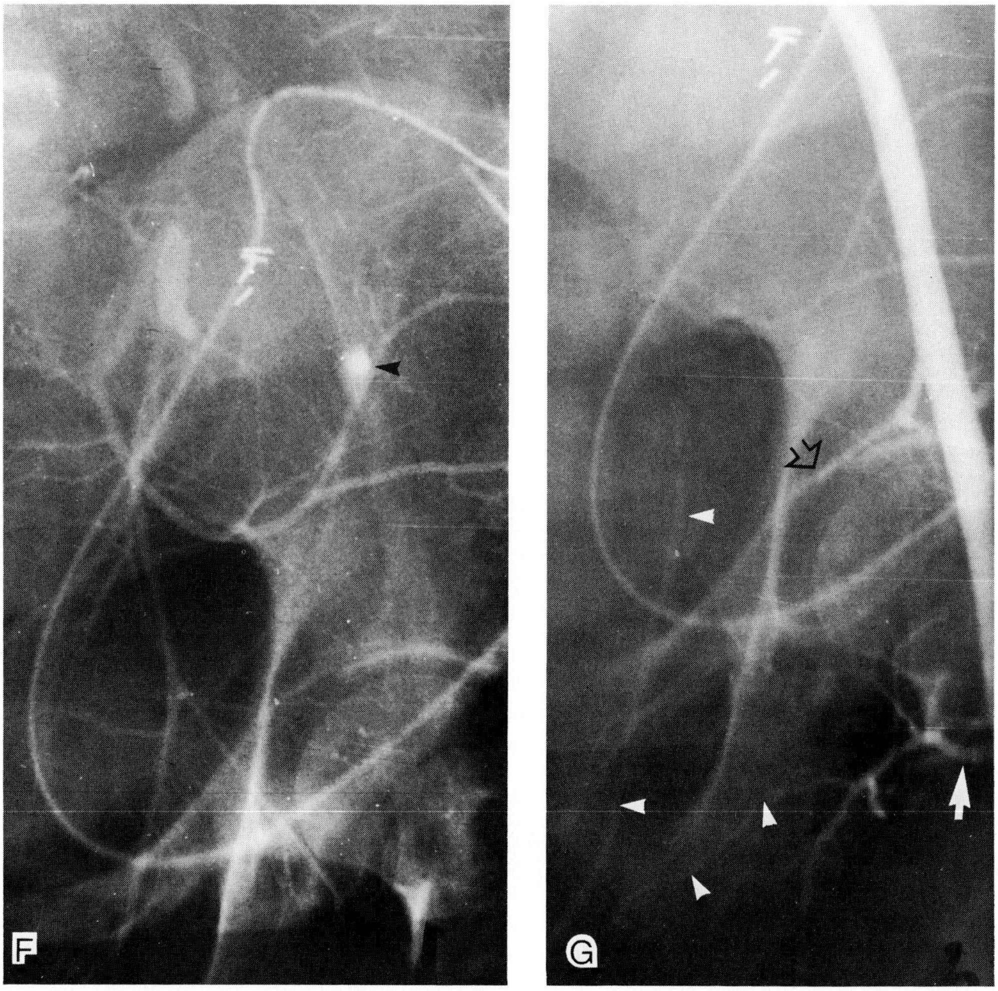

Fig. 7-4 (continued) (F) At 3 s after the end of injection, contrast medium is no longer present in the central arteries, but the left internal iliac artery branches have again been reconstituted, this time via the inferior epigastric and pudendal arteries. The extravasation from the inferior epigastric artery (arrowhead) overlies a branch of the superior gluteal artery. The relationships of some of the vessels and the surgical drain to the bones and the surgical clips have changed slightly because of patient movement between (E) and (F). The inferior epigastric artery was selectively catheterized and embolized with Gelfoam pledgets. (G) Injection of the left external iliac artery shows that the inferior epigastric artery has been obstructed about 2 cm distal to its origin (open arrow). The pudendal branch (white arrow) of the superficial femoral artery, however, has dilated and reconstitutes the obturator artery (white arrowheads).

Fig. 7-4 (continued) (H) After another 2 s, the internal iliac artery branches (arrows) distal to the surgical ligation have been reconstituted via the obturator artery (arrowheads). However, neither the uterine nor the vesical arteries are opacified and no extravasation is present. Aortography and superior mesenteric arteriography showed that only the inferior mesenteric artery provided additional collateral supply to the pelvic viscera. (I) Selective inferior mesenteric artery injection shows the superior rectal artery and its branches that surround the rectum (white arrowheads). Collateral circulation via the hemorrhoidal arteries has reconstituted several pelvic arteries, but no extravasation is present. This injection documents a collateral route by which the viscera in the right hemipelvis can be perfused until the embolized arteries recanalize or new collaterals from internal iliac branches develop. Although the patient's postoperative course was stormy as a result of complications of prolonged shock, the pelvic bleeding was clinically controlled and did not recur. The patient survived and has suffered no detectable long-term sequelae from this procedure. (Reprinted from Pais, S.O., Glickman, M.G., Schwartz, P. et al.: Embolization of pelvic arteries for control of postpartum hemorrhage. Obstet. Gynecol., 55, 754, 1980, by permission of the American College of Obstetricians and Gynecologists.

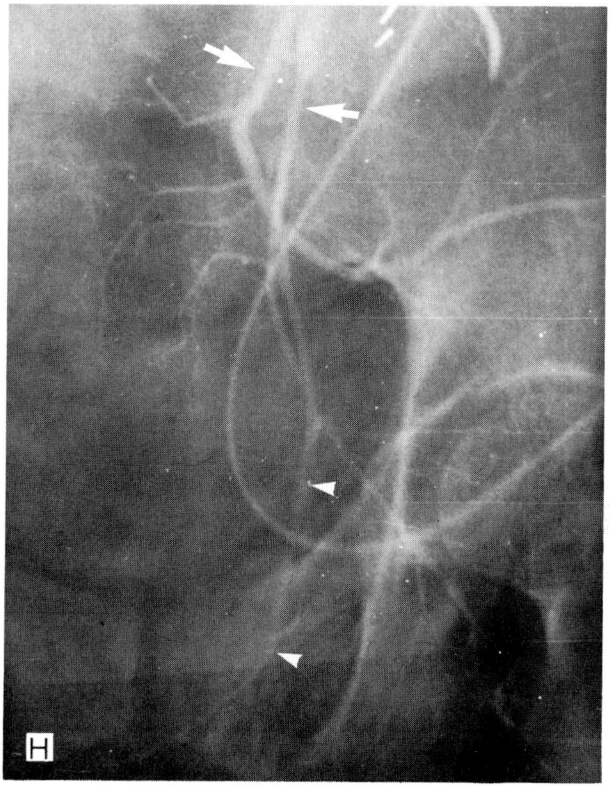

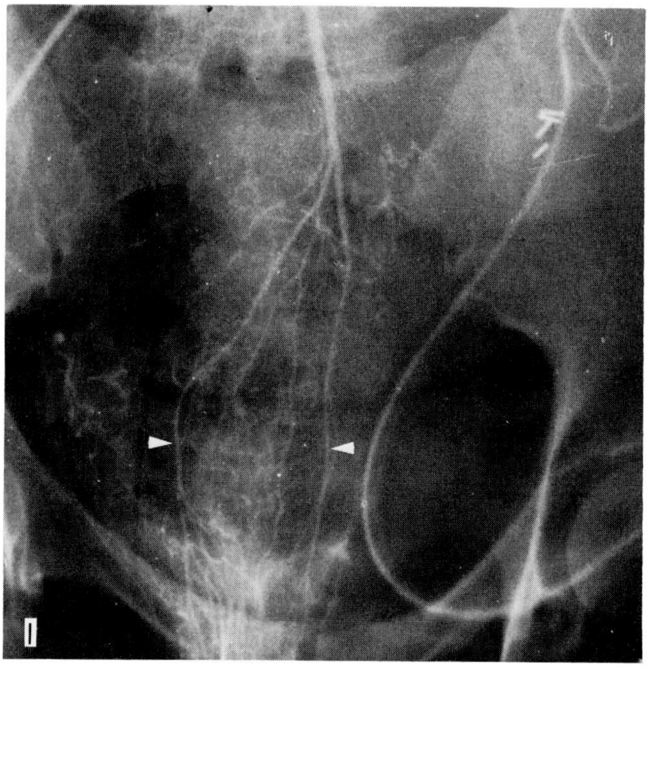

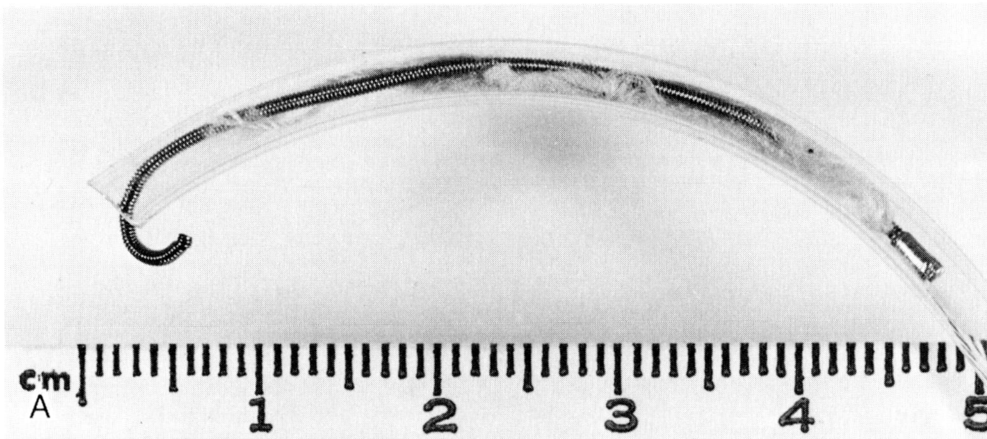

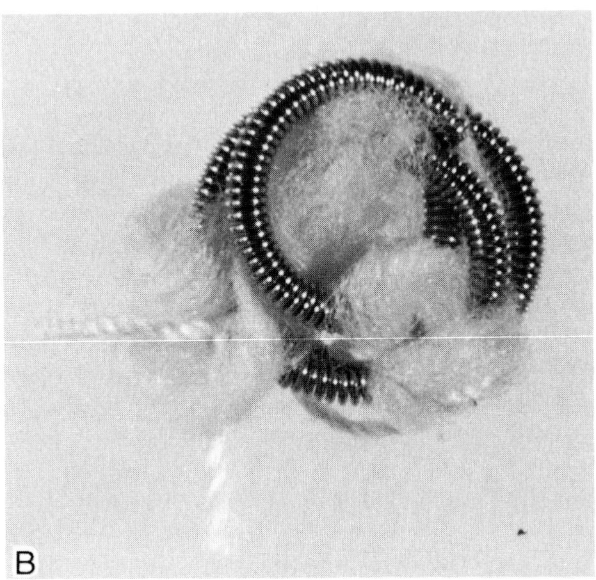

Fig. 7-5 Stainless steel coil embolus consisting of a 3 cm length of an arteriographic guidewire to which Dacron strands have been attached. The guidewire has been treated so that it assumes a coil shape 8 mm in diameter. (A) For purposes of illustration the device has been threaded into a transparent plastic catheter. In practice the straightened embolus is pushed through an arteriographic catheter with a guidewire. (B) After emerging from the arteriographic catheter into the artery to be embolized, the device assumes a coiled shape. The Dacron strands interweave the coil and induce thrombosis.

larger catheter. The inner catheter tip is advanced beyond the tip of the outer catheter. After embolization the inner catheter is removed, leaving the outer one in place. Even if the lumen of the inner catheter is obstructed by premature polymerization of adhesive, it can be removed and replaced by a new catheter with a minimum of manipulation.[10]

The major disadvantage of cyanoacrylate embolization in nonmalignant disease is that its long-term fate in human tissue has not been established.[15,31] Consequently it should only be used in emergency situations for which more thoroughly tested materials are not suitable. At the date of this writing it is regulated as an experimental agent and is only available by special arrangement with the manufacturer.

Since permanent vascular occlusion is usually not necessary to control hemorrhage in obstetrical patients, the best device for obstructing arteries larger than the diameter of the angiographic catheter may be a double-lumen balloon catheter.[32] These commercially available catheters have a latex balloon attached to a polyethylene arteriographic catheter which has two parallel lumina. One channel communicates with the balloon and is used for inflation and deflation. The other lumen opens at the catheter tip for injection of contrast medium into the artery distal to the balloon. The polyethylene catheter has excellent curve memory and can be shaped to permit arteriographic manipulation and catheterization of the vessel to be obstructed (Fig. 7-6).

Once in place, the balloon is inflated, and the catheter is taped or sutured to the skin of the groin. After 2 or 3 days the balloon is deflated and the catheter removed. Depending on the length of time that the catheter is left in place, the resultant thrombus may undergo lysis and recanalization may occur. An indwelling arterial catheter is usually well tolerated for 2 or 3 days. Although infection may occur, the frequency of this complication with indwelling catheters is low. If infection does occur, the catheter should be immediately removed; the response to antibiotic therapy is usually prompt.[7]

RESULTS

Arteriographic embolization was first introduced as a means of controlling gastrointestinal arterial hemorrhage in 1972.[25] The technique was soon applied to hemorrhage in the pelvis, and a few months later successful embolic control of pelvic hematomas resulting from trauma was reported.[18] Thereafter, small series and case reports described successful control of hemorrhage in various organ systems, as well as occasional complications. Most of these early reports suggested that because of lack of extensive experience with this technique and the potential risk of ischemic complications, embolization should only be attempted in patients who were poor surgical risks or as a last resort after all other measures failed. It is only recently that large enough series have been published to begin to truly judge the merits of this technique.

Jander et al.[14] reported successful control of arterial hemorrhage by embolization in 51 of 55 patients (92.7 percent). Nineteen of these patients were bleeding from the gastrointestinal tract, but most of the remainder were bleeding into the pelvis as a result of trauma or tumors. Two patients (3.6 percent) died of necrosis of bowel segments, apparently as a direct result of the embolization procedure. Four patients (7.2 percent) suffered significant morbidity, including one with necrosis of a portion of the jejunum, which required surgical resection. Embolization in the gastrointestinal tract is more hazardous than in the pelvis because of more limited collateral circulation. Among those patients treated with embolization of pelvic arteries in the series by Jander et al., the reported complications were one case of femoral artery thrombosis, one patient with decreased quality of erections, and one case of sciatic pain. There were no deaths associated with embolization of pelvic arteries. In their review of the literature these authors found 288 patients with arterial hemorrhage treated by embolization, with successful control of hemorrhage in 265 (92 percent), 5 deaths (1.7 percent), and 7 other complications (2.4 percent).

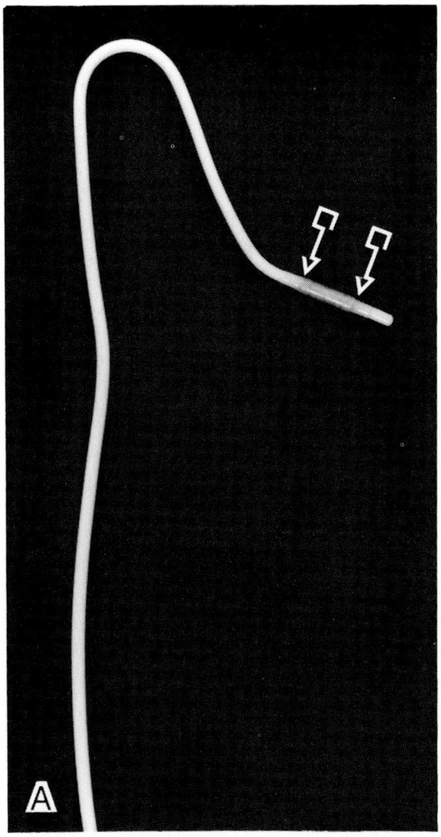

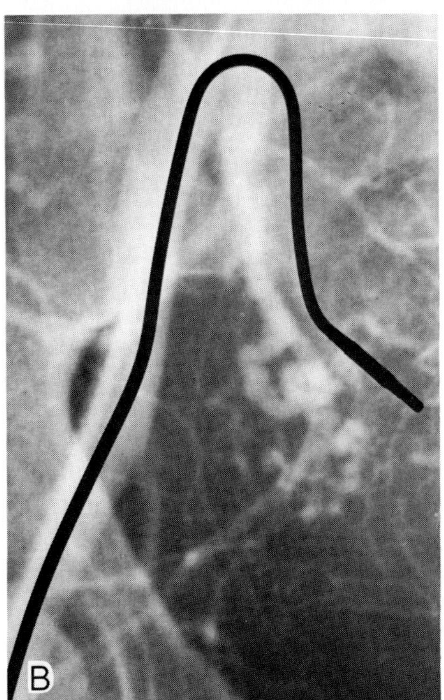

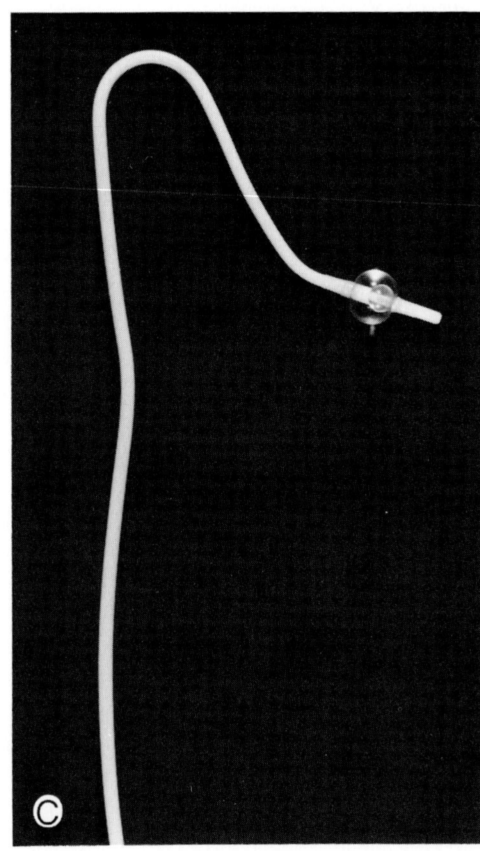

Fig. 7-6 Double-lumen balloon catheter. (A) The catheter has been curved by using steam to the appropriate shape for catheterization of an ipsilateral uterine artery. The uninflated balloon lies flat against the shaft of the catheter to permit percutaneous insertion. (B) The balloon catheter is superimposed on a radiograph showing opacified external and internal iliac arteries. The carefully shaped catheter will permit selective catheterization of the uterine artery with minimum manipulation and radiation exposure. (C) Balloon inflated. Once the catheter is properly positioned in the artery, the inflated balloon obstructs the lumen. Its position can be documented by injecting contrast medium through the catheter, since the catheter tip is distal to the balloon.

Control of hemorrhage was achieved in 26 of 28 patients treated with embolization of pelvic arteries at Massachusetts General Hospital.[2,19] These patients were bleeding as a result of trauma or following surgery for total hip replacement. In this group there were two complications, both a result of reflux of particulate emboli back along the catheter into nontarget arteries, but no deaths. The authors reported that both complications resulted from inexperience in the use of emboli. The frequency of complications due to reflux of emboli can be minimized by awareness of the likelihood of reflux and careful attention to a few technical precautions (see below).

Lang[16] reported 46 patients treated by arteriographic embolization for hemorrhage in the pelvis. The bleeding was controlled in all, but two had later recurrence of hemorrhage, one from a recurrent arteriovenous malformation and one from a recurrent tumor. Four patients in this series developed renal failure, two presumably as a result of contrast medium toxicity related to the arteriographic procedure. Contrast medium toxicity is also a potentially avoidable complication.

Thus, massive pelvic hemorrhage can be controlled by arteriographic embolization in experienced hands with a very high likelihood of success. Simple catheter manipulation techniques have been developed to the point that physicians well trained in arteriography can successfully catheterize the internal iliac arteries and pelvic collateral arteries relatively quickly in virtually all patients.

Although no obstetrical patients are included in the series quoted above, three case reports have documented that arteriographic embolization can successfully control postpartum hemorrhage.[12,23] Catheterization of pelvic arteries should be easier in obstetrical patients than in those with pelvic trauma or tumors because of the absence of significant atherosclerosis and the enlargement of vessels due to pregnancy. Therefore, selective catheterization of uterine arteries should be possible in most cases, and this should minimize both the volume of tissue rendered ischemic and the frequency of reflux of emboli into nontarget vessels. If this proves to be true, the frequency of complications in the treatment of postpartum hemorrhage will probably be shown to be less than that in the treatment of hemorrhage from trauma or tumors.

Although the series reviewed above document significant complications, in view of the life-threatening nature of postpartum hemorrhage the small number of adverse sequelae associated with embolization seems to be acceptable. The low complication rate can be further reduced by careful choice of embolic material and particle size and by placing the catheter as close to the bleeding site as possible before injecting emboli.

RADIATION EXPOSURE

The amount of radiation exposure during an embolization procedure is difficult to estimate since it varies with the number of vessels that require catheterization, the degree of difficulty in catheterizing specific arteries, the number of films required to verify that the bleeding has been controlled, the degree to which the patient is able to cooperate, and numerous other factors. However, at best arteriography involves the use of more radiation than any other diagnostic radiographic procedure, with exposures measured in rads rather than millirads. Although life-threatening problems such as postpartum hemorrhage justify the relatively high radiation exposure, a number of measures can be taken to reduce this as much as possible.

All image intensifiers and x-ray tubes are equipped with collimators that reduce the volume of tissue exposed to the x-ray beam and control the size of the field of view. Tight collimation, reducing the field size as much as is compatible with diagnostic accuracy, limits scattered radiation, reduces patient exposure, and improves the level of resolution of the image. The following precautions will further reduce patient exposure: (1) use of a 6-in fluoroscopic field wherever possible; (2) use of individual spot films rather than rapid-sequence filming to document proper catheter position; (3) intermittent rather than continuous fluoroscopy during catheter manipulation (this requires a high level of skill and experience on the part of the radiologist); (4) use of videotape to record fluoroscopic test injections, which permits immediate playback at slow speed and often avoids the necessity for repeated injections and fluoroscopic viewing to document accurate catheter placement.

COMPLICATIONS

The complications of arteriographic embolization in patients with arterial hemorrhage are caused by one of three mechanisms: (1) Embolization may cause ischemia or necrosis of the tissue in the distribution of the obstructed artery, especially if the collateral circulation has been previously compromised or if emboli are deposited in capillaries or precapillary arterioles distal to collateral arteries. (2) Emboli may reflux back along the shaft of the catheter to reach critical, nontarget arteries, causing ischemia or necrosis of tissue distant from the bleeding site. (3) Contrast medium in excessive amounts is toxic to the kidneys.[14,16]

Necrosis in the distribution of embolized pelvic arteries occurs rarely. The bladder and the distal portion of the rectum are the two organs in the pelvis most susceptible to ischemia from pelvic artery embolization. Although bladder and rectal ischemia have resulted on rare occasions from internal iliac artery ligation, clinically significant rectal ischemia has not been reported following pelvic arterial embolization, and bladder necrosis has been reported only once.[4] In that patient the bladder functioned normally for more than 30 days after pelvic artery embolization. Then, after an episode of pulmonary embolism, the bladder perforated, and at surgery bladder necrosis was confirmed. Pulmonary embolism was presumed to have resulted from pelvic thrombophlebitis. The long latent period between pelvic artery embolization and necrosis suggests that the bladder might have remained viable had not pelvic venous thrombosis supervened.

Evaluation of the adequacy of potential collaterals by aortography prior to embolization and careful choice of embolic material and particle size should minimize the frequency of ischemic complications in the distribution of the embolized vessels. Selective catheterization and embolization of only the arterial branches from which hemorrhage arises reduces the volume of tissue rendered ischemic and should further diminish the potential for ischemic complications. The use of absorbable emboli whenever possible permits recanalization of embolized arteries and should reduce the likelihood that delayed ischemia may occur.

Thrombosis of the femoral and popliteal arteries and digital ischemia have been reported as complications of embolization procedures.[19,33] This results from reflux of emboli in a direction opposite to that of normal blood flow. In this situation the emboli may escape from the internal iliac artery into the external iliac and its peripheral branches. In the presence of active hemorrhage, rapid linear blood flow toward the bleeding site makes reflux of emboli extremely unlikely. However, when emboli have obstructed the arterial lumen, forward flow stops. If additional emboli are then injected, the force of injection creates turbulence. Introduction of emboli in the presence of turbulent flow permits their reflux.

This complication can be avoided if the emboli are injected slowly, in small aliquots, and if the blood flow rate is monitored fluoroscopically by injection of 1 or 2 ml of contrast medium after injection of each aliquot of emboli. Stasis of contrast medium indicates complete obstruction and a risk of reflux if additional emboli are injected.

An attempt should be made to advance the catheter tip as close to the bleeding site as possible. The placement of emboli is more accurately controlled and reflux into critical arteries is less likely to occur if the emboli are introduced into small peripheral vessels rather than large central ones. Some authors have suggested injecting emboli through a double-lumen balloon catheter to reduce the likelihood of reflux.[11] With this technique the emboli are introduced distal to an inflated balloon which obstructs the lumen of the artery and are driven peripherally by injection of saline prior to its deflation.

Renal toxicity from contrast medium is volume related. Doses of 250 to 300 ml of standard arteriographic contrast medium over a period of 1 or 2 h are well tolerated by normal kidneys. However, compromised renal function, as measured by elevated blood creatinine levels prior to the procedure, increases the risk of renal failure following the administration of large volumes of this material.[13]

Separate injections of contrast medium are necessary for the various steps in the diagnostic arteriogram, for selective catheter placement, and for documentation of the degree of obstruction following introduction of each aliquot of emboli. Consequently, the entire embolization procedure requires volumes of contrast medium that approach toxic limits. Therefore, the volume administered during each injection should be carefully noted and should be limited to the minimum amount necessary.

The risk of renal toxicity is reduced if fluid and electrolyte balance are maintained and the patient is kept well hydrated, since all the contrast media used for arteriography are excreted primarily by glomerular filtration. Contrast media produce an osmotic diuresis, which may aggravate intravascular volume depletion. Careful hydration results in dilution of the contrast medium in renal blood and glomerular filtrate and increases its rate of excretion.[13] Adequate hydration may be difficult to maintain in a patient with active hemorrhage but should be attempted. In experienced hands clinically successful diagnostic and therapeutic arteriography can be completed without using high enough volumes of contrast medium to compromise the kidneys, and significant renal toxicity rarely occurs.[13]

Although the likelihood of complications can be minimized by these maneuvers, some risk must be accepted. Arteriographic embolization should be reserved for those patients with severe, life-threatening hemorrhage, and in this clinical setting the complication rate associated with embolization is probably acceptable. Since prolonged hemorrhage and shock reduce perfusion of the pelvis and extremities and increase the likelihood of ischemic complications, arteriography should always be considered early in the course of severe hemorrhage and unnecessary delays should be avoided.

REFERENCES

1. Anderson, J.H., Wallace, S., Gianturco, C., and Gerson, L.P.: "Mini" Gianturco stainless steel coils for transcatheter vascular occlusion. Radiology, *132:*301, 1979.
2. Athanasoulis, C.A.: Therapeutic applications of angiography. N. Engl. J. Med., *302:*1117, 1980.
3. Barth, K.H., Strandberg, J.D., White, R.I., Jr.: Long-term followup of transcatheter embolization with autologous clot, Oxycel, and gelfoam in domestic swine. Invest. Radiol., *12:*273, 1977.
4. Braf, Z.F. and Coontz, W.W., Jr.: Gangrene of the bladder. Complication of hypogastric artery embolization. Urology, *9:*670, 1977.
5. Brown, B.J., Heaston, D.K., Poulson, A.M. et al.: Uncontrollable postpartum bleeding: A new approach to hemostasis through angiographic arterial embolization. Obstet. Gynecol., *54:*361, 1979.
6. Burchell, R.C.: Physiology of internal iliac artery ligation. J. Obstet. Gynecol. Br. Commonw., *75:*642, 1968.
7. Conn, H.O., Rambsy, G.R., and Storer, E.H.: Selective intraarterial vasopressin in the treatment of upper gastrointestinal hemorrhage. Gastroenterology, *63:*643, 1972.
8. Freeny, P.C., Mennemeyer, R., Kidd, C.R., and Bush, W.H.: Long-term radiographic-pathologic followup of patients treated with visceral transcatheter occlusion using isobutyl 2-cyanoacrylate (bucrylate). Radiology, *132:*55, 1979.
9. Gianturco, C., Anderson, J.H., and Wallace, S.: Mechanical devices for arterial occlusion. AJR, *124:*428, 1975.
10. Goldman, M.L., Freeny, P.C., Tallman, J. et al.: Transcatheter vascular occlusion therapy with isobutyl 2-cyanoacrylate (bucrylate) for control of massive upper gastrointestinal bleeding. Radiology, *129:*41, 1978.
11. Greenfield, A.J., Athanasoulis, C.A., Waltman, A.C., and LeMoure, E.R.: Transcatheter embolization: Prevention of embolic reflux using balloon catheters. AJR, *131:*651, 1978.
12. Heaston, D.K., Mineau, D.E., Brown, B.J., and Miller, F.J., Jr.: Transcatheter arterial embolization for control of persistent massive puerperal hemorrhage after bilateral surgical hypogastric artery ligation. AJR, *133:*152, 1979.
13. Hessel, S.J., Adams, D.F., and Abrams, H.L.: Complications of angiography. Radiology, *138:*273, 1981.
14. Jander, H.P. and Russinovich, N.A.E.: Transcatheter gelfoam embolization in abdominal, retroperitoneal, and pelvic hemorrhage. Radiology, *136:*337, 1980.
15. Kunstlinger, F., Brunelle, F., Chaumont, P., and Doyon, D.: Vascular occlusive agents. AJR, *136:*151, 1981.
16. Lang, E.K.: Transcatheter embolization of pelvic vessels for control of intractable hemorrhage. Radiology, *140:*331, 1981.

17. Light, R.U. and Prentice, H.R.: Surgical investigation of a new absorbable sponge derived from gelatin for use in hemostasis. J. Neurosurg., *2:*435, 1945.
18. Margolies, M.N., Ring, E.J., Waltman, A.C. et al.: Arteriography in the management of hemorrhage from pelvic fractures. N. Engl. J. Med., *287:*317, 1972.
19. Matalon, T.S.A., Athanasoulis, C.A., Margolies, M.N. et al.: Hemorrhage with pelvic fractures: Efficacy of transcatheter embolization. AJR, *133:*859, 1979.
20. Mengert, W.F., Burchell, R.C., Blumstein, R.W., and Daskal, J.L.: Pregnancy after bilateral ligation of the internal iliac and ovarian arteries. Obstet. Gynecol., *34:*664, 1969.
21. Nusbaum, M. and Baum, S.: Radiographic demonstration of unknown sites of gastrointestinal bleeding. Surg. Forum, *14:*374, 1963.
22. Osterman, F.A., Jr., Bell, W.R., Montali, R.I. et al.: Natural history of autologous blood clot embolization in swine. Invest. Radiol., *11:*267, 1976.
23. Pais, S.O., Glickman, M.G., Schwartz, P. et al.: Embolization of pelvic arteries for control of postpartum hemorrhage. Obstet. Gynecol., *55:*754, 1980.
24. Ravitch, M.M.: Hypogastric artery ligation in acute pelvic trauma (editorial). Surgery, *56:*601, 1964.
25. Rosch, J., Dotter, C.T., and Brown, M.J.: Selective arterial embolization: A new method for control of acute gastrointestinal bleeding. Radiology, *102:*303, 1972.
26. Rosenthal, D.M., Harkins, J.L., Garzo, G. et al.: The management of postoperative vaginal hemorrhage. Obstet. Gynecol., (in press).
27. Schwartz, P.E., Goldstein, H.M., Wallace, S., and Rutledge, F.N.: Control of arterial hemorrhage using percutaneous arterial catheter techniques in patients with gynecologic malignancies. Gynecol. Oncol., *3:*276, 1975.
28. Seavers, R., Lynch, J., Ballard, R. et al.: Hypogastric artery ligation for uncontrollable hemorrhage in acute pelvic trauma. Surgery, *55:*516, 1964.
29. Shinagawa, S.: Extraperitoneal ligation of the internal iliac arteries as a life- and uterus-saving procedure for uncontrollable postpartum hemorrhage. Am. J. Obstet. Gynecol., *88:*130, 1964.
30. Sniderman, K.W., Sos, T.A., and Alonso, D.R.: Transcatheter embolization with gelfoam and avitene: The effect of Sotradecol on the duration of arterial occlusion. Invest. Radiol., *16:*501, 1981.
31. White, R.I., Jr., Strandberg, J.V., Gross, G.S., and Barth, K.H.: Therapeutic embolization with long-term occluding agents and their effects on embolized tissue Radiology, *125:*677, 1977.
32. Wholey, M.H.: The technology of balloon catheters in interventional angiography. Radiology, *125:*671, 1977.
33. Woodside, J., Schwarz, H., and Bergreen, P.: Peripheral embolization complicating bilateral renal infarction with gelfoam. AJR, *126:*1033, 1976.

8

Maternal Sepsis

Patrick Duff, M.D.
Ronald S. Gibbs, M.D.

BACTEREMIA IN OBSTETRICS

Genital tract infection is one of the most common clinical problems encountered by the obstetrician. It is now estimated that 0.5 to 1 percent of all pregnant patients develop chorioamnionitis.[26] Of patients experiencing vaginal delivery, 1 to 4 percent develop postpartum endomyometritis.[28] The incidence of endomyometritis after cesarean section is even higher, ranging from approximately 15 percent in middle-class patients undergoing elective abdominal delivery to 85 percent in indigent patients undergoing operative delivery after a period of labor and ruptured membranes.[13,16]

Several serious complications may develop as a result of primary operative-site infections. Such complications include incisional infection and/or dehiscence, abdominopelvic abscess or phlegmon, and septic pelvic vein thrombophlebitis. The frequency of such serious sequelae varies widely depending upon the patient population being surveyed. In middle-class populations less than 2 percent of patients develop such complications. In indigent populations, however, the incidence of these complications is higher, ranging from 4 to 30 percent.[13,27]

Another potentially serious complication of operative-site infection is the development of bacteremia. Again, the frequency of bacteremia depends upon the patient population being examined (Table 8-1).[4,12,14,16,23,27,86] The principal pathogens responsible for bacteremia in obstetric patients are coliform organisms, particularly *Escherichia coli*; Group B streptococci; anaerobic streptococci; and *Bacteroides* species.[4,19,25] Other significant causative organisms include *Clostridia* species, enterococci and, rarely, *Staphylococcus aureus* and *Streptococcus pneumoniae*.[4,58] In certain patients, multiple aerobic and anaerobic organisms may be responsible for bacteremia.[64]

Table 8-1. Incidence of Bacteremia in Association with Endomyometritis

Author	Institution	Percent of Infected Patients with Bacteremia
Sweet[86]	University of Michigan	8
Gibbs[27]	University of Texas, San Antonio	8
diZerega[14]	University of Southern California	25
Blanco[4]	University of Texas, San Antonio	9.7
Gall[23]	Duke University, North Carolina	4.2
Cunningham[2]	University of Texas, Dallas (Parkland Hospital)	11.7
Duff[16]	Walter Reed Army Medical Center, Washington, D.C.	0

Most obstetric patients with bacteremia respond promptly to intravenous antibiotic therapy, and their ultimate prognosis is certainly much better than that of medical or general surgery patients with bacteremia. In isolated instances, however, even the parturient may develop the life-threatening complication of bacteremia which we recognize as septic shock. Septic shock is an acute medical and surgical emergency with an alarmingly high mortality rate. Accordingly, the remainder of this chapter is devoted to an intensive discussion of the pathophysiology, diagnosis, and management of septic shock.

PREDISPOSING FACTORS FOR SEPTIC SHOCK

The shock state represents a severe derangement of the normal circulatory system, characterized by decreased cardiac output and decreased tissue perfusion. Sepsis is the third most common cause of shock in the general hospital population; it is exceeded only by acute hemorrhage and myocardial infarction.

Any organism capable of infecting a human host may cause septic shock. The principal organisms responsible for this disorder, however, are the endotoxin-producing aerobic gram-negative bacilli. In most clinical series, *E. coli* is implicated in approximately 50 percent of cases of septic shock. Infection due to members of the *Klebsiella-Enterobacter-Serratia* group, *Proteus* species, and *Pseudomonas aeruginosa* account for an additional 30 percent of cases. The remaining cases result from infections with atypical organisms such as viruses, rickettsiae, gram-positive aerobic bacteria, and gram-negative anaerobic bacteria.[18]

Septic shock occurs almost exclusively in hospitalized patients. The microorganisms responsible for sepsis usually are part of the patient's endogenous flora or are acquired during hospitalization. Patients at particular risk for developing septicemia include individuals of advanced age; those with chronic debilitating diseases such as cirrhosis, heart failure, and diabetes; those with disseminated malignancies; and those with immune deficiency disorders. Those patients receiving immunosuppressive drugs, cytotoxic agents, and parenteral hyperalimentation also may be unusually susceptible to the development of bacteremia. Moreover, certain surgical procedures clearly predispose the patient to increased risk of septicemia. These procedures include biliary, urinary, intestinal, and genital tract surgery.[22]

Because septic shock usually occurs in debilitated, hospitalized patients, the prognosis for survival is markedly affected by the patient's underlying medical illness. In selected series, the mortality associated with bacteremia alone is 40 percent; once clinical shock supervenes, the proportion of fatalities increases to 50 to 80 percent. In a study of 270 patients with gram-negative bacteremia, Freid and Vosti emphasized the importance of underlying disease as a determinant of prognosis. These investigators classified their patients as having "rapidly fatal," "ultimately fatal," and "nonfatal" underlying diseases and observed fatality ratios of 86, 46, and 16 percent, respectively.[22]

The vast majority of obstetric patients with septic shock would be included in the latter category of "no underlying fatal disease." Because their prognosis is so favorable relative to other patients with more serious underlying diseases, these individuals will derive the most benefit from prompt, effective treatment of septic shock. Freid and Vosti have shown clearly that prognosis is adversely affected in this specific group of patients when initial medical and surgical therapy is imprecise.[22] Successful management of septic shock requires thorough understanding of its intricate pathophysiology and aggressive application of complex medical and surgical techniques.

PATHOPHYSIOLOGY OF SEPTIC SHOCK

Endotoxin is a complex lipopolysaccharide which is present in the cell wall of gram-negative bacteria. The critical component of endotoxin is a substituent termed lipid A, which has a β-1,6-diglucosamine backbone joined in an ester and amide linkage to long-chain fatty acids.[3] Endotoxin is released into the host's circulation at the time of the bacterium's death; once in the bloodstream, endotoxin initiates the intricate series of pathophysiologic derangements summarized in Figure 8-1.

One of the first effects of endotoxin is direct activation of Hageman factor (XII), which in turn initiates the intrinsic clotting cascade. Hageman factor also directly activates factor VII, thus stimulating the extrinsic coagulation pathway. Activation of the coagulation system leads to concurrent activation of the fibrinolytic system. Plasmin, the active component of the latter system, then acts upon Hageman factor to produce fragments termed prekallikrein activators. These substances activate prekallikrein to form kallikrein. Kallikrein causes conversion of plasminogen to plasmin and also directly activates Hageman factor. This results in enhanced coagulation and accelerated fibrinolysis and precipitates the phenomenon of disseminated intravascular coagulation. Another major effect of kallikrein activation is the production of a variety of inflammatory mediators such as hydrogen peroxide, free radicals, and bradykinin. These substances cause intense inflammatory injury to vital organs.[59]

Inflammatory injury also occurs as a result of endotoxin-induced activation of the complement cascade. This activation occurs through the classic pathway, through the alternate (properdin) pathway, and through direct activation of the first component of complement.[20,60] In the classic activation sequence (Fig. 8-2), bacteria-antibody complexes combine to activate C1, which activates C4, and this in turn

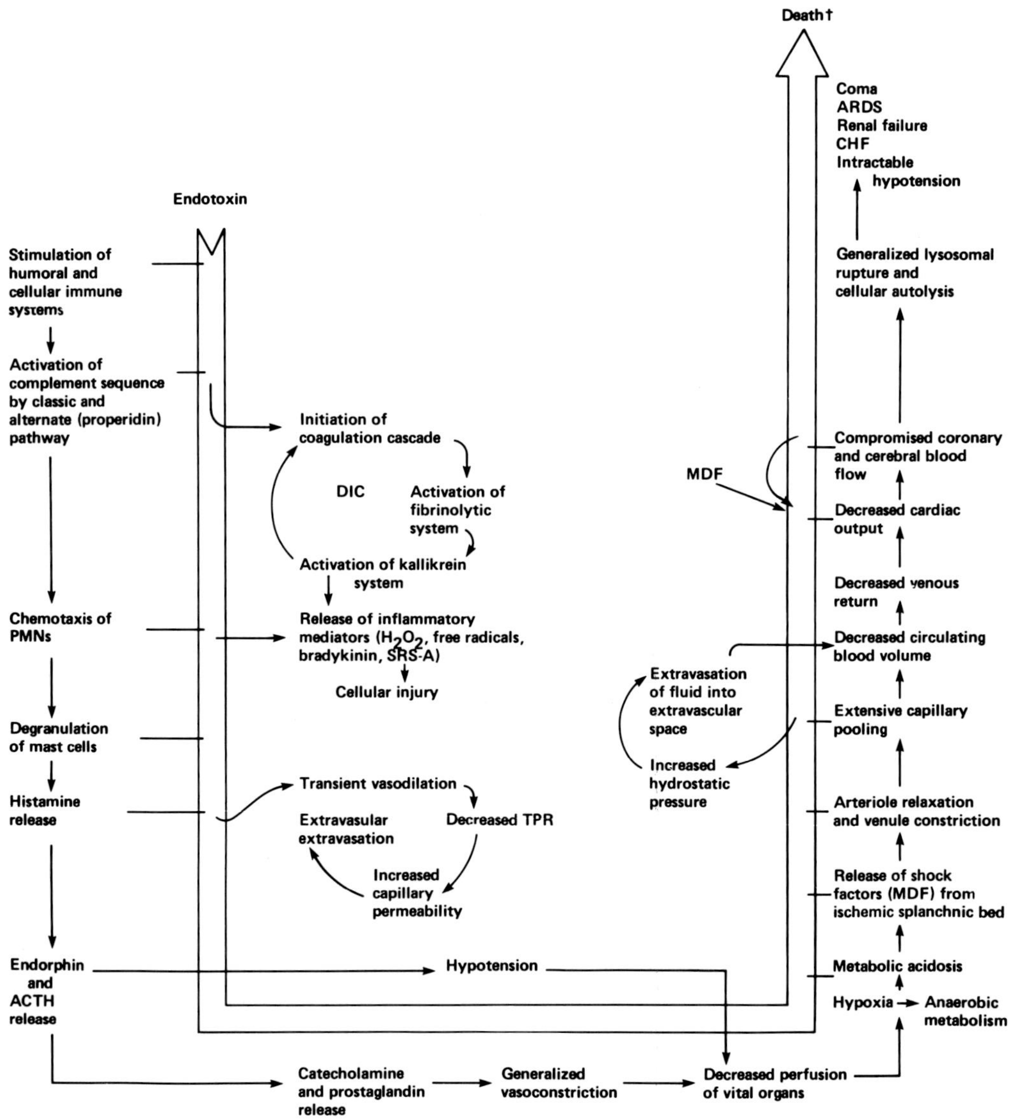

Fig. 8-1 Pathophysiology of endotoxic shock.

combines with C2 to form the $C\overline{42}$ complex. The $C\overline{42}$ activates the third component of complement (C3), which then activates the terminal sequence of the pathway C5 to C9.[60]

In the alternate activation sequence (Fig. 8-3), endotoxin interacts with properdin, a proesterase termed factor D, and other unidentified plasma factors to create activated properdin and an active esterase factor $\overline{D}$. Factor $\overline{D}$ then cleaves the third component of complement to produce C3b, which in turn cleaves activated properdin; this results in activation of a substance termed factor B, which functions as a proactivator of C3. Activation of factor B generates a minor fragment Ba and a major

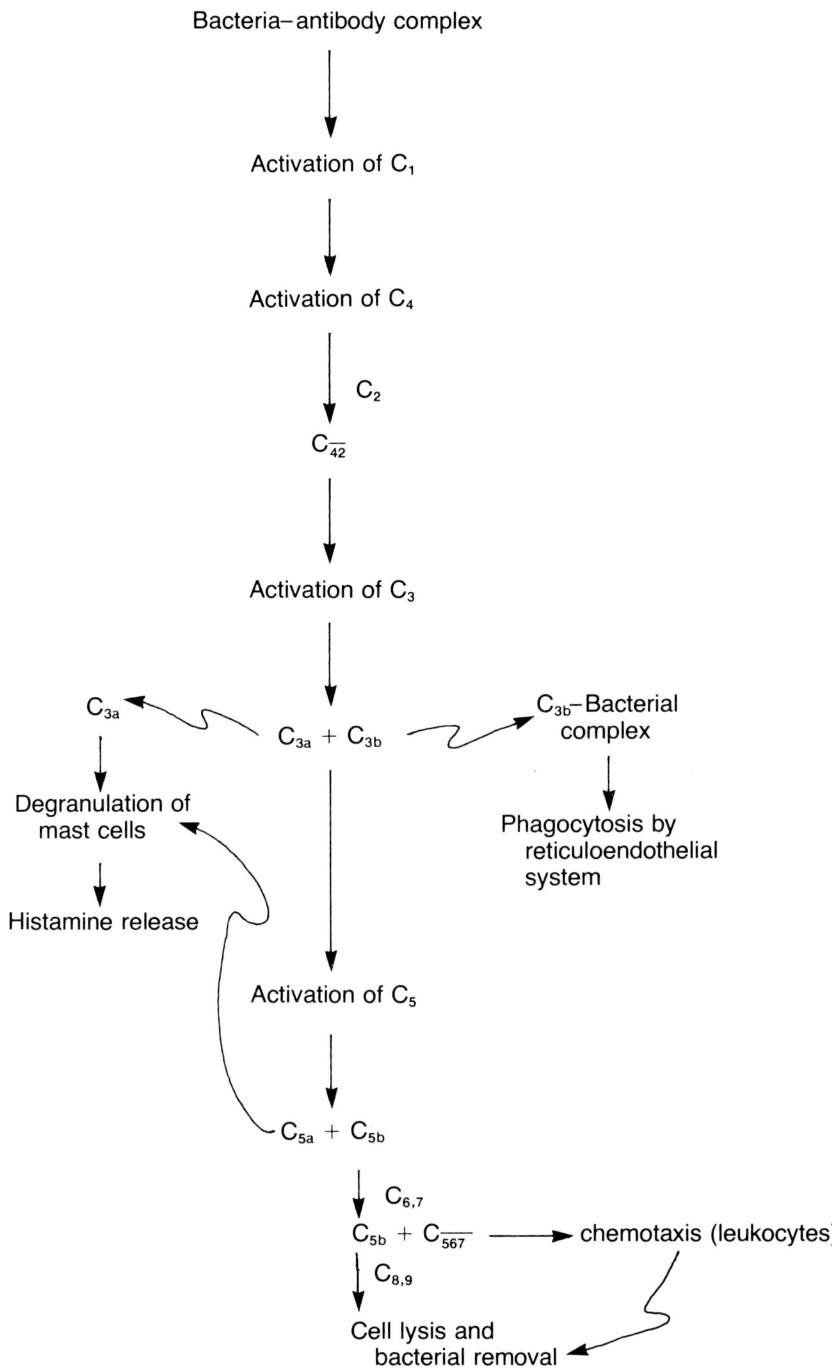

Fig. 8-2 Classic pathway of complement activation.

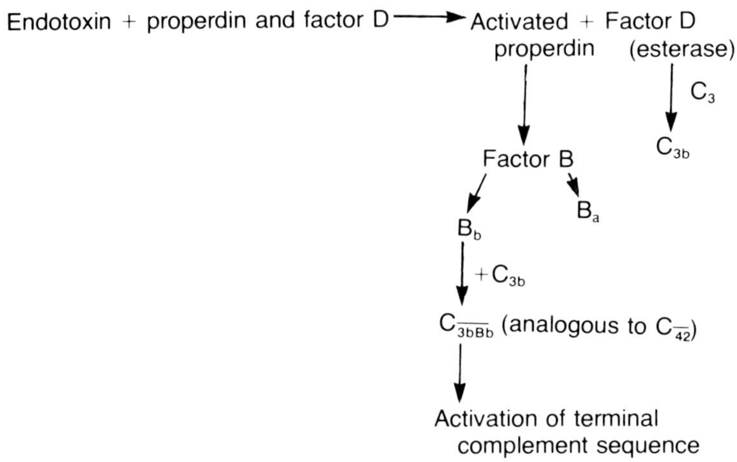

Fig. 8-3 Alternate (properdin) pathway of complement activation.

fragment Bb. The latter substance combines with C3b to form C3bBb, which is functionally analogous to $C\overline{42}$ in its ability to activate the remainder of the complement sequence.[20]

There are three major effects of complement activation. First, C5a and the $C\overline{5,6,7}$ complex interact to exert a chemotactic effect, promoting migration of leukocytes into injured tissue, with accelerated inflammation, bacterial lysis, and enhanced release of endotoxin. Second, release of inflammatory mediators by leukocytes causes injury to vascular endothelium with resultant platelet aggregation, release of platelet factor 3, and intensification of the coagulation cascade. Third, components C3a and C5a interact to cause degranulation of mast cells and release of histamine.

Histamine release has several major pathophysiologic effects, including disruption of endothelial integrity, increase in capillary permeability, decrease in plasma volume, vasodilation, and hypotension. In response to this initial state of hypotension, there is an increase in the host's heart rate and cardiac output. Accordingly, in this early stage of sepsis, the patient appears to be warm, flushed, and maximally vasodilated, and it is for this reason that septic shock is referred to as "warm shock."[20,22,60]

It is important to recognize that this early stage of vasodilation, decreased peripheral resistance, and increased cardiac output usually is short-lived. As sepsis evolves, there is intense activation of the sympathetic nervous system manifested by increased catecholamine release from peripheral nerves and the adrenal medulla. The principal effect of this sympathetic discharge is generalized vasoconstriction in virtually every vascular bed.[1,68,69,75,81] This vasoconstrictive process is intensified by the localized constrictive effects of prostaglandins released from injured endothelial tissue.[21]

The most serious effect of generalized vasoconstriction is profound diminution in perfusion of vital organs, resulting in localized tissue hypoxia and acidosis and ultimately in systemic metabolic acidosis. As acidosis evolves, there is a marked change in circulatory hemodynamics, characterized by relaxation of smooth muscle in the wall of arterioles and constriction of smooth muscle in the wall of venules. This process leads to extensive pooling in most capillary beds, increased hydrostatic pressure, and transudation of intravascular fluid into the extravascular space.[18,29,37,39,40,68,75,85]

Generalized capillary pooling causes significant decrease in effective circulating blood volume, with resultant decrease in venous return to the heart and progressive decrease in cardiac output and systemic blood pressure.[1,29,37,39,40,68,69,81,85] Kwaan and Weil have emphasized that this process is much more likely to occur in the presence of gram-negative bacteremia than gram-positive bacteremia.[52]

Although decreased venous return is the single most important cause of decreased cardiac output, there are at least two other factors that contribute to impaired myocardial performance. In the shock state, levels of endogenous beta endorphins are increased significantly. These peptides are released from the pituitary gland along with adrenocorticotropic hormone (ACTH) in response to stress, and their principal hemodynamic effect is to lower blood pressure.[36,42,63]

In addition, several studies in both laboratory animals and humans have identified the presence of a specific shock factor, termed myocardial depressant factor (MDF), which apparently is released from the ischemic pancreas during evolution of the shock state (Fig. 8-4).[6,33,54,73,76,93] Although MDF has only been partially characterized, it is thought to be a peptide or glycopeptide with a molecular weight of 500 to 1,000.[33] Lefer has shown that during shock in experimental animals, MDF gradually accumulates in the plasma in direct proportion to the severity of splanchnic ischemia. MDF has several biologic effects, principally a direct depressant effect on myocardial contractility. It does not alter heart rate, rhythm, or coronary blood flow. It enhances vasoconstriction within splanchnic blood vessels, thus accelerating its own production, and it directly depresses the phagocytic capacity of the reticuloendothelial system, resulting in impaired clearance of lysosomal enzymes and MDF from the circulation.[54]

As cardiac output initially begins to fall, local regulatory changes occur in an attempt to preserve perfusion of the coronary and cerebral vascular beds. If the

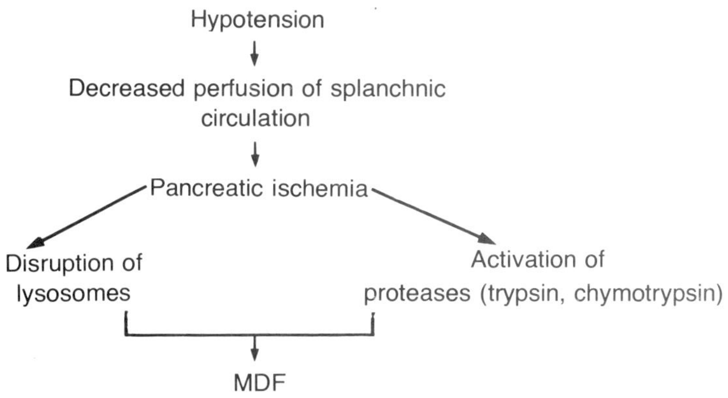

Fig. 8-4 Formation of myocardial depressant factor (MDF). (Modified from Lefer, A.M.: Role of a myocardial depressant factor in shock states. Mod. Concepts Cardiovasc. Dis., *42*:59, 1973.)

hemodynamic changes precipitated by septicemia are not corrected, however, there is progressive diminution in cardiac output and ultimately compromise of both coronary and cerebral blood flow. Weisel and associates have demonstrated a direct correlation between maintenance of cardiac output and ultimate survival.[93]

At the end point in evolution of the shock state, there is development of irreversible circulatory failure, characterized by intractable hypotension, severe metabolic acidosis, and extensive cellular autolysis. Clinically, this end state is manifested by complete vasomotor collapse, coma, renal failure, and cardiopulmonary failure.

Although the major effects of endotoxin are on the cardiovascular system, this substance also has other significant pathophysiologic effects. Endotoxin adheres to the cell membrane of circulating leukocytes, causing these cells to be sequestered in the reticuloendothelial system. As a result, the early shock state may be distinguished by neutropenia. As cell-mediated immunologic defenses are mobilized, however, rebound leukocytosis usually ensues.[18] This rebound effect, of course, may not occur in immunosuppressed patients, who are precisely those at greatest risk for developing septic shock.

Endotoxin also exerts a prominent effect on the temperature-regulating center of the hypothalamus. In the early phase of sepsis, the hypothalamic center may be depressed. As a result, hypothermia may be present. As shock evolves, however, the principal effect of endotoxin is activation of the hypothalamic center and elevation of body temperature, an effect mediated by endogenous pyrogen released from host leukocytes.[3]

Finally, endotoxin frequently causes severe damage to the host's pulmonary system. As outlined in Figure 8-5, endotoxin directly damages the endothelium of the pulmonary vasculature. As disruption of capillaries occurs, fragmented collagen is exposed; platelets then adhere to the area of injury. Release of platelet factor 3 activates the intrinsic coagulation cascade, resulting in microembolization and stasis of blood flow in the pulmonary microcirculation.[18] Prostaglandins are released from platelets and injured endothelium, and these substances cause pulmonary vasoconstriction, with subsequent increase in pulmonary vascular resistance. The net effect of these processes is impairment of pulmonary perfusion and ischemic and progressive injury to the vascular endothelium.[7] Moss and coworkers,[67] utilizing a dog model, also have suggested that the cerebral ischemia resulting from hypotension intensifies pulmonary vasoconstriction.

Endotoxin-mediated endothelial injury also leads to activation of the complement cascade. Complement activation causes further damage to the lung by enhancing leukocyte migration into the pulmonary parenchyma, with resultant release of additional inflammatory mediators.[38] Lee and associates have documented increased activity of the proteolytic enzyme elastase in bronchoalveolar lavage fluid obtained from patients with adult respiratory distress syndrome (ARDS).[53]

Continued inflammation in turn results in increased capillary permeability, transudation of protein-rich fluid into the interstitium and alveolus, and destruction of surfactant. In a baboon model, Moss and DasGupta have presented excellent histochemical and electron microscopic evidence of disruption of the surfactant lining of the alveolus.[66] Sibbald et al., in a clinical study of patients with septic shock and ARDS, have documented the marked changes in capillary permeability occur-

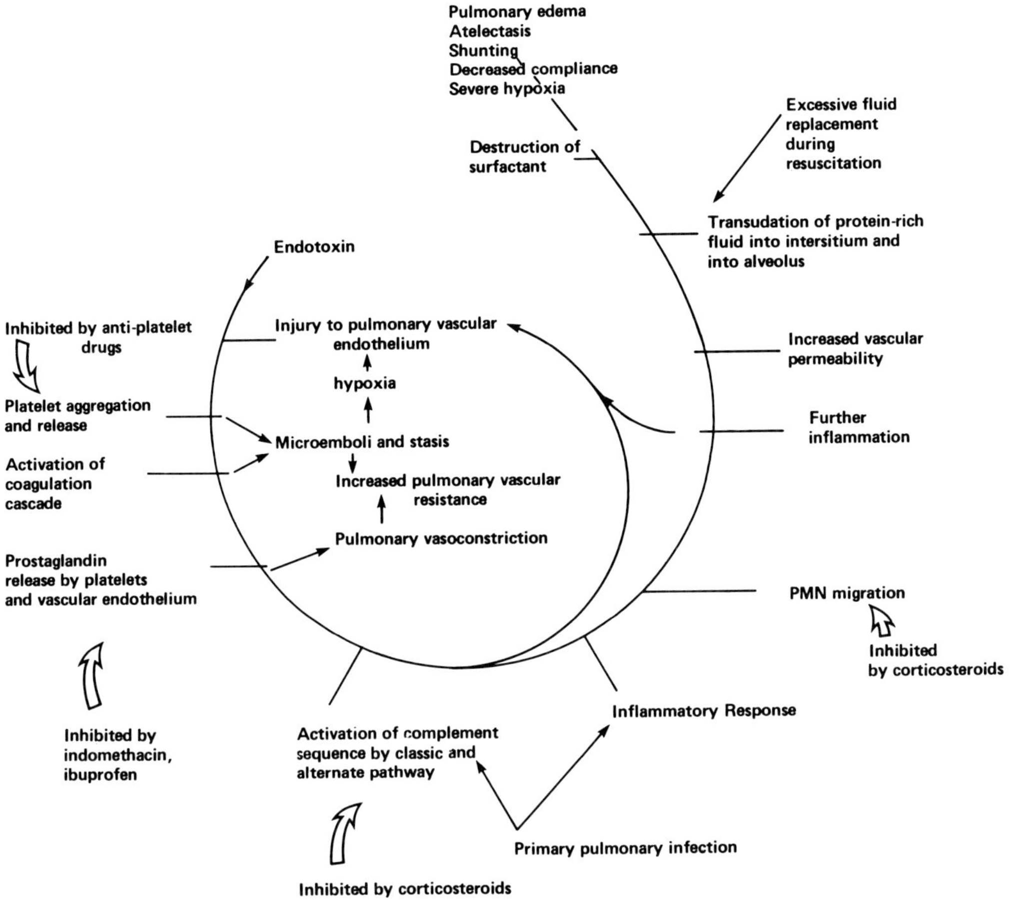

Fig. 8-5 Pathophysiology of pulmonary injury in septic shock.

ring in this disease process.[83] The functional consequence of these events is a state characterized by extensive atelectasis, perfusion-ventilation imbalance, decreased compliance, interstitial and intra-alveolar edema, severe hypoxemia and, ultimately, respiratory failure (Fig. 8-6).

CLINICAL MANIFESTATIONS OF SEPSIS

One of the earliest manifestations of septic shock is an alteration in the patient's sensorum, characterized by restlessness, anxiety, confusion, disorientation, and impaired intellect and judgment. Other early signs of evolving septicemia include temperature instability, flushing, and peripheral vasodilation.[1]

The most prominent pathophysiologic alterations induced by septicemia are

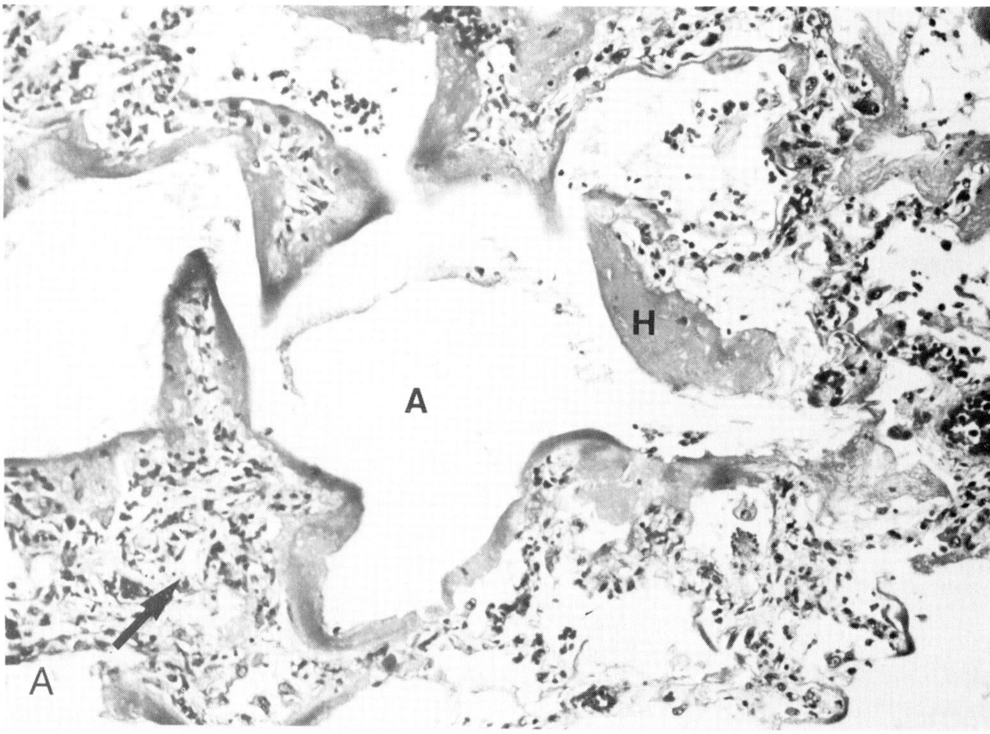

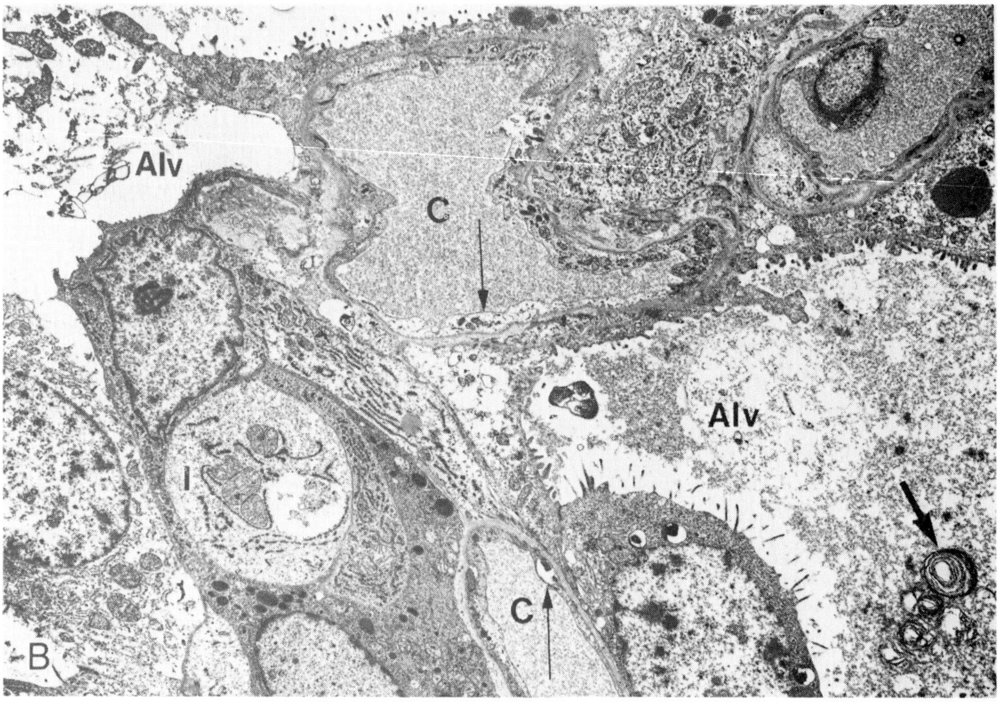

Fig. 8-6 (A) Photomicrograph of lung tissue from patient with ARDS. Diffuse alveolar damage is characterized by presence of prominent hyaline membranes (H), microatelectasis (arrow), and inflammatory exudate. Air space (A). Hematoxylin and eosin, × 220. (Courtesy of J. Coalson.) (B) Electron micrograph of lung tissue from patient with ARDS secondary to streptococcal septicemia. Proteinaceous debris and cellular fragments (thick arrow) are seen within the alveolar space (Alv). The interstitium (I) is edematous and contains numerous cells, including macrophages and fibroblasts. The endothelium of the capillaries (c) shows focal edema (thin arrows). Uranyl acetate and lead citrate, × 5,200. (Courtesy of J. Coalson.)

those affecting the cardiovascular system. In the early stage of septicemia, a hyperdynamic state prevails. Cardiac output is increased significantly, oxygen consumption by the myocardium and peripheral tissues is increased, and total peripheral resistance is decreased. These early findings of increased cardiac output and peripheral vasodilation usually are followed by a state of intense vasoconstriction, leading to progressive decrease in cardiac output and blood pressure and decrease in perfusion of vital organs.[8,18,55,56,69,81,89,91] Diminished tissue perfusion leads to progressive impairment of myocardial performance, which is manifested clinically by tachycardia, tachyarrhythmia, myocardial ischemia, and even infarction and biventricular failure, with associated jugular venous distension, pulmonary edema, and hepatic congestion.

The respiratory system may be either the primary focus of infection leading to septic shock or one of the principal target organs affected by the shock state. Approximately 50 percent of patients with septic shock develop ARDS. The most frequent manifestations of this disorder include tachypnea, dyspnea, stridor, cyanosis, lobar consolidation, and pulmonary edema.[46]

The abdominopelvic examination is critically important in evaluation of the patient with septic shock, since most obstetric patients have either a gastrointestinal or genitourinary focus as the site of primary infection. For example, examination of the upper abdomen may demonstrate evidence of hepatobiliary disease such as cholecystitis or ascending cholangitis or renal parenchymal disorders such as acute pyelonephritis. Alternatively, there may be evidence of an intestinal obstruction, wound infection, evisceration, or even necrotizing fasciitis that is responsible for the evolving septicemia. Demonstration of generalized peritonitis may suggest intra-abdominal problems such as perforated viscus, appendicitis, diverticulitis, or inflammatory bowel disease as the etiology for septicemia. Finally, palpation of enlarged or tender pelvic viscera or a pelvic mass will direct the physician's attention to diagnoses such as septic abortion, intra-amniotic infection, endomyometritis, ruptured uterus, and pelvic abscess.

Other clinical manifestations that may be helpful in localizing the site of infection or in identifying organs compromised by shock include oliguria or anuria, hematuria or pyuria, jaundice, nausea, and vomiting. Development of a coagulopathy may be heralded by spontaneous hemorrhage from the gastrointestinal or genitourinary tract and by bleeding from venipuncture sites. Figure 8-7 summarizes the principal manifestations of septic shock.

DIAGNOSIS

Several disorders must be considered in the differential diagnosis of septic shock. These conditions include cardiogenic and hypovolemic shock, acute pulmonary embolus, cardiac tamponade, dissection of the aorta, hemorrhagic pancreatitis, diabetic ketoacidosis, and amniotic fluid embolus. Distinction between septic shock and these other entities usually can be made on the basis of history, physical examination, and a limited number of laboratory tests (Table 8-2).

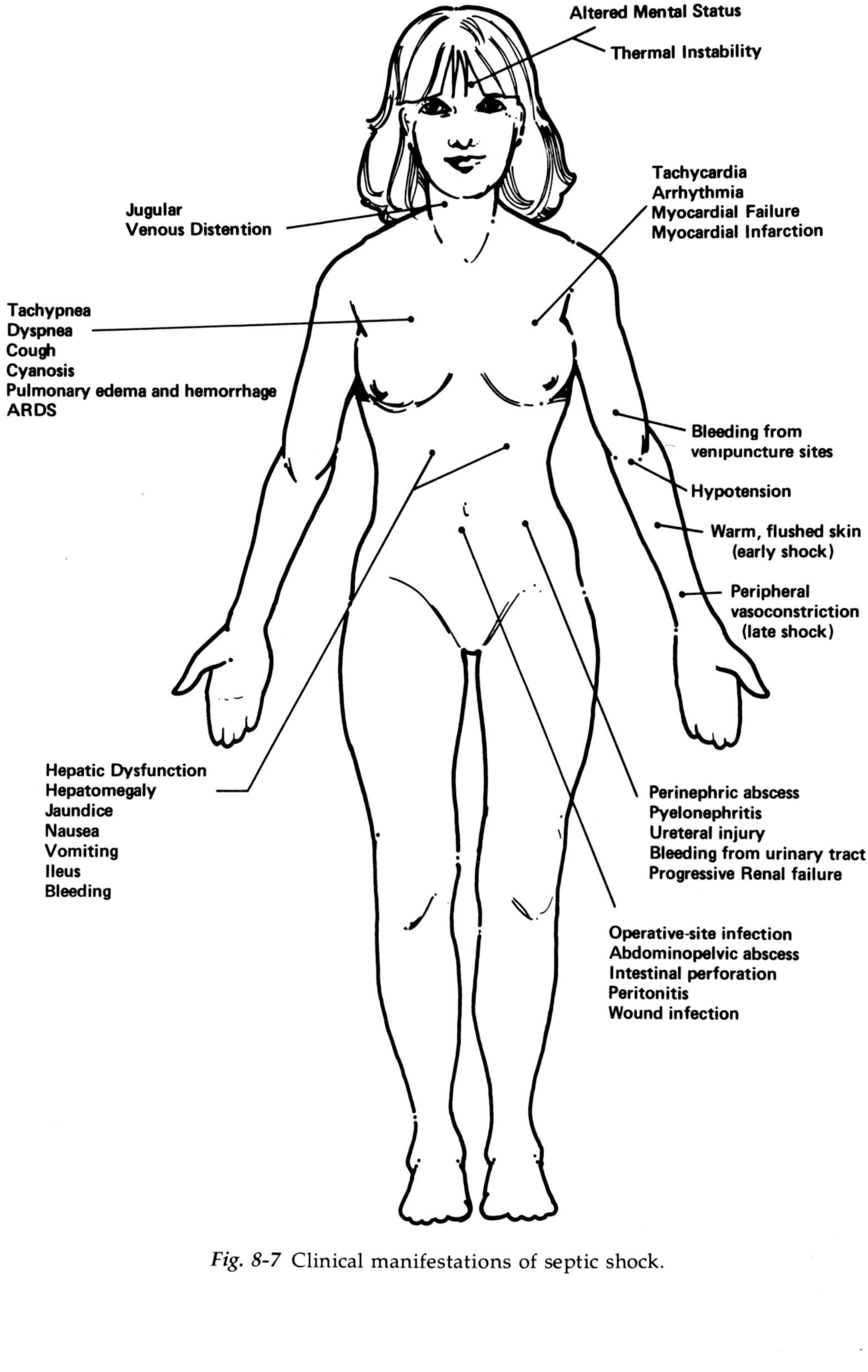

Fig. 8-7 Clinical manifestations of septic shock.

Table 8-2. Laboratory Studies in Septic Shock

Laboratory Test	Results
1. White blood cell count (WBC)	Initially ↓, then ↑
2. Hematocrit (HCT)	Variable, depending on blood loss and plasma volume
3. Platelet count	↓ with DIC
4. Fibrinogen	↓ with DIC
5. Fibrin degradation products (FDP)	↑ with DIC
6. Prothrombin time (PT), activated partial thromboplastin time (aPTT), thrombin time (TT)	↑ with DIC
7. pH	Initially ↑ due to respiratory alkalosis, then ↓ due to metabolic and respiratory acidosis
8. Lactic acid	↑
9. Arterial pO_2	↓
10. Arterial pCO_2	↑
11. Bicarbonate	↓
12. Potassium	May be ↑ in response to evolving acidosis
13. Glucose	↑, but impaired utilization
14. Insulin	Initially ↑, then ↓
15. Blood urea nitrogen (BUN)	↑ with onset of oliguria
16. Creatinine	↑ with onset of oliguria
17. Creatinine clearance	↓
18. Urine culture	Determine source of infection
19. Sputum culture	Determine source of infection Evaluation of ARDS
20. Aerobic and anaerobic blood culture	Determine organism responsible for septicemia
21. Blood culture for fungal organisms	Rule out infection due to opportunistic organisms
22. Operative-site culture (endometrium), wound culture, culture of abscess cavity	Determine source of infection
23. Chest x-ray	Evaluate for pneumonia, ARDS
24. Abdominal films	Evaluate for intestinal obstruction, perforated viscus, abscess
25. CT scan or ultrasound	Delineate abscess
26. Excretory urography [Intravenous pyelogram (IVP)]	Rule out perinephric abscess, ureteral fistula, ureteral injury
27. Electrocardiogram	Detect ischemic changes or arrhythmia
28. Swan-Ganz catheter studies	Determine CVP, pulmonary artery pressure, PCWP

In the early stage of septic shock, the white blood cell count may be low owing to sequestration of leukocytes in the reticuloendothelial system. Neutropenia almost invariably is followed by a prominent leukocytosis, with a distinct shift toward more immature granulocyte forms. If acute blood loss accompanies sepsis, the hematocrit may be low. Alternatively, the hematocrit may be elevated as a result of the decreased effective circulating plasma volume resulting from pooling in the capillary bed. A diminished platelet count, decreased fibrinogen level, and elevated level of fibrin degradation products are the earliest and most sensitive indicators of disseminated intravascular coagulation (DIC).[1,8,18,55,56,81,89]

Acid-base changes in septic shock tend to occur in a characteristic pattern. In the early stage of septicemia, the patient may have a transient respiratory alkalosis due to hyperventilation. Respiratory alkalosis is quickly superseded by a profound metabolic acidosis, as hypoxia leads to an increase in anaerobic metabolism, with a concomitant increase in plasma levels of lactic acid.[1] Peretz and associates[71] have demonstrated that lactate is the major organic acid responsible for the metabolic acidosis that accompanies the shock state. These investigators and others have shown that lactate levels correspond to the severity of circulatory failure in shock and have confirmed that patients with the highest levels of lactate have the worst prognosis for ultimate survival. In a clinical study of 56 patients with shock of various types, Broder and Weil[5] found that no individual survived when the excess lactate level exceeded 4 mmol/L.

In the septic patient with concurrent ARDS, respiratory failure also contributes to the severe metabolic derangement. These patients will have both a metabolic and a respiratory acidosis, and this acute state will be manifested by decreased arterial pH, decreased serum bicarbonate, diminished arterial pO_2, and increased arterial PCo_2.[46] Serum potassium concentrations may increase as intracellular potassium flows from the cell in exchange for hydrogen ion.

Measures of renal function may be altered in the patient with septic shock. With severe compromise in renal blood flow resulting from generalized vasoconstriction, urine output will first diminish and then cease. With the onset of oliguria, creatinine clearance will decrease. Serum concentrations of substances normally filtered by the glomerulus or actively secreted by tubular epithelium, such as urea, creatinine, and uric acid, will then increase.[1,18]

Plasma glucose levels in septic shock usually are normal or high. In the early stage of septic shock, when cardiac output is high and peripheral resistance is low, both plasma glucose and plasma insulin levels are elevated. Despite the presence of high concentrations of insulin, however, glucose uptake by peripheral cells is impaired, reflecting a state of at least partial insulin antagonism. As septic shock progresses and a low cardiac output state develops, plasma insulin levels decrease below those of uninfected controls and glucose utilization is impaired even further.[11]

Microbiologic studies are essential in establishing the diagnosis of septic shock and determining the origin of infection. A sample of urine should be obtained aseptically through the urethral catheter for microscopic examination and bacteriologic culture. Sputum culture and gram stain should be performed in patients with symptoms suggestive of pneumonia or ARDS. At least two sets of aerobic and anaerobic blood cultures should be obtained to determine the pathogenic organism responsible for septicemia. Blood specimens also should be evaluated for fungi, especially in patients receiving parenteral hyperalimentation and those receiving immunosuppressive drugs, since these individuals are at increased risk for fungal septicemia. Finally, cultures of the operative site, wound, or abscess cavity should be obtained, when appropriate, in order to isolate the microorganism responsible for infection.

Selected radiographic procedures may be helpful in the evaluation of the patient with septic shock. Posteroanterior and lateral films of the chest may indicate whether a primary respiratory infection is present and may also permit early detection of septic pulmonary emboli, cardiomegaly, pulmonary edema, or the diffuse interstitial infiltrates characteristic of ARDS (Fig. 8-8).[46] Immediate recognition of the pulmonary changes associated with ARDS is essential in view of the fact that the disorder so adversely affects the prognosis in septic shock. In this regard, it is critically important to realize that these radiographic changes may develop after clinical

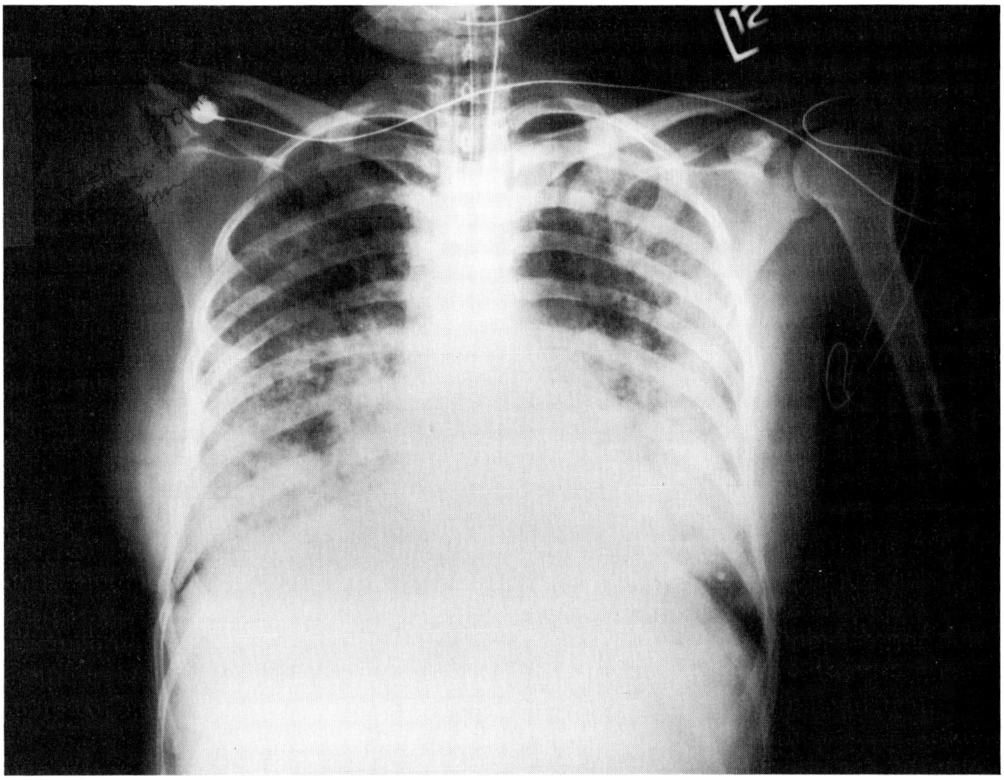

Fig. 8-8 Chest radiograph of a 20-year-old woman with ARDS. Note characteristic diffuse bilateral infiltrates reflecting extensive intra-alveolar and interstitial edema. (Courtesy of E. Greenberg.)

changes such as increasing tachypnea, dyspnea, cyanosis, and stridor already have become apparent.

Abdominal films should be obtained if there is suspicion of intestinal obstruction, perforated viscus, foreign body, or abdominopelvic abscess. In selected instances, computerized tomography (CT) and ultrasonography may be helpful in delineating the presence of an abscess, particularly in morbidly obese patients in whom pelvic examination alone is imprecise (Figs. 8-9 and 8-10). In addition, excretory urography [intravenous pyelogram (IVP)] may be indicated in certain patients when there is a need to establish the presence or absence of perinephric abscess, ruptured renal pelvis, ureteral fistula, or operative ureteral injury.

Accurate monitoring of cardiovascular performance is of paramount importance in the patient with septic shock.[68,91] Standard electrocardiography should be utilized to detect evidence of myocardial ischemia and disturbances in cardiac rhythm. In the septic patient with endocarditis, echocardiography may be indicated to detect valvular dysfunction. Finally, Swan-Ganz catheter studies provide invaluable data in assessing adequacy of venous return and determining pulmonary artery systolic and diastolic pressures, pulmonary vascular resistance, pulmonary capillary wedge pressure (PCWP), and cardiac output.

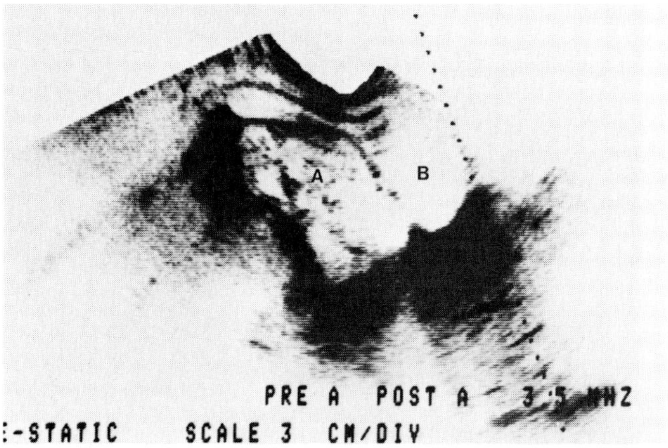

Fig. 8-9 Sonogram of pelvis, demonstrating a right tuboovarian abscess. Longitudinal section, 2 cm to right of midline. Bladder (B); abscess (A). (Courtesy of N.C. Dornbluth.)

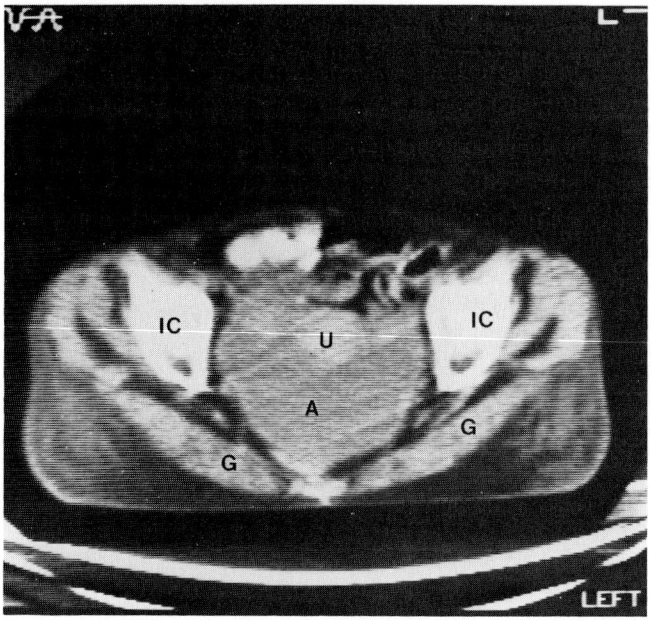

Fig. 8-10 CT scan of pelvis, demonstrating a normal-size uterus (U) and a large pelvic abscess (A). Ischium (IC); gluteus maximus (G). (Courtesy of J. Potter.)

MANAGEMENT

Correction of Hemodynamic Abnormalities

The first priority in treating septic shock (Table 8-3) is correction of the hemodynamic abnormalities outlined above. Immediate attention should be directed to establishment of reliable means for monitoring the septic patient.[68,91] Ideally, a Swan-Ganz catheter should be inserted to evaluate cardiac function. If this is not possible,

Table 8-3. Treatment of Septic Shock

A. Correct hemodynamic abnormalities
   1. Establish reliable methods for physiologic monitoring
   2. Restore intravascular volume
   3. Consider use of shock trousers as an adjunct to fluid resuscitation
   4. Improve perfusion of vital organs by administering dopamine
      a. 5-ml ampule, 40 mg/ml (total 200 mg)
      b. Dilute four ampules in 500 ml of sterile saline or 5% dextrose to give a concentration of 1,600 μg/ml
      c. Begin infusion at the rate of 2 μg/kg/min
      d. Titrate dosage to achieve adequate tissue perfusion
   5. Digitalize patient if overt congestive heart failure develops
   6. Administer pharmacologic doses of glucocorticoids
      a. Methylprednisolone (30 mg/kg) or dexamethasone (3 mg/kg)
      b. Administer as an intravenous bolus at the time fluid resuscitation is initiated. Repeat in 4 h if necessary.

B. Treat the underlying infection
   1. Initially, administer antibiotics covering entire range of potential pelvic pathogens
   2. Surgery, if indicated

C. Support the respiratory system
   1. Administer oxygen
   2. Monitor arterial blood gases frequently to detect onset of respiratory failure
   3. Early use of mechanical ventilation with volume-cycled respirator

D. Restore body temperature to normal

E. Correct coagulation abnormalities

F. Administer white cell transfusions to severely immunosuppressed patients with *Pseudomonas* septicemia

a central venous pressure (CVP) catheter should be positioned to provide at least some information about intracardiac filling pressures. An arterial line should be inserted to provide continuous assessment of blood pressure and arterial oxygenation. A urethral catheter should be placed to monitor urine output, and a large-bore intravenous catheter should be inserted to administer medications and fluid replacement.

The next goal of therapy is to restore the patient's effective circulating blood volume. If the patient has experienced acute blood loss, this objective may be accomplished by administering either packed red cells or whole blood. In the absence of blood loss, plasma volume loss may be corrected by infusion of isotonic crystalloids such as normal saline or lactated Ringer's solution or colloid solutions such as plasmanate or albumin. Fluid resuscitation should be started, of course, even though all the aforementioned physiologic monitors have not been inserted. Initial fluid replacement should be administered in small increments of 150 to 200 ml over 10 min, with adjustments made on the basis of measurements of clinical parameters such as blood pressure, pulse, jugular venous pulse, and urine output.

Continued restoration of intravascular volume should be guided by measurements of the patient's PCWP. Optimally, PCWP should be maintained at a level of 10 to 12 mmHg. Lower levels do not provide adequate filling pressures for the left atrium and left ventricle, while higher levels may overload the cardiovascular system and result in pulmonary edema.[18] Shubin and associates have proposed the "7-3" rule for fluid replacement in patients with septic shock.[81] They recommend administration of a bolus of 5 to 20 ml/min for 10 min with continuous monitoring of PCWP. If PCWP increases more than 7 mmHg above the patient's baseline, then the infusion should be discontinued temporarily. If the PCWP does not rise more than 3 mmHg above baseline, then a second fluid challenge should be given, and the 7-3 rule reapplied. If CVP rather than PCWP is used as a guideline, the upper and lower decision points are 5 cmH_2O and 2 cmH_2O, respectively.

Clowes and coworkers[11] have suggested that fluid resuscitation in septic shock also should include administration of glucose, potassium, and insulin. In experimental studies of pigs, these investigators demonstrated that in the late stage of septic shock characterized by decreased cardiac output and markedly diminished tissue perfusion, insulin levels and peripheral utilization of glucose are significantly decreased. Infusion of intravenous fluids containing glucose, insulin, and potassium improved glucose uptake in tissue, resulting in decreased serum lactate levels and improved myocardial performance.

In an uncontrolled clinical trial in 10 patients with sepsis and systemic hypotension unresponsive to intravenous fluids, ionotropic agents, and corticosteroids, these same authors administered intravenously, over a 10-min period, a solution containing 1 g glucose and 1.5 units regular insulin per kilogram of body weight, 10 mg potassium chloride, and 1 g albumin. Each patient experienced a prompt increase in cardiac output and a decrease in PCWP as a result of the infusion. In spite of these encouraging results, however, the ultimate value of such therapy must be established in additional controlled clinical trials.

While fluid resuscitation is being initiated, application of shock trousers to the septic patient may result in immediate improvement in cardiac function.[62,70,90] The principal effect of the pneumatic trousers is to mobilize blood that has pooled in the lower extremities and lower abdomen and return it to the heart-brain-lung circulation, thereby preventing myocardial and cerebral ischemia due to hypotension. McSwain estimates that 750 to 1,000 ml of autologous blood is returned to the circulation by this maneuver. This autotransfusion effect occurs without compromising the arterial supply to the lower abdomen and lower extremities. Early use of the shock trousers may decrease the amount of fluid needed for resuscitation, thereby reducing the subsequent risk of pulmonary edema due to excessive fluid replacement. Use of the pneumatic trousers is a temporary measure only, however, and the unit should be gradually deflated as normal perfusion pressure is reestablished by intravenous fluid therapy. The only absolute contraindications to use of the shock trousers are congestive heart failure and cerebral edema resulting from head trauma.[62,70,90]

If fluid resuscitation alone does not restore adequate tissue perfusion, persistent vasoconstriction may be alleviated by administration of dopamine, an agent with unique pharmacologic properties that make it invaluable in the management of septic shock.[34] In low doses, dopamine has a weak betamimetic effect on the heart that increases myocardial contractility and heart rate without causing a disproportionate increase in myocardial oxygen consumption. The drug also stimulates special dopaminergic receptors in the renal, mesenteric, coronary, and cerebral vasculature to cause vasodilation. Unlike pure beta stimulants, dopamine causes vasoconstriction in skeletal muscle. Its net effect, then, is to peserve renal, splanchnic, coronary, and cerebral blood flow.

These actions of dopamine are uniquely dose-dependent. In doses exceeding 15 to 20 $\mu g/kg/min$, the principal effect of dopamine is stimulation of alpha receptors with resultant vasoconstriction, an effect also noted with use of conventional vasopressors such as metaraminol and ephedrine. The ultimate result of this vasoconstriction is a transient increase in cardiac output followed by a sustained decrease in tissue perfusion, clearly an undesirable phenomenon in the shock state.

Dopamine should be administered by continuous intravenous infusion. The solution for infusion may be prepared by mixing four 5-ml ampules (200 mg/ampule) in 500 ml of sodium chloride, 5 percent dextrose, 5 percent dextrose and 0.9 percent sodium chloride, lactated Ringer's solution, or 5 percent dextrose and lactated Ringer's solution. Dopamine should not be mixed with bicarbonate solution since it is inactivated in an alkaline medium. When prepared in the manner described, the concentration of dopamine will be 1,600 μg/ml. The recommended starting dose for intravenous infusion is 2 to 5 μg/kg/min; the infusion then should be titrated upward in order to achieve the desired hemodynamic response.

In patients with overt congestive heart failure complicating septic shock, digitalization is indicated. This may be accomplished by administering a loading dose of 0.75 mg of digoxin in three divided doses, 4 to 6 h apart, followed by a daily maintenance dose calculated to provide a serum digoxin level of 0.5 to 2.5 ng/ml. Usual maintenance doses will be in the range of 0.125 to 0.375 mg/day.[15] The dosage of digoxin, however, must be adjusted in the presence of impaired renal function.

Treatment of Infection

As hemodynamic parameters are being corrected, attention also must be directed toward elimination of the underlying source of infection. Treatment of life-threatening septicemia requires administration of broad-spectrum antibiotics directed against the pathogens most likely to be present at the site of infection. In obstetric and gynecologic patients, the major organisms responsible for bacteremia and soft-tissue pelvic infections are the aerobic gram-negative rods, Group B streptococci, anaerobic streptococci, and *Bacteroides species*.[30] Although it is not the only acceptable regimen, the antibiotic combination of penicillin (5 million units every 6 h), tobramycin, or gentamicin (3 to 5 mg/kg/day in divided doses), and clindamycin (600 mg every 6 h) will provide effective coverage against virtually all potential pelvic pathogens. Therapy with this or another appropriate antibiotic combination should be initiated promptly after sputum, urine, blood, and operative-site cultures have been obtained.

Each of these antibiotics has potentially serious side effects.[18] In very high doses, penicillin may cause impairment of central nervous system function, including generalized seizures. For this reason, dosage of penicillin must be modified in the presence of renal dysfunction. In susceptible patients, penicillin also may precipitate a life-threatening allergic reaction. Gentamicin and the other aminoglycosides may cause both ototoxicity and nephrotoxicity. In the seriously ill patient, particularly the individual with evidence of renal dysfunction, aminoglycoside dosage should be determined on the basis of measurements of peak and trough drug levels in the serum. Ototoxicity appears to be associated with excessive peak serum levels, while nephrotoxicity seems to be associated with high trough levels. Risk of toxicity is minimized when peak serum levels are maintained in the range of 6 to 10 μg/ml and trough levels are maintained at less than 2 μg/ml. Dosage adjustments are particularly difficult, yet critically important, in the obstetric patient because of wide interpatient variation in rates of elimination and volume of distribution of the antibiotic.[94]

The most common side effect related to use of clindamycin is diarrhea, but the most worrisome complication is the development of psuedomembranous enterocolitis.[2] Although rare, this disorder may be responsible for major morbidity and even death in the affected patient. Pseudomembranous enterocolitis results from destruction of the normal anaerobic colonic flora, with resultant overgrowth of a clindamycin-resistant strain of clostridia, *Clostridium difficile*. This organism then elaborates an exotoxin, which initiates an intense inflammatory reaction in the mucosa of the colon. Diagnosis of this complication may be confirmed by demonstration of characteristic grayish white plaques on the colonic mucosa during sigmoidoscopic examination.

While simple drug-induced diarrhea may respond to discontinuation of the antibiotic, pseudomembranous enterocolitis may require treatment with vancomycin, 500 mg orally every 6 h, until the diarrhea resolves. Relapses after discontinuation of vancomycin have been described.[24] Relapse does not appear to be due to development of resistance to vancomycin, but rather to persistence of *Clostridium difficile* spores in the bowel or to reinfection with *Clostridium difficile*. Relapse may be treated by administration of binding resins, specific antitoxin, or other antibiotics active against *Clostridium difficile*, such as bacitracin, miconazole, or metronidazole.

In addition, there are certain unique situations in which the obstetrician may need to utilize different antibiotic combinations. For example, immunosuppressed patients with neutropenia may require use of carbenicillin or ticarcillin in conjunction with amikacin in treating infections due to resistant *Pseudomonas* organisms.[18] Antifungal agents such as amphotericin or miconazole may be necessary to eliminate fungal septicemia in a patient receiving parenteral hyperalimentation or in an immunosuppressed patient. A semisynthetic penicillin should be substituted for aqueous penicillin G when *Staphylococcus aureus* is suspected or actually isolated.[18] Finally, specialized antimicrobial therapy with pentamidine or trimethoprimsulfamethoxazole may be indicated for management of *Pneumocystis carinii* infections in severely immunocompromised patients.[43]

In addition to administration of broad-spectrum antibiotics, elimination of the source of infection may also require surgery—for example, to drain an abdominopelvic abscess, to remove infected products of conception, to extirpate grossly contaminated pelvic organs, or to debride devitalized subcutaneous and fascial tissue in the abdominal wall.[32,57] It is essential for the obstetrician-gynecologist to recognize that surgical intervention may, in fact, be the single most important step in stabilization of the critically ill patient. Definitive surgical therapy should not be delayed simply because the patient's blood pressure and tissue perfusion respond initially to fluid resuscitation.

The management of the gravid patient with septic shock due to chorioamnionitis presents a particularly difficult problem for the obstetrician. Several investigators have demonstrated that the maternal and fetal prognosis in chorioamnionitis has improved remarkably in recent years, presumably owing to early diagnosis and aggressive use of potent broad-spectrum antibiotics.[26,48] Chorioamnionitis alone no longer is an indication for cesarean section unless other obstetric complications develop, such as cephalopelvic disporportion, malpresentation, or fetal distress.[26]

The maternal and fetal prognosis may not be so favorable, however, when chorioamnionitis and septic shock coexist. In a study of pregnant baboons, Morishima and associates noted that several omnious pathophysiologic changes occurred after administration of endotoxin to the mother.[65] Uterine activity increased significantly, and uterine blood flow decreased. Maternal and fetal temperature increased. The baseline fetal heart rate decreased in all subjects, and all fetuses developed persistent late decelerations. All the mothers and fetuses developed metabolic acidosis, and all the fetuses died in utero 2 to 6 h after injection of endotoxin.

Given these experimental observations, we would recommend prompt delivery of the fetus, by cesarean section if necessary, if the parturient's cardiovascular dysfunction does not improve with the measures outlined above. If maternal blood pressure, cardiac output, and tissue perfusion do improve, trial of labor may be acceptable provided that the fetus is continuously monitored. Immediate delivery by the most expeditious route is indicated if there is any evidence of deterioration in the condition of the fetus or worsening of maternal cardiovascular performance.

Surgery in the presence of deteriorating maternal cardiovascular function clearly is hazardous. It may be necessary, however, precisely because surgical removal of the focus of infection is the only way to stabilize the critically ill patient. Most investigators recommend endotracheal intubation and general anesthesia for emergency abdominal delivery, particularly in a patient with hemodynamic dysfunction.[80] Regional anesthetics, which often require more time to administer, may aggravate maternal hypotension, which in turn may result in further decrease in uterine blood flow and progressive fetal hypoxia and acidosis. Furthermore, epidural or spinal anesthesia is contraindicated in septic patients because of the possibility of creating an intraspinal abscess secondary to hematoma.

The preferred agents for general anesthesia are those that produce the least depressive effect on the cardiovascular system of the mother and fetus. Inhalation gases that result in marked uterine relaxation, such as halothane and enflurane, should be avoided in patients with chorioamnionitis and septic shock since such patients already are particularly susceptible to uterine atony and postoperative hemorrhage. One anesthetic regimen that has been widely advocated for emergency cesarean section is the combination of thiopental (2 to 4 mg/kg) for induction, followed by 50 percent nitrous oxide with oxygen until delivery of the bably. In the presence of hypotension, ketamine (1.0 mg/kg) may be preferred to thiopental for induction because of its sympathomimetic properties. Following delivery, anesthesia may be deepened with intravenous narcotics and diazepam as tolerated. Adequate muscle relaxation can be provided with a continuous succinylcholine infusion (0.1 to 0.2 percent) or incremental doses of pancuronium.

It is essential to recognize that even light or moderate degrees of inhalation anesthesia may depress the fetus when induction-to-delivery time is prolonged.[80] Accordingly, surgery should be performed as rapidly as is consistent with maternal safety. In addition, the delivery must be attended by an individual skilled in resuscitation of the newborn.

Administration of Corticosteroids

Many investigators also advocate the use of glucocorticoids in the treatment of septic shock.[9,50,51,77,78,82,84,87] Several recent laboratory and clinical studies have demonstrated improvement in both circulatory hemodynamics and survival in subjects treated with these agents. Other investigators have failed to document improved survival in patients receiving corticosteroids.[47,49]

There are several reasons for the apparently discordant conclusions reached by different study groups.[79] First, it is very difficult to separate the effect of corticosteroid administration from the effect of other treatment modalities such as fluid resuscitation, ventilatory support, and timing of surgical intervention. In essence, no two patients will ever be treated exactly the same, except for the administration of steroids. Second, the dosages of steroids used in different studies often are not comparable, thus making valid conclusions about relative efficacy difficult. Finally, not only the dosage but also the timing of corticosteroid administration appears to be critically important in determining whether the drugs have a beneficial effect on survival. In most of the investigations reporting lack of success with steroid administration, the medication was not given until the shock state was already fully developed.

If corticosteroids are to be of value in treatment of septic shock, it is clear that they must be given in pharmacologic doses very early in the evolution of the shock state. We recommend that corticosteroids be administered at the time fluid resuscitation is begun. We follow the regimen originally proposed by Shumer,[82] who utilized methylprednisolone (30 mg/kg) or dexamethasone (3 mg/kg) as a single intravenous bolus. The infusion may be repeated in 4 h if necessary. Other investigators have recommended continuing corticosteroids for 24 to 48 h.[84] Even after 48 h of use, the drugs may be discontinued abruptly without precipitating adrenal crisis.

When given early in the disease state and in proper dosage, corticosteroids appear to have several beneficial effects in improving the pathophysiologic derangements precipitated by sepsis. They exert a positive inotropic effect on the heart and thereby increase cardiac output.[9,77–79,82,87] They dilate the peripheral vasculature and cerebral vasculature and improve tissue perfusion. They promote gluconeogenesis and thus enhance the availability of glucose to the central nervous system.[17] They suppress the release of myocardial depressant factor from the ischemic pancreas.[31] Finally, and most importantly, glucocorticoids inhibit the intense inflammatory reaction mediated by initiation of the complement cascade and leukocyte aggregation.[38,45] Accordingly, their net effect on an ultrastructural level is to stabilize lysosomal membranes and preserve the integrity of capillary endothelium, thus preventing cellular autolysis and transudation of intravascular fluid into the interstitial spaces. This latter effect of glucocorticoids is particularly important in preventing serious inflammatory injury to the pulmonary vasculature.[10,45,50,83]

Serious side effects occur in approximately 6 percent of patients receiving pharmacologic doses of corticosteroids for the treatment of septic shock. Complications of steroid therapy include gastrointestinal bleeding, hyperosmolar diabetes, and acute psychosis.

Support of the Respiratory System

The most common cause of death in septic shock is respiratory failure due to ARDS. Of patients with septic shock, 25 to 50 percent will develop ARDS. Kaplan and associates have demonstrated that the mortality rate in septic shock complicated by respiratory failure may be as high as 90 percent, almost twice that in septic shock without ARDS.[46] Clowes and coworkers have confirmed the poor prognosis in patients with septic shock who develop ARDS.[10]

A major objective in the management of the critically ill patient is *prevention* of respiratory failure. Patients with septicemia and shock are, by definition, hypoxic and acidotic; therefore, oxygen therapy with nasal cannula or face mask should be instituted immediately. Arterial blood gases should be monitored frequently to detect early onset of respiratory failure. Excessive fluid replacement should be avoided. Most importantly, the patient should be managed with mechanical ventilation at the earliest manifestation of decreased pulmonary compliance, thereby preventing irreversible hypoxic damage to the pulmonary vasculature. Clowes and associates have provided valuable clinical confirmation of the importance of effective ventilatory support in the treatment of the septic patient and have emphasized the unique application of volume-cycled respirators and positive-end expiratory pressure in this clinical setting.[10]

Additional Supportive Measures

It is essential to prevent wide fluctuations in the patient's temperature, since thermal instability may aggravate existing cardiovascular dysfunction. Coagulation abnormalities should be identified promptly and corrected by administration of cryoprecipitate, fresh frozen plasma, fresh whole blood, or platelets.[18] Only in rare circumstances should it be necessary to consider use of heparin for management of a consumption coagulopathy. In immunosuppressed patients, especially those with infections due to *Pseudomonas* organisms, transfusion of compatible white blood cells may be indicated. Graw and associates,[35] in a controlled study of neutropenic patients with gram-negative bacteremia, have documented improved survival in individuals receiving white cell transfusions in addition to appropriate antimicrobial therapy.

Future Directions in Treatment

At the present time there are several experimental modalities that ultimately may have more widespread clinical application in management of patients with septic shock. McCabe[61] and associates have demonstrated that mortality in gram-negative bacteremia is reduced significantly in patients who develop antibodies directed against certain common antigens shared by the Enterobacteriaceae. In a study of 175 patients with bacteremia due to gram-negative bacilli, these investigators noted that both shock and death were one-third as frequent in patients with high titers of antibody directed against an antigen present in the cell wall of rough mutant strains of bacteria (RE antibody). This discovery raises the intriguing possibility of passively immunizing debilitated hospitalized patients prior to the development of septicemia.

Several investigators have documented elevated plasma levels of prostaglandin in experimental animals receiving injections of endotoxin. Fletcher and Ramwell[21] have demonstrated that increases in prostaglandin levels correlate with disturbances in hemodynamic parameters such as cardiac output, mean arterial pressure, heart rate, and pulmonary artery pressure. They also have shown that pretreatment with indomethacin, a nonsteroidal anti-inflammatory agent, prevents these hemodynamic derangements in the dog subjected to endotoxic shock.

Similarly, Cefalo and coworkers[7] have suggested that increased prostaglandin levels are specifically responsible for vasoconstriction of the pulmonary vasculature, with resultant development of pulmonary hypertension, pulmonary edema, and respiratory failure. Using a sheep model, these authors have confirmed that the increase in prostaglandins E and $F_2\alpha$ can be blocked by pretreatment of the animals with indomethacin or ibuprofen. Rao and associates,[74] utilizing a primate model, have demonstrated that pretreatment of experimental subjects with aspirin reduces platelet aggregation in the small vessels of the kidney and presumably also of the lung, thereby minimizing stasis, microembolization, and release of inflammatory mediators such as prostaglandins and complement. Based upon these experimental observations, clinical trials of antiplatelet drugs and prostaglandin inhibitors would appear to be warranted.

Finally, there now is impressive experimental evidence implicating endogenous beta-endorphin in the pathophysiology of septic shock. In a rat model, Moberg[63] has shown that endotoxin has a direct effect on the hypothalamus, resulting in the release of corticotropin-releasing hormone (CRH), which in turn causes the pituitary gland to secrete ACTH. Both ACTH and beta-endorphin are polypeptides which form part of a larger glycoprotein molecule. Therefore, release of ACTH during endotoxic shock also results in the release of beta-endorphin.

In laboratory animals, endorphin exerts a profound depressant effect on the cardiovascular system, leading to decreased heart rate and hypotension. Holaday and Faden[41] have shown that this hypotensive effect of endorphin can be reversed by administration of the narcotic antagonist naloxone (Narcan). These same investigators also have demonstrated that administration of thyrotropin-releasing hormone (TRH) increases blood pressure, heart rate, and pulse pressure in rats subject to endotoxic shock. This effect occurs because TRH functions as a physiologic opiate antagonist without directly attaching to opiate receptor sites.[41]

There now are at least two reports describing the use of endorphin antagonists in patients with seemingly irreversible septic shock. Tiengo[88] administered naloxone subcutaneously to an 8-year-old child with fulminant meningococcemia and noted an immediate increase in blood pressure and decrease in the degree of tachycardia. After three separate injections, the patient's cardiovascular indices stabilized and the shock state resolved. In a larger, although uncontrolled, trial, Peters and associates[72] administered naloxone intravenously to eight patients with septicemia and prolonged hypotension. Each of these individuals experienced a significant increase in blood pressure within minutes of receiving the drug, and the increases were sustained for an average of 45 min. Despite the apparent efficacy of these experimental modalities of treatment, however, additional clinical research is needed to establish their value in the management of septic shock.

PREVENTIVE MEASURES

The most effective treatment of maternal sepsis is prevention. Preventive measures that may be employed in the preoperative period include stabilization of the patient's preexisting medical disease prior to surgery and avoidance of unnecessarily prolonged preoperative hospitalization, a factor which increases the patient's risk of being colonized by multiply resistant pathogenic bacteria. Precautions that may be applied in the intraoperative and immediate perioperative period include effective hemostasis, judicious use of operative-site drains in selected patients, aseptic wound and catheter care, aseptic placement of peripheral and central venous and arterial catheters, and consistent hand washing by medical personnel between patient examinations.[44]

In the postoperative period, the physician's attention should be directed primarily toward early identification of patients with infection-related complications. There now is some evidence that prompt diagnosis of operative-site infections combined with precise antimicrobial therapy can prevent many of the serious sequelae of soft-tissue pelvic infections.

Specifically, recent work by diZerega and associates[14] demonstrates that treatment of operative-site infections with agents highly effective against both anaerobic organisms and coliform organisms markedly reduces the risk of life-threatening complications of pelvic infections, such as pelvic abscess, septic pelvic vein thrombophlebitis, and septic shock. The clinical experience of these investigators is consistent with the laboratory studies of Weinstein and associates,[92] who demonstrated that most serious abdominopelvic infections occur in two phases: a peritonitis-septicemia stage caused by the coliform organisms and a later abscess formation stage mediated by anaerobic organisms, particularly *Bacteroides* species.

None of the preventive measures outlined above, however, is a substitute for frequent, personalized bedside monitoring of the parturient. Optimal obstetric care requires unrelenting attention on the part of the clinican to every detail of the patient's perioperative course.

REFERENCES

1. Barnett, J.A. and Sanford, J.P.: Bacterial shock. JAMA, *209:*1514, 1969.
2. Bartlett, J.G., Charg, T.W., Gurwith, M. et al.: Antibiotic-associated pseudomembranous colitis due to toxin-producing Clostridia. N. Engl. J. Med., *298:*531, 1978.
3. Bernheim, H.A., Block, L.H., and Atkins, E.: Fever: pathogenesis, pathophysiology, and purpose. Ann. Intern. Med., *91:*261, 1979.

4. Blanco, J.D., Gibbs, R.S., and Castaneda, Y.S.: Bacteremia in obstetrics: clinical course. Obstet. Gynecol., *58*:621, 1981.
5. Broder, G. and Weil, M.H.: Excess lactate: an index of reversibility of shock in human patients. Science, *143*:1457, 1964.
6. Bruni, F.D., Komwatana, P., Soulsby, M.E., and Hess, M.L.: Endotoxin and myocardial failure: role of the myofibril and venous return. Am. J. Physiol., *235*:H150, 1978.
7. Cefalo, R.C., Lewis, P.E., O'Brien, W.F. et al.: The role of prostaglandins in endotoxemia. Am. J. Obstet. Gynecol., *137*:53, 1980.
8. Cherry, J.W.: Endotoxin shock. Surg. Clin. North Am., *50*:403, 1970.
9. Christy, J.H.: Treatment of gram-negative shock. Am. J. Med., *50*:77, 1971.
10. Clowes, G.H.A., Hirsch, E., Williams, L. et al.: Septic shock and shock lung in man. Ann. Surg., *181*:681, 1975.
11. Clowes, G.H.A., O'Donnell, T.F., Ryan, N.T., and Blackburn, G.L.: Energy metabolism in sepsis. Am. Surg., *179*:684, 1974.
12. Cunningham, F.G., Hauth, J.C., Strong, J.D., and Kappus, S.S.: Infectious morbidity following cesarean section. Obstet. Gynecol., *52*:656, 1978.
13. DePalma, R.T., Leveno, K.J., Cunningham, F.G. et al.: Identification and management of women at high risk for pelvic infection following cesarean section. Obstet. Gynecol., *55*:185, 1980.
14. DiZerega, G., Yonekura, L., Roy, S. et al.: A comparison of clindamycin-gentamicin and penicillin-gentamicin in the treatment of post–cesarean section endomyometritis. Am. J. Obstet. Gynecol., *134*:238, 1979.
15. Doherty, J.E.: Digitalis glycosides. Ann. Intern. Med., *79*:229, 1973.
16. Duff, P., Smith, P.N., and Keiser, J.F.: Antibiotic prophylaxis in low risk cesarean section. J. Reprod. Med., *27*:133, 1982.
17. Emerson, T.E. and Raymond, R.M.: Methylprednisolone in the prevention of cerebral hemodynamic and metabolic disorders during endotoxin shock in the dog. Surg. Gynecol. Obstet., *148*:361, 1979.
18. Eskridge, R.A.: Septic shock. Crit. Care Q., *2*:55, 1980.
19. Faro, S.: Group B beta-hemolytic streptococci and puerperal infection. Am. J. Obstet. Gynecol., *139*:686, 1981.
20. Fearon, D.T., Ruddy, S., Schur, P.H., and McCabe, W.R.: Activation of the properdin pathway of complement in patients with gram-negative bacteremia. N. Engl. J. Med., *292*:937, 1975.
21. Fletcher, J.R., Ramwell, P.W., and Herman, C.M.: Prostaglandins and the hemodynamic course of endotoxin shock. J. Surg. Res., *20*:589, 1976.
22. Freid, M.A. and Vosti, K.L.: The importance of underlying disease in patients with gram-negative bacteremia. Arch. Intern. Med., *121*:418, 1968.
23. Gall, S.A.: The efficacy of prophylactic antibiotics in cesarean section. Am. J. Obstet. Gynecol., *134*:506, 1979.
24. George, W.L., Volpicelli, N.A., Stiner, D.B. et al.: Relapse of pseudomembranous colitis after vancoymcin therapy. N. Engl. J. Med., *301*:414, 1979.
25. Gibbs, R.S. and Blanco, J.D.: Streptococcal infection in pregnancy: A study of 48 bacteremias. Am. J. Obstet. Gynecol., *140*:405, 1981.
26. Gibbs, R.S., Castillo, M.S., and Rodgers, P.J.: Management of acute chorioamnionitis. Am. J. Obstet. Gynecol., *136*:709, 1980.
27. Gibbs, R.S., Jones, P.M., and Wilder, C.J.: Antibiotic therapy of endometritis following cesarean section. Obstet. Gynecol., *52*:31, 1978.
28. Gibbs, R.S., Rodgers, P.J., Castaneda, Y.S., and Ramzy, I.: Endometritis following vaginal delivery. Obstet. Gynecol., *56*:555, 1980.
29. Gilbert, R.P.: Endotoxin shock in the primate. Proc. Soc. Exp. Biol. Med., *111*:328, 1962.

30. Gilstrap, L.C. and Cunningham, F.G.: The bacterial pathogenesis of infection following cesarean section. Obstet. Gynecol., *53*:545, 1979.
31. Glenn, T.M. and Lefer, A.M.: Anti-toxic action of methylprednisolone in hemorrhagic shock. Eur. J. Pharmacol., *13*:230, 1971.
32. Golde, S. and Ledger, W.J.: Necrotizing fasciitis in postpartum patients. Obstet. Gynecol., *50*:670, 1977.
33. Goldfarb, R.D. and Weber, P.: The chemical nature of a pancreatic cardiodepressant factor. (Brief Communication.) Circ. Shock, *4*:95, 1977.
34. Goldberg, L.I.: Dopamine—Clinical uses of an endogenous catecholamine. N. Engl. J. Med., *291*:707, 1974.
35. Graw, R.G., Herzig, G., Perry, S., and Henderson, E.S.: Normal granulocyte transfusion therapy. N. Engl. J. Med., *287*:367, 1972.
36. Guillemin, R., Vargo, T., Rossier, J. et al.: β-Endorphin and adrenocorticotropin are secreted concomitantly by the pituitary gland. Science, *197*:1367, 1977.
37. Guntheroth, W.G. and Kawabori, I.: The contribution of splanchnic pooling to endotoxin shock in the dog. Circ. Res., *41*:467, 1977.
38. Hammerschmidt, D.E., White, J.G., Craddock, P.R., and Jacob, H.S.: Corticosteroids inhibit complement-induced granulocyte aggregation. J. Clin. Invest., *63*:798, 1979.
39. Hinshaw, L.B. and Brake, C.M.: The mechanism of endotoxin shock. Okla. State Med. Assoc. J., *57*:421, 1964.
40. Hinshaw, L.B., Emerson, T.E., and Reins, D.A.: Cardiovascular responses of the primate in endotoxin shock. Am. J. Physiol., *210*:335, 1966.
41. Holaday, J. W., D'Amato, R. J., and Faden, A. I.: Thyrotropin-releasing hormone improves cardiovascular function in experimental endotoxic and hemorrhagic shock. Science, *213*:216, 1981.
42. Holaday, J. W. and Faden, A. I.: Naloxone reversal of endotoxin hypotension suggests role of endorphins in shock. Nature, *275*:450, 1978.
43. Hughes, W.T.: *Pneumocystis carinii* pneumonia. N. Engl. J. Med. *297*:1381, 1977.
44. Iffy, L., Kaminetzky, H.A., Maidman, J.E. et al.: Control of perinatal infection by traditional preventive measures. Obstet. Gynecol., *54*:403, 1979.
45. Jacob, H.S.: Role of complement and granulocytes in septic shock. Monograph. The Upjohn Company, 1978.
46. Kaplan, R.L., Sahn, S.A., and Petty, T.L.: Incidence and outcome of the respiratory distress syndrome in gram-negative sepsis. Arch. Intern. Med., *139*:867, 1979.
47. Klastersky, J., Cappel, R., and Debusscher, L.: Effectiveness of betamethasone in management of severe infections. N. Engl. J. Med., *284*:1248, 1971.
48. Koh, K.S., Chan, F.H., Monfared, A.H. et al.: The changing perinatal and maternal outcome in chorioamnionitis. Obstet. Gynecol., *53*:730, 1979.
49. Kreger, B.E., Craven, D.E., and McCabe, W.R.: Gram-negative bacteremia. Am. J. Med., *68*:344, 1980.
50. Krober, M.: Use of corticosteroids in the treatment of infectious diseases. South. Med. J., *67*:728, 1974.
51. Kusajima, K., Wax, S., and Webb, W.R.: Effects of methylprednisolone on pulmonary microcirculation. Surg. Gynecol. Obstet., *139*:1, 1974.
52. Kwaan, H.M. and Weil, M.H.: Differences in the mechanism of shock caused by bacterial infections. Surg. Gynecol. Obstet., *128*:37, 1969.
53. Lee, C.T., Fein, A.M., Lippmann, M. et al.: Elastolytic activity in pulmonary lavage fluid from patients with adult respiratory distress syndrome. N. Engl. J. Med., *304*:192, 1981.
54. Lefer, A.M.: Role of a myocardial depressant factor in shock states. Mod. Concepts Cardiovasc. Dis., *42*:59, 1973.

55. Lillehei, R.C., Dietzman, R.H., Motsay, G.J. et al.: The pharmacologic approach to the treatment of shock. I. Geriatrics, *27*:73, 1972.
56. Lillehei, R.C., Dietzman, R.H., Motsay, G.J. et al.: The pharmacologic approach to the treatment of shock II. Geriatrics, *27*:81, 1972.
57. Lowthian, J.T. and Gillard, L.J.: Postpartum necrotizing fasciitis. Obstet. Gynecol., *56*:661, 1980.
58. Mariona, F. G. and Ismail, M. A.: *Clostridium perfringens* septicemia following cesarean section. Obstet. Gynecol., *56*:518, 1980.
59. Mason, J.W., Kleeberg, U., Dolan, P., and Colman, R.W.: Plasma kallikrein and Hageman factor in gram-negative bacteremia. Ann. Intern. Med., *73*:545, 1970.
60. McCabe, W.R.: Serum complement levels in bacteremia due to gram-negative organisms. N. Engl. J. Med., *288*:21, 1973.
61. McCabe, W.R., Kreger, B.E., and Johns, M.: Type-specific and cross-reactive antibodies in gram-negative bacteremia. N. Engl. J. Med., *287*:261, 1972.
62. McSwain, N.E.: Pneumatic trousers and the management of shock. J. Trauma, *17*:719, 1977.
63. Moberg, G.P.: Site of action of endotoxins on hypothalamic-pituitary-adrenal axis. Am. J. Physiol., *220*:397, 1971.
64. Monif, G.R.G. and Baer, H.: Polymicrobial bacteremia in obstetric patients. Obstet. Gynecol., *48*:167, 1976.
65. Morishima, H.O., Niemann, W.H., and James, L.S.: Effects of endotoxin on the pregnant baboon and fetus. Am. J. Obstet. Gynecol., *131*:899, 1978.
66. Moss, G.S. and DasGupta, T.K.: The normal electron histochemistry and the effect of hemorrhagic shock on the pulmonary surfactant system. Surg. Gynecol. Obstet., *140*:53, 1975.
67. Moss, G., Staunton, C., and Stein, A.A.: Cerebral etiology of the shock lung syndrome. J. Trauma, *12*:885, 1972.
68. Motsay, G.J., Dietzman, R.H., Ersek, R.A., and Lillehei, R.C.: Hemodynamic alterations and results of treatment in patients with gram-negative septic shock. Surgery, *67*:577, 1970.
69. Nishijima, H., Weil, M.H., Shubin, H., and Cavanilles, J.: Hemodynamic and metabolic studies on shock associated with gram-negative bacteremia. Medicine, *52*:287, 1973.
70. Paris, P.M.: Antishock garments. N. Engl. J. Med., *305*:960, 1981.
71. Peretz, D.I., McGregor, M., and Dossetor, J.B.: Lacticacidosis: A clinically significant aspect of shock. Can. Med. Assoc. J., *90*:673, 1964.
72. Peters, W.P., Friedman, P.A., Johnson, M.W., and Mitch, W.E.: Pressor effect of naloxone in septic shock. Lancet, *1*:529, 1981.
73. Raffa, J. and Trunkey, D.D.: Myocardial depression in sepsis. J. Trauma, *18*:617, 1978.
74. Rao, P.S., Cavanagh, D., and Lamont, W.G.: Endotoxic shock in the primate: Effects of aspirin and dipyridamole administration. Am. J. Obstet. Gynecol., *140*:914, 1981.
75. Roberts, J.M. and Laros, R.K.: Hemorrhagic and endotoxic shock: A pathophysiologic approach to diagnosis and management. Am. J. Obstet. Gynecol., *110*:1041, 1971.
76. Rogel, S. and Hilewitz, H.: Cardiac impairment and shock factors. Fed. Proc., *37*:2718, 1978.
77. Rosenbaum, R.W., Hayes, M.F., and Matsumoto, T.: Efficacy of steroids in the treatment of septic and cardiogenic shock. Surg. Gynecol. Obstet., *136*:914, 1973.
78. Sambhi, M.P., Weil, M.H., and Udhoji, V.N.: Acute pharmacodynamic effects of glucocorticoids. Circulation *31*:523, 1965.
79. Sheagren, J.N.: Septic shock and corticosteroids. N. Engl. J. Med., *305*:456, 1981.
80. Shnider, S.M.: Choice of anesthesia for labor and delivery. Obstet. Gynecol. *58*:24S, 1981.
81. Shubin, H., Weil, M.H., and Carlson, R.W.: Bacterial shock. Am. Heart J. *94*:112, 1977.
82. Shumer, W.: Steroids in the treatment of clinical septic shock. Ann. Surg. *184*:333, 1976.

83. Sibbald, W.J., Anderson, R.R., Reid, B. et al.: Alveolar-capillary permeability in human septic ARDS. Chest, *79:*133, 1981.
84. Sladen, A.: Methylprednisolone—pharmacologic doses in shock lung syndrome. J. Thorac. Cardiovasc. Surg., *71:*800, 1976.
85. Swan, K.G., Barton, R.W., and Reynolds, D.G.: Mesenteric hemodynamics during endotoxemia in the baboon. Gastroenterology, *61:*872, 1971.
86. Sweet, R.L. and Ledger, W.J.: Puerperal infectious morbidity: A two year review. Am. J. Obstet. Gynecol., *117:*1093, 1973.
87. Thomas, C.S. and Brockman, S.K.: The role of adrenal corticosteroid therapy in *Escherichia coli* endotoxin shock. Surg. Gynecol. Obstet., *143:*61, 1968.
88. Tiengo, M.: Naloxone in irreversible shock. Lancet, *2:*690, 1980.
89. Tramont, E.C.: The diagnosis and treatment of septic shock. Milit. Med., *144:*153, 1979.
90. Waeckerle, J.F.: Antishock garments. Crit. Care Q., *2:*15, 1980.
91. Weil, M.H. and Nishijima, H.: Cardiac output in bacterial shock. Am. J. Med., *64:*920, 1978.
92. Weinstein, W.M., Onderdonk, A.B., Bartlett, J.G., and Gorbach, S.L.: Experimental intra-abdominal abscesses in rats: Development of an experimental model. Infect. Immun., *10:*1250, 1974.
93. Weisel, R.D., Vito, L., Dennis, R.C. et al.: Myocardial depression during sepsis. Am. J. Surg., *133:*512, 1977.
94. Zaske, D.E., Cipolle, R.J., Strate, R.G. et al.: Rapid gentamicin elimination in obstetric patients. Obstet. Gynecol., *56:*559, 1980.

9

The Management of Acquired Hemostatic Failure during Pregnancy

Roberto Romero, M.D.

INTRODUCTION

The objective of the hemostatic mechanism is to maintain blood within the circulatory system by sealing vascular leaks without compromising blood fluidity.[107] This goal is accomplished by the complex and balanced interaction of four main components: the vessel wall, the platelets, the coagulation system, and the fibrinolytic system. Hemostatic disorders such as hemorrhage or thrombosis are two of the more serious hazards of pregnancy. This chapter will review the basic physiology and laboratory testing of the hemostatic mechanism and will focus on the clinical management of acquired hemostatic failure during pregnancy.

BASIC PHYSIOLOGY OF THE HEMOSTATIC SYSTEM

Overview of the Hemostatic System

Vascular injury activates all the components of the hemostatic system. Blood vessel damage leads to vasoconstriction, which decreases blood flow and favors more effective contact activation of platelets and coagulation factors. Platelets adhere to the subendothelial connective tissue, spread to cover the damaged surface, and induce further thrombocyte deposition to form a platelet plug or primary hemostatic plug. This platelet plug is only temporary and unless secured with fibrin will disintegrate, resulting in rebleeding. Activation of the coagulation cascade results in the transformation of fibrinogen into fibrin, which when deposited onto the platelet plug imparts solidity to it and allows initiation of the tissue repair process. Finally, the fibrinolytic system removes the excess of hemostatic material and reestablishes vascular patency after healing.[107]

The relative participation of the four components of the hemostatic system varies with the size of the injured vessel. Capillaries, once severed, seal essentially by adhesion of the endothelial cells, without vasoconstriction or significant participation of the rest of the hemostatic system.[107,253] Injuries to arterioles and venules are sealed essentially by the formation of a platelet hemostatic plug. Damage to medium-size vessels requires vasoconstriction and active participation of all the components of the hemostatic system. Injury to larger vessels cannot be repaired by platelet and fibrin deposition alone. Other mechanisms such as vasoconstriction, blood shunting, and inflammatory reactions of the vessel wall decrease blood flow through the damaged vessels and increase the effectiveness of participation of the hemostatic system. If the vessel is large enough, however, these mechanisms may be insufficient to arrest bleeding until either surgical repair occurs or bleeding produces hypotension, frequently associated with fatal blood loss.

Platelets and Vessel Wall

Vascular injury with endothelial disruption exposes subendothelial collagen to circulating blood. Platelets passing by will *adhere* to the raw collagen fibers. Platelet adhesion involves the interaction of von Willebrand's factor, platelet surface glycoprotein Ib (GPIb), and connective tissue. The hereditary absence of GPIb (Bernard-Soulier syndrome) or Von Willebrand's factor produces a defect in platelet adhesion and consequent abnormal bleeding in response to vessel injury.[111,199] Injury of the vessel wall exposes plasma to collagen, which results in the activation of both the intrinsic and extrinsic pathway of the coagulation system and local generation of thrombin (Fig. 1).

Following the interaction of platelets with subendothelial collagen, and possibly in the presence of thrombin, the platelets undergo a change in shape and secrete a number of substances that act synergistically in recruiting additional circulating platelets by aggregation to form an enlarging platelet mass or primary hemostatic plug.[111,104,199] This secretory process, whereby substances stored in platelet granules are expelled from the platelet, is known as the platelet release reaction. The release reaction can occur through either an arachidonic-dependent or an independent pathway[104] (Fig. 9-2). The arachidonic-independent pathway is activated by high-dose thrombin, concentrated collagen, and divalent cation ionophores. Any of these agents can activate the phospholipase C enzyme, which generates phosphatidic acid from membrane phospholipid and leads to mobilization of calcium and to granule release.[88]

The arachidonic acid–dependent pathway is initiated by activation of the phospholipase A_2 enzyme in response to adenosine diphosphate (ADP), epinephrine, dilute collagen, or low-dose thrombin. Phospholipase A_2 cleaves arachidonic acid from the membrane phospholipids: phosphatidylcholine and phosphatidylethanolamine.[26,38] Arachidonic acid is transformed by cyclooxygenase or prostaglandin synthetase into the labile prostaglandin endoperoxides PGG_2 and PGH_2. These compounds have a short half-life and may undergo nonenzymatic transformation into PGE_2, PGF_2, or PGD_2. The main pathway of platelet endoperoxide metabolism is the conversion by thromboxane synthetase to thromboxane A_2, which is a vasoconstrictor and the most potent platelet aggregatory agent known (Fig. 9-3).

Increased concentrations of thromboxane A_2 in the platelet inhibit adenylate cyclase, decrease levels of cyclic adenosine monophosphate (cAMP) and result in mobilization of calcium from intracellular storage sites. Elevation of free calcium leads to phosphorylation of platelet myosin, triggering contraction and initiating secretion of compounds such as ADP, serotonin, and other substances which induce further platelet aggregation[199] (Fig. 9-2).

Aspirin inhibits the platelet release reaction in vitro and prolongs the bleeding time in vivo. This effect is due to the irreversible acetylation of the cyclooxygenase enzyme and consequent inhibition of the formation of endoperoxides and thromboxane A_2 in platelets.[252,272]

Vascular injury leads to platelet adhesion and aggregation but not necessarily to thrombus formation. The generation of prostacyclin (PGI_2) by the vessel wall appears to be one of the physiologic mechanisms responsible for vascular thrombus resistance by preventing the continuous enlargement of the platelet plug. Prostacyclin is the major product of the cyclooxygenase cascade in the vessel wall. It is a vasodilator and the most potent platelet antiaggregatory agent yet described. It seems to work by stimulting platelet adenyl cyclase, which increases the concentration of cyclic adenosine monophosphate (cAMP). This in turn restores calcium inside the cellular stores. The net effect of these changes is depression of platelet aggregation[199] (Fig. 9-1 and 9-2).

It has been postulated that a balance between the synthesis of thromboxane A_2 and prostacyclin permits the physiologic participation of platelets in endothelial repair without thrombus formation. An imbalance in the activity of these substances could lead to dramatic consequences.[185]

Coagulation System

Coagulation consists of a series of chemical reactions that culminate in the transformation of a soluble protein (fibrinogen) into an insoluble one (fibrin). The coagulation component of the hemostatic mechanism is organized as a biological amplification system that permits multidirectional and sequential activation of plasma clotting factors and has for that reason been called the coagulation cascade (Fig. 9-4).

An international committee has established a nomenclature system that utilizes roman numerals rather than names to designate the clotting factors (Table 9-1). It

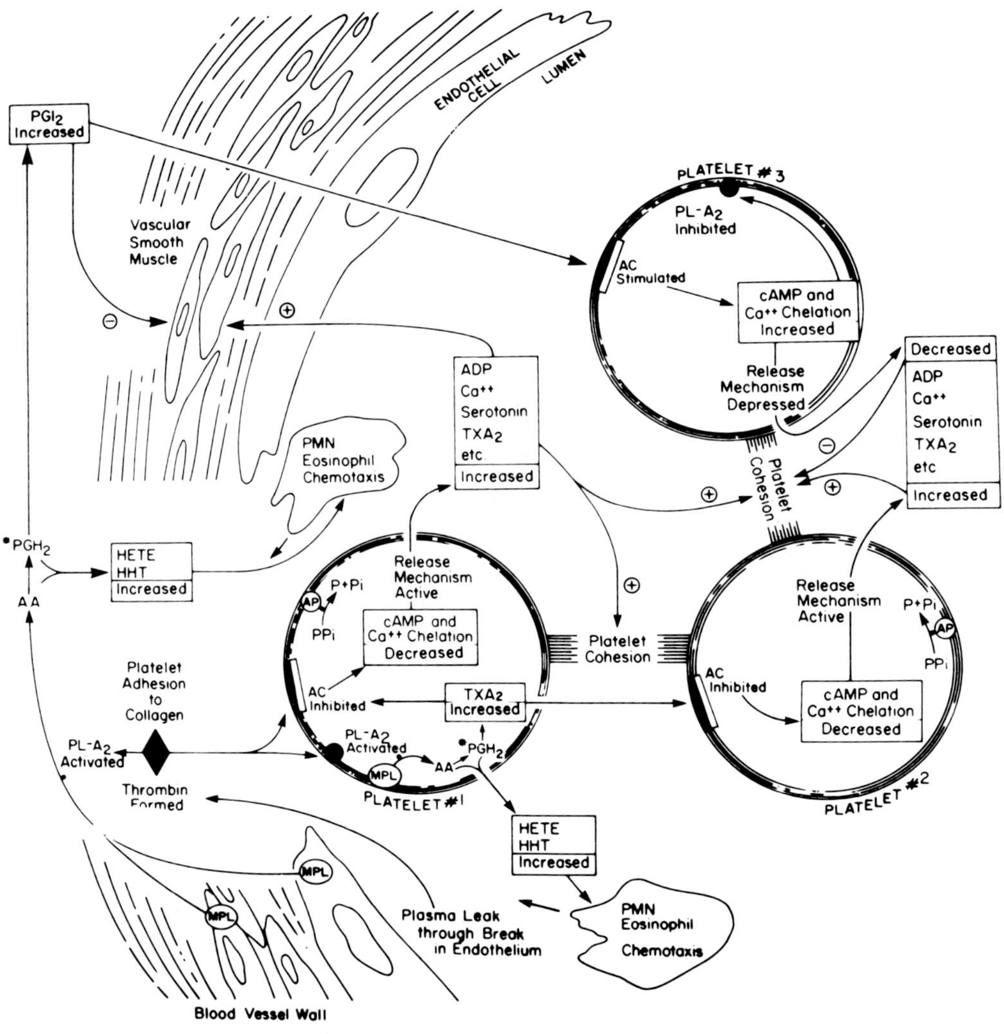

should be noted that the numerals were assigned in order of discovery and not in order of chemical reaction and that there is no factor VI. Some coagulation factors circulate in an inactive form; their active form is indicated by the letter "a" following the roman numeral, e.g., XIIa is the active form of XII. An exception to the latter is the active form of prothrombin (factor II), which is called thrombin rather than factor IIa.[10,301,303]

The reactions of the coagulation cascade can be divided into two major overlapping pathways, intrinsic and extrinsic. Blood collected in a glass tube generates thrombin slowly through the intrinsic pathway and clots in 5 to 15 min. The addition of tissue extracts results in a more rapid generation of thrombin through the extrinsic pathway, and clot formation occurs in 12 to 15 s.

Although the intrinsic and extrinsic mechanisms have been described as independent pathways, growing evidence supports their biochemical interdependence at

◄ *Fig. 9-1* Three platelets are shown in hemostatic response to a break in the blood vascular endothelium. Platelet 1 is responding to collagen and other subendothelial substances by adhesion. Thrombin is also formed at the site by exposure of plasma to tissue thromboplastin. Phospholipase-A_2 ($PL.A_2$) is activated both in vessel wall and in platelet 1. Membrane phospholipids (MPL) in the platelet and the vessel-wall endothelium and media are acted upon to form arachidonic acid (AA), and endoperoxide (PGH_2) is formed. Chemotactic factors (HETE and HHT) are formed from AA and PGH_2 to attract polymorphonuclear leukocytes (PMN) and eosinophils to the area. In platelet 1 thromboxane (TXA_2) is formed, resulting in inhibition of adenylate cyclase (AC) in that platelet and in platelet 2. The result of AC inhibition is decreased cyclic adenosine monophosphate (cAMP) and decreased calcium chelation, which allows an active release mechanism to form. With the release of ADP, calcium ions, serotonin, thromboxane, etc., there occurs platelet cohesion (for example between platelets 1 and 2 or between platelets 2 and 3). In addition, vascular smooth muscle contraction is stimulated. Prostacyclin (PGI_2) is formed from PGH_2 in the vessel wall. PGH_2 formed in platelet 1 is also starred (*) because upon release it migrates to the vessel wall to enhance formation of PGI_2. Prostacyclin stimulates AC of platelet 3, resulting in depression of the release mechanism, with ultimate lack of platelet cohesion. In addition, PGI_2 inhibits vascular smooth muscle. In the platelets, phosphorylated protein (PPi) complexes with calcium and this complex is continuously being broken down by alkaline phosphatase (AP). In platelets 1 and 2 a more complete breakdown with calcium ion release occurs since cAMP is decreased, while in platelet 3 calcium ion chelation is increased. (AA) arachidonic acid, (AC) adenylate cyclase (membrane-bound), (ADP) adenosine diphosphate, (AP) alkaline phosphatase (membrane-bound), (cAMP) cyclic adenosine 3′,5′-monophosphate, (HHT) chemotactic agent, (HETE) chemotactic agent, (MPL) membrane phospholipid, (P) protein (cAMP-dependent), (PGH_2) endoperoxide, (PGI_2) prostacyclin, (Pi) phosphorus, inorganic ($PL.A_2$) phospholipase A_2, (PMN) polymorphonuclear leukocyte, (PPi) phosphorylated protein, (TXA_2) thromboxane. (Reproduced from Nalbandian, R.M. and Henry, R.L.: Platelet endothelial cell interaction. Semin. Thromb. Haemotas., *5*:87, 1978.)

a stage subsequent to contact activation. Schematically, the coagulation cascade can be divided into separate initial phases and a common final phase. During the initial phase, both pathways form factor Xa. In the common terminal phase of blood coagulation, factor Xa generates thrombin, which catalyzes the conversion of fibrinogen into fibrin (Fig. 9-4).

The Intrinsic Pathway. The intrinsic pathway of blood coagulation begins with contact or surface activation of factor XII. This activation process occurs when plasma is exposed to negatively charged materials such as collagen, endotoxin, platelet phospholipids, glass, kaolin, and other substances. Binding of factor XII to any of these materials seems to make the molecule more susceptible to the proteolytic activation of kallikrein, or Fletcher factor, which catalyzes the activation of surface-bound factor XII.[102–104]

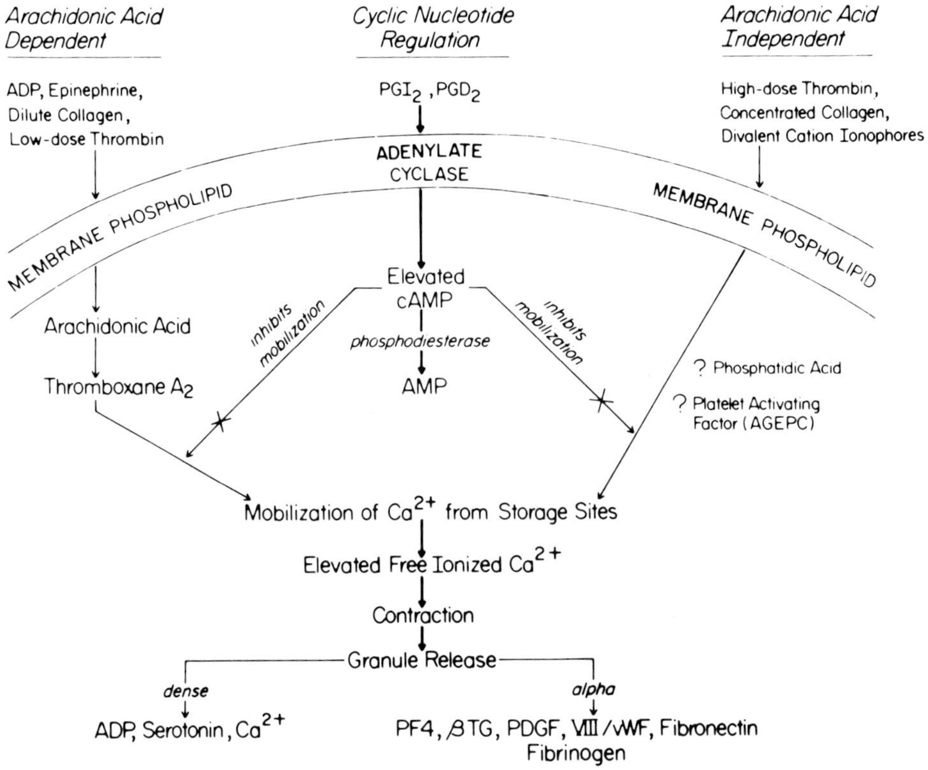

Fig. 9-2 Mechanisms of platelet release. In the arachidonic acid-dependent pathway ADP, epinephrine, dilute collagen, or low-dose thrombin initiate membrane phospholipase activity, leading to the liberation of arachidonic acid and the formation of thromboxane A_2. Thromboxane A_2 mobilizes divalent calcium (Ca^{2+}) from intracellular storage sites, producing an elevation of free ionized cytoplasmic Ca^{2+}. Elevated Ca^{2+} triggers contraction and initiates secretion. Alpha-granule contents, i.e., platelet factor 4 (PF4), beta-thromboglobulin (BTG), platelet-derived growth factor (PDGF), factor VIII von Willebrand's, fibrinogen, and fibronectin are most readily released. Dense granule contents (Ca^{2+}, serotonin, and ADP) are also released. Elevated Ca^{2+} also stimulates phospholipase, further amplifying the process and inhibits adenylate cyclase lowering cAMP. High-dose thrombin, divalent cation ionophore, and concentrated collagen initiate granule release by an arachidonic acid–independent pathway perhaps involving other phospholipase products, such as phosphatidic acid or platelet-activating factor acetyl glyceryl ether phosphorylcholine (AGEPC). Mobilization of Ca^{2+} again appears to be the final critical event triggering contraction and release. Binding of PGI_2 and PGD_2 to membrane receptor initiates adenylate cyclase activity elevating cyclic AMP (cAMP). Elevated cAMP inhibits Ca^{2+} mobilization from storage sites and this prevents granule release either by arachidonic acid–dependent or by independent pathways. (Reproduced from Harlan, J.M. and Harker, J.A.: Hemostasis, thrombosis, and thromboembolic disorders. Med. Clin. North Am., *65:*865, 1981.)

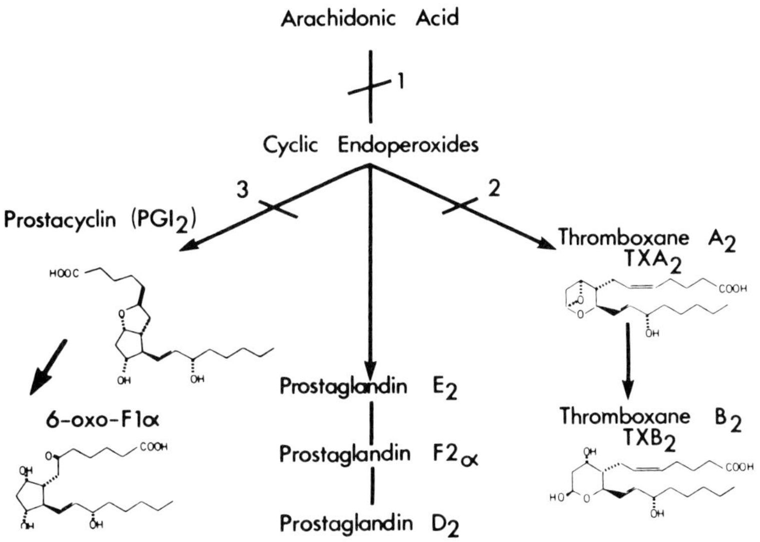

Fig. 9-3 The cyclooxygenase pathway of archidonic acid metabolism. The numbers 1, 2 and 3 represent the cyclooxygenase, thromboxane synthetase, and prostacyclin synthetase enzymes. Note that the endoperoxide intermediates are pivotal for the production of prostacyclin and thromboxane A_2. (Reprinted, by permission of the New England Journal of Medicine, from Monacada, S. and Vane, J.R.: Arachidonic acid metabolites and the interaction between platelets and blood vessel wall. N. Engl. J. Med., *300:*1142, 1979.)

Factor XIIa activates factor XI to factor XIa and prekallikrein to kallikrein. High-molecular-weight kininogen (HMW kininogen), or Fitzgerald factor, accelerates all the reactions mentioned.[103,104] This series of reactions is known as the contact phase of blood coagulation. Although the reactions are important in vitro, their physiologic role in coagulation in vivo remains to be established. Patients with a

Table 9-1. **Plasma Coagulation Factors**

Roman Numeral	Coagulation Factor
I	Fibrinogen
II	Prothrombin
IV	Ionic calcium
V	Proaccelerin
VII	Proconvertin
VIII	Antihemophilic factor A (AHF)
IX	Antihemophilic factor B (Christmas factor)
X	Stuart Prower factor
XI	Antihemophilic factor C
XII	Hageman factor
XIII	Fibrin-stabilizing factor
Not assigned	High molecular weight kininogen (HMG) Kininogen or Fitzgerald factor
Not assigned	Prekallikrein or Fletcher factor

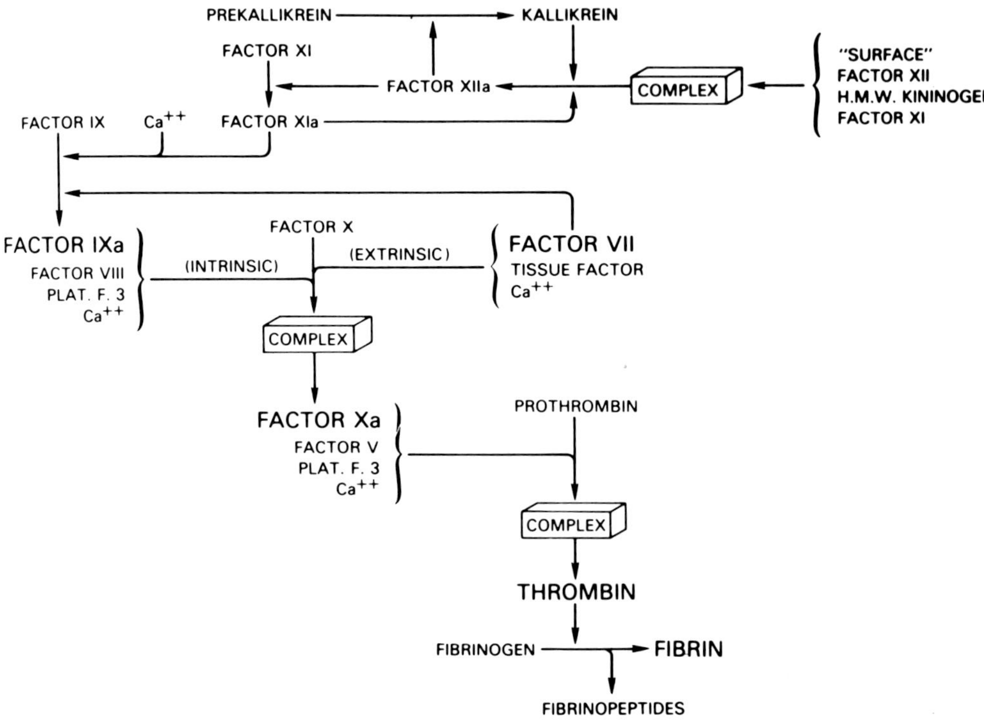

Fig. 9-4 The coagulation cascade. (Reproduced from Murano G.: A basic outline of blood coagulation. Semin. Thromb. Hemostas. *6:*140, 1980.)

deficiency in factor XII, kallikrein, or HMW kininogen have prolonged partial thromboplastin times but generally do not have a bleeding tendency. This suggest either that alternative mechanisms exist for activation of the hemostatic system in vivo or that the contact phase of the blood coagulation is tangential to the process of clotting in vivo.

Recent evidence suggests the existence of a platelet dependent pathway for the generation of factor XIa in the absence of factor XII.[292] This could explain the asymptomatic nature of factor XII, kallikrein, and HMW kininogen deficiencies.

Contact-phase proteins participate in physiologic processes other than activation of the intrinsic pathway of the coagulation system (e.g., activation of the fibrinolytic system and complement cascade). Their relative participation and importance in the control of these functions has not been established.

All the contact-phase proteins are depressed in hepatic disease, which implies that the liver is a major site of their production. A congenital deficiency of each of these factors can be inherited as an autosomal recessive trait[103]; however only deficiency of factor XI is associated with a significant bleeding tendency.

Factor XIa catalyzes the conversion of factor IX to factor IXa, which in turn participates in the activation of factor X to factor Xa. Factor IXa, along with the other vitamin K–dependent factors (II, VII, IX, and X) is synthesized in the liver. Its congenital deficiency is inherited as an X-linked recessive disease and is known as hemophilia B.

The formation of Xa through the intrinsic pathway involves the participation of factor VIII, factor IXa, platelet phospholipids, and calcium. These four components have different roles in the complex responsible for activation of factor X. Factor IXa is the enzyme, factor VIII is a regulatory protein, platelet phospholipids provide the surface for the reaction, and calcium forms bridges between the coagulation factors.[192]

Platelet-membrane phospholipids, also known as platelet factor 3 (PF3),[136] are made available when platelets are activated by trauma, aggregation, thrombin, kaolin, or other stimuli. In the absence of PF3, factor IXa activity is significantly retarded.

Factor VIII seems to be synthesized by endothelial cells. It has a complex structure, and three major properties have been attributed to its molecule:

1. Shortening of the clotting time (factor VIII Coag)
2. Precipitation with rabbit antibody (factor VIII Ag)
3. Correction of the defect in platelet aggregation associated with von Willebrand's disease (factor VIII VWF)

The portion of the molecule that participates in the activation of factor X is factor VIII Coag. A congenital deficiency of this factor produces the serious hemostatic disorder known as hemophilia A and is inherited as an X-linked recessive trait. Factor VIII Coag is activated to factor VIIIa by the action of thrombin prior to its participation in the reaction with factor IXa and calcium. Factor VIII VWF is important in the process of platelet adhesion to the vessel wall. Its deficiency is inherited as an autosomal dominant disease and is known as von Willebrand's disease.[192]

The Common Terminal Pathway of Blood Coagulation. Factor Xa forms a complex with factor V, calcium, and phospholipids that is responsible for the transformation of prothrombin to thrombin. The mechanism for this reaction is similar to the one previously described in the activation of factor X. Factor Xa functions as the enzyme, factor V functions as a cofactor, platelet phospholipids provide a surface for the reaction, and calcium allows binding of the different proteins participating in the reaction. This complex of factors is frequently referred to as prothrombinase. Reduction in the concentration of any of its components results in significant slowing of the reaction. Like factor VIII, factor V is activated by thrombin (to factor Va) prior to its participation in the generation of thrombin.[17,192] A congenital deficiency of factor V is known as parahemophilia and is transmitted as an autosomal recessive disorder. Factor X deficiency is transmitted in an autosomal recessive pattern and may also be associated with significant hemorrhagic symptoms.

The net effect of the reaction catalyzed by the prothrombinase complex is the transformation of prothrombin (factor II) to thrombin. Thrombin is a proteolytic enzyme with the following functions:

1. It transforms fibrinogen into fibrin.
2. It catalyzes the conversion of factor XIII to factor XIIIa.
3. It promotes platelet aggregation.
4. It activates factors V and VIII.

The transformation of fibrinogen into fibrin is the central event of the coagulation process. Thrombin catalyzes the removal of two pairs of peptides (fibrinopeptides A and B) from fibrinogen. The resulting molecule is known as a soluble fibrin monomer. Fibrin monomers undergo spontaneous polymerization to form the fibrin polymer designated as fibrin s. The letter "s" refers to its solubility in 5 *M* urea solution suggesting that the linkage between monomers is produced by noncovalent bonds. Factor XIIIa introduces covalent bonds within the polymerized fibrin, which is then transformed into fibrin i. The letter *i* refers to the polymer's insolubility in 5 *M* urea solutions.[192]

Factor XIII is activated by thrombin and factor Xa. A congenital deficiency of factor XIII is inherited as an autosomal recessive trait and is associated with bleeding from the umbilical cord at birth, delayed wound healing, and irregular scar formation. Congenital disorders in the quantity or quality of the fibrinogen molecule have been described and recently reviewed by Beck.[21]

Extrinsic Pathway. The extrinsic pathway of blood coagulation is activated when blood is exposed to tissue thromboplastin or to tissue factor (TF), a membrane-bound lipoprotein present in a variety of tissues, including brain, kidney, endothelial cells, leukocytes, and placenta.[305] Disruption of cells by mechanical trauma or proteolysis seems to be necessary to make TF available for initiation of the extrinsic pathway.

In the presence of calcium ions TF reacts with factor VIIa to activate factor X, which then initiates the common pathway of blood coagulation. Factor VIIa seems to act as an enzyme with TF as its cofactor. Activation of factor VII can also occur by the action of XIIa, kallikrein, IXa, and the prothrombinase complex. A deficiency of factor VII may be inherited as an autosomal recessive trait and is associated with significant hemorrhagic problems.[201,305]

Control of Coagulation Reactions. Vascular injury activates the intrinsic and extrinsic pathways of blood coagulation and results in the generation of thrombin. Fibrin deposition, however, remains localized at the injured site. The following mechanisms are all instrumental in the prevention of generalized intravascular clotting[298]:

1. Blood flow through the injured site: this can dilute the procoagulants formed in the vicinity of the thrombogenic focus.
2. Absorption of thrombin by deposited fibrin: this is also known as antithrombin I and can lead to sequestration of thrombin from the systemic circulation.
3. Restriction of the availability of platelet phospholipid: activation of platelets at the site of injury by trauma or thrombin is necessary for the membrane phospholipids to become available for surface support of the interaction of coagulation factors. Inactive circulating platelets do not execute this function.
4. Removal of activated coagulation factors by the reticuloendothelial system.[67,153,293]

5. Neutralization of some coagulation factors by plasma inhibitors, the most important of which is antithrombin III (AT-III).

AT-III is a glycoprotein, manufactured in the liver, whose main function is the inactivation of thrombin. It can also inhibit other coagulation factors such as factor XIIa, XIa, Xa, IXa, and kallikrein.[56,265] The rate of inhibition of these activated factors by AT-III is increased by the addition of heparin. AT-III also inhibits thrombin-induced platelet aggregation,[73] plasmin formation, and complement activation. A congenital deficiency of AT-III has been associated with a high incidence of recurrent thromboembolism, often during pregnancy, the puerperium, or postoperative periods.[212] Acquired AT-III deficiency may occur as a consequence of liver disease, administration of oral contraceptive agents, venous thromboembolism, disseminated intravascular coagulation (DIC), and preeclampsia.[212,265,295]

Other proteins with similar activity include α_1-antitrypsin and α_2-macroglobulin. AT-III, however, is the major biochemical inhibitor of blood coagulation in the nonpregnant patient.

Fibrinolysis

Fibrinolysis is the process by which insoluble fibrin is broken down into soluble fibrin degradation products (FDPs). This may occur in either a cellular or fluid phase. The cellular phase is mainly conducted by the polymorphonuclear leukocytes, which contain the enzymes necessary for the degradation of fibrin.[276] This phase may be responsible for fibrinolysis in extravascular areas or in places where the components of the soluble phase are unavailable.[170] The fluid phase is conducted by plasmin, a soluble plasma enzyme, whose main function is to digest fibrin. Although it has been recently suggested that the cellular phase can account for a significant amount of fibrinolytic activity, most of the literature on the subject has concentrated on the fluid phase.[189] Clearly, more investigation is necessary to establish the role of these two participants in normal and pathologic fibrinolysis. This section will focus on the physiology of the soluble phase, which will be referred to as the "fibrinolytic system."

The fibrinolytic enzymatic system consists of three components (Fig. 9-5):

1. Plasminogen, which is the inactive precursor of plasmin
2. Plasminogen activators, which are responsible for the transformation of plasminogen into plasmin
3. Inhibitors which can interfere with the activation of plasminogen or neutralize plasmin

Plasminogen and Plasminogen Activators. Plasminogen is manufactured in the liver and its plasma concentration parallels changes in fibrinogen concentrations. It is transformed into plasmin by the action of activators. Plasminogen activators are classified according to their origin into three groups: extrinsic, intrinsic, and exogenous.[170]

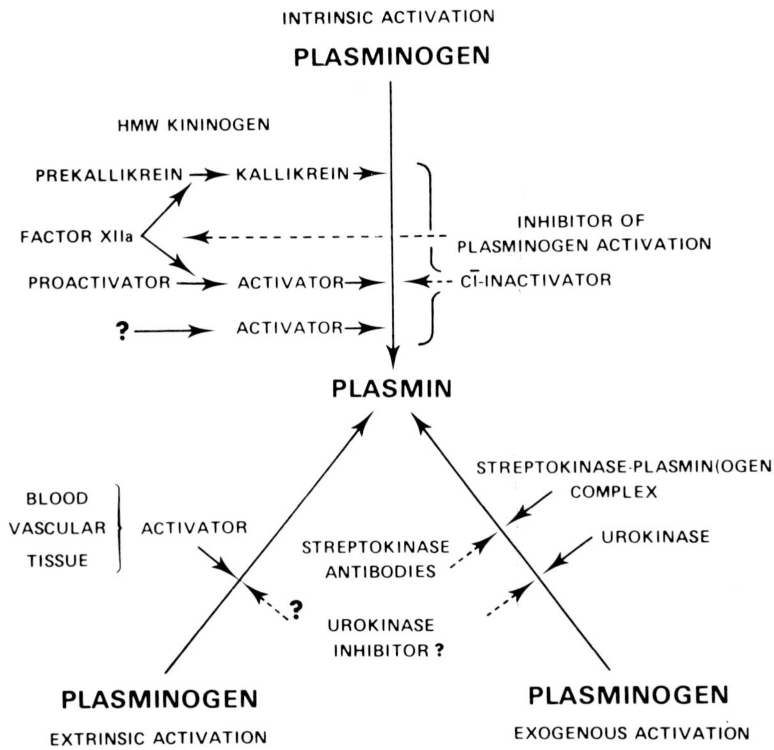

Fig. 9-5 Schematic representation of activation pathways of plasminogen and site of action of inhibitors. (Reproduced from Collen D.: Inhibitors in fibrinolysis. In Thomson, J.M.: Blood Coagulation and Haemostasis. 2nd Ed., Churchill Livingstone, Edinburgh, 1980.)

Extrinsic Activation occurs by the liberation of plasminogen activator from tissues or blood vessel walls. It is termed extrinsic to differentiate it from activation which originates within plasma.

Intrinsic Activation can occur through factor XII–dependent or independent pathways. Activation of the contact phase of blood coagulation generates factor XIIa, which promotes transformation of plasminogen proactivator into plasminogen activator. Prekallikrein and HMW kininogen have been implicated in this reaction. Little information is available about the factor XII–independent pathway. The existence of a factor XII–dependent mode of activation of the fibrinolytic system is important because it provides a linkage between activation of the coagulation cascade and the mechanisms for fibrin removal.

Exogenous Activation can occur during the administration of streptokinase, urokinase, and other nonphysiologic activators, such as chloroform and glycerol.

Plasmin. Plasmin is an endopeptidase whose main function is to break down fibrin into fibrin degradation products. Plasmin is, however, relatively nonspecific and may attack other substrates such as fibrinogen (fibrinogenolysis) prothrombin, factor V, and factor VIII. Since the degradation products of fibrinogen and fibrin are similar, they have been frequently referred to as fibrinogen/fibrin degradation products (FDPs) or split products.

Fibrinogen/Fibrin Degradation Products. Plasmin digests fibrinogen to produce progressively smaller fibrinolytic fragments (Fig. 9-6). The initial reaction splits a fibrinogen molecule into fragments A, B, C, and X. The first three of these products have low molecular weight. Fragment X is much larger and retains the ability to engage in clot formation after exposure to thrombin. Subsequently, fragment X is further split into fragments Y and D. Fragment Y is then degraded into one molecule of fragment D and one of fragment E. Each molecule of fibrinogen is therefore eventually split into two molecules of fragment D, one of fragment E, and a number of small peptide molecules.[5,168,170]

Fibrinogen/fibrin degradation products are removed from the circulation by the reticuloendothelial system and have a half-life of 9 h.[107] Their detection in peripheral blood signifies that fibrinolysis has occurred. FDPs can inhibit normal fibrin mono-

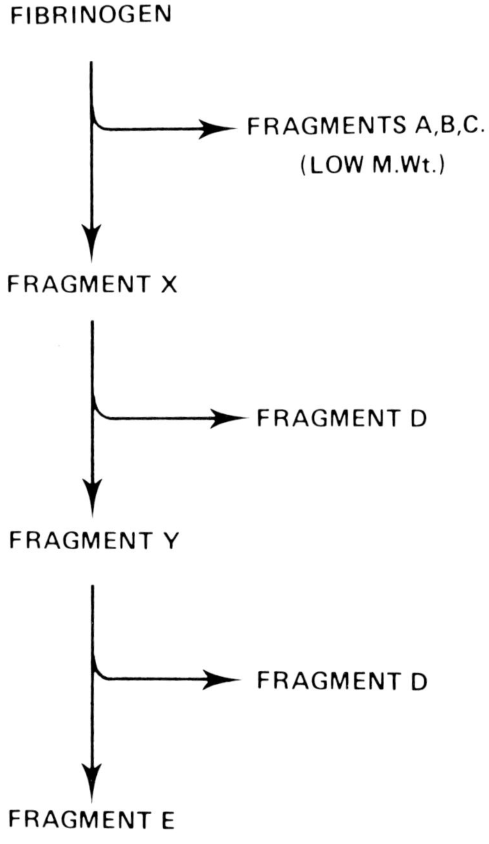

Fig. 9-6 Conversion of fibrinogen to fibrinogen degradation products by the action of plasmin. (Reproduced from Lowe, G.D.O. and Prentice, C.R.N.: The laboratory investigation of fibrinolysis. In Thomson, J.M.: Blood Coagulation and Haemostasis. 2nd Ed., Churchill Livingstone, Edinburgh, 1980.)

mer polymerization and platelet aggregation. These effects can aggravate the coagulation defects which are already present in DIC.[6,82,139,273]

Inhibitors of Fibrinolysis. Inhibition of the fibrinolytic process can take place either by interference with plasminogen activation or by direct inactivation of plasmin.

Inhibitors of Plasminogen Activators. Inhibitors of the intrinsic pathway include C1 inactivator,[153] heparin–antithrombin III complex,[274] α_2-macroglobulin,[174] and an inhibitor of factor XIIa–induced fibrinolysis.[116] Inhibitors of the extrinsic pathway have been postulated but not yet identified.[56] Antistreptokinase antibodies can inactivate exogenous streptokinase.

Inhibitors of Plasmin. Inhibitors of plasmin include:

1. α_2-Antiplasmin is the principal physiological inhibitor of plasmin in plasma. It reacts quickly and in a nonreversible form with plasmin.
2. α_2-Macroglobulin functions to inactivate plasmin after α_2-antiplasmin has been saturated.
3. α_1-Antitrypsin, C1 inactivator, and antithrombin III can inactivate plasmin but to a lesser extent than α_2-antiplasmin and α_2-macroglobulin.

Fibrinolysis in Vivo. Activation of the fibrinolytic system is mediated through the formation of plasmin. This enzyme can digest fibrin and fibrinogen. The unselective digestion of both substrates could lead to thrombus dissolution and systemic fibrinogenolysis. Under physiologic circumstances, however, activation of the fibrinolytic system results in fibrin dissolution without significant fibrinogenolysis. Several hypotheses have been advanced to explain this observation. All of them propose local activation of plasmin at the site of fibrin deposition and systemic inhibitors of circulating plasmin.[5,7,51]

An accepted overall model for fibrinolysis in vivo involves the following sequence: After a fibrin clot is formed, plasminogen is absorbed onto its surface. Plasminogen activator is produced either by the extrinsic pathway (vessel wall) or the intrinsic pathway (plasma) and is sequestered into the clot. Plasminogen activator transforms plasminogen into plasmin, which is generated on the clot surface and begins fibrin digestion. Any plasmin formed in the plasma will be bound and inactivated by plasmin inhibitors, primarily α_2-antiplasmin.[51,86,170]

CHANGES IN THE HEMOSTATIC SYSTEM DURING PREGNANCY

During pregnancy blood vessels become more prominent. This phenomenon is probably due to the combination of increased blood volume and vasodilation normally observed during gestation. A specialized regional circulation (the placental vascular bed) develops to ensure adequate supply of maternal blood to the conceptus.

The platelet count tends to decrease with advancing gestational age. This has been attributed to hemodilution and placental trapping. Nevertheless, the platelet count during pregnancy remains within the limits of the normal adult range (150,000 to 350,000 per cubic millimeter). Platelet life span during pregnancy is similar to that in nonpregnant females.[225,239,249,291]

During pregnancy there is activation of the coagulation components of the hemostatic system. Evidence of such an activation are the increased concentrations of fibrinopeptide A[98] and high-molecular-weight fibrinogen complexes[81] as pregnancy progresses. This hypercoagulable state seems to be related to the participation of the hemostatic system in the modeling of the placental bed and spiral arteries and to maternal preparation for the eventual separation of the placenta.

Fibrin is deposited in the placental bed as pregnancy progresses, and it can be found in the floor of the placenta (Nitabuch's layer), lining the intervillous space, and on the surface of the villi.[176] The spiral arteries undergo important morphologic changes during pregnancy. Some of these changes are the replacement of the elastic lamina and the smooth muscle of the vascular wall by a matrix containing fibrin. Physiologic consequences of these changes include[32]: (1) The spiral arteries are transformed into large, distended, nonresponsive vessels known as uteroplacental arteries, which are able to accommodate the increased blood flow to the conceptus as pregnancy progresses. Removal of the elastic lamina also reduces the variations in pressure in the blood flowing to the placenta. (2) Fibrin replacement of the tunica media also facilitates the severance of the terminal part of the spiral arteries at the time of separation of the placenta and their occlusion by the action of the myometrial contractions.

McKay has proposed that normal pregnancy is a state of chronic intravascular coagulation localized to the placental bed. This state would result in a compensatory increase in the synthesis of coagulation factors and a decrease in the platelet count.[176]

The changes in the coagulation factors during pregnancy are presented in Table 9-2.[25,60,83,90,149,206,208,221,242] It should be noted that the activity of all coagulation factors except factors XI and XIII is increased. The decreased level in factor XIII is, however, consistent with the increased deposition of fibrin at the end of pregnancy, since recent evidence suggests that the concentration of factor XIII decreases during the acute phase of thromboembolism.[81]

The activity of coagulation inhibitors has been the subject of contradictory reports but it does not seem to be substantially altered with pregnancy.[32,279,294] The traditional concept has been that fibrinolysis is depressed during pregnancy. Evidence to support that view includes the detection during gestation of[12,35,115,266,267]:

1. Falling levels of plasminogen activator
2. Decreased fibrinolytic activity of plasma
3. Decreased fibrinolytic capacity in response to venous occlusion
4. The presence of an inhibitor of urokinase-induced fibrinolysis
5. Increased concentration of plasmin inhibitors such as macroglobulin and antiplasmin, with no change in inhibitors of plasminogen activator

Table 9-2. Coagulation Factor and Inhibitors in Late Pregnancy

Fibrinogen	4.0–6.5 g/l
Factor II	100–125%
Factor V	100–150%
Factor VII	150–250%
Factor VIII	200–500%
Factor IX	100–150%
Factor X	150–250%
Factor XI	50–100%
Factor XII	100–200%
Factor XIII	35– 75%
Antithrombin III	75–100%
Antifactor Xa	75–100%

Reproduced from Brownar, J.: Haemostasis and coagulation disorders. In Bloom, A.L. and Thomas, eds.: Pregnancy. Haemostasis and Thrombosis. Churchill Livingstone, Edinburgh, 1981.

Fletcher et al., using studies of fibrinogen catabolism,[82] have challenged this concept of depression of fibrinolysis during pregnancy. They have proposed that there is an appropriate fibrinolytic response but that the levels of plasminogen activator are depressed because of its sequestration in sites of fibrin deposition.

LABORATORY EVALUATION OF THE HEMOSTATIC SYSTEM

The laboratory evaluation of the hemostatic system should be conducted in a stepwise fashion. Screening tests are first used to establish whether or not an abnormality is present. If one is found, more specific tests are then employed to identify and characterize the defect.

A wide variety of methods are available to test the hemostatic system. This section will discuss the principles and interpretation of the screening tests frequently used in the management of obstetric patients. The reader is referred to specialized texts for information in regard to more sophisticated laboratory techniques.

Indications for Hemostatic Testing in the Obstetric Patient

Screening tests are indicated whenever there is a significant risk of hemostatic failure. The most frequent reasons for testing in the obstetric patient are:

1. To evaluate the relative contributions of the different components of the hemostatic system to the causation of excessive spontaneous or surgical hemorrhage

2. To test for subclinical activation of the hemostatic system in patients with obstetrical complications which may be associated with DIC (e.g., preeclampsia, fetal death, abruptio placentae). Detection of significant activation of the hemostatic system could change clinical management in these conditions
3. For laboratory monitoring of the progress of hemostatic therapy in cases of coagulation failure or of anticoagulation in patients with thromboembolic disease
4. For antepartum or preoperative hemostatic testing of the patient with a history suggestive of a bleeding diathesis or medical disorder associated with hemostatic problems

Abnormalities in any of the four components of the hemostatic system may cause an increased bleeding tendency. Screening tests should include evaluation of vascular integrity, platelet number and function, the different pathways of the coagulation cascade, and fibrinolytic activity. Table 9-3 discloses a battery of tests that allow screening of all these components.

Specific Tests of Hemostatic Competence

Vascular Integrity. Any time a patient has significant bleeding, vascular integrity should be examined, as its loss is the most common cause of hemostatic failure. A loss of vascular integrity should be strongly considered if the bleeding is profuse and localized, and testing of the other three components of the hemostatic system has produced normal results. Uterine atony and the resulting relaxation of the intramyometrial Pinard's ligatures is the most frequent cause of hemostatic failure in the obstetric patient.

Evaluation of vascular integrity is best performed by inspection of the surgical field or bleeding area. Inadequate surgical hemostasis is often found to be the cause of continued bleeding. On occasion auxiliary techniques such as pelvic angiography will be necessary to exclude unusual causes of vessel disruption such as those caused by a uterine aneurysm or an arteriovenous malformation.

Specific screening tests for the vascular component alone are not currently used. Capillary fragility tests (e.g., Rumpel-Leede test or Hess test) essentially assess the capacity of blood vessels to retain blood when they are stressed by increased capillary pressure. They examine the competence of blood vessel wall–platelet interactions at the arteriolar level rather than vessel wall function alone. These tests have

Table 9-3. Screening Tests of the Hemostatic System

Platelet count
Bleeding time
Fibrinogen
Prothrombin time
Partial thromboplastin time
Thrombin time
Fibrinogen degradation products

been abandoned in most laboratories because of their high incidence of false positive and negative results.

Platelets. Platelet number and function are important for adequate hemostasis. The platelet count and bleeding time are the mainstays of platelet screening tests.

Platelet Count. A rapid estimation of the number of platelets in circulating blood can be made by examination of a peripheral smear. The presence of 10 to 15 platelets per high power field generally correlates well with a platelet count of 150,000 to 300,000/mm.[3] The peripheral smear can also provide some indication of the thrombokinetic state of the patient. The number of large, young platelets (megathrombocytes) in the peripheral circulation correlates well with the megakaryocytic mass in the marrow and is an index of platelet production.[87] Many megathrombocytes in a smear would suggest that platelet production within the marrow is being stimulated and by implication that platelets are being excessively destroyed. The laboratory techniques routinely used to enumerate platelets are phase-contrast microscopy in a hemocytometer chamber and electronic counting systems. A low count should be verified by direct examination of the peripheral smear. Generally, a platelet count between 150,000 and 350,000 should be considered normal.

Bleeding Time. This is a test for platelet plug formation in precapillary arterioles and postcapillary venules. The test is almost entirely dependent on platelet number and function.[163] It measures the elapsed time between the infliction of a standard skin incision and the cessation of bleeding. Several techniques have been described. The Duke method involves puncturing the patient's earlobe. This technique, however, was not considered to be sufficiently sensitive and reliable for assessing hemostatic effectiveness of platelets and has been superseded by more standardized techniques. The Ivy method consists of a 3-mm puncture wound in the forearm after capillary pressure has been elevated by inflating a blood-pressure cuff to 40 mmHg in the upper arm. The reliability of this technique has been improved by substituting for the skin puncture a standard incision performed with a template. This modification is known as the Mielke technique or template bleeding time (TBT).[182] A disposable bleeding time device has become commercially available and has replaced the template system. Upper limits of normal for these techniques are: Ivy, <5 min; template, <7.5 min; and the disposable device method, <9.5 min. The last two techniques have the disadvantage of requiring an incision that can leave a faint scar or on occasion lead to keloid formation. Because of this problem some laboratories still prefer the Ivy method, particularly in patients who will require successive studies.[280]

A bleeding time can be prolonged because of a decreased number of platelets or platelet dysfunction. The study will be normal when normal platelets circulate at levels of 100,000/mm^3 or higher. Between platelet counts of 100,000 and 10,000/mm^3 the expected TBT can be calculated by the formula[108]:

$$\text{TBT (min)} = 30.5 - \frac{\text{platelet count}}{3{,}850}$$

In patients with abnormal platelet function, such as those with von Willebrand's disease, uremia, dysproteinuria, or following aspirin consumption, the bleeding time will be prolonged beyond that predicted for a given platelet count. Conversely, some patients with immune thrombocytopenic purpura (ITP) whose peripheral platelet population has a significant number of megathrombocytes, which are hemostatically more competent, will have a shorter bleeding time than that predicted from the numerical value of their platelet count.[108,145]

Platelet aggregation studies are indicated in the presence of longer bleeding times than are expected from the platelet count. A detailed account of these specialized tests is beyond the scope of this chapter.

Coagulation. It would be ideal to measure the activity and concentration of each one of the coagulation factors. However, this is not done in practice because of the difficulties in the functional or chemical isolation of most factors.[299] Instead, screening tests have been designed to examine the functional integrity of the different pathways. The prothrombin time test (PT) evaluates the extrinsic pathway, the partial thromboplastin time test (PTT) the intrinsic pathway, and the thrombin time test (TT) the effectiveness of the conversion of fibrinogen into fibrin.

The following general principles must be taken into account when testing the coagulation system[80]:

1. A clean venipuncture must be performed to avoid contamination of the specimen with tissue thromboplastin, as this will alter the test results.
2. Blood is collected into tubes containing a calcium chelating agent (sodium citrate). This prevents blood from clotting prior to testing. Calcium must then be added to the plasma in order to induce coagulation in the laboratory. Coagulation tests are performed with platelet-poor plasma, which is prepared by centrifugation at 2,000 g for 15 min or longer.
3. The basis for all screening tests is the reactivation of the coagulation system under controlled laboratory conditions. The elapsed time between activation of the system and clot formation is dependent upon an adequate fibrinogen concentration. Regardless of the test, clotting studies will be prolonged in the presence of severe hypofibrinogenemia.
4. The difference among PT, PTT, and TT is the point at which activation of the clotting system is induced.

Prothrombin Time (PT). This test is designed to detect abnormalities in the extrinsic pathway. It is performed by adding tissue factor from human or animal brain tissue along with calcium to platelet-poor plasma. The TF will interact with factor VII and Ca^{2+} to initiate the extrinsic pathway of blood coagulation. When the elapsed time between recalcification and clot formation of the patient's sample is more than 2 s longer than that of a normal control, the test is generally considered to be abnormal. Variability of the test's results depends upon the source of TF and other technical details.

The PT will detect deficiencies in factors V, VII, and X when their levels fall below 0.20 to 0.25 units/ml. Prothrombin concentrations below 0.10 units/ml or fibrinogen concentrations of 50 to 100 mg/dl can also produce prolongation of the PT.[89,126,229]

Partial Thromboplastin Time (PTT). This test is used to detect abnormalities in the intrinsic pathway. The test is performed by adding platelet phospholipids and calcium to platelet-poor plasma. Coagulation is initiated by glass contact activation of the intrinsic pathway. The time elapsed between recalcification and clot formation of the patient's plasma is compared with a normal control. This test has been superseded in most laboratories by the activated partial thromboplastin time test (APTT). The APTT is a modification of the PTT designed to correct for variability in contact activation. In the APTT, maximal surface activation is produced by exposure of the plasma to kaolin, Celite, or other agent prior to its recalcification. When the elapsed time between recalcification and clot formation of the patient's plasma is more than 5 s longer than that of a sample from a normal control, the test is generally considered abnormal. Variability of results is mainly due to the source of phospholipid employed. It is therefore important to be familiar with the technique and normal values used in the local laboratory.

These tests (PTT and APTT) are prolonged in deficiencies of the following factors: factor XII; Fletcher factor; Fitzgerald factor; factors XI, IX, X, VIII, and V; prothrombin; and fibrinogen. They are not sensitive to deficiencies of factors VII and XIII. The presence of heparin, FSP, or other circulating anticoagulants can also prolong the results of these tests. Shortening of the test times can be observed in association with a hypercoagulable state or when technical problems have led to activation of the coagulation system (e.g., poor venipuncture technique or inadequate preparation of platelet-poor plasma). The PTT and APTT are most sensitive to deficiencies in the early stages of the coagulation cascade. Deficiencies of up to 0.20 or 0.25 units/ml of factors, XII, XI, X, IX, VIII, or V can give prolonged test results while prothrombin deficiencies up to 0.10 units/ml or fibrinogen levels of 50 to 100 mg/dl are necessary to alter the test.[39,68,125,238]

Thrombin Time (TT). This is designed to test the reaction that converts fibrinogen into fibrin. The test is performed by adding an excess of thrombin to a sample of platelet-poor plasma and measuring the time necessary for clot formation. Calcium may be added to accelerate the reaction but this is not an indispensable part of the test. A prolongation of 5 seconds over the control is considered abnormal in most laboratories.[127]

A prolonged TT can be observed in the following circumstances:

1. When the fibrinogen concentration is below 100 mg/dl
2. In the presence of qualitative disorders of fibrinogen.
3. In the presence of high concentration of fibrin degradation products because they interfere with fibrin polymerization.

4. In the presence of significant quantities of thrombin inhibitors such as heparin.

Fibrinogen Concentration. An estimation of the fibrinogen concentration is helpful to screen for hemostatic disorders due to hypofibrinogenemia and to guide replacement therapy during fibrinopenic states.

The fibrinogen level gradually increases during the second and third trimester of pregnancy to reach levels of 400 to 650 mg/100 ml in the third trimester. Because of this wide range, a single determination has limited value unless the fibrinogen level is clearly in the pathologic range. Serial determination can provide insight into the intensity of a consumptive process.

Fibrinolysis. The end result of the action of plasmin on fibrin or fibrinogen is the formation of fibrin or fibrinogen degradation products (FDP). Their presence in serum indicates activity of the fibrinolytic system. The most frequently used technique to detect FDPs is the latex particle agglutination test. Following an atraumatic venipuncture, 2 ml of blood is collected in a tube containing thrombin and epsilon-aminocaproic acid (EACA). The thrombin converts fibrinogen into fibrin and the EACA prevents in vitro fibrinolysis and generation of FDPs. The serum obtained from this sample is then incubated with latex particles that have been coated with antibody to fragments D and E. Clumping will occur in the presence of FDPs. The test is run with both positive and negative controls. Normal human plasma diluted to a fibrinogen concentration of 5 to 10 μg/dl functions as a positive control. Human serum with an FDP concentration of less than 2 mg/ml functions as a negative control. The test is performed in dilutions of the patient's sample in order to obtain a semiquantitative determination. An FDP concentration of less than 10 μg/ml is considered normal. Higher levels indicate active fibrinolysis.[128]

As has been mentioned, the fibrinolytic system has four components: plasminogen, plasmin, plasminogen activators, and inhibitor. Different tests have been designed to examine the activity and concentration of each component, but a discussion of these tests is beyond the scope of this chapter.

BLOOD REPLACEMENT THERAPY IN COAGULATION FAILURE

The most common indications for transfusion therapy in the obstetric patient are hypovolemia, anemia, and the need to replace hemostatic components. The use of crystalloid or colloid fluid therapy to correct a deficiency in circulating volume is discussed in Chapter 3. The optimal use of blood component therapy for hemostatic replacement requires familiarity with the composition of the different available preparations.

Whole Stored Blood

When a unit of blood is drawn, it can be kept as whole blood or separated into its individual components. Whole blood is collected into an anticoagulant preservative solution and stored at 4°C. These conditions are designed to maintain viability of red blood cells but are not optimal for preservation of platelets or coagulation factors.

Table 9-4 describes the stability of different coagulation factors in stored blood, plasma concentrations required for hemostasis, and other important kinetic parameters of clotting factors in whole blood.

Under storage conditions, platelets deteriorate rapidly; there is a 50 percent loss of function within 24 h and an almost complete loss of function after 72 h despite the fact that the platelets may have a normal appearance on light microscopy. Factor V levels fall to 50 percent of the initial value within 3 to 5 days. Factor VIII falls to 50 percent of the original value within 24 h and thereafter decreases more slowly. The rest of the coagulation factors are not significantly changed during the routine shelf life of stored blood.[16,47,113,188,193]

In general, deterioration of the hemostatic function of whole blood begins 6 h after collection and this, along with volume considerations, limits the usefulness of stored whole blood for replacement of hemostatic components.

Whole stored blood or the combination of red blood cells and crystalloid solution is appropriate therapy for replacement of volume and oxygen-carrying capacity in the acutely hemorrhaging obstetric patient without a coagulopathy. However, when the amount transfused within a 24-h period exceeds the patient's circulating blood volume, a bleeding disorder due in part to loss and dilution of platelets and plasma coagulation factors can occur.[131,154,300] Because of this possibility some authors have suggested that during massive transfusions, one-third of the blood administered should be fresh. A more practical alternative is the administration of fresh frozen plasma and/or platelet concentrates.

Fresh Whole Blood

The term "fresh blood" is generally used to designate blood that has been collected less than 6 to 24 h prior to administration. This preparation has an acceptably minimal loss of hemostatic factors, it is less expensive than blood component therapy, and its use is not associated with the problems of microaggregates of platelets, white blood cells, and fibrin formed during storage of whole blood. The major disadvantages of using fresh blood are the risk of hepatitis because there may be insufficient time to complete hepatitis screening and the risk of circulatory overload if fresh blood is administered to replace factors in a patient who is not actively bleeding. At present, the use of fresh whole blood is being actively discouraged by blood bank services in the United States. Insufficient time for hepatitis screening, limited availability of donors, and more efficient utilization of blood components are the reasons for this policy. The use of fresh blood will probably be limited to those parts of the world where transfusion services are not appropriately developed.[47]

Table 9-4. Coagulation Factors in Whole Blood

Factor	Synonym	Plasma Concentration Required for Haemostasis (% normal)	Half-Life of Transfused Factor under Optimal Conditions	Recovery in Blood (as % of Dose Transfused under Optimal Conditions)	Stability in Whole Blood at 4°C
I	Fibrinogen	10–25	4 days	50	Stable
II	Prothrombin	40	3 days	40–80	Stable
V	Proaccelerin	10–15	12–15 h	?80	Unstable
VII	Proconvertin	5–10	4–6 h	70–80	Stable
VIII	Antihaemophilic factor (AHF)	10–40	12–15 h	50–80	Unstable
IX	Christmas factor	10–40	20 h	25–50	Stable
X	Stuart-Prower factor	10–15	2 days	50	Stable
XI	Plasma Thromboplastin antecedent (PTA)	?30	3 days	90–100	Stable
XII	Hageman factor	?	?	?	Stable
XIII	Fibrin-stabilizing factor	1–5	6 days	?5–100	Stable
Platelets		5–10	4 days	29–45	Unstable

Modified from Rizza, C.R.: Coagulation factor therapy. Clin. Haematol. 5:113–133, 1976.

Reproduced from Cash, J.: Blood replacement therapy. In Bloom, A.L. and Thomas, D.P., Eds.: Haemostasis and Thrombosis. Churchill Livingstone.

Fresh Frozen Plasma

Fresh frozen plasma (FFP) is obtained by separation and freezing of the plasma derived during the preparation of red blood cells and platelet concentrates from a unit of whole blood. The plasma must be frozen within 6 h of donation and stored at temperatures lower than −18°C. The product is available in 200- to 250-ml bags.

FFP is devoid of platelets but contains all the other coagulation factors, including factors V and VIII. Its concentration of clotting factors is similar to that found in an equivalent volume of circulating plasma in a normal person. It carries the same risk of hepatitis as a unit of whole blood. The product should be administered to ABO-compatible recipients.

FFP is a good source of coagulation components and is frequently used to administer these factors, along with volume, to the obstetric patient with hemorrhage and DIC.

Since none of the factors are concentrated, large volumes of FFP are usually needed to achieve hemostatic levels of depleted coagulation components. The risk of circulatory overload is therefore the most important limiting factor in the use of FFP for hemostatic replacement. For this reason, most congenital factor deficiencies are best treated with concentrates of specific factors.

Indications for the use of FFP include[9,270]:

1. Documented deficiencies of isolated coagulation factors for which no concentrate is available, such as factor XI
2. Coumadin overdose, when it is unsafe to wait for the time required for correction by parenteral vitamin K
3. Liver disease complicated by significant bleeding in the presence of a prolonged PT or PTT
4. Disseminated intravascular coagulation

Cryoprecipitate

Cryoprecipitate is the term used to designate the white gelatinous precipitate produced by thawing of fresh frozen plasma at 1 to 6°C. A unit of cryoprecipitate has a volume of 15 to 25 ml and is an excellent source of fibrinogen and factors VIII and XIII.[2,202,230,231]

Once prepared, cryoprecipitate can be stored at −20°C for up to 1 year. When needed for transfusion, cryoprecipitate is thawed at 37°C. Several units of cryoprecipitate are generally pooled into one bag for ease of administration. Once pooled, cryoprecipitate must be used or discarded in 6 h because of the danger of bacterial contamination. It is preferable to administer this preparation to ABO-compatible recipients.[297]

The main indication for administering cryoprecipitate in the obstetric patient is the need to replace fibrinogen. Each unit contains about 250 mg of fibrinogen, so that significant amounts of this protein can be delivered in a relatively small volume.

Ten units of cryoprecipitate generally increase the circulating fibrinogen in an average-sized person by 50 mg/dl. Other uses of cryoprecipitate are for replacement of factors VIII and XIII and in the management of bleeding in Von Willebrand's disease. The risk of hepatitis with a unit of cryoprecipitate is the same as with one unit of whole blood.

Platelets

Platelets can be administered in fresh whole blood, platelet-rich plasma (PRP), and platelet concentrates. The use of fresh blood and PRP as a source of platelets should be discouraged because a large volume will generally be necessary to achieve a platelet hemostatic level and circulatory overload is likely to arise before such a level is reached.

Platelet-rich plasma is obtained by low-speed centrifugation of a unit of fresh whole blood. Platelets remain in the plasma phase whereas red blood cells (RBCs) and white blood cells (WBCs) precipitate because of their higher specific gravity. A unit of platelet concentrate is obtained from a unit of PRP by centrifugation at a higher speed to precipitate platelets. Each unit is suspended in 30 to 50 ml of donor plasma and its platelet content is dependent upon the donor's platelet count and the blood volume from which the platelets were extracted.[132] Platelet concentrates are stored at room temperature (22°C) for a maximum of 72 to 120 h depending upon the types of bag used. Storage for longer periods of time or at 4°C results in platelets having a shortened life span.[78,193,194]

The response to platelet concentrate transfusions is expressed in terms of the increment in platelet count per square meter of body area. This method permits evaluation of the effectiveness of platelet transfusions independently of blood volume and allows comparison between individuals. One unit of transfused platelets generally raises the platelet count by 5,000 to 10,000 per cubic centimeter per square meter of body surface.[131,159] Fever, infection, alloimmunization, and drug-induced platelet antibodies can shorten the life span of transfused platelets. Platelets are contaminated with red blood cells, and Rh sensitization can occur after the administration of platelets from Rh-positive donors to Rh-negative recipients.[92] Therefore, an effort should be made to obtain Rh-negative platelet concentrates for the Rh-negative obstetric patient. If this is not possible, Rh immunoglobulin (50 μg) should be administered to prevent the development of antibodies when platelets from an Rh-positive donor are given to an Rh-negative recipient. Although platelets have ABO antigens, they can be transfused to ABO-incompatible recipients if compatible platelets are not available. Episodes of mild hemolysis can occur if large amounts of group O platelet concentrates (with anti-A and anti-B plasma) are administered to group A or B recipients. Shortened and normal life spans of nonallogenic platelets with respect to the ABO group have been reported but this does not seem to be a significant clinical problem.[13,161]

Indications for the use of platelet transfusions include prophylaxis against and treatment of excessive bleeding caused by thrombocytopenia and platelet dysfunction. The combined use of platelet counts and bleeding times permits assessment of the contribution of platelet abnormalities to hemostatic failure. Platelet concentrate therapy is indicated in the following circumstances:

1. Prophylaxis of bleeding in surgical or antepartum patients with a platelet count below 60,000/mm^3
2. Prophylaxis of spontaneous bleeding in patients with platelet counts below 20,000/mm^3 and prolonged bleeding times
3. Prophylaxis and treatment of excessive bleeding in patients with known platelet dysfunction
4. Therapy of excessive bleeding in the patient who has been subjected to massive transfusion therapy and has developed dilutional thrombocytopenia

Six to ten units of platelet concentrate are usually administered at one time. The optimal dose will naturally depend upon the cause of the thrombocytopenia, the initial platelet count, the level that needs to be reached, the presence of known platelet dysfunction, and alloimmunization or other factors that increase platelet dysfunction.[4]

Platelet concentrates are more effective in treating patients with impaired platelet production than in those with increased destruction. A notable example of the latter is the patient with immune thrombocytopenic purpura in whom transfused platelets may be destroyed in hours or minutes.

Occasionally, patients receiving frequent transfusions of platelet concentrates may become refractory to random-donor platelets. The underlying mechanism for this phenomenon is the development of alloantibodies to platelet-associated human-leukocyte antigens (HLAs). Under those circumstances, HLA-compatible concentrates can be used if platelet transfusions are necessary.[152,161]

Plasma Fractions (Fibrinogen and Factor IX Complexes)

Plasma obtained from whole blood or plasmapheresis can be used as fresh frozen plasma or pooled and fractionated into different components such as fibrinogen, antihemophilic factor (AHF or factor VIII), factor IX complex, gamma globulin, and albumin. Pooling of several units of plasma is performed to allow efficient large-scale preparation of the plasma fractions. However, the act of mixing plasma from many donors increases the risk of hepatitis transmission. Heat treatment can inactivate the hepatitis virus. This procedure is used in the preparation of albumin and gamma globulin, rendering these products virtually free of hepatitis risk. Coagulation fractions, however, cannot be heated and therefore these pooled preparations are associated with a significant risk of hepatitis transmission. For this reason fibrinogen concentrates are no longer a licensed product in the United States. Cryoprecipitate is the preparation of choice for efficient fibrinogen replacement.[36]

Factor IX complex (Proplex or Konyne) is a stable, dried, purified plasma fraction that contains factors II, VII, IX, and X.[131] It is available in vials whose contents are reconstituted with sterile pyrogen-free water. The concentration of factors II, VII, IX, and X is roughly equivalent to 500 ml of FFP. Factor IX complex is prepared from large pools of plasma and therefore carries a substantial risk of hepatitis. It is preferable to administer FFP to replace the factors contained in the IX complex and reserve this complex for those cases in which time and volume considerations prevent therapy with vitamin K and/or FFP. The administration of factor IX complex has been associated with the production of venous thrombosis or DIC in the recipient. These side effects are possibly due to the presence of procoagulant activity in most factor IX preparations.[27,50,64,135]

The other plasma fraction with hemostatic value is factor VIII concentrate. This preparation is rarely used in the obstetrical patient except in the occasional instance of a specific factor deficiency or a circulating inhibitor.

DISSEMINATED INTRAVASCULAR COAGULATION

Disseminated intravascular coagulation is a pathologic state caused by excessive thrombin activity. It is kinetically and pathologically characterized by increased thrombin generation, increased turnover of platelets and coagulation factors, formation of thrombi in the microcirculation, and secondary activation of the fibrinolytic system. These events are manifested clinically by varying degrees of bleeding and ischemic tissue damage.

Many synonyms have been applied to this process. Terms such as defibrination syndrome and hypofibrinogenemia allude to the consumption of fibrinogen during DIC. The term consumption coagulopathy describes the acquired coagulation defect caused by decreased levels of coagulation factors and platelets in the course of the process. The designation intravascular coagulation and fibrinolysis (ICF) is more accurate than DIC because it recognizes that fibrinolysis is an integral part of the pathologic process. In practice these two terms are used interchangeably.[37,191,215,216,262]

DIC is not a specific disease but rather a sequence of pathologic events that can be associated with many different conditions. It has been considered by McKay[175] as an intermediate mechanism of disease.

Familiarity with the pathophysiology, diagnosis, and management of DIC is important, since this condition is the most frequent cause of acquired coagulopathy in the obstetric patient. Inappropriate handling of this pathological process can lead to serious and potentially fatal complications.

Generation of Thrombin

The hemostatic system functions as a local mechanism of defense against blood vessel injury. Mechanisms reviewed earlier in this chapter are responsible for limiting the spread of hemostatic reactions. When these mechanisms are overwhelmed, thrombin activity is no longer confined to areas of vascular injury but becomes generalized, and intravascular coagulation occurs.

An excessive generation of thrombin is therefore the hallmark of DIC. Any disease agent or pathologic process able to activate the coagulation cascade and hence to generate thrombin can lead to DIC.

There are three major mechanisms for activation of the coagulation sequence:[191]

1. Activation of the intrinsic pathway of blood coagulation. Agents able to activate the contact phase of blood coagulation include antigen-antibody complexes, viruses, and particulate matter.
2. Activation of the extrinsic pathway. This can occur by intravascular liberation of tissue factor (TF) in conditions such as abruptio placentae, retained dead fetus syndrome, or gram-negative sepsis in which endotoxin promotes leukocyte release of TF.
3. Direct activation of factor X. Bypass of the initial phase of blood coagulation and direct activation of factor X at the beginning of the common pathway of blood coagulation can occur in cases of amniotic fluid embolus or bites of some poisonous snakes.

This classification of the mechanisms of initiation of DIC is a compartmentalized view, which may not correspond to the in vivo pathological process. Frequently, activation of the coagulation cascade occurs at more than one point. For example, circulating endotoxin can cause endothelial injury and activation of factor XII (in-

Table 9-5. Causes of Disseminated Intravascular Coagulation

Obstetrical causes:
Abruptio placentae
Pregnancy-induced hypertension
Intrauterine fetal death
Chorioamnionitis
Septic abortion
Saline-induced abortion
Hydatidiform mole
Nonobstetrical causes:
Infections (viral, bacterial, mycotic, rickettsial)
Intravascular hemolysis
Hemolytic transfusion reaction
Drug-induced
Sickle-cell anemia
Neoplasm (acute leukemia and solid tumors)
Trauma
Fat embolism
Burns
Major surgery
Immunologic
Anaphylactic shock
Immune complexes
Vascular disorder
Hypertensive crisis
Vascular malformations (hemangiomas, aneurysms)

trinsic pathway)[171,172,203,204] and also induce the release of TF by leukocytes (extrinsic pathway). In amniotic fluid embolus, activation of the coagulation cascade may occur by the release of TF (extrinsic pathway), substances able to activate factor X directly (common pathway), and/or particulate matter able to activate the intrinsic pathway.[223,275,276,302]

DIC can complicate the course of many obstetrical, medical, and surgical disorders. Table 9-5 summarizes the most frequent causes of this pathologic process.

Consequences of Thrombin Generation

Acute or chronic activation of the coagulation cascade results in the generation of excessive amounts of thrombin, which is the central event in DIC. Thrombin has multiple actions, including transformation of fibrinogen into fibrin; activation of factors V, VIII, and XIII; induction of platelet aggregation; and activation of plasminogen. The kinetic and pathologic characteristics of DIC can be deduced if these properties of thrombin are taken into account.

1. Transformation of fibrinogen into fibrin is responsible for the increased turnover of fibrinogen and the formation of fibrin in the microcirculation.
2. An excess of thrombin will lead to increased utilization of the factors consumed during normal coagulation, i.e., factors V, VIII, and XIII.
3. Intravascular platelet aggregation may be induced by a thrombin concentration lower than that needed to transform fibrinogen into fibrin. The net result of this will be removal of platelets from the circulation to sites of clot formation and thus an increased turnover of platelets.
4. Transformation of plasminogen into plasmin leads to secondary activation of the fibrinolytic process and lysis of formed microthrombi.

It is better to express the effect of thrombin on its substrates in terms of turnover changes than in terms of absolute levels because the latter depend upon the rate of production and destruction of a specific factor. In massive and decompensated DIC, the levels of all consumable factors will be depressed (platelets, fibrinogen, V, VIII, and XIII). In compensated DIC the rate of production of some or all of these factors may compensate or overcompensate for their increased consumption and peripheral levels may be normal or elevated.[215–217]

Platelet and fibrinogen turnover studies permit the identification of three different kinetic and pathologic states: DIC, selective platelet consumption, and primary fibrinolysis. DIC is characterized by an increase in both platelet and fibrinogen turnover. Selective platelet consumption such as that occurring in ITP and thrombotic thrombocytopenic purpura (TTP) is manifested by an increased platelet turnover but normal fibrinogen turnover. Primary fibrinolysis is characterized by an increased destruction and turnover of fibrinogen but no change in platelet turnover.[109]

Thrombi Formation in the Microcirculation

Both platelets and fibrin participate in the formation of thrombi in the microcirculation. During the initial phase of DIC, platelet aggregates form platelet-rich microthrombi. In later stages fibrin is deposited into the platelet thrombi, which are transformed into fibrin-rich microthrombi.[28]

The distribution of fibrin microthrombi is not homogenous. The frequency and extent of microclot formation vary from one organ to another. The proximity of the organ to the source of thrombin and the anatomy of its circulation seem to be important determining factors in its being affected by this process. This probably explains the high frequency of involvement of the lung and kidney, which act as sieves for fibrin in the venous and arterial circulations, respectively.[28,191]

Other factors that may play a role in determining the severity of thrombus formation include blockade of the reticuloendothelial system, concentration of coagulation inhibitors, altered vasomotor tone, and degree of activation of the fibrinolytic system.

The reticuloendothelial system (RES) exerts a protective effect by clearing activated clotting factors, fibrin monomers, and in some cases the specific trigger of DIC (e.g., endotoxin). Blockade of the RES may explain the frequent association between DIC and liver disease.[66,158] A depressed level of coagulation inhibitors, in particular antithrombin III, may also predispose to increased thrombin activity. Alterations in vasomotor tone, such as the vasoconstriction produced by alpha-adrenergic stimulation, can increase the deposition of fibrin in specific organs such as the kidney.[39,191]

All these factors can result in increased deposition of fibrin. Appropriate activation of the fibrinolytic system, however, can remove the formed clots and reduce ischemic damage to the affected organ.

Secondary Fibrinolysis

The fibrinolytic system can be activated during DIC through one or more of the following mechanisms[49,302]:

1. Release of plasminogen activator by the vascular endothelium where fibrin is being deposited.
2. Release of plasminogen activator by tissue extracts or leukocytes participating in the generation of thrombin.
3. Conversion by factor XIIa of a plasminogen proactivator present in the circulation into plasminogen activator. If activation of the coagulation cascade has occurred through the intrinsic pathway of blood coagulation, factor XII provides a connection between the coagulation and the fibrinolytic systems.
4. Transformation by thrombin of plasminogen into plasmin.

The end result of activation of the fibrinolytic system is the formation of fibrinogen-fibrin degradation products. Inhibition of this process during the course of DIC could have dramatic consequences, since removal of the microthrombi would be impaired and the risk of irreversible ischemic damage would be increased.

Clinical Consequences of DIC

In general, the clinical manifestations of DIC are bleeding and ischemic tissue damage. The bleeding tendency arises as a result of the consumption of coagulation factors and platelets and of the antihemostatic effect of fibrin degradation products, which they can exert by competing with the action of thrombin, by interfering with fibrin polymerization, and by becoming incorporated into the fibrin clot and thereby weakening it. Bleeding manifestations of DIC can be generalized (bleeding from venipuncture sites, petechia ecchymosis, etc) or localized.[55,117,171,172]

Ischemic tissue damage is due to the formation of thrombi in the microcirculation. The distribution of microthrombi may be generalized or restricted to one or more organs. The clinical manifestations depend on the severity of the process and the organs affected by the pathologic process.

Generalized or disseminated thrombosis can lead to multiple organ failure. Preferential or single organ involvement will result in signs and symptoms of target organ ischemia. Renal involvement can vary from mild dysfunction to bilateral cortical necrosis. Pulmonary involvement may result in ARDS. Ischemia of the adrenals, liver, pancreas, and pituitary can result in adrenal insufficiency, acute liver necrosis, pancreatitis, pituitary infarction, and neurologic manifestations of central nervous system involvement. The passage of red blood cells through partially thrombosed vessels results in traumatic hemolysis known as microangiopathic hemolytic anemia.[22,98,241,248,277]

When activation of thrombin has occurred through the intrinsic pathway, factor XIIa can stimulate the production of kinins, which are potent vasodilators. It is believed that vasodilation and blockade of the microcirculation are responsible for the hypotension and shock associated with some forms of DIC.[55,117,171,172]

DIC Course: Acute or Chronic

DIC is a pathologic process that can occur either acutely or chronically. The acute process is frequently seen in patients with abruptio placentae and is characterized by depletion of the coagulation-sensitive factors and platelets, along with fibrinolysis. These patients will therefore have thrombocytopenia, hypofibrinogenemia, low concentrations of factors V and VIII, and high levels of FDPs.

Chronic DIC is due to a low-grade generation of thrombin. The levels of plasma coagulation factors and platelets will depend upon their relative rate of production and destruction. Their rate of consumption is related to the intensity of thrombin generation and the mechanism of DIC initiation. The rate of production is determined by the ability of the liver and bone marrow to respond to the reduction in plasma coagulation factors and platelets.[39,215–217]

In chronic DIC, compensation or overcompensation for the destruction of clotting factors may occur and then the concentration of platelets, fibrinogen, and factors V and VIII can be normal or even elevated. The PT and PTT may be normal, shortened, or prolonged, and the TT may be normal or slightly prolonged. Since the liver and the bone marrow may not provide the same degree of compensation, thrombocytopenia and normal or high fibrinogen concentration can be present in a patient with chronic DIC. In these cases, the diagnosis of compensated or overcompensated chronic DIC depends upon a high index of suspicion, the detection of elevated FDPs indicating active fibrinolysis, and evidence of excessive thrombin activity (e.g., elevated plasma fibrinopeptide A levels or detectable fibrin monomer complexes).[57,58,215–217,222]

Diagnosis of DIC

The evaluation of an obstetric patient suspected to have DIC can be performed by testing for serum fibrinogen and FDP levels, platelet count, PTT, PT, and TT and inspection of the peripheral smear.

An elevated concentration of FDPs reflects active fibrinolysis. Since primary fibrinolysis is such a rare event, it can be generally assumed that an elevated level of FDP (>10 μg/ml) indicates secondary fibrinolysis in response to intravascular coagulation. Detection of FDPs by the latex technique (Thrombo-Wellcome test) is currently the most sensitive clinically available method to screen obstetric patients for DIC.[59,74] Although the TT test can also detect FDPs, a concentration of 35 μg/ml is necessary for it to be prolonged.[166] It must be stressed that the use of FDPs as a screening test in DIC is an indirect approach that relies on the presence of secondary fibrinolysis as a consequence of this process. When more direct tests of thrombin activity, such as fibrinopeptide A measurements, become available, it will be possible to directly detect the presence and degree of intravascular clotting.

The distinction between primary fibrinolysis and DIC may be difficult. Plasmin can destroy fibrinogen, factor V, and factor VIII and produce elevated levels of FDPs. However, the platelet count should be normal in primary fibrinolysis and low in acute DIC. The differential diagnosis between low-grade primary fibrinolysis and chronic DIC (with a normal or elevated platelet count) can be made by demonstrating soluble fibrin monomer complexes in the case of chronic DIC and their absence in primary fibrinolysis (Table 9-6).

Once the diagnoses of excessive fibrinolysis and DIC have been made, the state of compensation can be determined by measurement of the serum levels of fibrinogen, platelets, factor V, and factor VIII. Since quantification of factor V and VIII require time-consuming specialized techniques, a rapid screening can be performed by PT, PTT, and fibrinogen level determinations and a platelet count.

Acute decompensated DIC generally results in a low platelet count and fibrinogen concentration and prolonged PT, PTT, and TT. Patients with chronic compensated DIC may have normal or elevated platelet counts and fibrinogen concentration

Table 9-6. Laboratory Findings in DIC and Primary Fibrinolysis

	Acute Decompensated DIC	Chronic DIC	Primary Fibrinolysis
Platelets	Low	Low-normal-elevated	Normal
Fibrinogen	Low	Low-normal-elevated	Low
FDP	Elevated	Elevated	Elevated
Factor V	Low	Low-normal-elevated	Low
Factor VIII	Low	Low-normal-elevated	Low
Paracoagulation test	Positive	Positive	Negative

and generally have normal PT, PTT, and TT. Although the platelet count may be normal, platelet function can be altered by high concentration of circulating FDPs. A bleeding test to screen for platelet dysfunction is indicated in the presence of bleeding manifestations with normal clotting studies or prior to surgery in patients with chronic DIC.

Evaluation of the effects of DIC on target organs is assessed by special function tests. A peripheral smear, quantitation of plasma hemoglobin, and lactic dehydrogenase (LDH)-RBC isoenzyme determination provide information about the degree of traumatic hemolysis due to fibrin deposition in the microcirculation. Renal (blood urea nitrogen, creatinine, urinalysis), pulmonary (arterial blood gas determination), and liver [serum glutamic-oxaloacetic transaminase (SGOT), liver LDH isoenzyme] function tests can screen for organ dysfunction during the course of the disease.

When a patient is receiving heparin therapy and the diagnosis of DIC is being considered, the laboratory should be alerted because both the TT and FDP test (Thrombo-Wellcotest) can be abnormal in this setting. In both tests the circulating heparin can inhibit the added thrombin. If informed, however, the clinical laboratory can add reptilase, which is a thrombinlike enzyme that will clot fibrinogen even in the presence of heparin or other antithrombin agents. The reptilase time test is then performed in a fashion similar to that used for the TT and will be prolonged in cases of reduced fibrinogen or elevated FDP concentrations.

Management of DIC in the Obstetric Patient

General Principles

1. DIC is always secondary to a disease that causes excessive thrombin generation. The most effective treatment for DIC is to eliminate the cause of activation of the hemostatic system. This implies therapy of the primary disease and in obstetrics frequently indicates the need for delivery.

2. The association of DIC with any obstetric entity (abruptio placentae, chorioamnionitis, etc.) transforms a local disorder into a systemic disease and introduces the risk of multiple organ failure. Therefore, the presence of DIC magnifies the severity of the underlying disease.

3. As a mode of delivery the vaginal route is preferable to cesarean section or hysterotomy in a patient with a decompensated coagulopathy. The vaginal approach places less stress on the hemostatic mechanism than an abdominal operation in which there is a significant risk of bleeding from the uterine and abdominal wall incisions. It would be ideal if an episiotomy or any other obstetric operative intervention could be safely avoided during the course of a vaginal delivery.

4. The administration of conduction anesthesia (caudal, epidural, or spinal) is contraindicated in a patient with hemostatic failure because of the increased risk of formation of an epidural hematoma and subsequent permanent neurologic damage.

5. Replacement therapy of the depleted hemostatic components is indicated only in the presence of bleeding or to correct subnormal levels of hemostatic factors prior to surgical intervention or a vaginal delivery. If the fibrinogen level is above 100 mg/100 ml and the platelet count is more than 60,000/mm^3, replacement therapy is not generally required.

6. The rationale for the use of heparin in DIC is to decrease the excessive thrombin generation and activity. This would arrest coagulation factor consumption and fibrin deposition and reduce the risk of consumptive coagulopathy and ischemic damage. Although the most effective treatment for DIC is the elimination of the cause of activation of the hemostatic system, this cannot always be immediately accomplished (infections, neoplasia). Heparin has been used with some success under these circumstances to prevent the deleterious consequences of DIC. Heparin therapy, however, is rarely indicated in the obstetric patient because most episodes of DIC are self-limited and because detachment of the placenta at delivery or during abruption creates significant vascular disruption and heparin magnifies the potential for life-threatening hemorrhage. Its use should be limited to those cases in which there is an intact intravascular bed and delivery is not anticipated during the period of anticoagulation. Heparin has a high molecular weight and does not cross the placental barrier; therefore, it is an ideal anticoagulant for obstetric use.[32,117]

Abruptio Placentae. Abruptio placentae (AP) is the most frequent cause of acute decompensated DIC in the obstetric patient. The incidence of AP varies from 0.2 to 2.4 percent of all pregnancies,[1] and DIC with fibrinogen concentrations of less than 100 mg/dl complicates one-third to one-fourth of the cases.[235] The etiology of AP is usually unknown. Risk factors include a history of severe abruptio placentae in a previous pregnancy, high parity, hypertensive diseases of the mother, cigarette smoking, and external trauma. The role of other proposed causes, such as polyhydramnios, a short umbilical cord, uterine anomalies, and folate deficiencies remains obscure and is not likely to be significant.[198,219,233]

The initial event is likely to be an ischemic lesion of the decidua, leading to decidual necrosis, vascular disruption, and bleeding. As hemorrhage occurs, laceration and dissection along a decidual plane and placental separation take place. The latter produces more vascular rhexis, arterial hemorrhage, retroplacental accumulation of blood, and further placental separation.[198,234]

Following delivery, control of uterine bleeding is dependent upon myometrial contraction, which constricts the severed vessels at the placental implantation site. This mechanism cannot operate efficiently in AP because the uterine cavity remains distended by the presence of the fetus. Since maternal venous sinuses are opened, thromboplastic material can be infused into the maternal circulation. Bleeding stops following delivery of the fetus and placenta or, less frequently, by self-limitation of the precipitating event.

The clinical manifestations of AP depend upon the site of placental implantation, the type and degree of separation, the amount of blood loss, and the presence of DIC. It has been suggested that abruption of posteriorly implanted placentas tends to be less symptomatic than that occurring with anterior placentas.[209,210] The site of separation also has clinical importance, as it may determine the intensity of blood loss. Central detachments involve disruption of the spiral arteries, and the resulting high-pressure arterial bleeding causes an expanding retroplacental hemorrhage. On the other hand, marginal separations produce bleeding from veins at the edge of the placental disk or from the intervillous space. In either case, the bleeding is not of arterial origin and therefore less serious than that seen with central separations.[76,240]

Not all central detachments lead to total separation of the placenta and fetal death. If a hematoma can form before the separation and hemorrhage becomes extensive, the process may stop and only be detected at the time of delivery as an organized thrombus in an area of infarcted placenta.[240]

It must be remembered that the amount of vaginal bleeding is not a reliable indicator of the degree of placental separation. Significant amounts of blood can be concealed within the uterus until delivery. When fetal death occurs blood loss commonly amounts to 2,500 ml[234] and may be more than 5,000 ml. Therefore, anemia and hypovolemic shock can be present with little evidence of major vaginal bleeding.

Older studies have reported the maternal mortality in AP to be 1.0 to 2.8 percent.[1,164] Maternal complications include anemia, hypovolemic shock, acquired consumptive coagulopathy, renal failure, postpartum hemorrhage, and the sequelae of ischemic damage to distant organs.

The occurrence of DIC seems to be related to the degree of placental separation and retroplacental bleeding. The greater the separation, the higher the likelihood of significant bleeding and acquired coagulopathy.[32]

The fetal mortality in AP has been reported to be over 50 percent, and a significant number of perinatal deaths occur prior to hospital admission.[1] The fetal complications in this disorder are related to hyoxemia and occasionally to anemia. Hypoxemia results from maternal hypovolemia, anemia, and reduction of the available placental interface for fetal-maternal exchange. When fetal anemia occurs, it is probably due to bleeding from lacerated villi.[1,197,240]

Three main theories have been proposed to explain the fibrinogen depletion and the hemorrhagic diathesis associated with AP:[20,35,235]

1. Release of tissue thromboplastin into the maternal circulation, with the production of DIC.[85,257–262]

2. Intrauterine consumption of fibrinogen and other coagulation factors during the formation of the retroplacental clot.

3. Primary fibrinolysis, with digestion of the circulating fibrinogen.[224]

The first theory seems to provide the most plausible explanation for the occurrence of a coagulopathy in AP. The placenta and decidua are rich in thromboplastic material. DIC has been experimentally induced by injecting placental extracts into animals.[258–260] It has been postulated that thromboplastic material is introduced through the maternal venous sinuses and that activation of the extrinsic mechanism of blood coagulation results in DIC.

It must be stressed that the bleeding diathesis associated with AP is due not only to fibrinogen consumption but also to depletion of other coagulation factors such as factors V and VIII and to the anticoagulant effects of fibrin degradation products.[18] The incidence of postpartum hemorrhage has been better correlated with a high level of circulating FDPs than with the fibrinogen concentration.[20] This underlines the importance of fibrinolysis in the production of clinical manifestations of bleeding in DIC.[20,34,61,62]

The clinical course and laboratory findings of the coagulopathy of AP are those of decompensated acute DIC. Fibrinogen and factor V and VIII levels are low, while FDPs are elevated. Platelets are either low or normal, and frequently the degree of thrombocytopenia is less than that expected from the hypofibrinogenemia. It has been suggested that a very active fibrinolytic system lyses the clots and avoids excessive traumatic destruction of platelets and red blood cells.[234,235]

A patient with a placental abruption should be cared for in the labor and delivery unit. Women with extensive placental separations usually present complaining of abdominal pain and vaginal bleeding. The uterus is often tetanically contracted and fetal heart tones may be absent. Initial evaluation includes recording of vital signs, assessment of vaginal bleeding, electronic fetal heart rate monitoring, and blood drawing for baseline studies (hematocrit, platelet count, fibrinogen, PT, PTT, TT, FSPs, and clot observation test). A secure intravenous route for administration of blood and fluid should be started by using a 16- or 18-gauge cannula. Because fluid can be administered more rapidly under pressure than by gravity alone, it would be ideal to use plastic fluid bags rather than glass bottles. Fluid bags can be compressed by a pressor infusion set to increase the rate of infusion.[228] The infusion should be initiated with a crystalloid solution such as Ringer's lactate. A Foley catheter should be inserted to follow urinary output; 30 ml/h is indicative of adequate renal perfusion.

Tests that can be performed in the labor-floor laboratory include hematocrit, a clot observation test, and a peripheral smear for platelet enumeration. The clot observation test is done by collecting 5 ml of maternal venous blood in a glass tube and inverting it four or five times. An abnormality should be suspected if a clot fails to form in 6 min. If the clot forms in less than 6 min, the concentration of fibrinogen is likely to be more than 150 mg/dl. When a clot is not formed in 30 min, the fibrinogen concentration is likely to be less than 100 mg/dl. This test is simple and should be performed in every patient suspected of having an abruptio placentae.[1,48]

Rapid clot formation essentially makes the possibility of severe hypofibrinogenemia unlikely, and under these circumstances surgical intervention can be undertaken for fetal indications. If a clot has not formed in 30 min, however, a serious disruption of the hemostatic mechanism is likely to exist. In institutions where blood components are immediately available upon request, surgery for fetal distress may be started and replacement therapy begun during the procedure. If a delay in obtaining blood products is anticipated, however, it is best to delay surgery until they are available because of the possibility of maternal exsanguination during the operation. A Wright stain of a peripheral smear can be used to quickly screen for a platelet deficiency. If less than four platelets per high power field are seen, thrombocytopenia should be strongly suspected.

The management of individual cases of severe AP depends upon gestational age, fetal status, severity of the abruption, feasibility of vaginal delivery, and presence of shock and DIC. If the fetus is previable or dead, every effort should be made to accomplish vaginal delivery because this imposes less severe demands on the hemostatic system than hysterotomy or cesarean section. If fetal distress is present in a viable infant, delivery should be accomplished in the most expeditious way. If fetal distress is not present and vaginal delivery is anticipated within 6 to 8 h, the vaginal delivery may be attempted provided that electronic and biochemical means of fetal assessment, anesthesia, blood, and operating room access are continuously available to perform an emergency cesarean section if this becomes necessary. If these conditions are not present, cesarean section is likely to improve perinatal salvage.[218]

Induction of labor should begin with amniotomy. The loss of amniotic fluid decreases intrauterine volume and allows more effective hemostasis at the placental site. Oxytocin administration by intravenous infusion should be started immediately following the amniotomy.

If there are signs of circulatory collapse in association with DIC, rapid volume replacement is necessary in order to prevent acute renal failure. Replacement with Ringer's lactate solution is initiated pending availability of blood. When fetal death has occurred, a deficit of at least 1,000 to 2,000 ml of blood can be estimated. A central venous pressure (CVP) line should be placed to assess the effectiveness of intravascular volume replacement. The average CVP in the third trimester should be 10 cm H_2O and this value can be used as a guide to follow the progress of fluid replacement.

Packed red cells are indicated if anemia is present. The goal is to maintain the hematocrit around 30 percent. Each unit of red blood cells can be expected to increase the hemoglobin by 1 to 1.5 g and the hematocrit by 3 points. Fresh frozen plasma can be used as a plasma expander or to replace the hemostatic components consumed in DIC, such as fibrinogen, factor V, factor VIII, and antithrombin III. Cryoprecipitate is the most volume-efficient form of fibrinogen replacement. Its use is indicated when fibrinogen concentrations are below 100 mg/dl. Each unit of cryoprecipitate contains approximately 250 mg per bag and raises the fibrinogen concentration by approximately 5 mg/dl.

If the fibrinogen level is above 100 mg/dl, volume replacement therapy can be given as whole blood, packed red cells and fresh frozen plasma, or packed red cells and crystalloid solutions. The best combination is packed red cells and fresh frozen plasma because it provides more labile coagulation factors than whole blood and avoids crystalloid-induced dilution of circulating coagulation factors.

Heparin therapy has been advocated by some authors to arrest coagulation factor consumption in AP.[62] However, in the presence of a disruption of the vascular integrity it is likely to increase the risk of severe hemorrhage; therefore its use in this setting is not recommended.

Since fibrinolysis in AP is a protective mechanism against intravascular coagulation, interfering with its natural course by the use of fibrinolytic inhibitors is potentially dangerous. A recent publication, however, has associated uterine inertia refractory to amniotomy and oxytocin with hyperfibrinolysis, and reported resolution of the hypodynamia after the administration of the fibrinolytic inhibitor Trasylol. Although the explanation for these observations remains speculative, their confirmation could create an indication for fibrinolytic inhibitors in AP complicated by refractory uterine inertia.[268,269]

Occasionally, severe bleeding from the placental site occurs several hours after delivery. Bonnar[32] has proposed that active local fibrinolysis may be responsible for this phenomenon. He has suggested that if a surgical cause for the hemorrhage is excluded and bleeding cannot be controlled by manual or pharmacological stimulation of the myometrium, ϵ aminocaproic acid or other inhibitors of fibrinolysis might be used. This should rarely be necessary, however, and consultation with a hematologist is advised prior to starting a patient on these agents.

Prolonged Retention of a Dead Fetus. The association between prolonged retention of a dead fetus and hemostatic failure has been recognized for many years. The coagulopathy seems to be due to the slow release of tissue thromboplastin from the fetoplacental unit into the maternal circulation. The resultant activation of the extrinsic pathway of blood coagulation leads to excessive generation of thrombin and DIC. This pathologic process is initially low-grade, but the progressively increased and sustained generation of thrombin may eventually transform an early compensated DIC into a decompensated state.[106,138,141,237,285]

The frequency of DIC associated with fetal demise is related to the length of time the fetus has been retained in the uterine cavity and to the laboratory criteria employed to diagnose DIC. Pritchard studied over 100 patients with a dead fetus retained for more than 1 week and found that no patient demonstrated a fibrinogen concentration below 150 mg/dl less than 5 weeks after detection of fetal death. When more than 5 weeks had elapsed, one-third of the patients had fibrinogen concentrations below 150 mg/dl.[141] The factors responsible for the development of hypofibrinogenemia in some patients and not in others are not known.

Aggressive management of the patient with a fetal demise has made prolonged retention of a dead fetus a rare cause of coagulopathy in modern obstetrics. The availability of ultrasonography and of effective means to induce premature labor have virtually eliminated the delay in uterine evacuation due to diagnostic uncertainty or fear of induction failure. All patients with a fetal demise should be screened with coagulation studies prior to pregnancy termination because clinical manifestations of DIC are often minimal and the first sign of hemostatic failure may be a dangerously severe postpartum hemorrhage.[141,205]

The initial changes in the coagulation profile of a patient with a retained dead fetus are an elevation in the circulating levels of FDPs and a fall in the concentration of fibrinogen. These changes precede the development of abnormalities in the PTT and PT. The fall in platelet count is less marked than that in fibrinogen levels.

The management of a patient with DIC due to a retained dead fetus depends upon the state of hemostatic compensation and whether or not the patient is in labor. If the DIC is either compensated or overcompensated (elevated FDPs, normal or elevated fibrinogen and platelets), the risk of hemostatic failure is small. The management goal in this setting is to accomplish delivery of the dead infant in order to eliminate the source of thromboplastic material and suppress the excessive generation of thrombin. The duration of pregnancy and the state of cervical ripeness will determine whether oxytocin or prostaglandin preparations should be used for induction of labor.

If the patient has decompensated DIC (low fibrinogen or platelets), the management objective should be to decrease the risk of peripartum hemorrhage by restoring hemostatic levels of the consumed coagulation components prior to delivery. This can be accomplished by the administration of heparin if the patient is not in labor or by supplying the consumed factor with blood component therapy if labor is in progress.

When the patient is in labor, potential areas of vascular disruption and injury are likely to develop (e.g., placental implantation site, episiotomy, or lacerations). Under these circumstances the administration of heparin is contraindicated because it may increase the bleeding tendency by reducing the ability to form clots in areas of vascular injury. Management should be directed at replacing the deficient hemostatic components. Fibrinogen is the most frequently depleted coagulation factor in this setting. Platelet counts and factor V and VIII levels are frequently within a safe hemostatic range (platelets $>$ 60,000/mm^3; factor V 10 to 20 percent and factor VIII 25 to 30 percent). Fibrinogen replacement is best accomplished by administration of cryoprecipitate. Approximately 10 units of this product will be necessary to increase the circulatory level of plasma fibrinogen by 50 mg/dl. Cryoprecipitate is preferred to fresh frozen plasma because the correction of hypofibrinogenemia with the latter product will require the administration of large volumes of colloids, placing the patient at risk for circulatory overload.

If the patient is not in labor, the administration of heparin can arrest the consumption of coagulation factors, permit restoration of hemostatic competence, and obviate the need for blood replacement therapy. Heparin is best administered by continuous intravenous infusion. This reduces the risk of bleeding which may accompany intermittent bolus administration. A recommended program for heparin therapy is to give an initial bolus of 5,000 units and then start an infusion at 1,000 units/h. Modification of the maintenance rate may be necessary to avoid bleeding complications and achieve therapeutic goals.

Heparin therapy is monitored with serial fibrinogen levels, platelet counts, and PTTs. The objective of therapy is to increase the concentrations of fibrinogen, coagulation factors, and circulating platelets above safe hemostatic levels. A reasonable goal is to achieve a fibrinogen concentration between 200 and 300 mg/dl and a platelet count above 60,000/mm^3. The PTT is performed to assess the risk of excessive anticoagulation and should not be prolonged over more than 2.5 times the normal range.

Patients should be cautioned to avoid trauma and to report any episode of bleeding during heparin administration. Treatment goals can usually be accomplished in 24 to 48 h, after which heparin can be stopped. Induction of labor can begin 6 h after discontinuation of therapy since heparin's anticoagulant activity is virtually gone 4 h after the infusion has been stopped.

Another indication for heparin therapy is the mangement of a multiple gestation complicated by decompensated DIC secondary to the death of one of the infants.[271] If the gestation is at term and the mother is not in labor, heparin therapy should be administered in order to achieve safe levels of hemostatic factors. The anticoagulant should then be stopped and labor induced. If the gestation is preterm, however, significant prolongation of the pregnancy can be achieved by anticoagulation of the mother. This can be accomplished initially with intravenous administration of heparin until the fibrinogen concentration has reverted to acceptable levels and then by subcutaneous therapy. The dose of subcutaneous heparin used for maintenance therapy is 5,000 units every 6 h. Modification of the treatment plan will depend upon changes in plasma fibrinogen concentration. Platelet counts should be monitored during heparin therapy because thrombocytopenia can be a side effect of heparin administration. Heparin therapy should be discontinued prior to elective induction when the living twin has been shown to be pulmonically mature. Total discontinuation of heparin therapy weeks prior to delivery without a recurrence of the coagulopathy was possible in one case (Romero, R., unpublished observation).

Pregnancy-Induced Hypertension. Pregnancy-induced hypertension (PIH), also known as toxemia of pregnancy, is a common cause of chronic DIC in the pregnant patient.

The mechanism of activation of the hemostatic system in PIH is unknown. Several authors have proposed that such an activation occurs prior to the clinical onset of hypertension and is an integral part of the pathophysiology of the disease.[94,95,112,134,243] Evidence for excessive thrombin activity is provided by the increased concentration of fibrinopeptide A and soluble fibrin complexes in preeclamptic patients as compared with normal pregnant women.[70,72,177,250] The kinetic consequences of excessive thrombin, namely thrombocytopenia, decreased fibrinogen concentrations, and a decreased factor VIII C/VIII Ag ratio have been well documented in the course of the disease.[129,130] Thrombi in the microcirculations of the liver,[11] kidney,[190] and placental bed of patients with PIH have been identified and may account for the multiorgan manifestations of the disease.

Elevated levels of FDPs are consistent with secondary activation of the fibrinolytic system. The presence of thrombotic lesions in the microcirculation in PIH, however, may be due to a relative impairment of fibrinolytic activity. Activation of the hemostatic system is important in this disease because a correlation has been demonstrated between the severity of hypertension and proteinuria and the degree of coagulation abnormality.[130,250]

The most frequent manifestations of DIC in PIH are thrombocytopenia and elevated circulatory levels of fibrin degradation products. Platelet counts of less than

150,000 mm^3 have been reported in as many as 15 percent of patients with preeclampsia and 30 percent of those with eclampsia.[236] This thrombocytopenia is due to intravascular consumption of platelets. In preeclamptic women with thrombocytopenia, fibrinogen levels are usually normal or may even be elevated. This may be due to a greater degree of compensation afforded by the liver as compared with the bone marrow. Alternatively, it is possible that platelets participate in the process of initiation of DIC in PIH and therefore are consumed to a greater degree than fibrinogen and other coagulation factors.[247,250]

The typical hemostatic profile of a patient with chronic DIC associated with PIH includes thrombocytopenia; normal PT, PTT, and TT; normal, low, or high fibrinogen levels; elevated FDPs; and microangiopathic hemolytic changes of the red blood cells. Bone marrow aspiration typically demonstrates normal or elevated number of megakaryocytes. Serum levels of LDH can be elevated, reflecting the release of LDH from mechanical destruction of RBCs. Patients with these laboratory findings frequently present with epigastric pain and elevation of the SGOT.[151,250,296] On occasion the triad of abdominal pain, thrombocytopenia, and liver dysfunction may precede the development of hypertension.[94,95,250]

The process of chronic DIC invariably resolves after delivery of the infant. Antepartum resolution of thrombocytopenia and correction of the liver dysfunction have been observed to occur spontaneously or after the administration of antiplatelet agents such as aspirin and dipyridamole.[140,250] Spontaneous antepartum resolution of the thrombocytopenia does not mean that the DIC process has resolved. Frequently, elevated levels of FDP can still be demonstrated despite a normal platelet count. This evidence of fibrinolysis is generally accepted to indicate a state of chronic compensated DIC. The consequences of ongoing compensated DIC have not been established, but worsening of the hypertension and the delivery of growth-retarded infants has been observed in patients managed conservatively after resolution of their thrombocytopenia.[250]

Although the thrombocytopenia associated with acute PIH can be severe, antepartum bleeding is rare. Frequently, the nadir platelet count is reached during the first postpartum day, with spontaneous resolution occurring 72 h after delivery in most cases.

Patients with PIH and thrombocytopenia should be considered to have a severe form of toxemia regardless of the degree of systemic hypertension. These mothers are at risk for multiple organ ischemic involvement and their infants are at risk for intrauterine growth retardation (IUGR).[250,286] The mechanism responsible for IUGR has been postulated to be suboptimal placental perfusion and poor fetal-maternal exchange due to platelets and fibrin deposits in the uteroplacental microcirculation.

Delivery of the infant is the treatment of choice for patients with PIH and DIC. Platelet transfusions are not indicated unless the platelet count is less than 50,000/mm^3, there is severe hypertension or active bleeding, or the patient is being prepared for surgery. A reasonable goal is to raise the platelet count to 50,000/mm^3 prior to any surgical intervention. Fibrinogen replacement with cryoprecipitate is rarely necessary because serum fibrinogen levels generally exceed 100 mg/dl.

The role of heparin and antiplatelet agents in the treatment of DIC associated with toxemia has not been definitely established. Their use in patients with severe hypertension is contraindicated because of the risk of cerebral hemorrhage. On the other hand, they may prove to be useful in prolonging an early gestation in patients with mild hypertension but significant activation of the hemostatic system.[31,250]

PRESENCE OF CLOTTING INHIBITORS

Circulating Anticoagulants

Circulating anticoagulants are endogenous blood components that inhibit the action of clotting factors. They may be directed against a specific coagulation factor or interfere with a phase of blood coagulation. Specific inhibitors have been identified against factors V, VIII, IX, XI, XII, and XIII. Circulating inhibitors that interfere with a phase of blood coagulation were originally described in association with disseminated lupus erythematosus and are frequently referred to as "lupus-type inhibitors."

Specific Inhibitors

Specific inhibitors can occur in patients with congenital coagulation defects or in individuals with previously normal hemostasis. Most specific inhibitors are thought to be antibodies. Their appearance has been suggested to be due to an immunologic response of the host to a transfused factor (e.g. factor VIII in hemophilia A) although spontaneous inhibitors have also been reported. Among specific inhibitors the most frequent one is that directed against factor VIII. The inhibitor generally inactivates factor VIII irreversibly by means of a time-dependent and temperature-dependent reaction.[24,29,40] The clinical manifestations of this condition are similar to those of hemophilia A except for a lower frequency of hemarthroses and a higher prevalence of ecchymosis, muscle bleeds, hematuria, and menorrhagia.[72,84,101,120,169,181,290] The inhibitor may appear at any time during pregnancy but its most frequent occurrence is in the puerperal period. The hemorrhagic diathesis associated with this circulating anticoagulant may be severe and difficult to treat. The diagnosis is usually made by the presence of a prolonged PTT which is not corrected by the addition of normal plasma; PT and TT are typically normal. On occasion, demonstration of the inhibitor may require incubation of the mixture of plasmas for 1 h at 37°C. It is possible to quantitate the activity of the inhibitor, and standardized inhibitor units (Bethesda or Oxford) have been described.

Therapeutic modalities employed in the management of patients with acquired inhibitors to factor VIII include replacement of factor VIII alone (human, porcine, or bovine) or in combination with plasmapheresis, exchange transfusions, corticosteroids, antimetabolites, alkylating agents, and/or Autoplex, an anti-inhibitor coagulation complex.[77,181] While the traditional approach to the management of the acute crisis has been administration of factor VIII, encouraging results have been recently reported with Autoplex. This preparation contains activated clotting factors and its postulated mechanism of action is to bypass the site of action of factor VIII in the coagulation cascade. The recommended dose is 76 units/kg over 15 to 20 min. Therapy can be followed by observing the clinical response and by serial PTTs. This preparation is extremely expensive and should not be used without a precise diagnosis. Patients with an acute hemorrhagic diathesis due to a coagulation inhibitor represent serious management problems. They should be treated in conjunction with an expert hematologist and the blood bank service.

The prognosis of patients with factor VIII inhibitor is good provided they survive the acute stage of the disease. Most anticoagulants disappear in months or years after detection. Although most infants born to mothers with circulating anticoagulants have been clinically normal, an inhibitor has been detected in two neonates. The significance of this finding remains speculative. Coller et al. recently reviewed the hemostatic performance in successive pregnancies of 12 patients with a factor VIII inhibitor, 9 of whom were found to have uneventful pregnancies and to be in remission at the time of the subsequent delivery. These subjects included two patients with inhibitors present at the onset of their second pregnancies but whose antifactor VIII titers continued to decrease and finally disappeared before the second delivery. Bleeding manifestations persisted in three patients in their subsequent pregnancies and in one of them the disease became worse.[54,181]

It must be stressed that pregnancy or surgery in a patient with a high titer of a factor VIII inhibitor is a potentially life-threatening condition. It seems wise to follow patients who are known to have this problem with serial inhibitor titers and to advise them to wait until they are in remission to conceive. If the disease is detected during pregnancy or if patients become pregnant before remission is achieved, they should be advised as to their risk and followed with serial inhibitor titers. Consideration should be given to the use of steroids in the event of high or rising inhibitor titers.

Lupus-Type Inhibitors. This inhibitor was originally described in patients with systemic lupus erythematosus (SLE) but now has been observed in association with other conditions and in patients without any demonstrable disease.[45,46] The presence of this inhibitor may be the first manifestation of SLE.

The inhibitor seems to be an immunoglobulin of the IgG or IgM type. Its mechanism of action has not been completely established but most evidence suggests that it interferes with the reaction in which factor Xa, factor V, and phospholipid form a complex (prothrombinase) that transforms prothrombin into thrombin. It has been proposed that this inhibitor occupies the binding site of the phospholipid molecule, which is generally available for the coagulation factor.[232]

Bleeding is uncommon despite the significant abnormalities in in vitro coagulation. Thrombosis, on the other hand, seems to be a more significant problem in these patients. To explain this paradox, it has been proposed that bleeding does not occur because after saturation of the inhibitor molecule with phospholipid, enough phospholipid is still available to react with the coagulation factors and accomplish effective hemostasis. The tendency in some patients to develop thromboembolic accidents could be related to the presence of a plasma molecule able to inhibit the production of prostacyclin by the vessel wall. The presence of a circulating anticoagulant is generally discovered by the detection of a prolonged PTT that is not corrected by the addition of normal plasma. The reaction is instantaneous rather than time-dependent, as is the case with the inhibitor to factor VIII. The PT and TT are frequently prolonged. The reasons for the prolongation of the TT are unclear. Thrombocytopenia is occasionally present. Excessive platelet destruction due to a relative deficiency of prostacyclin or to platelet antibodies could be the mechanism responsible for the low platelet count. Spontaneous remission of a lupus-type inhibitor is rarely observed but patients generally respond to steroids.

Recently two patients with lupus-type anticoagulants were found to have a syndrome characterized by repeated thromboembolic accidents and recurrent fetal loss. The plasma of these patients contained an inhibitor of prostacyclin. Pathologic examination of the placental bed demonstrated extensive atheromatous lesions.[45,46,65] These observations are important because they provide a link between systemic lupus and reproductive wastage and provide new possibilities for therapeutic interventions.

IMMUNE THROMBOCYTOPENIC PURPURA (ITP)

Immune thrombocytopenic purpura (ITP)* can be defined as a syndrome characterized by a low platelet count, a normal or increased number of megakaryocytes in the bone marrow, shortened platelet survival, and the presence of platelet-bound immunoglobulin.

In ITP, shortened platelet life span due to increased platelet destruction is the mechanism of thrombocytopenia. A circulating antibody, which is frequently an IgG, is produced against an unidentified platelet antigen. This antibody coats the platelets, which are then destroyed at an increased rate in the RES, mainly in the spleen.[178] The severity of the disease correlates with the quantity of platelet-bound IgG and not with serum antiplatelet IgG.[143] The antibody can cross the placenta, coat fetal platelets, and enhance their destruction by the fetal RES.[150] The antibody may be present in women who are in remission; therefore their fetuses remain at risk for neonatal thrombocytopenia even though they have normal platelet counts.[52,53,146,150,183,254,288,289]

ITP is not uncommon during pregnancy, as the disease predominantly affects young women during their reproductive years. The consequences of this disorder are related solely to the thrombocytopenia and to the disruption of the normal hemostatic mechanism that a low platelet count can produce. The ever-present threat of hemorrhage poses special problems to both the mother and her fetus during pregnancy, and the aim of management is to minimize that threat. The risks for antepartum, intrapartum, and postpartum hemorrhage present in all obstetrical patients are

* The abbreviation ITP is conventionally used for "idiopathic thrombocytopenic purpura," a term here reserved for a condition similar to immune thrombocytopenic purpura but not involving demonstrable platelet-bound IgG.

magnified in women with ITP, as is the potential for increased surgical bleeding during cesarean section. The main risk to the infant is intracranial hemorrhage secondary to transplacentally acquired thrombocytopenia.

The signs and symptoms of this disease are directly related to the platelet count and are not specific for ITP. Capillary bleeding generally occurs when the platelet count is less than $30{,}000/mm^3$ and is predominately dermal or mucosal (petechia, ecchymosis, epistaxis, hematuria, etc). Retinal hemorrhages are particularly important to recognize because they are signs of impending intracranial hemorrhage. With the exception of these findings, the physical examination is usually normal. An enlarged spleen suggests that the thrombocytopenia is secondary to another disorder, such as systemic lupus erythematosus, infectious mononucleosis, or a lymphoproliferative disorder.

The clinical course of the disease may be acute (associated with drug reactions or viral infections) or chronic. Chronic ITP usually has an insidious course, with episodes of intermittent exacerbations and remissions.

The following criteria have to be fulfilled to establish the diagnosis[135]:

1. Platelet count less than $100{,}000/mm^3$.
2. Presence of megathrombocytes on the peripheral smear, indicating that increased platelet destruction is occurring.
3. Normal or increased number of megakaryocytes in the bone marrow, indicating an adequate or increased platelet production and excluding the presence of a lymphoproliferative disorder.
4. Normal clotting studies, indicating the absence of intravascular coagulation.
5. Absence of splenomegaly. Significant sequestration of platelets is extremely unlikely with a normal-size spleen.
6. Demonstration of platelet-bound IgG in the absence of other conditions in which platelets may bind IgG, such as sepsis or hypergammaglobulinemia.[135,278] The term "idiopathic thrombocytopenic purpura" should probably be reserved for those patients who fulfill the rest of the criteria but do not have demonstrable platelet-bound IgG.

In the absence of another disease (lupus erythematosus, infectious mononucleosis, lymphoproliferative disorders, etc.) or exposure to a drug associated with immune thrombocytopenia, the condition can be referred to as "primary immune thrombocytopenic purpura" or simply "immune thrombocytopenic purpura." Some authors refer to it as "autoimmune thrombocytopenic purpura," but this designation seems premature since characterization of the platelet antigen(s) has not been performed. At the present time a heterologous antigen cannot be excluded as a causative agent.[178]

"Secondary immune thrombocytopenia" purpura is the term used to refer to ITP associated with another disease. Identification of an associated disorder may have significant prognostic implications. The immune thrombocytopenia associated with mononucleosis invariably resolves spontaneously. The prognosis for the patient with an immune thrombocytopenia associated with chronic lymphocytic leukemia or lymphoma, on the other hand, will be that of her primary disease. The workup of patients with ITP should also include thyroid function tests because of the association between immunologic thyroid disorders and ITP.

When the diagnois of ITP is made in a female of reproductive age, family planning and contraception should be discussed. Since medical therapy and splenectomy during pregnancy are not without risk, patients should be advised to postpone childbearing until a remission of the disease is obtained and steroid or immunosupressive therapy is not required. Splenectomy may be necessary to achieve this state. Occasionally, however, this goal may not be accomplished, because some patients require medical therapy even following splenectomy. If this is the case, patients who desire to become pregnant should be made aware of the potential risks of steroids or immunosupressants to the fetus. Patients should also be informed that they may need a cesarean section for fetal indications and that there is an increased risk to both the fetus and the mother with this disease. However, ITP is by no means an absolute contraindication to pregnancy.[249]

Regarding contraception, it is not wise to use intrauterine devices because, in addition to the risks of menorrhagia and uterine perforation, there is an increased failure rate of this method in patients taking steroids. There is no specific contraindication to the use of birth control pills in women with ITP.[249]

Once the patient with ITP is pregnant, the management goals are to decrease the risk of antepartum, intrapartum, and postpartum maternal hemorrhage and to prevent intracranial hemorrhage in the neonate. Treatment programs for patients with ITP during pregnancy largely reflect personal bias since most of the management recommendations have not been evaluated in well-designed clinical trials.[93,148,183,195,207,256]

Management of ITP in Pregnancy

The management of ITP is directed towards preventing platelet underproduction, platelet consumption, and impairment of platelet function. The mainstays of treatment are steroids and splenectomy.[3]

General Measures. Iron, folic acid, and vitamin B_{12} deficiency impair platelet production.[3,144] Therefore, identification of a deficiency, as well as adequate supplementation of the deficient substances during pregnancy is important. Myelotoxic agents such as alcohol should be avoided. Fever and infection should be identified and treated since they shorten platelet survival.[123] Drugs that impair platelet function or cause thrombocytopenia should be avoided.[105,124] (Table 9-7).

Steroid Therapy. Therapy in ITP always begins with steroids. The immediate effects of steroid administration are inhibition of antibody attachment to platelets and suppression of platelet phagocytosis by the RES. The long-term effect is inhibition of antibody synthesis.[53,178–180]

Table 9-7. Drugs that Produce Platelet Disorders

	Thrombocytopenia	Thrombopathia
Antibacterial agents		
Penicillin, cephlothin	+	
Sulfonamides	+	
Chloramphenicol	+	
Streptomycin, novobiocin	+	
Isoniazid, rifampicin	+	
p-Aminosalicylic acid	+	
Anticoagulants		+
Antidepressants		
Imidobenzyl derivatives		+
Monoamine oxidase inhibitors		+
Antihistamines		+
Anti-inflammatory nonsteroids	+	+
Barbiturates	+	
Cytotoxic agents	+	
Digitalis	+	
Glycerol guaiacolate		+
Local anesthetics		+
Oral hypoglycemic agents	+	
Phenothiazine	+	+
Quinine, quinidine	+	
Sympatholytic agents		
Propranolol		+
Phentolamine		+
Thiazide diuretics	+	
Tranquilizers		
Chlordiazepoxide		+
Diazepam		+

Reproduced from Horger, E.O. and Keane, M.W.D.: Platelet disorders in pregnancy. Clin. Obstet. Gynecol. 22:843, Harper & Row, 1979.

The objective of steroid therapy during pregnancy is not only to increase the platelet count to the level at which spontaneous hemorrhage is unlikely to occur (generally above 20,000/mm³) but also to provide an adequate reserve so that hemostatic failure will not occur in the case of an unforeseen maternal hemorrhage. Although the ideal goal is to bring the platelet count to normal levels, this frequently is difficult to achieve or requires the use of prohibitive doses of steroid therapy. A more reasonable goal is to maintain a platelet count above 50,000/mm³, since excessive surgical hemorrhage rarely occurs above this level if platelet function is normal. If platelet dysfunction is identified by a prolonged bleeding time, the goal should be to normalize the bleeding time.

Therapy with steroids usually begins with prednisone at a dose of 0.5 to 1 mg/kg/day in divided doses. Because the placental transfer of prednisone is less than that of other glucocorticoids (e.g., betamethasone, dexamethasone), this has been the steroid of choice in the therapy of ITP complicating pregnancy. Some authors have recently suggested the use of corticosteroids that readily cross the placenta with the aim of delivering steroids to the fetus, in which they might have the same therapeutic effect as in the mother.[146,157] A short course of steroids prior to delivery has been proposed for this purpose.

The effect of steroids on the mother is usually noted within the first 24 to 48 h but may take as long as 2 to 3 weeks. The therapeutic plan is to give the shortest course of steroids that will bring the platelet count to a safe level. Once the platelet count is above 80,000/mm^3, the steroids should be continued for 1 week and then tapered slowly. If on the other hand, the platelet count has not reached 50,000/mm^3 in 3 weeks, the dose of prednisone should be increased to 1.5 to 2 mg/kg/day. If continued steroid therapy is needed, it should consist of the smallest dose that will maintain the platelet count above 50,000/mm^3. This parameter must be checked during reduction and after termination of steroid therapy because a fall in the platelet count is the earliest indication of relapse in nonsymptomatic patients. Most pregnant women will respond to steroids so that the performance of a splenectomy can be deferred until the postpartum period.

The potential risks of steroid administration during pregnancy are difficult to assess. However, the risk of maternal hemorrhage outweighs the potential hazards of the judicious use of these drugs. Although animal studies have shown an increased incidence of cleft palate,[75] this has not been substantiated by the limited studies done in humans.[255] Other potential complications of steroids which are rarely reported include: transient adrenal insufficiency in the neonate,[30,122] neonatal hypoglycemia, and IUGR.[245]

Estriol production can be decreased if the equivalent of 75 mg of cortisol is administered daily because at this level transplacental steroids can depress the fetal adrenal production of estriol precursors.[211] Prednisone is secreted into the breast milk, but provided the dose is less than 30 mg/day, it is unlikely to cause any problems in the breast-fed neonate.[147]

Splenectomy. Removal of the spleen eliminates the major site of platelet destruction and an important site of antibody production.[135] Furthermore, since 40 percent of the platelets are normally sequestered in the spleen, this operation increases the number of platelets available for circulation.[14] Splenectomy is usually performed electively in patients with ITP because it may either eliminate the need for steroids or allow a significant reduction in their dosage. During pregnancy, however, splenectomy is indicated only in those women who have life-threatening hemorrhage and in whom primary therapy with steroids has failed to increase the platelet count and bleeding manifestations continue to occur. The major risks of performing a splenectomy in an obstetrical patient are premature labor and the occurrence of a surgical accident when ligating the splenic pedicle. During pregnancy all the blood vessels in the abdomen dramatically increase in size. The technical difficulties of operating on these dilated vessels are compounded by the presence of a gravid uterus, which make access to the splenic pedicle difficult to attain during the second half of pregnancy. However, the operation can be performed immediately following a cesarean section with few additional complications.

Splenectomy has been reported to produce permanent remission in 60 to 70 percent of patients, temporary remission in 20 percent, and no response in 10 percent.[3,165,214] The older literature reports a 9 to 10 percent maternal and a 25 percent perinatal mortality rate when splenectomy was performed during pregnancy.[121,124,142] These figures are likely to be different today because of the availability of platelet transfusions and improvements in surgical technique. At present the maternal operative risk of elective splenectomy during pregnancy is probably similar to that of a nonpregnant patient.

Immunosuppressive Therapy. Immunosuppressive agents (vinca alkaloids, cyclophosphamide, and azathioprine) have been used with some success to treat nonpregnant patients who are refractory to steroid therapy and splenectomy.[69,143] The rationale for their use is to depress the production of antiplatelet antibodies and the host's cellular immunity. Their role in the management of a pregnant patient with ITP has not been established, and concern exists about fetal side effects.[249] There is, however, at least one report in which a woman was successfully treated with cyclophosphamide in the early third trimester without obvious neonatal sequelae.[124]

Platelet Transfusions. Platelet transfusions have no place in the maintenance therapy of ITP. Transfused platelets are not only rapidly destroyed but they also become progressively less effective in raising the platelet count because the antigenic load they provide induces the production of antiplatelet antibodies. Platelet transfusions are indicated in the face of life-threatening hemorrhage, to maintain hemostasis during surgery, and in severe preeclampsia because of the added risk of intracranial hemorrhage. A rule of thumb is to transfuse platelets until the bleeding time is normalized in cases of severe preeclampsia and to provide a platelet count above 60,000/mm^3 and a normal bleeding time prior to surgery. High-dose corticosteroid therapy (prednisone 2 mg/kg or an intravenous preparation of equivalent dose) should be administered with platelet transfusions to prolong platelet survival.[148]

Mode of Delivery. The most serious perinatal problem associated with ITP is fetal thrombocytopenia, which makes the neonate susceptible to hemorrhages and particularly to intracranial bleeding.[214] It is believed that the trauma associated with delivery is a determining factor in the production of intracranial hemorrhage. Since most trauma to the fetal head occurs during its passage through the birth canal, cesarean section has been proposed as the method of choice for delivering these infants. Although this is a logical assumption, it must be noted that the protective effect of cesarean section has not been, and probably will never be, demonstrated in clinical trials. However, adherence to a policy of routine cesarean section as the mode of delivery for patients with ITP will expose the mothers to the risks of defective intra- and postoperative hemostasis. Since 77.5 percent[264] of infants born to thrombocytopenic mothers have no detectable clinical bleeding, a significant number of unnecessary cesarean sections will be performed for putative fetal indications. A more logical approach would be to assess the neonatal risk of thrombocytopenia antenatally. Maternal platelet counts have been proposed to detect the infants at greater risk for thrombocytopenia. However, in one series 27 percent of thrombocytopenic neonates were born to mothers with platelet counts above 100,000/mm^3.[281] This observation invalidates the maternal platelet count as a reliable predictor of fetal thrombocytopenia.

Ayromlooi[15] and Scott et al.[264] have proposed that a platelet count be performed in fetal scalp capillary blood obtained at the beginning of spontaneous or induced labor, and the result be used to select the mode of delivery. The technique of scalp platelet count determination has been validated by its good correlation with umbilical cord and heel capillary platelet counts.

Scott et al.[264] have retrospectively reviewed the incidence and extent of neonatal bleeding in relationship to the neonatal platelet count. They found no bleeding manifestations with counts above 100,000/mm^3 and only mild cutaneous manifestations with platelet counts above 50,000/mm^3. Serious bleeding requiring treatment was confined to infants with counts of less than 50,000/mm^3. These authors have therefore proposed that a platelet count of 50,000/mm^3 in a scalp sample be used as a cutoff value for selecting the mode of delivery. Cesarean section would be indicated only for those infants with platelet counts below 50,000/mm^3.

It must be stressed that these recommendations are based upon a retrospective study and the possibility exists that some infants had had subclinical bleeds with platelet counts above 50,000/mm^3. A study including ultrasonographic examination and neurologic follow-up of infants born to mothers with ITP will be necessary to assess the prevalence of asymptomatic bleeds and to establish the long-term significance of these findings.

The technique for scalp platelet count is simple but must be mastered before it is used in a patient with ITP. The scalp platelet count should be performed at the beginning of labor or after elective amniotomy in patients with a dilated cervix at term. Ideally, the patient should be in the cesarean section room in lithotomy position. A plastic cone is placed in the vagina and directly applied to the fetal scalp. A stab wound scalp incision is then created similar to that used for scalp pH capillary collection. A Unopette test 5855 system (Becton-Dickinson) is used to collect the sample. This is a plastic pipette that fills by capillary action to 0.02 ml. This pipette is held in an Allis clamp to collect the sample. Once the pipette has been filled, it is emptied into a reservoir containing 1.98 ml of diluent and mixed. Platelet count determination is performed by an automated technique or a standard manual hemocytometer method. A critical part of the scalp platelet determination technique is the speed with which the procedure is performed. If the blood is collected slowly, it tends to clot, giving falsely low results. It is wise to confirm the machine results with a smear of capillary blood. Blood collection technique for smear preparation is similar to that previously described. Heparinized tubes should not be used for sample collection because of platelet clumping, which can produce abnormally low results.

Complications with the use of this technique have not yet been reported. Compression of the scalp incision should be maintained until bleeding has stopped completely. The capability of performing an emergency cesarean section is essential when this technique is used, as continued fetal bleeding could become a problem.

It has recently been suggested that the administration of a short course of steroids (10 to 20 mg prednisone) be given to the mother for 14 days prior to the estimated delivery date with the objective of reducing thrombocytopenia in the fetus. This program has been reported to be effective in increasing neonatal platelet counts. However, severe neonatal thrombocytopenia has been reported in steroid-treated mothers; therefore, even if this therapy has been specifically administered for its transplacental effect, a fetal scalp platelet count should be performed to ensure the adequacy of the infant's platelet count.

THROMBOTIC THROMBOCYTOPENIC PURPURA

Pathophysiology and Laboratory Findings

Thrombotic thrombocytopenic purpura (TTP) is a syndrome characterized clinically by thrombocytopenia, microangiopathic hemolytic anemia, neurologic abnormalities, renal dysfunction, and fever, and pathologically by the presence of intravascular hyaline thrombi consisting of platelets and fibrin.

The pathophysiology of this disease has not been definitively established; however, increasing evidence suggests that TTP is a disorder of the mechanism that regulates the blood vessel wall–platelet interaction. The following pathophysiologic model is based upon the observations of Kwaan and other investigators.[155,156,200] The initial event may be injury to discontinuous segments of the endothelium of small arteries and capillaries. The nature of the insult has not been determined but is likely to be diverse. Damage of the endothelial cell impairs the production of a platelet antiaggregatory agent, possibly prostacyclin, and leads to the segmental intravascular deposition of platelets and platelet-derived fibrin. Hyaline microthrombi so formed are not lysed because of local failure of the fibrinolytic system. The impairment of local fibrinolysis may be due to direct injury of the endothelial cell which is an important source of plasminogen activator and to plasmin inhibition by aggregated platelets. The end result of this process is the formation of extensive microthrombi which occlude the circulation and lead to the multiple organ involvement that characterizes TTP.

Although TTP has been confused with DIC, it should be noted that the operational mechanisms of these two processes are different. DIC is a thrombin-driven disorder characterized by an increased turnover of both platelets and fibrinogen and accompanied by a secondary fibrinolytic response. TTP is a platelet-driven process in which there is increased platelet consumption, normal fibrinogen turnover, and absent local fibrinolysis.[109,155]

The clinical and laboratory manifestations of TTP can be inferred from the proposed pathophysiologic model. Disseminated intravascular platelet aggregation will lead to platelet consumption and thrombocytopenia. This may be clinically manifested by petechiae, ecchymosis, and/or bleeding from mucous membranes. Vaginal bleeding may be the first evidence of the disease. The passage of red blood cells through areas of the microcirculation partially occluded with microthrombi will produce a microangiopathic hemolytic anemia, which can result in pallor and jaundice. Microthrombi may cause ischemic changes in multiple organs such as kidney, brain, and pancreas and can lead to renal failure, neurologic abnormalities, fever, pancreatitis, etc.[63,91]

The peripheral blood smear contains schistocytes, and urinalysis may show hematuria and proteinuria. Bone marrow aspirates reveal a normal or increased number of megakaryocytes. Fibrinogen levels and clotting studies are within normal limits unless DIC complicates the disease.[137] Pathologic examination of the gingiva, skin, spleen, and lymph nodes can demonstrate the presence of microthrombi in small-caliber vessels without evidence of vasculitis or peripheral clot lysis.[23,147]

TTP In Pregnancy

TTP is an uncommon disorder but it affects women more frequently than men and is seen predominantly between the ages of 10 and 40. It is therefore not surprising to see this disorder in association with pregnancy. More than 350 cases have been reported, of which 30 have been associated with pregnancy. Twenty-nine biopsy-proven cases of TTP associated with pregnancy have been reviewed by May, Harbert, and Thornton,[173] who found a 7 percent 2-year maternal survival rate and approximately 65 percent perinatal mortality. This, however, was prior to the more recent therapeutic approaches to this disease.[18,186,226]

When TTP presents prior to or during the first trimester of pregnancy, the diagnosis is relatively easy to make, and some successful pregnancies after therapy have been reported. When the onset of the disease takes place in the third trimester of pregnancy, the diagnostic problem is more difficult because of the striking similarities between eclampsia and TTP. Both diseases may present with thrombocytopenia, microangiopathic hemolytic anemia, renal dysfunction, fever, and coma and/or seizures.[263]

It is important to differentiate between TTP and eclampsia because the latter responds dramatically to delivery while the former requires therapy with exchange transfusions and antiplatelet agents. It has been recently suggested that gingival biopsies may provide a diagnostic tool to differentiate the two entities.[282] Biopsy specimens of patients with TTP should show microthrombi in small vessels without evidence of vasculitis and peripheral clot lysis, while patients with toxemia have been assumed to have no thrombotic lesions. The problem with this approach is that gingival biopsies have been reported to be negative in as many as 40 percent of patients with TTP, and the experience with gingival biopsies in women with toxemia is limited.[23] Furthermore, it is possible that toxemic patients with decompensated DIC have thrombotic fibrin deposits in small vessels similar to those found on light microscopy in cases of TTP. Differentiation between the thrombotic lesions of TTP and DIC currently require the histochemical identification of plasminogen activator activity. DIC lesions have increased fibrinolytic activity, while this is absent in TTP lesions. Unfortunately, this technique is still a research tool and is not generally available for clinical practice.[155]

Management of TTP in Pregnancy. Therapy for TTP has been empirical and has involved many different regimens, including steroids, splenectomy, heparin, heparin and urokinase, antiplatelet agents, immunosuppressive agents, hemodialysis, and plasma transfusions. Evaluation of the success of different therapeutic modalities is very difficult because they have frequently been used in combination. Furthermore, it is possible that several disorders with different pathophysiologic mechanisms have been inappropriately labelled as TTP. This, of course, will result in variable results to different therapeutic modalities.

The management of TTP complicating pregnancy depends upon the gestational age at the time of presentation. If a patient presents with the typical TTP pentad in the first or early second trimester, the diagnosis can be established with reasonable certainty because toxemia of pregnancy is unlikely to occur at this gestational age. Therapy should be directed towards inducing a hematologic remission with plasma exchange transfusions and antiplatelet agents. If the patient presents in the third trimester, however, it is very difficult to distinguish between TTP and eclampsia. Since eclampsia is the more prevalent condition, it should be assumed to be present if clinical and pathological data are not helpful in differentiating these disorders, and the patient should be delivered. Every effort should be made to accomplish a vaginal delivery since this imposes less stress on the hemostatic system than a cesarean section. Failure to improve following delivery suggests that the correct diagnosis is TTP and specific therapy for that disease can then be initiated.

Obstetric patients with TTP are best managed in conjunction with the hematology and blood bank services. Therapy should begin with plasma exchange transfusions and antiplatelet agents.[8,19,41–44,97,252] The current rationale for the use of exchange transfusions is based on the demonstration that patients with TTP are deficient in a factor that is present in normal plasma and can inhibit platelet aggregation.[37,156,160,287] The patient's status should be monitored with serial platelet counts, serum creatinine, LDH, and bilirubin determinations, as well as with frequent neurological examinations. Daily plasma transfusions should be instituted until a spontaneous increase in platelet count to near normal values is obtained and neurologic manifestations have disappeared. The volume of the transfusion should be sufficient to maintain the LDH concentration below 300 units/ml. The initial volume for exchange plasmapheresis has been recommended as 35 to 40 ml/kg. Response rates to plasma exchange transfusions have been reported to be as high as 82 percent.[42] The choice of the antiplatelet agent is arbitrary. Aspirin, 600 to 1,200 mg/day, dipyridamole 400 to 600 mg/day, and dextran 75 in 250 ml every 12 h have been recommended.[8] The response to antiplatelet agents has varied between 50 and 75 percent. Patients who have failed to respond to the initial therapy can be empirically treated with steroids, splenectomy, or immunosuppressive agents with varying degrees of response.[42] The choice of therapy after initial failure is arbitrary and reflects in most cases the personal experience and preference of the physicians managing the case. The administration of platelet concentrates has been associated with worsening of intravascular thrombus formation. They should only be used in cases of life-threatening hemorrhage and in conjunction with plasma exchange transfusions.[103]

REFERENCES

1. Abdul-Karim, R.W. and Chevli, R.N.: Antepartum hemorrhage and shock. Clin. Obstet. Gynecol., *19*:533, 1976.
2. Aggeler, P.M.: Physiological basis for transfusion therapy in hemorrhagic disorders: A critical review. Transfusion, *1*:71, 1961.
3. Ahn, Y.S. and Harrington, W.J.: Treatment of idiopathic thrombocytopenic purpura (ITP). Ann. Rev. Med., *28*:299, 1977.
4. Aisner, J.: Platelet transfusion therapy. Med. Clin. North Am. *61*:1133, 1977.
5. Alkjaersig, N., Fletcher, A.P., and Sherry, S.J.: The mechanism of clot dissolution by plasmin. J. Clin. Invest., *38*:1086, 1959.
6. Alkjaersig, N., Fletcher, A. P., and Sherry, S.: Pathogenesis of the coagulation defect developing during pathological plasma proteolytic ("fibrinolytic") states. II. The signifi-

cance, mechanism and consequences of defective fibrin polymerization. J. Clin. Invest. *41:*917, 1962.
7. Ambrus, C.M. and Marcus, G.: Plasmin antiplasmin complex as a reservoir of fibrinolytic enzyme. Am. J. Physiol., *199:*491, 1960.
8. Amorosi, E.L. and Karpakin, S.: Antiplatelet treatment of thrombotic thrombocytopenic purpura. Ann. Intern. Med. *86:*102, 1977.
9. Anonymous. Lab News, Yale-New Haven Medical Center, July 1981.
10. Anonymous. Introduction to the plasma coagulation factors. p. 1225. In Williams, W.J., Beutler, E., Erslev, A.J., and Rundles, R.W., Eds.: Hematology. McGraw-Hill, New York, 1977.
11. Arias, F. and Mancilla-Jimenez, R.: Hepatic fibrinogen deposits in pre-eclampsia. N. Engl. J. Med. *295:*578, 1976.
12. Astedt, B.: On fibrinolysis. A. In pregnancy, labour, puerperium and during treatment with sex hormones. B. In human ontogenesis and in human organ culture. Acta Obstet. Gynaecol. Scand., *51:* suppl. 18, 1972.
13. Aster, R.H.: Effect of anticoagulant and ABO incompatibility on recovery of transfused human platelets. Blood, *26:*732, 1965.
14. Aster, R.H.: Splenic platelet pooling as a cause of "hypersplenic" thrombocytopenia. Trans. Assoc. Am. Physicians, *78:*362, 1965.
15. Ayromlooi, J.: A new approach to the management of immunologic thrombocytopenic purpura in pregnancy. Am. J. Obstet. Gynecol. *130:*235, 1978.
16. Baldini, M., Costea, N., and Dameshek, W.: The viability of stored human platelets. Blood, *16:*1669, 1960.
17. Banton, P.G., Jackson, C.M., and Hanahan, D.J.: Relationship between factor V and activated factor X in the generation of prothrombinase. Nature, *214:*923, 1967.
18. Barbaro, C. and Hirsh, J.: Severe post-partum bleeding in abruptio placentae: failure to respond to fibrinogen infusion. Med. J. Aust. *2:*1182, 1968.
19. Barrett, C. and Marshall, J.R.: Thrombotic thrombocytopenic purpura. Obstet. Gynecol. *46:*231, 1975.
20. Basu, H.K.: Fibrinolysis and abruptio placentae. J. Obstet. Gynaecol. Br. Commonw., *76:*481, 1969.
21. Beck, E.A.: Congenital abnormalities of fibrinogen. Clin. Haematol., *8:*169, 1979.
22. Beischer, N.A.: Intravascular defibrination in pregnancy with associated pituitary and kidney damage. Am. J. Obstet. Gynecol., *82:*625, 1981.
23. Berkowitz, L.R., Daliforf, F.G., and Blatt, P.M.: Thrombotic thrombocytopenic purpura. JAMA, *241:*1709, 1979.
24. Biggs, R., Austen, D.E.G., Denson, K.W.E. et al.: The mode of action of antibodies which destroy factor VIII. I. Antibodies which have second-order concentration graphs. Br. J. Haematol., *23:*125, 1972.
25. Biland, L. and Duckert, F.: Coagulation factors of the newborn and his mother. Thromb. Diath. Haemorrh., *29:*644, 1973.
26. Billah, M.M., Lapetina, E.G., and Cuatrecasas, P.: Activity of platelets, differential substrate specificity, Ca^{++} requirement, pH dependence and cellular location. J. Biol. Chem., *255:*10227, 1980.
27. Blatt, P.M., Lundblad, R.L., Kingdon, H.S. et al.: Thrombogenic materials in prothrombin complex concentrates. Ann. Intern. Med., *81:*766, 1974.
28. Bleyl, U.: Morphologic diagnosis of disseminated intravascular coagulation: histologic, histochemical and electronmicroscopic studies. Semin. Thromb. Hemostas., 3(4):247, 1977.
29. Bloom, A.L., Davies, A.J., and Res, J.K.: A clinical and laboratory study of a patient with an unusual factor VIII inhibitor. Thromb. Diath. Haemorrh., *15:*12, 1966.

30. Bongiovanni, A.M. and McPadden, A.J.: Steroids during pregnancy and possible fetal consequences. Fertil. Steril. *11:*181, 1960.
31. Bonnar, J.: Haematological problems. Coagulation disorder. J. Clin. Pathol. [Suppl.], 29(10):35, 1976.
32. Bonnar, J.: Haemostasis and coagulation disorders in pregnancy. p. 454. In, Bloom, A.L. and Thomas, D.P., Eds.: Haemostasis and Thrombosis. Edinburgh, Churchill Livingstone, 1981.
33. Bonnar, J., McNicol, G.P., and Douglas, A.S.: Fibrinolytic enzyme system and pregnancy. Br. N.J., *3:*387, 1969.
34. Bonnar, J., McNicol, G.P., and Douglas, A.S.: The behaviour of the coagulation and fibrinolytic mechanisms in abruptio placentae. J. Obstet. Gynaecol., *76:*799, 1969.
35. Bonnar, J., McNicol, G.P., and Douglas, A.S.: Coagulation and fibrinolytic mechanisms during and after normal childbirth. Br. Med. J., *2:*200, 1970.
36. Bove, J.R.: Fibrinogen—is the benefit worth the risk? Transfusion, *18:*129, 1978.
37. Bowie, E.J.W. and Owen, C.A., Jr.: Hemostatic failure in clinical medicine. Semin. Hematol., *14:*341, 1977.
38. Broekman, M.J., Ward, J.W., and Marcus, A.J.: Phospholipid metabolism in stimulated human platelets. J. Clin. Invest. *66:*275, 1980.
39. Brozovic, M.: Acquired disorders of blood coagulation. In Bloom, A.L., and Duncan, D.P., Eds.: Haemostasis and Thombosis. Churchill Livingstone, Edinburgh, 1981.
40. Bruno, M.S. and Brody, H.S.: Hypothromboplastinemia associated with a circulating anticoagulant and hemorrhagic diathesis. Am. J. Med., *7:*756, 1954.
41. Bukowski, R.M., Hewlett, J.S., Harris, J.W. et al.: Exchange transfusions in the treatment of thrombotic thrombocytopenic purpura. Semin. Hematol., *13:*219, 1976.
42. Bukowski, R.M., Hewlett, J.S., Reimer, R.R. et al.: Therapy of thrombotic thrombocytopenic purpura: An overview. Semin. Thromb. Hemostas. *7:*1, 1981.
43. Byrnes, J.J. and Khurana, M.: Treatment of thrombotic thrombocytopenic purpura with plasma. N. Engl. J. Med., *297:*1386, 1977.
44. Byrnes, J.J. and Lian, E.C.Y.: Recent therapeutic advances in thrombotic thrombocytopenic purpura. Semin. Thromb. Hemostas., *5:*199, 1979.
45. Carreras, L.O., Machin, S.J., Deman, R. et al.: Arterial thrombosis, intrauterine fetal death and lupus anticoagulant detection of immunoglobulin interfering with prostacycline formation. Lancet *1:*244, 1981.
46. Carreras, L.O., Spitz, B., Vermylen, J., and Van Assche, A.: Lupus anticoagulant and inhibition of prostacycline formation in patients with repeated abortion, intrauterine growth retardation and intrauterine fetal death. Br. J. Obstet. Gynaecol., *88:*890, 1981.
47. Cash, J.: Blood replacement therapy. p. 472. In Haemostasis and Thrombosis. Bloom, A.L., and Thomas, D.P., Eds.: Churchill Livingstone, Edinburgh, 1981.
48. Cavanagh, D.: Clotting disorders in pregnancy. Ch. 2, p. 7. In Cavanagh, D., Woods, R.E., O'Connor, T.C.F., and Knuppel, R.A., Eds.: Obstetric Emergencies. 3rd Ed., Harper & Row, Philadelphia, 1981.
49. Cavanagh, D., Rao, P.S., Sutton, D.M.C. et al.: Pathophysiology of endotoxin shock in the primate. Am. J. Obstet. Gynecol., *108:*705, 1970.
50. Cederbaum, A.I., Blatt, P.M., and Roberts, H.R.: Intravascular coagulation with use of human prothrombin complex concentrates. Ann. Intern. Med., *84:*683, 1976.
51. Chesterman, C.N., Allington, M.J., and Sharp, A.A.: Relationship of plasminogen activator to fibrin. Nature, *238:*15, 1972.
52. Cines, D.B., Dusak, B., Tomaski, A. et al.: Immune thrombocytopenic purpura and pregnancy. N. Engl. J. Med., *306:*826, 1982.
53. Cines, D.B. and Schreiber, A.D.: Immune thrombocytopenia. N. Engl. J. Med., *300:*106, 1979.

54. Coller, B.S., Hultin, M.B., Hoyer, L.W. et al.: Normal pregnancy in a patient with a prior postpartum factor VIII inhibitor: with observations on pathogenesis and prognosis. Blood, *58:*619, 1981.
55. Colman, R.W., Robboy, S.J., and Minna, J.D.: Disseminated intravascular coagulation (DIC): An approach. Am. J. Med., *52:*679, 1972.
56. Conrad, J.: Inhibitors of blood coagulation. In Thomson, J.M., Ed., Blood Coagulation and Haemostasis. A Practical Guide. Churchill Livingstone, Edinburgh, 1900.
57. Cooper, H.A., Bowie, E.J.W., Didisheim, P., and Owen, C.A. Jr.: Paradoxic changes in platelets and fibrinogen in chronically induced intravascular coagulation. Mayo Clin. Proc., *46:*521, 1971.
58. Cooper, H.A., Bowie, E.J.W., and Owen, C.A., Jr.: Chronic induced intravascular coagulation in dogs. Am. J. Physiol., *225:*1355, 1973.
59. Cooper, H.A., Bowie, E.J.W., and Owen, C.A., Jr.: Evaluation of patients with increased fibrinolytic split products (FSP) in their serum. Mayo Clin. Proc., *49:*654, 1974.
60. Coopland, A.T., Alkjaersig, N., and Fletcher, A.P.: Reduction in plasma factor XIII (fibrin stabilizing factor) concentration during pregnancy. J. Lab. Clin. Med., *73:*144, 1969.
61. Coopland, A.T., Israels, E.D., Zipursky, A., and Israels, L.G.: The pathogenesis of defective hemostasis in abruptio placentae. Am. J. Obstet. Gynecol. *100:*311, 1968.
62. Coopland, A.T. and Livingstone, R.A.: Heparin treatment in abruptio placentae. Can. Med. Assoc. J. *103:*377, 1970.
63. Crain, S.M. and Choudhury, A.M.: Thrombotic thromboctyopenic purpura. JAMA, *246:*1243, 1981.
64. Davey, R.J., Shashaty, G.G., and Rath, C.E.: Acute coagulopathy following infusion of prothrombin complex concentrate. Am. J. Med., *60:*719, 1976.
65. DeWolf, F., Carreras, L.O., Moerman, P. et al.: Decidual vasculopathy and extensive placental infarction in a patient with repeated thromboembolic accidents, recurrent fetal loss, and a lupus anticoagulant. Am. J. Obstet. Gynecol., *142:*829, 1982.
66. Deykin, D.: The clinical challenge of disseminated intravascular coagulation. Sherwood, L.M. and Parris, E.E., Eds.: Seminars in Medicine of the Beth Israel Hospital. N. Engl. J. Med., *283:*636, 1970.
67. Deykin, D., Cochios, F., DeCamp, G., and Lopez, A.: Hepatic removal of activated factor X by the perfused rabbit liver. Am. J. Physiol., *214:*414, 1968.
68. Didisheim, P.: Tests of blood coagulation and hemostasis. III. The partial thromboplastin time. JAMA, *199:*169, 1967.
69. DiFino, S.M., Lachant, N.A., Kirschner, J.J., and Gottlieb, A.J.: Adult idiopathic thrombocytopenic purpura. Clinical findings and response to therapy. Am. J. Med., *69:*430, 1980.
70. Douglas, J.T., Shah, M., Lowe, G.D.O. et al.: Plasma fibrinopeptide A and beta-thromboglobulin in pre-eclampsia and pregnancy hypertension. Thromb. Haemost., *47:*54, 1982.
71. Dreskin, O.H. and Rosenthal, N.: A hemophilia-like disease with prolonged coagulation time and a circulating anticoagulant. Blood *5:*46, 1950.
72. Edgar, W., McKillop, C., Howie, P.W., and Prentice, C.R.M.: Composition of soluble fibrin complexes in pre-eclampsia. Thromb. Res. *10:*567, 1977.
73. Eika, C. and Abildgaard, U.: Inhibition of thrombin induced aggregation of human platelets by antithrombin III. Scand. J. Haematol., *7:*460, 1970.
74. Ellman, L., Carvalho, A., and Colman, R.W.: The thrombo-wellcotest as a screening test for disseminated intravascular coagulation. N. Engl. J. Med., *288:*633, 1973.
75. Fainstat, T.: Cortisone-induced congenital cleft palate in rabbits. Endocrinology, *55:*502, 1954.

76. Ferguson, J.H. and Hatton, R.L.: Abruptio placentae and rupture of the marginal sinus of the placenta: some relationships. Am. J. Obstet. Gynecol., *78:*947, 1959.
77. Files, J.C., Morrison, F.S., and Halbrook, J.: Post-partum treatment of a patient with a factor VIII inhibitor. N. Engl. J. Med., *305:*1650, 1981.
78. Filip, D.J. and Aster, R.H.: Relative hemostatic effectiveness of human platelets stored at 4° and 22°C. J. Lab. Clin. Med., *91:*618, 1978.
79. Firkin, B.G., Howard, M.A., and Radford, N.: Possible relationship between lupus inhibitor and recurrent abortion in young women. Lancet, *2:*366, 1980.
80. Fischbach, D.P. and Fogdall, R.P.: Coagulation: The Essentials. Williams & Wilkins, Baltimore, 1981.
81. Fletcher, A.P., Alkjaersig, N.K., and Burstein, R.: The influence of pregnancy upon blood coagulation and plasma fibrinolytic enzyme function. Am. J. Obstet. Gynecol., *134:*743, 1979.
82. Fletcher, A.P., Alkjaersig, N., and Sherry, S.: Pathogenesis of the coagulation defect developing during pathological plasma proteolytic ("fibrinolytic") states. I. The significance of fibrinogen proteolysis and circulating fibrinogen breakdown products. J. Clin. Invest., *41:*896, 1962.
83. Fresh, J.W., Ferguson, J.H., and Lewis, J.H.: Blood-clotting studies in parturient women and the newborn. Obstet. Gynecol. *7:*117, 1956.
84. Frick, P.G.: Hemophilia-like disease following pregnancy with transplacental transfer of an acquired circulating anticoagulant. Blood, *8:*598, 1953.
85. Fulton, L.D. and Page, E.W.: Nature of the refractory state following sublethal dose of human placental thromboplastin. Proc. Soc. Exp. Biol. Med., *68:*594, 1948.
86. Gaffney, P.J.: The fibrinolytic system. p. 198. In Bloom, A.L. and Thomas, D.P., Eds.: Haemostasis and Thrombosis. Churchill Livingstone, Edinburg, 1981.
87. Garg, S.K., Amorosi, E.L., and Karpatkin, S.: Use of the megathrombocyte as an index of megakaryocyte number. N. Engl. J. Med. *284:*11, 1971.
88. Gerrard, J.M., Butler, A.M., Peterson, D.A. et al.: Phosphatidic acid releases calcium from platelet membrane *in vitro*. Prostaglandins Med., *1:*387, 1978.
89. Giddings, J.C.: The investigation of hereditary coagulation disorders. In Thomson, J.M., Ed.: Blood Coagulation and Haemostasis. A Practical Guide. Churchill Livingstone, Edinburgh, 1980.
90. Gilabert, J., Aznar, J., Parrilla, J.J. et al.: Alterations in the coagulation and fibrinolysis system in pregnancy, labour and puerperium, with special reference to a possible transitory state in intravascular coagulation during labour. Thromb. Haemost., *40:*387, 1978.
91. Goldenfarb, P.B. and Finch, S.C.: Thrombotic thrombocytopenic purpura. JAMA, *226:*644, 1973.
92. Goldfinger, D. and McGinniss, M.H.: RH-incompatible platelet transfusions—risks and consequences of sensitizing immunosuppressed patients. N. Engl. J. Med., *284:*942, 1971.
93. Goldsweig, H. and Chediak, J.: Quantitative and qualitative platelet disorders that complicate pregnancy. J. Reprod. Med., *19:*205, 1977.
94. Goodlin, R.C.: Severe pre-eclampsia: Another great imitator. Am. J. Obstet. Gynecol., *125:*747, 1976.
95. Goodlin, R.C. and Holdt, D.: Impending gestosis. Obstet. Gynecol. *58:*743, 1981.
96. Gordon, Y.B., Ratky, S.M., Sola, C.M. et al.: Circulating levels of fibrin/fibrinogen degradation fragment E in normal pregnancy, and in association with intrauterine growth retardation and perinatal asphyxia. Br. J. Obstet. Gynaecol., *82:*958, 1975.
97. Gottschall, J.L., Pisciotta, A.V., Darin, J. et al.: Thrombotic thrombocytopenic purpura: Experience with whole blood exchange transfusion. Semin. Thromb. Hemostas., *7:*25, 1981.
98. Graeff, H. and Kuhn, W.: Coagulation Disorders in Obstetrics. Vol. 13. In Friedman,

E.A., Ed.: Major Problems in Obstetrics and Gynecology. W.B. Saunders, Philadelphia, 1980.
99. Graeff, H. and von Hugo, R.: Fibrinogen derivatives in a case of abruptio placentae. Am. J. Obstet. Gynecol., *120:*335, 1974.
100. Green, D. and Lechner, K.: A survey of 215 non-hemophilic patients with inhibitors to factor VIII. Thromb. Haemost., *45:*200, 1981.
101. Greenwood, R.J. and Rabin, S.C.: Hemophilia-like postpartum bleeding. Obstet. Gynecol., *30:*362, 1967.
102. Griffin, J.H.: Role of surface in surface-dependent activation of Hageman factor (blood coagulation factor XII). Proc. Natl. Acad. Sci. USA, *75:*1998, 1978.
103. Griffin, J.H.: The contact phase of blood coagulation. p. 84. In Bloom, A.L. and Thomas, D.P., Eds.: Haemostasis and Thrombosis. Churchill Livingstone, Edinburgh, 1981.
104. Griffin, J.H. and Cochrane, C.G.: Recent advances in the understanding of contact activation reactions. Semin. Thromb. Hemostas., *5:*254, 1979.
105. Hackett, T., Kelton, J.G., and Powers, P.: Drug-induced platelet destruction. Semin. Thromb. and Hemostas., *8:*116, 1982.
106. Hafter, R. and Graeff, H.: Molecular aspects of defibrination in a reptilase-treated case of "dead fetus syndrome." Thromb. Res. *7:*391, 1975.
107. Harker, L.A.: Hemostasis Manual, 2nd Ed. F.A. Davis, Philadelphia, 1974.
108. Harker, L.A. and Slichter, S.J.: The bleeding time as a screening test for evaluation of platelet function. N. Engl. J. Med., *287:*155, 1972.
109. Harker, L.A. and Slichter, S.J.: Platelet and fibrinogen consumption in man. N. Engl. J. Med., *287:*999, 1972.
110. Harkness, D.R., Byrnes, J.J., Lian, E.C-Y et al.: Hazard of platelet transfusion in thrombotic thrombocytopenic purpura. JAMA, *246:*1931, 1981.
111. Harlan, J.M. and Harker, L.A.: Hemostasis, thrombosis, and thromboembolic disorders. Med. Clin. North Am. *65:*855, 1981.
112. Hathaway, W.E. and Bonnar, M.D.: Physiology of Coagulation in Pregnancy. p. 27. In: Perinatal Coagulation. Grune & Statton, New York, 1978.
113. Hathaway, W.E. and Bonnar, M.D.: Hemorrhagic disorders during pregnancy. p. 81. In: Perinatal Coagulation. Grune & Stratton, New York, 1978.
114. Hathaway, W.E. and Bonnar, M.D.: Coagulation changes in preeclampsia, eclampsia, and fetal growth retardation. p. 201. In: Perinatal Coagulation. Grune & Stratton, New York, 1978.
115. Hedner, U. and Astedt, B.: Studies on fibrinolytic inhibitors during pregnancy. Acta Obstet. Gynaecol. Scand., *50:*99, 1971.
116. Hedner, U. and Martinsson, G.: Inhibition of activated Hageman factor (factor XIIa) by an inhibitor of the plasminogen activation (PA inhibitor). Thromb. Res., *12:*1015, 1978.
117. Heene, D.L.: Disseminated intravascular coagulation: Evaluation of therapeutic approaches. Semin. Thromb. Hemostas. *3:*291, 1977.
118. Heimark, R.L., Kurachi, K., Fujikawa, K., and Davie, E.W.: Surface activation of blood coagulation, fibrinolysis and kinin formation. Nature *286:*456, 1980.
119. Herbst, K.D., Rapaport, S.I., Kenoyer, D.G. et al.: Syndrome of an acquired inhibitor of factor VIII responsive to cyclophosphamide and prednisone. Ann. Intern. Med. *198:*575, 1981.
120. Hewlett, J.S. and Haden, R.L.: Hemophilia-like disease in women. J. Lab. Clin. Med., *34:*151, 1949.
121. Heys, R.F.: Child bearing and idiopathic thrombocytopenic purpura. J. Obstet. Gynaecol. Br. Commonw. *73:*205, 1966.
122. Heys, R.F.: Steroid therapy for idiopathic thrombocytopenic purpura during pregnancy. Obstet. Gynecol., *28:*532, 1966.

123. Higby, D.J., Cohen, J.E., Holland, J.F., and Sinks, L.: The prophylactic treatment of thrombocytopenic leukemic patients with platelets: a double blind study. Transfusion, *14:*440, 1974.
124. Horger, E.O. III and Keane, M.W.D.: Platelet disorders in pregnancy. Clin. Obstet. Gynecol. *22:*843, 1979.
125. Hougie, C.: Recalcification time test and its modifications (partial thromboplastin time, activated partial thromboplastin time, and expanded partial thromboplastin time). Ch. A.30, p. 1642. In Williams, W.J., Beutler, E., Erslev, A.I., and Rundles, R.W., Eds.: Hematology. 2nd Ed. McGraw-Hill, 1977.
126. Hougie, C.: One-stage prothrombin time. Ch. A31, p. 1645. In Williams, W.J., Beutler, E., Erslev, A.I., and Rundles, R.W., Eds.: Hematology. 2nd Ed. McGraw-Hill, 1977.
127. Hougie, C.: Methods for estimating fibrinogen concentration. p. 1650. In Williams, W.J., Beutler, E., Erslev, A.J., and Rundles, R.W., Eds.: hematology. 2nd Ed. McGraw-Hill, New York, 1977.
128. Hougie, C.: Latex particle agglutination test for fibrin or fibrinogen degradation products. Chap. A34, p. 1651. In Williams, W.J., Beutler, E., Erslev, A.I., and Rundles, R.W., Eds.: Hematology. 2nd Ed. McGraw-Hill, 1977.
129. Howie, P.W.: The haemostatic mechanisms in pre-eclampsia. Clin. Obstet. Gynaecol., *4:*595, 1977.
130. Howie, P.W., Begg, C.B., Purdie, D.W., and Prentice, C.R.M.: Use of coagulation tests to predict the clinical progress of pre-eclampsia. Lancet, *1:*323, 1976.
131. Huestis, D.W., Bove, J.R., and Busch, S.: Blood transfusion. p. 217. In: Practical Blood Transfusion. Little, Brown, Boston, 1981.
132. Huestis, D.W., Bove, J.R., and Busch, S.: Blood components, fractions, and derivatives. p. 285. In: Practical Blood Transfusion. Little, Brown, Boston, 1981.
133. Hultin, M.B. and Nemerson, Y.: Activation of factor X by factors IXa and VIII; a specific assay for factor IXa in the presence of thrombin-activated factor VIII. Blood, *52:*928, 1978.
134. Imrie, A.H. and Raper, C.G.L.: Severe intravascular coagulation preceding severe pre-eclampsia. Br. J. Obstet. Gynaecol. *84:*71, 1977.
135. Iwarson, S., Kjellman, H., and Teger-Nilsson, A-C.: Incidence of viral hepatitis after adminsitration of factor IX concentrates. Vox Sang., *31:*136, 1976.
136. Jackson, C.M., Owen, W.G., Gitel, S.N., and Esmon, C.T.: The chemical role of lipids in prothrombin activation. Thromb. Diath. Hemorr., (Suppl) *57:*273, 1974.
137. Jaffe, E.A., Nachman, R.L., and Merskey, C.: Thrombotic thrombocytopenic purpura—coagulation parameters in twelve patients. Blood, *42:*499, 1973.
138. Jennison, R.F. and Walker, A.H.C.: Foetal death in utero with hypofibrinogenaemia managed conservatively. Lancet, *2:*607, 1956.
139. Jerushalmy, Z. and Zucker, M.B.: Some effects of fibrinogen degradation products (FDP) on blood platelets. Thromb. Diath. Haemorr., *25:*414, 1966.
140. Jespersen, J.: Disseminated intravascular coagulation in toxaemia of pregnancy. Correction of the decreased platelet counts and raised levels of serum uric acid and fibrin(ogen) degradation products by aspirin. Thromb. Res., *17:*743, 1980.
141. Jimenez, J.M. and Pritchard, J.A.: Pathogenesis and treatment of coagulation defects resulting from fetal death. Obstet. Gynecol., *32:*449, 1968.
142. Jones, W.R., Storey, B., Norton, G., and Neische, F.W. Jr.: Pregnancy complicated by acute idiopathic thrombocytopenic purpura. A report of two patients treated by simultaneous caesarean section and splenectomy. J. Obstet. Gynaecol. Br. Commonw. *81:*330, 1974.
143. Karpatkin, S.: Autominnune thrombocytopenic purpura. Blood, *56:*329, 1980.
144. Karpatkin, S., Garg, S.K., and Freedman, M.L.: Role of iron as a regulator of thrombopoiesis. Am. J. Med., *57:*521, 1974.

145. Karpatkin, S., Khan, Q. and Freedman, M.: Heterogeneity of platelet function. Am. J. Med., *64:*542, 1978.
146. Karpatkin, M., Porges, R.F., and Karpatkin, S.: Platelet counts in infants of women with autoimmune thrombocytopenia. N. Engl. J. Med., *305:*936, 1981.
147. Katz, F.H. and Duncan, B.R.: Entry of prednisone into human milk. N. Engl. J. Med., *293:*1154, 1975.
148. Kelton, J.G. and Gibbons, S.: Autoimmune platelet destruction: Idiopathic thrombocytopenic purpura. Semin. Thromb. Hemostas., *8:*83, 1982.
149. Kennan, A.L. and Bell, W.N.: Blood coagulation during normal pregnancy, labor, and the puerperium. Am. J. Obstet. Gynecol., *73:*57, 1957.
150. Kernoff, L.M., Malan, E. and Gunston, K.: Neonatal thrombocytopenia complicating autoimmune thrombocytopenia in pregnancy. Ann. Intern. Med., *90:*55, 1979.
151. Killam, A.P., Dillard, S.H., Patton, R.C., and Pederson, P.R.: Pregnancy-induced hypertension complicated by acute liver disease and disseminated intravascular coagulation. Am. J. Obstet. Gynecol., *123:*823, 1975.
152. Klein, C.A. and Blajchman, M.A.: Alloantibodies and platelet destruction. Semin. Thromb. Hemostas., *8:*105, 1982.
153. Kluft, C.: Occurrence of C_1 inactivator and other proteinase inhibitors in euglobulin fraction and their influence on fibrinolytic activity. Haemostasis 5*:*136, 1976.
154. Krevens, J.R. and Jackson, D.P.: Hemorrhagic disorder following massive whole blood transfusions. JAMA, *159:*171, 1955.
155. Kwaan, H.C.: The pathogenesis of thrombotic thrombocytopenic purpura. Semin. Thromb. Hemostas., *5:*184, 1979.
156. Kwaan, H.C.: A relational, unified approach to the problem of thrombotic thrombocytopenic purpura. Semin. Thromb. Hemostas. *5:*241, 1979.
157. Laros, R.K. Jr. and Sweet, R.L.: Management of idopathic thrombocytopenic purpura during pregnancy. Am. J. Obstet. Gynecol., *122:*182, 1975.
158. Lee, L.: Reticuloendothelial clearance of circulating fibrin in the pathogenesis of the generalized Shwartzman reaction. J. Exp. Med. *115:*1065, 1962.
159. Levin, R.H., Pert, J.H., and Freireich, E.J.: Response to transfusion of platelets pooled from multiple donors and the effects of various technics of concentrating platelets. Blood, *5:*54, 1965.
160. Lian, E.C-Y., Harkness, D.R., Byrnes, J.J. et al.: Presence of a platelet aggregating factor in the plasma of patients with thrombotic thrombocytopenic purpura (TTP) and its inhibition by normal plasma. Blood, *53:*333, 1979.
161. Lohrmann, H-P., Bull, M.I., Decter, J.A. et al.: Platelet transfusions from HL-A compatible unrelated donors to alloimmunized patients. Ann. Intern. Med., *80:*9, 1974.
162. Lollar, P., Hoak, J.C., and Owen, W.G.: Binding of thrombin to cultured human endothelial cells. J. Biol. Chem., *255:*10,278, 1980.
163. Ludlam, C.A.: Assessment of platelet function. p. 775. In Bloom, A.L., and Thomas, D.P., Eds.: Haemostasis and Thrombosis. Churchill Livingstone, Edinburgh, 1981.
164. Lunan, C.B.: The management of abruptio placentae. J. Obstet. Gynaecol. Br. Commonw., *80:*120, 1973.
165. MacPherson, A.I.S. and Richmond, J.: Planned splenectomy in treatment of idiopathic thromboctyopenic purpura. Br. Med. J. *1:*64, 1975.
166. Marder, V.J., Natchett, M.O., and Sherry, S.: Detection of serum fibrinogen and fibrin degradation products: comparison of six techniques. Am. J. Med., *51:*71, 1971.
167. Marder, V.J., Shulman, N.R., and Carroll, W.R.: High molecular weight derivatives of human fibrinogen produced by plasmin. Physicochemical and immunological characterization. J. Biol. Chem., *244:*2111, 1969.
168. Marder, V.J. and Shulman, N.R.: High molecular weight derivatives of human fibrinogen

produced by plasmin. II. Mechanism of their anticoagulant activity. J. Biol. Chem. *244:*2120, 1969.
169. Marengo-Rowe, A.J., Murff, G., Leveson, J.E., and Cook, J.: Hemophilia-like disease associated with pregnancy. Obstet. Gynecol., *40:*56, 1972.
170. Marsh, N.: Fibrinolysis. John Wiley & Sons, New York, 1981.
171. Mason, J.W. and Colman, R.W.: The role of Hageman factor in disseminated intravascular coagulation induced by septicemia, neoplasia, or liver disease. Thromb. Diath. Haemorr., *26:*325, 1971.
172. Mason, J.W., Kleeberg, U., Dolan, P., and Colman, R.W.: Plasma kallikrein and Hageman factor in gram-negative bacteremia. Ann. Intern. Med., *73:*545, 1970.
173. May, H.V. Jr., Harbert, G.M., and Thornton, W.N. Jr.: Thrombotic thrombocytopenic purpura associated with pregnancy. Am. J. Obstet. Gynecol., *126:*452, 1976.
174. McConnell, D.J.: Inhibitiors of kallikrein in human plasma. J. Clin. Invest., *51:*1611, 1972.
175. McKay, D.G.: Disseminated intravascular coagulation: An intermediary mechanism of disease. Harper Hoeber, New York, 1965.
176. McKay, D.G.: The clinical spectrum and management of acquired coagulopathy in pregnancy. p. 285. In Reid, D.E. and Christian, C.D., Eds.: Controversy in Obstetrics and Gynecology. II. W.B. Saunders, 1974, p. 285.
177. McKillop, C., Forbes, C.D., Howie, P.W., and Prentice, C.R.M.: Soluble fibrinogen/fibrin complexes in pre-eclampsia. Lancet, *1:*56, 1976.
178. McMillan, R.: Chronic idiopathic thrombocytopenic purpura. N. Engl. J. Med., *304:*1135, 1981.
179. McMillan, R., Longmire, R.L., Tavassoli, M. et al.: *In vitro* platelet phagocytosis by splenic leukocytes in idiopathic thrombocytopenic purpura. N. Engl. J. Med., *290:*249, 1974.
180. McMillan, R., Longmire, R., and Yelenosky, R.: The effect of corticosteroids on human IgG synthesis. J. Immunol., *116:*1592, 1976.
181. Michiels, J.J., Bosch, L.J., van der Plas, P.M., and Abels, J.: Factor VIII inhibitor postpartum. Scand. J. Haematol., *26:*97, 1978.
182. Mielke, C.H. Jr., Kaneshiro, M.M., Maher, I.A. et al.: The standardized normal Ivy bleeding time and its prolongation by aspirin. Blood, *34:*204, 1969.
183. Minchinton, R.M., Dodd, N.J., O'Brien, H. et al.: Autoimmune thrombocytopenia in pregnancy. Br. J. Haematol., *44:*451, 1980.
184. Moloney, W.C., Egan, W.J., and Gorman, A.J.: Acquired afibrinogenemia in pregnancy. N. Engl. J. Med., *240:*596, 1949.
185. Moncada, S. and Vane, J.R.: Arachidonic acid metabolites and the interactions between platelets and blood-vessel walls. N. Engl. J. Med., *300:*1142, 1979.
186. Moon, E.C. and Kitay, D.Z.: Hematologic problems in pregnancy. II. Thrombotic (thrombohemolytic) thrombocytopenia purpura. J. Reprod. Med., *9:*212, 1972.
187. Moore, C.M., McAdams, A.J., and Sutherland, J.: Intrauterine disseminated intravascular coagulation: A syndrome of multiple pregnancy with a dead twin fetus. J. Pediatr., *74:*523, 1969.
188. Mooreside, D.E., Graybeal, F.Q. Jr., and Langdell, R.D.: Effects of adenine on clotting factors in fresh blood, stored blood, and stored fresh frozen plasma. Transfusion, *9:*191, 1969.
189. Moroz, L.: Increased blood fibrinolytic activity after aspirin ingestion. N. Engl. J. Med., *296:*525, 1977.
190. Morris, R.H., Vassalli, P., Beller, F.K., and McCluskey, R.T.: Immunofluorescent studies of renal biopsies in the diagnosis of toxemia of pregnancy. Obstet. Gynecol., *24:*32, 1964.

191. Muller-Berghaus, G.: Pathophysiology of generalized intravascular coagulation. Semin. Thromb. Hemostas., *3:*209, 1977.
192. Murano, G.: A basic outline of blood coagulation. Semin. Thromb. Hemostas., *6:*140, 1980.
193. Murphy, S. and Gardner, F.H.: Platelet preservation. Effect of storage temperature on maintenance of platelet viability—deleterious effect of refrigerated storage. N. Engl. J. Med., *280:*1094, 1969.
194. Murphy, S. and Gardner, F.H.: Platelet storage at 22°C; metabolic, morphologic, and functional studies. J. Clin. Invest., *50:*370, 1971.
195. Murray, J.M. and Harris, R.E.: The management of the pregnant patient with idiopathic thrombocytopenic purpura. Am. J. Obstet. Gynecol., *126:*449, 1976.
196. Mustard, J.F.: A study of changes in platelets, antihaemophilic globe factor V and factor VII during blood collection and storage by different techniques. Br. J. Pharmacol. *3:*202, 1977.
197. Myers, R.E. and Brann, A.W., Jr.: Abruptio placentae in rhesus monkey causing brain damage to the fetus. Am. J. Obstet. Gynecol., *126:*1048, 1976.
198. Naeye, R.L., Harkness, W.L., and Utts, J.: Abruptio placentae and perinatal death: A prospective study. Am. J. Obstet. Gynecol., *128:*740, 1977.
199. Nalbandian, R.M. and Henry, R.L.: Platelet-endothelial cell interactions. Metabolic maps of structures and actions of prostaglandins, prostacyclin, thromboxane and cyclic AMP. Semin. Thromb. Hemostas., *5:*87, 1978.
200. Nalbandian, R.M., Henry, R.L., and Bick, R.L.: Thrombotic thrombocytopenic purpura. An extended editorial. Semin. Thromb. Hemostas., *5:*216, 1979.
201. Nemerson, Y. and Pitlick, F.A.: The tissue factor pathway of blood coagulation. In Spaet, T.H., Eds., Progress in Hemostasis and Thrombosis. Vol. 1. Grune & Stratton, New York, 1972.
202. Ness, P.M. and Perkins, H.A.: Cryoprecipitate as a reliable source of fibrinogen replacement. JAMA, *241:*1690, 1979.
203. Niemetz, J. and Fani, K.: Role of leukocytes in blood coagulation and the generalized Shwartzman reaction. Nature, *232:*247, 1971.
204. Niemetz, J. and Marcus, A.J.: The stimulatory effect of platelets and platelet membranes on the procoagulant activity of leukocytes. J. Clin. Invest., *54:*1437, 1974.
205. Nilsson, I.M., Astedt, B., Hedner, U., and Berezin, D.: Intrauterine fetal death and circulating anticoagulant (antipthromboplastin). Acta Med. Scand., *197:*153, 1975.
206. Nilsson, I.M. and Kullander, S.: Coagulation and fibrinolytic studies during pregnancy. Acta Obstet. Gynecol. Scand., *46:*273, 1967.
207. Noriega-Guerra, L., Aviles-Miranda, A., de la Cadena, O.A. et al.: Pregnancy in patients with autoimmune thrombocytopenic purpura. Am. J. Obstet. Gynecol., *133:*439, 1979.
208. Nossel, H.L., Lanzkowsky, P., Levy, S. et al.: A study of coagulation factor levels in women during labour and in their newborn infants. Thromb. Diath. Haemorr., *16:*185, 1966.
209. Notelovitz, M.: Silent abruption of the posteriorly inserted placenta. S. Afr. Med. J., *48:*92, 1974.
210. Notelovitz, M., Bottoms, S.F., Dase, D.F., and Leichter, P.J.: Painless abruptio placentae. Obstet. Gynecol. *53:*270, 1979.
211. Oakey, R.E.: The interpretation of urinary oestrogen and pregnanediol excretion in pregnant women receiving corticosteroids. J. Obstet. Gynaecol. Br. Commonw., *77:*922, 1970.
212. Odegard, O.R. and Abilgaard, U.: Antithrombin III critical review of assay methods significance of variation in health and disease. Haemostasis, *7:*127, 1978.

213. Ogston, D., Ogston, C.M., Ratnoff, O.D., and Forbes, C.D.: Studies on a complex mechanism for the activation of plasminogen by kaolin and by chloroform: the participation of Hageman factor and additional cofactors. J. Clin. Invest., *48:*1786, 1969.
214. O'Reilly, R.A. and Taber, B-Z.: Immunologic thrombocytopenic purpura and pregnancy. Six new cases. Obstet. Gynecol., *51:*590, 1978.
215. Owen, C.A. Jr. and Bowie, E.J.W.: Chronic intravascular coagulation syndromes. A summary. Mayo Clin. Proc. *49:*673, 1974.
216. Owen, C.A. Jr. and Bowie, E.J.W.: Chronic intravascular coagulation and fibrinolysis (ICF) syndromes (DIC). Semin. Thromb. Hemostas., *3:*268, 1977.
217. Owen, C.A. Jr., Bowie, E.J.W., and Cooper, H.A.: Turnover of fibrinogen and platelets in dogs undergoing induced intravascular coagulation. Thromb. Res., *2:*251, 1973.
218. Page, E.W., King, E.B., and Merrill, J.A.: Abruptio placentae. Dangers of delay in delivery. Obstet. Gynecol., *3:*385, 1954.
219. Paterson, M.E.L.: The aetiology and outcome of abruptio placentae. Acta Obstet. Gynecol. Scand., *58:*31, 1979.
220. Paulus, J-M.: Platelet size in man. Blood, *46:*321, 1975.
221. Pechet, L. and Alexander, B.: Increased clotting factors in pregnancy. N. Engl. J. Med., *265:*1093, 1961.
222. Phillips, L.L.: Fibrin monomer as a test for intravascular coagulation. Obstet. Gynecol., *45:*129, 1975.
223. Phillips, L.L. and Davidson, E.C.: Procoagulant properties of amniotic fluid. Am. J. Obstet. Gynecol., *113:*911, 1972.
224. Phillips, L.L., Skrodelis, V., and Taylor, H.C. Jr.: Hemorrhage due to fibrinolysis in abruptio placentae. Am. J. Obstet. Gynecol., *84:*1447, 1962.
225. Pitkin, R.M. and Witte, D.L.: Platelet and leukocyte counts in pregnancy. JAMA, *242:*2696, 1979.
226. Piver, M.S., Lisker, S.A., Rowan, N. et al.: Thrombotic thromboctyopenic purpura during pregnancy. Am. J. Obstet. Gynecol., *100:*302, 1968.
227. Plow, E.F.: The major fibrinolytic proteases of human leukocytes. Biochim. Biophys. Acta, *630:*47, 1980.
228. Plumer, M.H.: Bleeding problems. In: Obstetric Anesthesia: The Complicated Patient. James, F.M. and Wheeler, A.S., Eds., F.A. Davis, Philadelphia, 1982.
229. Poller, L. and Thomson, J.M.: The interpretation of prothrombin results: A national survey. Int. J. Haematol., *16:*31, 1969.
230. Pool, J.G. and Hershgold, E.J.: High-potency antihaemophilic factor concentrate prepared from cryoglobulin precipitate. Nature, *203:*312, 1964.
231. Pool, J.G. and Shannon, A.E.: Production of high-potency concentrates of antihemophilic globulin in a closed-bag system. Assay *in vitro* and *in vivo*. N. Engl. J. Med., *273:*1443, 1965.
232. Prentice, C.R.M.: In Hoffbrand, A.V. and Lewis, S.M., Eds.: 2nd Ed. Acquired Disorders of Haemostasis in Postgraduate Haematology. Appleton-Century-Crofts, Norwalk, Conn., 1981.
233. Pritchard, J.A.: Genesis of severe placental abruption. Am. J. Obstet. Gynecol., *108:*22, 1970.
234. Pritchard, J.A.: Haematological problems associated with delivery, placental abruption, retained dead fetus and amniotic fluid embolism. Clin. Haematol. 2:562, 1973.
235. Pritchard, J.A. and Brekken, A.L.: Clinical and laboratory studies on severe abruptio placentae. Am. J. Obstet. Gynecol., 97:681, 1967.
236. Pritchard, J.A., Cunningham, F.G., and Mason, R.A.: Coagulation changes in eclampsia: Their frequency and pathogenesis. Am. J. Obstet. Gynecol., *124:*855, 1976.
237. Pritchard, J.A. and Ratnoff, O.D.: Studies of fibrinogen and other hemostatic factors in

women with intrauterine death and delayed delivery. Surg. Gynecol. Obstet., *101:*467, 1955.
238. Proctor, R.R. and Rapaport, S.I.: The partial thromboplastin time with kaolin. A simple screening test for first stage plasma clotting factor deficiencies. Am. J. Clin. Pathol., *36:*212, 1961.
239. Rakoczi, I., Tallian, F., Bagdany, S., and Gati, I.: Platelet life-span in normal pregnancy and pre-eclampsia as determined by a non-radioisotope technique. Thromb. Res., *15:*553, 1979.
240. Ramsey, E.M. and Donner, M.W.: Placental Vasculature and Circulation. W.B. Saunders, Philadelphia, 1980.
241. Rapaport, S.I.: Defibrination syndromes. Ch. 161, p. 1454. In Williams, W.J., Beutler, E., Erslev, A.J. and Rundles, R.W., Eds.: Hematology. 2nd Ed. McGraw-Hill, 1977.
242. Ratnoff, O.D., Colopy, J.E., and Pritchard, J.A.: The blood-clotting mechanism during normal parturition. J. Lab. Clin. Med., *44:*408, 1954.
243. Redman, C.W.G., Bonnar, J., and Beilin, L.: Early platelet consumption in preeclampsia. Br. Med. J., *1:*467, 1978.
244. Regoeczi, E. and Hobbs, K.R.: Fibrinogen turnover in pregnancy. Scand. J. Haematol., *6:*175, 1969.
245. Reinisch, J.M., Simon, N.G., Karow, W.G., and Gandelman, R.: Prenatal exposure to prednisone in humans and animals retards intrauterine growth. Science, *202:*436, 1978.
246. Renaud, S. and Lecompte, F.: Thrombosis prevention by coagulation and platelet aggregation inhibitors, in hyperlipemic rats. Thromb. Diath. Haemorr., *24:*577, 1970.
247. Roberts, J.M. and May, W.J.: Consumptive coagulopathy in severe preeclampsia. Obstet. Gynecol., *48:*163, 1976.
248. Rodriguez-Erdmann, F.: Bleeding due to increased intravascular blood coagulation. Hemorrhagic syndromes caused by consumption of blood-clotting factors (consumption-coagulopathies). N. Engl. J. Med., *273:*1370, 1965.
249. Romero, R. and Duffy, T.P.: Platelet disorders in pregnancy. Clin. Perinatol., *7:*327, 1980.
250. Romero, R., Snyder, E., Rickles, F. et al.: The clinical significance and mechanism of thrombocytopenia in pregnancy induced hypertension. (Abstract.) 29th Society for Gynecologic Investigation Annual Meeting, Dallas, March 24–27, 1982.
251. Rossi, E.C., del Greco, F., Kwaan, H.C., and Lerman, B.B.: Hemodialysis-exchange transfusion for treatment of thrombocytopenic purpura. JAMA, *244:*1466, 1980.
252. Roth, G.J., Stanford, G.J.N., and Majerus, P.W.: Acetylation of prostaglandin synthetase by aspirin. Proc. Natl. Acad. Sci. USA, *72:*3073, 1975.
253. Sanders, A.G.: *In vivo* observations on haemostasis in the hamster. Symp. Zool. Soc. London, *27:*109, 1970.
254. Scharfman, W.B., Babcock, R.B., and Rauch, A.E.: Letter to the editor. N. Engl. J. Med., *306:*745, 1982.
255. Schatz, M., Patterson, R., Zeitz, S. et al.: Corticosteroid therapy for the pregnant asthmatic patient. JAMA, *233:*804, 1975.
256. Schenker, J.G. and Polishuk, W.Z.: Idiopathic thrombocytopenia in pregnancy. Gynaecologia *165:*271, 1968.
257. Schneider, C.L.: The inactivation of placental toxin by human serum. Am. J. Physiol. *146:*140, 1945.
258. Schneider, C.L.: The active principle of placental toxin: thromboplastin; its inactivator in blood: antithromboplastin. Am. J. Physiol., *149:*123, 1947.
259. Schneider, C.L.: Complications of late pregnancy in rabbits induced by experimental placental trauma. Surg. Gynecol. Obstet., *90:*613, 1950.
260. Schneider, C.L.: "Fibrin embolism" (disseminated intravascular coagulation) with defibrination as one of the end results during placenta abruptio. Surg. Obstet. Gynecol., *92:*27, 1951.

261. Schneider, C.L.: Rupture of the basal (decidual) plate in abruptio placentae: A pathway of autoextraction from the decidua into the maternal circulation. Am. J. Obstet. Gynecol., *63*:1078, 1952.
262. Schneider, C.L.: Disseminated intravascular coagulation thrombosis versus fibrination, in clinical disease states. Thromb. Diath. Haemorr., *36*:1, 1969.
263. Schwartz, M.L. and Brenner, W.E.: The obfuscation of eclampsia by thrombotic thrombocytopenic purpura. Am. J. Obstet. Gynecol., *131*:18, 1978.
264. Scott, J.R., Cruikshank, D.P., Kochenour, N.K. et al.: Fetal platelet counts in the obstetric management of immunologic thrombocytopenic purpura. Am. J. Obstet. Gynecol., *136*:495, 1980.
265. Seegers, W.H.: Antithrombin III theory and clinical applications. Am. J. Clin. Pathol., *69*:367, 1978.
266. Shaper, A.G., MacIntosh, D.M., and Kyobe, J.: Fibrinolytic activity in pregnancy, during parturition, and in the puerperium. Lancet, *2*:874, 1966.
267. Sheppard, B.L. and Bonnar, J.: Fibrinolysis in decidual spiral arteries in late pregnancy. Thromb. Haemost. *39*:751, 1978.
268. Sher, G.: Pathogenesis and management of uterine inertia complicating abruptio placentae with consumption coagulopathy. Am. J. Obstet. Gynecol., *129*:164, 1977.
269. Sher, G.: A rational basis for the management of abruptio placentae. J. Reprod. Med. *21*:123, 1978.
270. Silbert, J.A., Bove, J.R., Dubin, S., and Bush, W.S.: Patterns of frozen plasma use. Conn. Med. *45*:507, 1981.
271. Skelly, H., Marivate, M., Norman, R. et al.: Consumptive coagulopathy following fetal death in a triplet pregnancy. Am. J. Obstet. Gynecol., *142*:595, 1982.
272. Smith, T.W. and Willis, A.L.: Aspirin selectively inhibits prostaglandin production in human platelets. J. Clin. Invest. *52*:965, 1973.
273. Stachurska, J., Latallo, Z., and Kopec, M.: Inhibition of platelet aggregation by dialyzable fibrinogen degradation products (FDP). Thrombosis et Diathesis Haemorrhagica *23*:91, 1970.
274. Stead, N., Kaplan, A.P., and Rosenberg, R.D.: Inhibition of activated factor XII by antithrombin heparin cofactor. J. Biol. Chem., *251*:6481, 1976.
275. Steiner, P.E. and Lushbaugh, C.C.: Maternal pulmonary embolism by amniotic fluid as a cause of obstetric shock and unexpected deaths in obstetrics. JAMA, *117*:1245, 1941.
276. Steiner, P.E. and Lushbaugh, C.C.: Maternal pulmonary embolism by amniotic fluid as a cause of obstetric shock and unexpected deaths in obstetrics. JAMA, *117*:1340, 1941.
277. Talbert, L.M. and Blatt, P.M.: Disseminated intravascular coagulation in obstetrics. Clin. Obstet. Gynecol., *22*:889, 1979.
278. Tate, D.Y., Sorenson, R.L., Gerrard, J.M. et al.: An immunoenzyme histochemical technique for the detection of platelet antibodies from the serum of patients with idiopathic (autoimmune) thrombocytopenic purpura (ITP). Br. J. Haematol., *37*:265, 1977.
279. Teisner, B., Davey, M.W., and Grudzinskas, J.G.: Circulating antithrombins in pregnancy. Br. J. Obstet. Gynaecol., *89*:62, 1982.
280. Ten Cate, J.W. and Jenkins, C.S.P.: Platelet function tests. In Thomson, J.M., Ed.: Blood Coagulation and Haemostasis. A Practical Guide. Churchill Livingstone, Edinburgh, 1980.
281. Territo, M., Finklestein, J., Oh, W. et al.: Management of autoimmune thrombocytopenia in pregnancy and in the neonate. Obstet. Gynecol., *41*:579, 1973.
282. Thiagarajah, S., Harbert, G.M. Jr., Caudle, M.R., and Sturgill, B.C.: Thrombotic thrombocytopenic purpura in pregnancy: A reappraisal. Am. J. Obstet. Gynecol., *141*:20, 1981.
283. Thomason, J.M.: Laboratory control of anticoagulant therapy. In: Blood Coagulation and Haemostasis. A Practical Guide. 2nd Ed. Churchill Livingstone, Edinburgh, 1980.

284. Todd, M.E., Thompson, J.H. Jr., Bowie, E.J.W., and Owen, C.A. Jr.: Changes in blood coagulation during pregnancy. Mayo Clin. Proc., *40:*370, 1965.
285. Tricomi, V. and Kohl, S.G.: Fetal death in utero. Am. J. Obstet. Gynecol., *74:*1092, 1957.
286. Trudinger, B.J.: Platelets and intrauterine growth retardation in pre-eclampsia. Br. J. Obstet. Gynecol., *83:*284, 1976.
287. Upshaw, J.D. Jr.: Congenital deficiency of a factor in normal plasma that reverses microangiopathic hemolysis and thrombocytopenia. N. Engl. J. Med., *298:*1350, 1978.
288. Van Leeuwen, E.G., Helmerhorst, F.M., Engelfriet, C.P., and von dem Borne, A.E.G., Jr.: Maternal autoimmune thrombocytopenia and the newborn. Br. Med. J., *283:*104, 1981.
289. Veenhoven, W.A., van der Schans, G.S., and Nieweg, H.O.: Platelet antibodies in idiopathic thrombocytopenic purpura. Clin. Exp. Immunol., *39:*645, 1980.
290. Voke, J. and Letsky, E.: Pregnancy and antibody to factor VIII. J. Clin. Pathol., *30:*928, 1977.
291. Wallenburg, H.C.S. and van Kessel, P.H.: Platelet lifespan in normal pregnancy as determined by a nonradioisotopic technique. Br. J. Obstet. Gynaecol., *85:*33, 1978.
292. Walsh, P.N.: The effects of collagen and kaolin on the intrinsic coagulant activity of platelets. Br. J. Haematol., *22:*393, 1972.
293. Walsh, R.T. and Barnhart, M.I.: Clearance of coagulation and fibrinolysis products by the reticuloendothelial system. Thromb. Diath. Hemorr., *36:*83, 1969.
294. Weiner, C.P. and Brandt, J.: Plasma antithrombin III activity in normal pregnancy. Obstet. Gynecol., *56:*601, 1980.
295. Weiner, C.P. and Brandt, J.: Plasma antithrombin III activity: An aid in the diagnosis of preeclampsia-eclampsia. Am. J. Obstet. Gynecol., *142:*275, 1982.
296. Weinstein, L.: Syndrome of hemolysis, elevated liver enzymes, and low platelet count: A severe consequence of hypertension in pregnancy. Am. J. Obstet. Gynecol., *142:*159, 1982.
297. Widmann, F.K., Ed.: Preparation of blood components. Ch. 3, p. 38. In: Technical Manual of the American Association of Blood Banks. 8th Ed. Williams & Wilkins, Baltimore.
298. Williams, W.J.: Control of coagulation reactions. Ch. 138, p. 1276. In Williams, W.J., Beutler, E., Erslev, A.J., and Rundles, R.W., Eds.: Hematology. 2nd Ed. McGraw-Hill, New York, 1977.
299. Williams, W.J.: Principles of coagulation tests. Ch. 139, p. 1285. In Williams, W.J., Beutler, E., Erslev, A.J., and Rundles, R.W., Eds.: Hematology. 2nd Ed. McGraw-Hill, New York, 1977.
300. Wilson, R.F., Bassett, J.S., and Alexander, J.W.: Five years of experience with massive blood transfusions. JAMA, *194:*851, 1965.
301. Wintrobe, M.: Blood coagulation. p. 409. In: Clinical Hematology. 8th Ed. Lea & Febiger, Philadelphia, 1981.
302. Wintrobe, M.M., Lee, G.R., Boggs, D.R. et al.: Diffuse intravascular coagulation. p. 1213. In: Clinical Hematology. 8th Ed. Lea & Febiger, Philadelphia, 1981.
303. Wright, I.S.: The nomenclature of blood clotting factors. Thromb. et Diath. Hemorr., *7:*301, 1962.
304. Zucker, M.B.: The functioning of blood platelets. Sci. Am., *242:*86, 1980.
305. Zur, M. and Nemerson, Y.: Tissue factor pathways of blood coagulation. p. 214. In Bloom, A.L. and Thomas, D.P. Eds.: Haemostasis and Thrombosis. Churchill Livingstone, Edinburgh, 1981.

10

The Surgical Approach to Severe Postpartum Hemorrhage

Peter E. Schwartz, M.D.

OBSTETRIC HEMORRHAGE

Hemorrhage remains an important cause of morbidity and mortality in obstetric patients. Postpartum bleeding accounts for most of these complications and was responsible for 24 percent of obstetric deaths in one recent study.[5] Advances in intervention radiology for the management of pelvic bleeding in association with trauma and malignancies are now being evaluated for controlling postpartum bleeding[2,15,17,18] and are discussed in Chapter 7. Prostaglandin administration is also being investigated for this problem.[7,8,19] This chapter will review the management of postpartum hemorrhage and will concentrate on indications for surgery and surgical techniques to control massive hemorrhage in the postpartum patients.

Definition of Postpartum Hemorrhage

Substantial blood loss is routine during the third stage of labor, but less than 500 ml is not considered to be hemorrhage.[12,21] When blood loss exceeds 1,500 ml, however, the hemorrhage is considered to be massive. Postpartum hemorrhage may be further subdivided into immediate postpartum hemorrhage, i.e., blood loss within the first 24 h postpartum and delayed postpartum hemorrhage, i.e., bleeding occurring more than 24 h postpartum.

CONSERVATIVE MANAGEMENT OF POSTPARTUM HEMORRHAGE

The most common causes of postpartum hemorrhage are uterine atony, genital lacerations, and retained placental fragments. Uterine atony may be secondary to an overdistended uterus resulting from a large fetus, multiple gestation, or polyhydramnios. It is also associated with grand multiparity, prolonged labor, and oxytocin stimulation of labor. The physician caring for patients with these conditions should routinely establish an intravenous line with a large-bore plastic cannula and have blood available for rapid transfusion if necessary. Proper management of the third stage of labor will minimize hemorrhage due to uterine atony (Table 10-1). Elevation of the uterus out of the pelvis in concert with fundal massage will readily control the bleeding but the effect may be temporary. Intravenous oxytocin administration will stimulate rhythmic contractions of the uterine musculature. Ergonovine or methylergonivine administration will also aide in controlling postpartum hemorrhage but must be used with caution, as each may induce significant hypertension. Intramyometrial injections of these uterotonic agents have been recommended for stimulation of atonic uteri at the time of cesarean section. Manual exploration of the uterine cavity will eliminate the possibilities of retained placental fragments or a uterine rupture. Careful inspection of the cervix and vagina will aid in identifying occult lacerations that can be readily sutured. A technique which is no longer routinely utilized to control postpartum hemorrhage secondary to uterine atony is intrauterine lavage with hot saline (40 to 55°C). This technique may occasionally be useful

Table 10-1. Treatment of Postpartum Hemorrhage

- I. Conservative management
  - A. Mechanical stimulation
    - 1. Massage
    - 2. Compression
  - B. Pharmacologic
    - 1. Oxytocin drugs
      - a. Parenteral administration (I.M., I.V.)
      - b. Intramyometrial injection
    - 2. Prostaglandins
      - a. Intravaginal
      - b. Parenteral
      - c. Intramyometrial
  - C. Repair Lacerations
- II. Intervention radiography
  - A. Selective transarterial embolization
  - B. Hypogastric artery Pitressin infusion
- III. Surgical management
  - A. Vascular Ligation
    - 1. Uterine artery
    - 2. Hypogastric artery
    - 3. Ovarian artery
  - B. Hysterectomy
    - 1. Supracervical
    - 2. Total

when hemorrhage persists which is unresponsive to oxytocic drugs in an intact uterus.[4]

Persistent uterine bleeding despite aggressive conservative mechanical and pharmacologic management would have routinely led to a surgical approach in the past. However, recent advances in prostaglandin (PG) therapy for induction of abortion have led to investigations of the role of these agents in the management of persistent uterine atony. Intravaginal prostaglandin E_2 suppositories and intramuscular and intramyometrial administration of prostaglandin $F_{2\alpha}$ analogues have been successfully employed in the management of severe postpartum hemorrhage secondary to uterine atony.[7,8,19] Side effects of prostaglandin E_2 and $F_{2\alpha}$ are significant and include nausea, vomiting, diarrhea, headache, fever, and chills. Most importantly, $PGF_{2\alpha}$ can cause transient diastolic hypertension, which may be particularly severe in toxemic patients. Eighteen of 20 patients were recently reported to be successfully treated with intramuscular injections of (15-S)-15-methyl-$PGF_{2\alpha}$-THAM for postpartum hemorrhage associated with uterine atony.[7] This prostaglandin $F_{2\alpha}$ analogue has 10-fold greater uterotonic activity than the parent compound, has a longer duration of action, and causes only moderate diastolic hypertension ($\leq$100 mmHg). The majority of patients in this series required only one or two injections. The two failures were associated with chorioamnionitis and were subsequently successfully treated surgically.

Uterine packing has been employed in the past to control postpartum hemorrhage.[9] It has also been suggested as a temporizing technique to control hemorrhage immediately prior to surgery.[10] Retention of a uterine pack may lead to infection, however, and its use as a temporizing measure may hide blood loss and lead to incorrect judgments regarding blood replacement. I therefore feel that uterine packing plays no role in the modern management of postpartum hemorrhage.

Massive immediate hemorrhage unresponsive to mechanical and pharmacologic techniques suggests the possibility of uterine rupture, abnormal placentation, or uterine inversion. However, a coagulopathy secondary to conditions such as severe toxemia, abruption, sepsis, or amniotic fluid embolization must also be considered in the differential diagnosis of massive postpartum hemorrhage (Ch. 9).

Patients with delayed postpartum hemorrhage[11] may often to be managed conservatively. Lee and associates have recently reported on ultrasonic evaluations of the uterus in 56 patients whose bleeding began more than 24 h after delivery. They were able to identify retained placental tissue in 9 women, large blood clots in 5, and an empty uterus in the remaining 42 patients. The latter group was successfully treated conservatively with intravenous oxytocin infusions without dilatation and curettage.

Pelvic hematomas occur approximately once in every 800 to 900 deliveries and may be readily diagnosed when they involve the vulva and vagina. These patients can be successfully managed with surgical evacuation, hemostasis, and vaginal packing when appropriate.[2] Retroperitoneal hematomas, on the other hand, can be occult and massive. They are usually managed by surgical evacuation and may require hypogastric artery ligation to help control bleeding. Retroperitoneal hematomas may be present in association with massive blood loss and replacement in patients with coagulopathies.

Selective Pelvic Artery Embolization

Surgery remains the treatment of choice for postpartum patients with massive hemorrhage if rapid deterioration occurs and stabilization cannot be achieved. However, in institutions where skilled arteriographers are readily available, selective pelvic artery embolization techniques are preferable because (1) the bleeding site is often extremely difficult or sometimes impossible to identify at the time of surgery; (2) injury to ureters, bladder, and bowel may occur while trying to surgically identify the site of bleeding; (3) the rich collateral circulation may negate the effect of hypogastric artery ligation; (4) a hysterectomy may be avoided; and (5) it is much easier to identify and embolize branches of the hypogastric artery before surgical intervention than after a hypogastric artery ligation has failed to control bleeding.[2,15] However, selective arterial catheterization techniques may take 1 to 2 h to be successfully accomplished and this may be an unacceptable delay for unstable patients.

It is important for obstetricians to be aware of the selective arterial catheterization techniques described in Chapter 7. If a community hospital is unable to offer these services, it may be appropriate to transfer the patient, after stabilization has been achieved, to a regional center where they can be provided. Furthermore, the services of skilled pelvic and vascular surgeons may be needed to perform the extremely difficult surgery that might be required to control massive hemorrhage, as well as intensive care specialists to manage complications such as pulmonary and renal failure. Recently gravity suits have been developed to diminish massive hemorrhage in trauma victims and they have been successfully used in the management of women with life-threatening bleeding from ectopic pregnancies. Those suits may be used to control major hemorrhage in the postpartum patient unresponsive to standard therapy in order to transfer her to a tertiary care facility.[6]

SURGICAL MANAGEMENT OF POSTPARTUM HEMORRHAGE

Indications for Surgery

Massive immediate postpartum hemorrhage unresponsive to conservative mechanical or pharmacologic techniques has traditionally been the major indication for surgery. Patients who have not been successfully managed medically or whose bleeding could not be arrested with intervention radiology techniques must now be added to the list of those for whom surgery is indicated to control postpartum hemorrhage.[15]

Uterine, ovarian, and hypogastric artery ligations have been advocated as means of controlling bleeding and avoiding hysterectomy.[1,3,20] Bilateral uterine artery ligation may readily control the hemorrhage in some patients with uterine atony.[3] The addition of bilateral ovarian artery ligation may help control persistent bleeding without sacrificing the adnexa or uterus.[1] Some surgeons prefer to go directly to hypogastric artery ligation, hoping to achieve more rapid coagulation by reducing the pulse pressure in the pelvic arteries.[3] However, the vasculature of the pelvis is supplied with a rich collateral circulation, which is particularly prominent in pregnancy, and hypogastric artery ligation has been demonstrated to reverse blood flow through its distal branches. The principal arterial anastomotic channels in the pelvis which immediately fill following hypogastric artery ligation are (1) lumbar–iliolumbar, (2) middle sacral–lateral sacral, and (3) superior hemorrhoidal–middle hemorrhoidal (Fig. 10-1).[3]

Ligation of the ascending branches of the uterine arteries is the easiest technique to employ for surgeons who do not routinely operate in the pelvic retroperito-

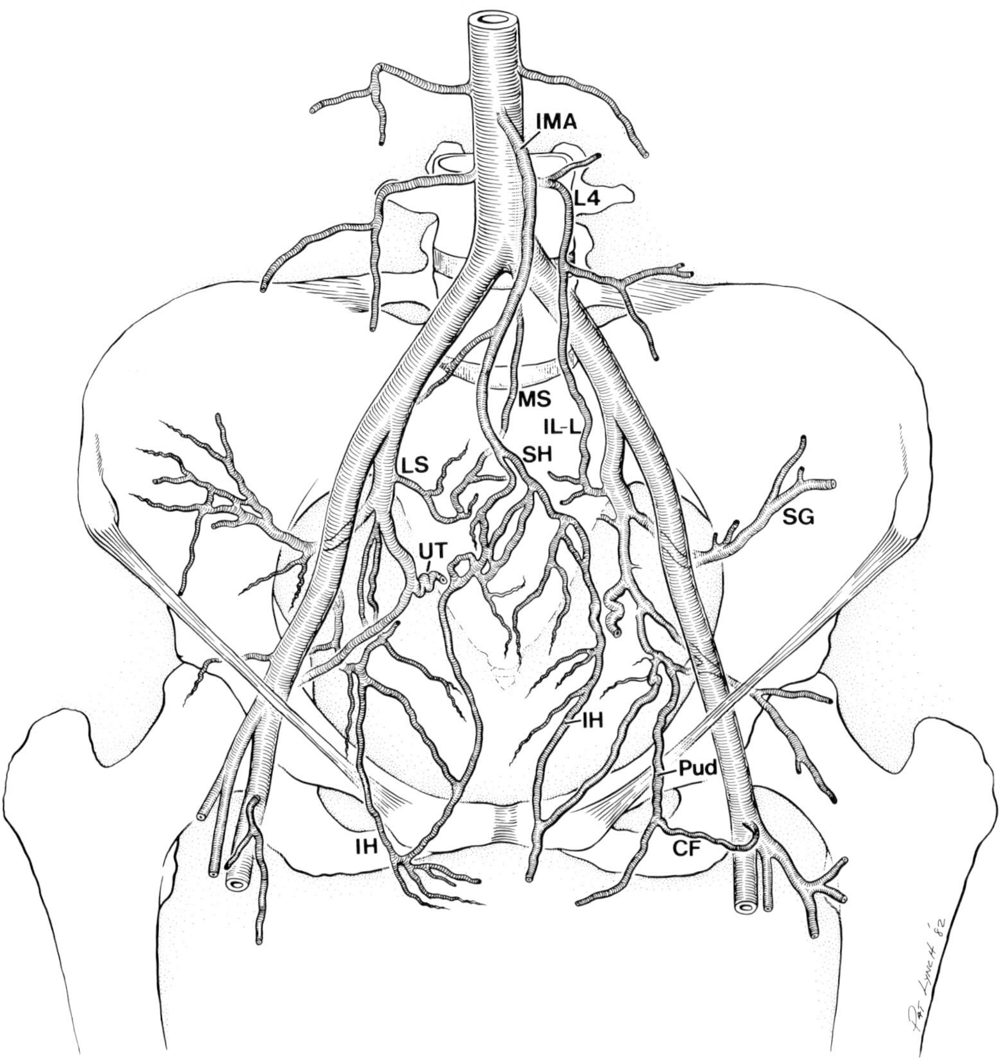

Fig. 10-1 Collateral arterial circulation in the pelvis during pregnancy: LS-MS, lateral sacral–median sacral arteries; IMA-SH-IH, inferior mesenteric–superior hemorrhoidal–inferior hemorrhoidal arteries; L4-IL-L, fourth lumbar-ileolumbar arteries; CF-PUD, circumflex femoral-pudendal arteries; UT, uterine artery; SG, superior gluteal.

neum. I prefer to go directly to bilateral hypogastric artery ligation when trying to control massive postpartum hemorrhage, particularly when the hemorrhage is a complication of an abnormal placentation. Successful pregnancies have been reported to occur following uterine, ovarian, and hypogastric artery ligations.[1,14] O'Leary[14] has recently reported 12 patients with successful term gestations in a group of 110 women who had previously undergone bilateral uterine artery ligations for treatment of post–cesarean section hemorrhage. Menstrual irregularities and infertility problems were not reported to have occurred in this group of women, but 3 of the 12 patients who subsequently became pregnant had recurrent hemorrhage, managed with a second bilateral uterine artery ligation at the time of repeat cesarean section.

Failure to control bleeding following arterial ligation requires a hysterectomy to be performed. A supracervical hysterectomy will usually suffice and can be readily performed in a postpartum patient. In my experience, however, total hysterectomy is necessary when persistent bleeding is secondary to abnormal placentation (e.g., placenta previa or low-lying placenta accreta, increta, or percreta), when there is an extensive cervical laceration which extends into the broad ligament, or in the rare situation of an abdominal pregnancy implanting on the pelvic organs. In these circumstances bilateral hypogastric artery ligations may also be necessary to control persistent deep pelvic bleeding following total hysterectomy.

Uterine Artery Ligation Technique

By advancing the vesicouterine peritoneum off the cervix, the contents of the broad ligament are exposed. The ascending branches of the uterine arteries are easily identified by palpation and should be suture-ligated bilaterally with a number 0 or 1 chromic catgut suture (Figure 10-2). It is unnecessary to divide the arteries after they have been ligated, and the uterine veins should not be included in the ligatures. The main branch of the uterine artery should not be ligated since it lies in close apposition to the ureter in patients whose cervix has recently been dilated.

O'Leary[14] has successfully employed a mass ligature incorporating the ascending branches of the uterine arteries and veins, as well as 2 to 3 cm of uterine musculature medial to the vessels to control post–cesarean section bleeding. The suture is directed through the avascular space of the broad ligament and then through the myometrium inferior to the transverse uterine incision and beneath the reflected vesicouterine peritoneal flap. No untoward effects were reported with this technique.

Hypogastric Artery Ligation Technique

It is axiomatic that successful exposure of the hypogastric arteries will be readily accomplished only when adequate steps are taken to displace the bowel and pelvic

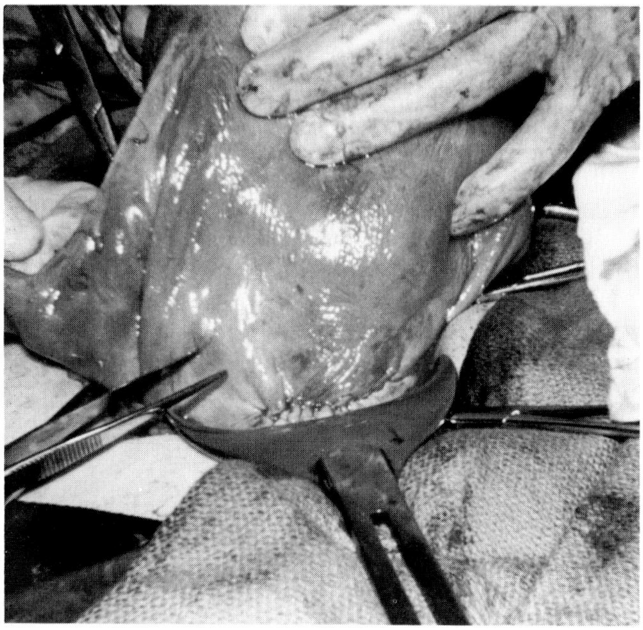

Fig. 10-2 Ligation of the uterine artery: the forceps indicate the site where the ascending branch of the uterine artery may be safely ligated.

organs away from the pelvic sidewalls. Large laparotomy pads are extremely useful for packing off the bowel as well as for compressing bleeding sites while the hypogastric artery ligation is being performed. I routinely ligate both hypogastric arteries even when bleeding is localized to one side of the pelvis because of the rich collateral circulation in the deep pelvis.

The hypogastric artery may be easily exposed and ligated by employing the following technique. First, the round ligament is doubly suture-ligated in its midportion, leaving approximately 1 cm between the ties (Fig. 10-3). The ligament is then divided in the area incorporated by the ties. Gentle traction on each tie will expose the loose areolar tissue of the broad ligament and the pelvic sidewall. A tonsil suction tip may then be inserted into this space and directed superior and lateral to the infundibulopelvic ligament. By using the tonsil suction as a guide, the peritoneum is incised 1 cm lateral to the infundibulopelvic ligament up to the pelvic sidewall (Fig. 10-4), thereby widely exposing the structures on the pelvic sidewall (Fig. 10-5).

Using the tonsil suction tip as a dissector, one can rapidly expose the external iliac artery and the bifurcation of the common iliac artery. The ureter will be identified crossing the common iliac artery immediately superior to the bifurcation of the artery (Fig. 10-6). It then courses inferior and medial and stays on the medial fold of the pelvic peritoneum. The tonsil suction tip or a cotton pledget on a clamp may be used to bluntly expose the hypogastric artery for a distance of 3 to 4 cm below the bifurcation of the common iliac artery. A Mixter clamp is then directed around the lateral and posterior aspect of the hypogastric artery about 2 cm distal to its takeoff from the common iliac artery (Fig. 10-7). It is necessary to gently open and close the

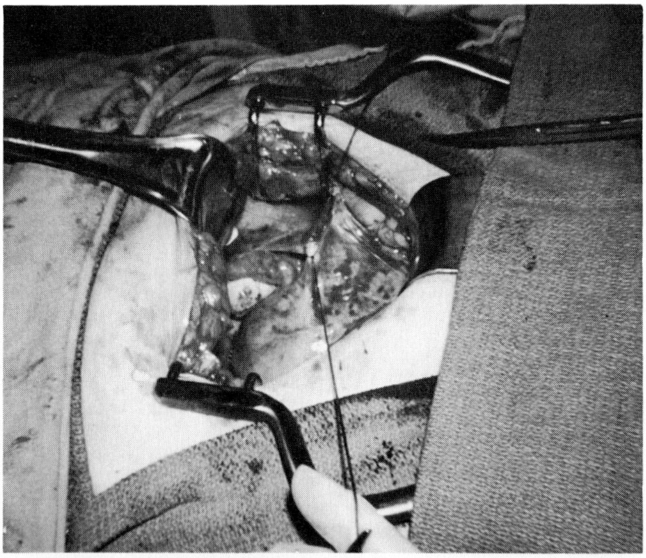

Fig. 10-3 The round ligament is doubly suture-ligated, leaving a distance of at least 1 cm between the ligatures.

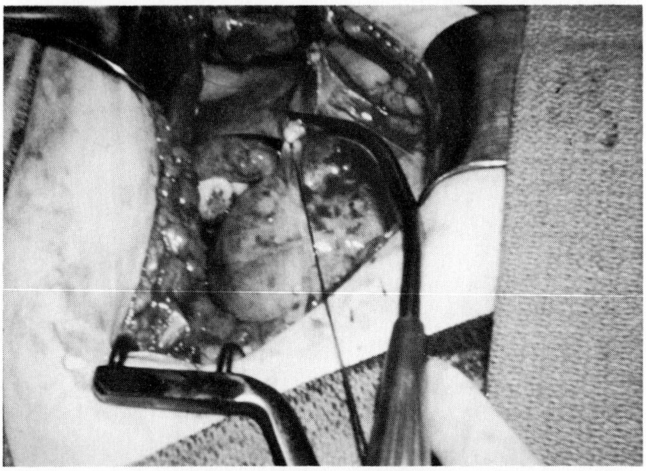

Fig. 10-4 The round ligament is divided between the ties; the tip of a tonsil suction has been introduced into the defect and is being advanced 1 cm lateral and parallel to the infundibulopelvic ligament.

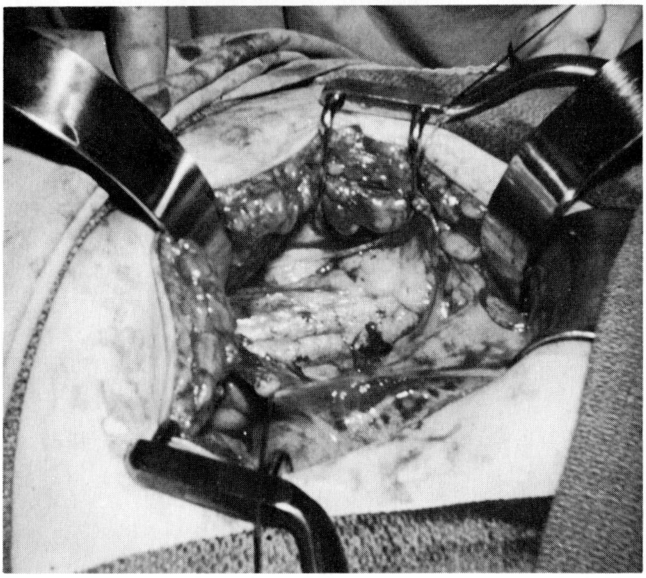

Fig. 10-5 The pelvic sidewall has been exposed by dividing the pelvic peritoneum 1 cm lateral to the infundibulopelvic ligament, using the tonsil suction (Fig. 10-4) as a guide. The external iliac artery and vein are easily identified under the adipose tissue.

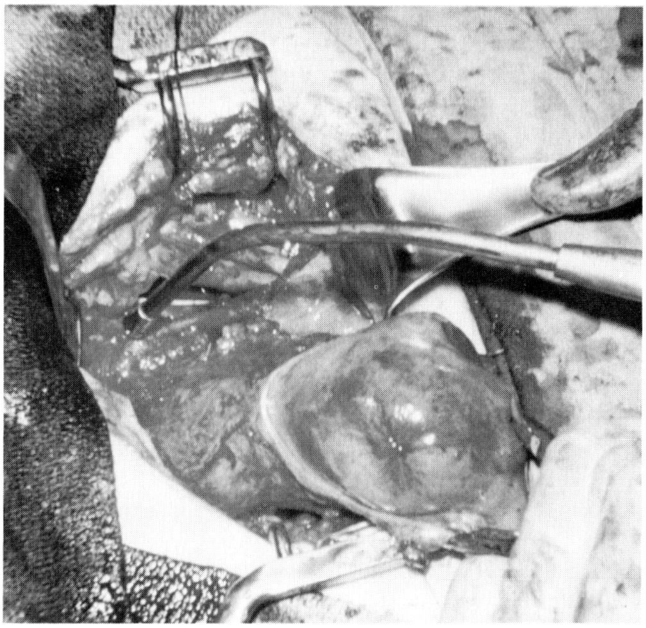

Fig. 10-6 Course of the ureter in the pelvis: the ureter (indicated by the tonsil suction) crosses the common iliac artery as it descends into the pelvis and stays on the medial leaf of the pelvic peritoneum. It then traverses the parametrium and enters into the urinary bladder. (This photograph was obtained during the performance of a radical hysterectomy.)

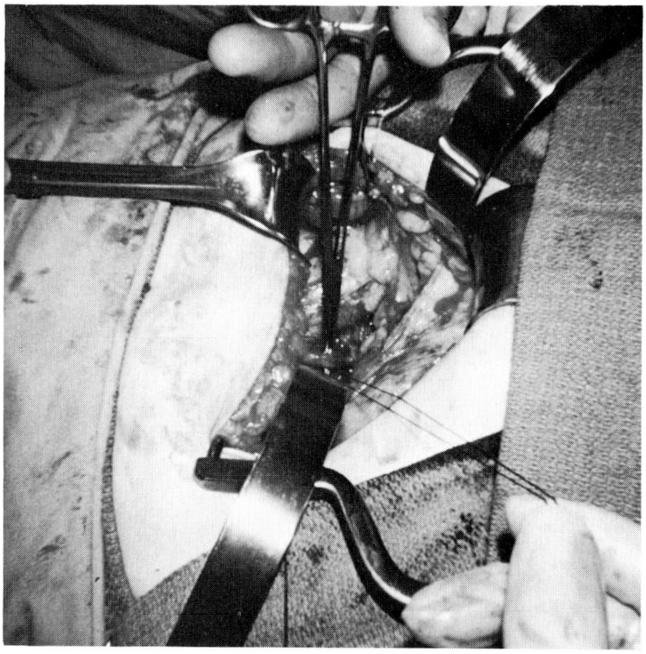

Fig. 10-7 The hypogastric artery has been exposed by using the tonsil suction tip as a dissector; a Mixter clamp has been gently advanced under the artery; and the midsegment of a 0-silk tie has been placed in the jaws of the clamp.

Mixter clamp as it is advanced around the artery to sweep away the loose connective tissue surrounding the vessel. Care must be taken not to be too vigorous in order to avoid injuring the hypogastric vein, which lies posterior and medial to the hypogastric artery. After the Mixter clamp has been passed around the vessel, the midsegment of a number zero silk tie is inserted into its jaws, the clamp is carefully withdrawn, the midsegment of the tie is divided, and the vessel is doubly ligated. It is not necessary to divide the artery.

Occasionally hemorrhage persists in the deep pelvis after a subtotal or total hysterectomy has been performed. In these cases access to the pelvic sidewalls may be obstructed by bundles of tissue incorporating the round and uteroovarian ligaments. In this situation it is advisable to redivide the round ligament closer to the pelvic sidewall and then to incise the peritoneum lateral to the infundibulopelvic ligament as indicated above. Valuable time may otherwise be wasted trying to displace the bundles of tissue containing the ligaments and ovary laterally and anteriorly in order to identify the pelvic sidewall vasculature.

Control of Bleeding Following Hypogastric Artery Ligation. Bilateral hypogastric artery ligation may dramatically reduce, but not entirely eliminate, pelvic hemorrhage following supracervical or total hysterectomy by diminishing the pulse pressure and local mean arterial blood flow. This is particularly true when placental implantation has involved the cervix; when there has been a placenta accreta, increta or percreta; or when tears have extended into the parametrium and broad ligament. Hypogastric artery ligation will also allow the surgeon to more readily inspect the bleeding site and control individual bleeders.

Patients receiving multiple transfusions with stored blood may develop a coagulopathy in addition to surgically controllable bleeding. Appropriate replacement therapy to avoid this problem in massively bleeding patients is discussed in Chapter 3. Persistent pelvic sidewall bleeding may respond to packing with hot pads or to topical anticoagulants in the form of Gelfoam pads, Surgicel, or Avitene. A decision may have to be made to close the retroperitoneum despite persistent oozing when it appears the patient's bleeding is due to a coagulopathy. Suction drains should be placed in the retroperitoneum of the pelvic sidewalls and brought out percutaneously in a retroperitoneal fashion. This permits removal of blood before it becomes a nidus for infection and allows for quantification of blood loss and therefore more accurate replacement.

Magrina and associates[13] have recently reported a case of postpartum hemorrhage persisting following a subtotal hysterectomy and bilateral hypogastric artery ligation which was successfully treated with a selective hypogastric artery infusion of Pitressin. Pitressin, a posterior pituitary extract, acts directly on vascular smooth muscle to cause vasoconstriction but has many other effects, including antidiuretic activity, myocardial depression resulting in bradycardia and decreased cardiac output, nausea, vomiting, and abdominal cramps. In addition, the infusion catheter must routinely be left in place for at least 24 h, thereby exposing the patient to complications from long-term arterial catheterization.[18] Selective arterial embolization techniques are clearly preferable to long-term intra-arterial Pitressin infusions.

Retroperitoneal Suction Catheter Placement Technique

Suction catheters (Hemovac, Jackson-Pratt) can be placed in the pelvic retroperitoneum while the sidewall is exposed. They are brought out percutaneously in retroperitoneal fashion by passing the trocar needle from the retroperitoneal space to the anterior abdominal wall. The path of the trocar is initiated from beneath the lateral segment of the divided round ligament superior to the external iliac artery. The tie on the lateral segment of the round ligament is placed on traction, the external iliac artery is palpated, and the trocar needle is carefully directed retroperitoneally under the round ligament and superior to the external iliac artery (Fig. 10-8). The trocar needle is then advanced laterally and anteriorly until the needle is observed to tent the skin. It is safest at this point to place the opened jaws of a Kelly clamp over the site where the needle tip will emerge and press the skin down while the trocar is being advanced. Upon exiting through the skin, the Kelley clamp is used to extract the trocar and its attached suction tubing. The catheters are then secured with stay sutures and are left in place until they drain less than 25 ml in 24 h. They are never irrigated once they are in place. Suction must be released prior to removing these catheters in order to avoid trauma to structures in the retroperitoneal space.

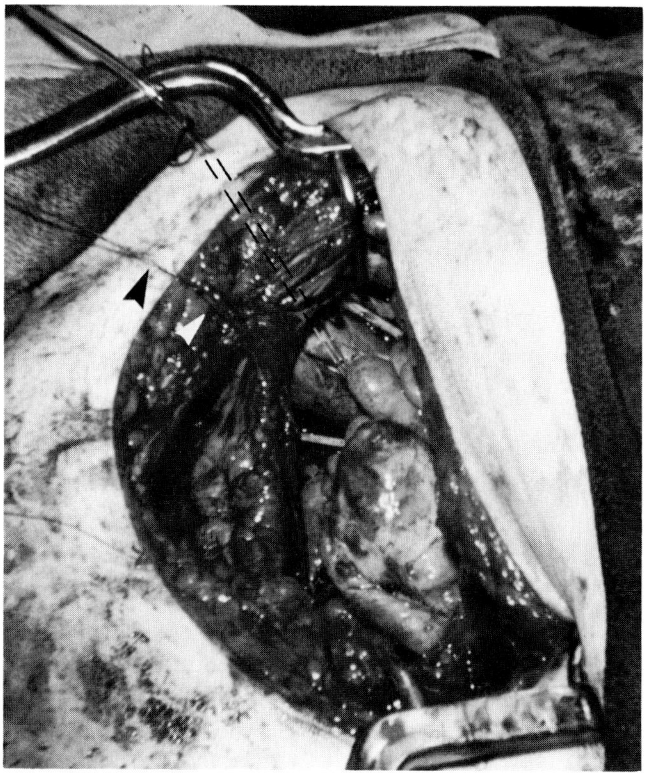

Fig. 10-8 Placement of retroperitoneal suction catheters: the round ligament (white arrow) has been placed on traction with a stay suture (black arrow). A suction catheter has been advanced retroperitoneally under the round ligament, superior to the external iliac artery, and brought out percutaneously. The dashed lines indicate the path of the catheter through the anterior abdominal wall.

Monitoring Patients with Massive Hemorrhage

Patients about to undergo surgery for control of postpartum hemorrhage must be carefully monitored for renal, pulmonary, and cardiovascular complications. Volume replacement can usually be adequately monitored with a central venous pressure line, but when massive hemorrhage occurs, Swan-Ganz catheter and arterial catheter monitoring may be invaluable (Ch. 1). Careful attention must be paid to urine output as renal failure may occur as a result of prolonged hypotension, complications of hemorrhage superimposed on toxemia, and coagulopathies. Patients treated for massive hemorrhage may also develop adult respiratory distress syndrome, an entity which is associated with mortality in 50 percent of patients.[16]

CONCLUSION

The overwhelming majority of patients at high risk for postpartum hemorrhage may be identified by history or physical examination. The alerted physician should routinely establish a peripheral intravenous line with a large-bore plastic cannula when these women are admitted to the labor suite. Blood should be made readily available in the event that transfusions are subsequently necessary. Routine conservative measures are usually all that are necessary for the management of uterine atony, retained placental fragments, and cervical and vaginal lacerations.

Successful management of massive postpartum hemorrhage requires first and foremost a clear understanding of the possible causes of the hemorrhage. A systematic evaluation of the patient should be made by the obstetrician in charge, who must be aware of new nonoperative techniques to control hemorrhage, such as prostaglandin therapy and intervention radiologic techniques. Surgery should be limited to those patients who are unresponsive to nonoperative intervention and those with ruptured uteri.

REFERENCES

1. Breen, J.L., Gregori, C.A., and Kindzierski, J.A.: Hemorrhage in gynecologic surgery. Editorial comments. p. 442. In Schaefer, G., and Graber, E.A., Eds.: Complications in Obstetric and Gynecologic Surgery. Harper & Row, Cambridge, 1981.
2. Brown, B.J., Heaston, D.K., Poulson, A.M. et al.: Uncontrollable postpartum bleeding: A new approach to hemostasis through angiographic arterial embolization. Obstet. Gynecol., *54:*361, 1979.
3. Burchell, R.C.: Physiology of internal iliac artery ligation. J. Obstet. Gynaecol. Br. Commonw., *75:*642, 1968.
4. Fribourg, S.R.C., Rothman, L.A., and Rovinsky, J.J.: Intrauterine lavage for control of uterine atony. Obstet. Gynecol., *41:*876, 1973.
5. Gibbs, D.E. and Locke, W.E.: Maternal deaths in Texas, 1969–1973. Am. J. Obstet. Gynecol., *126:*687, 1976.

6. Hall, M. and Marshall, J.R.: The gravity suit: A major advance in management of gynecologic blood loss. Obstet. Gynecol., *53:*247, 1979.
7. Hayashi, R.H., Castillo, M.S., and Noah, M.L.: Management of severe postpartum hemorrhage due to uterine atony using an analogue of prostaglandin $F_{2\alpha}$. Obstet. Gynecol., *58:*426, 1981.
8. Hertz, R.H., Sokol, R.J., and Dierker, L.J.: Treatment of postpartum uterine atony with prostaglandin E_2 vaginal suppositories. Obstet. Gynecol., *56:*129, 1980.
9. Hester, J.D.: Postpartum hemorrhage and reevaluation of uterine packing. Obstet. Gynecol., *45:*501, 1975.
10. Kelly, J.V.: Postpartum hemorrhage. p. 60. In Schaefer, G. and Graber, E.A., Eds.: Complications in Obstetric and Gynecologic Surgery. Harper & Row, Cambridge, 1981.
11. Lee, C.Y., Maorazo, B., and Drukker, B.H.: Ultrasonic evaluation of the postpartum uterus in the management of postpartum bleeding. Obstet. Gynecol., *581:*227, 1981.
12. Lucas, W.E.: Postpartum hemorrhage. Clin. Obstet. Gynecol., *23:*637, 1980.
13. Magrina, J.F., Moffat, R.E., Masterson, B.J., and Krantz, K.E.: Selective arterial infusion of Pitressin for the control of puerperal hemorrhage after hypogastric artery ligation. Obstet. Gynecol., *58:*646, 1981.
14. O'Leary, J.L.: Pregnancy following uterine artery ligation. Obstet. Gynecol., *55:*112, 1980.
15. Pais, S.O., Glickman, M., Schwartz, P. et al.: Embolization of pelvic arteries for control of postpartum hemorrhage. Obstet. Gynecol., *55:*754, 1980.
16. Rinaldo, J.E. and Roger, R.M.: Adult respiratory distress syndrome: Changing concepts of lung injury and repair. N. Engl. J. Med., *306:*900, 1982.
17. Schwartz, P.E.: Arterial hemorrhage in gynecologic malignancies. In Delgado, G. and Smith, J.P., Eds.: *Management of Complications in Gynecologic Oncology*. John Wiley & Sons, New York, 1982.
18. Schwartz, P.E., Goldstein, H.M., Wallace, S., and Rutledge, F.N.: Control of arterial hemorrhage using percutaneous arterial catheter techniques in patients with gynecologic malignancies. Gynecol. Oncol., *3:*276, 1975.
19. Takagi, S., Yoshida, T., Togo, Y. et al.: The effects of intramyometrial injection of prostaglandin $F_{2\alpha}$ on severe postpartum hemorrhage. Prostaglandins, *12:*565, 1976.
20. Waters, E.G.: Surgical management of postpartum hemorrhage with particular attention to ligation of uterine arteries. Am. J. Obstet. Gynecol., *64:*1143, 1952.
21. Watson, P.: Postpartum hemorrhage and shock. Clin. Obstet. Gynecol., *23:*985, 1980.

11

The Management of Hypertensive Crises during Pregnancy

Richard L. Berkowitz, M.D.

INTRODUCTION

A great deal remains unknown about pregnancy-induced hypertension (PIH) despite extensive investigative efforts. Considerable controversy exists regarding the optimal management of this condition alone or superimposed on chronic hypertension. Several recent reviews have discussed therapeutic options in the management of mild to moderate elevations of blood pressure during pregnancy.[55,74,82] This chapter will focus on the treatment of acute hypertensive crises in women with PIH.

Preeclampsia has traditionally been defined as the development of hypertension during pregnancy in association with proteinuria and edema. The addition of convulsions to this complex is referred to as eclampsia. Renal biopsy studies have demonstrated, however, that histopathological correlation between the classic lesions of preeclampsia and the typical clinical presentation are very poor, especially in multiparas.[22] On the other hand, a variety of atypical syndromes may represent prodromal aspects of preeclampsia or variants of that disorder.[33] All this makes it very difficult to accurately define severe preeclampsia and consequently to appreciate the true maternal and perinatal consequences of that disorder. Hypertension, however, is inevitably part of the picture when preeclampsia becomes severe and poses a threat to the life of the mother and her fetus regardless of any other abnormalities that may be present. In this chapter a diagnostic approach to the woman with severe PIH will be presented, but the reader is referred to the chapters on renal, hepatic, hematologic, and neurologic emergencies for management of the nonhypertensive complications of this disorder. Prior to presenting recommendations for therapy of a hypertensive crisis during pregnancy, the rationale for treatment will be discussed, the pharmacologic actions of major antihypertensive agents currently being used will be reviewed, and data obtained from invasive studies of the cardiovascular consequences of severe PIH will be considered.

RATIONALE FOR TREATMENT

In a study of 501 consecutive maternal deaths in Texas, "toxemia" was associated with approximately 25 percent of those cases felt to be due to direct obstetrical causes.[30] About one-third of the toxemic deaths were ascribed to cerebral vascular accidents and another one-third to cardiac failure. Hodgkinson et al.[40] state that in other studies of gestational hypertension, cerebral hemorrhage or edema has been responsible for 29 to 53 percent of the maternal deaths and cardiac failure for 10 to 30 percent. In a retrospective analysis of more than 41,000 births, Naeye and Friedman[60] reported that the perinatal mortality in women with gestational diastolic blood pressures of 85 mmHg or higher and proteinuria of 1+ or greater was more than 2 times greater than in normotensive, nonproteinuric controls. Of the total excess perinatal deaths in the pregnancies associated with hypertension, 42 percent were due to large placental infarcts, 15 percent to intrauterine growth retardation, and 13 percent to abruptio placenta.

Sudden rises in blood pressure (BP) above critical thresholds result in focal arteriolar damage in both experimental animals and humans, and if the hypertension is sustained, left ventricular overload will follow. In rats segmental dilatation of arterioles with associated endothelial tears can be demonstrated within 10 min of attaining mean arterial pressures of 150 mmHg, and these lesions become extensive after 1 h.[32] Redman[82] points out that the functional result of forced dilatation of arterioles is loss of the autoregulatory mechanism, which protects more peripheral vessels from the effects of high-pressure hyperfusion. He claims that this is responsible for hypertensive encephalopathy and that the threshold for forced dilatation of vessels is lower in previously normotensive patients than it is for women with chronically elevated BP. This process, if continued, may result in cerebral microaneurysms, which can be the source of an acute cerebral hemorrhage. While eclampsia is not simply a variant of malignant hypertension, there is a great deal of evidence to suggest that it is a form of hypertensive encephalopathy. This issue is discussed in greater depth in Chapter 13. Regardless of their views on the etiology of eclamptic seizures, however, virtually all authorities have advised that when they occur, blood pressure should be stabilized and the patient delivered as expeditiously as possible.

Additional target organs of concern when an acute hypertensive crisis occurs during pregnancy are the heart, kidneys, and uteroplacental circulation. The generalized increase in systemic vascular resistance (SVR) greatly increases the left ventricular work required to maintain an appropriate cardiac output. If significant elevations in SVR persist or the patient has preexisting cardiac disease, congestive heart failure may occur. The combination of reduced renal blood flow secondary to vascular spasm and the hypovolemia which invariably accompanies severe hypertensive crises in pregnancy may aggrevate intrinsic damage to the kidney caused by preeclampsia and result in profound oliguria. If not corrected, this has the potential to evolve into bilateral cortical necrosis. Finally, reduction in flow to the uteroplacental unit may cause fetal hypoxia, which results in acute fetal distress, or alternatively a placental abruption may occur which directly threatens the life of the fetus and may initiate a maternal coagulopathy.

Thus, it can be seen that an acute rise in BP above a critical threshold may set the stage for a variety of potentially life-threatening fetal and maternal problems. Redman et al.[83] state that a BP of 180/120 mmHg corresponds to values in animal experiments which result in rapid vascular damage. Treatment at that level is therefore mandatory for maternal indications, and by treating all women with values greater than 170/110 mmHg, the margin of safety is widened. For the remainder of this chapter I will refer to values in excess of 180/120 mmHg as severe hypertension and will assume that a reasonable therapeutic objective is to lower the BP in these women to at least 170/110 mmHg. One additional general comment is necessary. The actual values cited above are absolute upper limits and may be too high for some patients. A teenager whose BP is normally 110/60 mmHg may be very sick with values of 150/100 mmHg. The physician must therefore evaluate the entire clinical picture and not be lulled into a false sense of security by the patient's failure to achieve some arbitrarily chosen index of severity.

ANTIHYPERTENSIVE DRUGS

Diuretics

General Considerations. During most normal pregnancies, there is a gradual cumulative retention of between 500 and 900 mEq of sodium.[53] This is distributed between the products of conception and the maternal extracellular volume. A concomitant increase in plasma volume also occurs. Multiple conflicting regulatory factors control sodium metabolism during pregnancy. These include increased renal perfusion and glomerular filtration rate as well as the opposing actions of progesterone and aldosterone. Despite an increase in circulating aldosterone levels, the pregnant patient maintains the ability to respond to physiologic demands by further alterations in the production of this hormone. On the other hand, even though experimental evidence suggests that normal pregnant women handle acute and chronic sodium loads similarly to nonpregnant patients, 80 percent of normotensive women develop dependent or generalized edema at some time during their otherwise uncomplicated gestations. Marked sodium retention and edema may occur in PIH, but it is unclear what relationship this has with the etiology of that condition.

Thiazide Diuretics. When administered chronically to hypertensive patients, diuretics reduce arterial pressure by decreasing total peripheral resistance. The primary mode of action of thiazide diuretics is inhibition of electrolyte reabsorption in the distal collecting tubules. This results in an increase in sodium, chloride, and potassium excretion along with accompanying water. In addition, uric acid excretion is inhibited. The thiazides cause an initial reduction in extracellular and plasma volumes, along with a concurrent decrease in cardiac output (CO). The effect is transient, and in 1 to 2 weeks plasma volume and CO return to normal levels, but a reduction in peripheral resistance is maintained.[88,109] The persistent hypotensive effect may be secondary either to a direct action on the arteriolar smooth muscle or to changes of electrolyte concentration in its wall. The latter could influence the tone or pressor responsiveness of the vessel.[46] The autonomic reflex mechanisms essential for cardiovascular homeostasis are unimpaired. Consequently, a proportional decrease in both systolic and diastolic BP is seen in the absence of orthostatic changes or disturbances in regional circulation. Finally, plasmin renin increases in response to sodium depletion and may remain increased throughout the administration of the drug.

When patients become acutely toxemic, they have been demonstrated to have reduced plasma volumes.[53] Assali feels that this is secondary to constriction of the vascular bed and not a primary factor in causing the condition.[3] In any case, administration of a diuretic further depletes intravascular volume. This may compromise the fetus by decreasing uterine blood flow, in addition to placing the mother in jeopardy should bleeding occur.[45]

Gant et al.[28] have demonstrated a reduced MCR_{DS} [metabolic clearance rate (MCR) of dehydroepiandrosterone sulfate (DS)] in 9 out of 10 pregnant patients studied on the seventh day of thiazide therapy. They also found a rebound to control levels after therapy was discontinued. The MCR_{DS} represents a summation of placental conversion of DS to estradiol, as well as 16-α-hydroxylation in the maternal liver. Since approximately 40 to 50 percent of the total MCR_{DS} in pregnancy is secondary to the former route, this rate is felt to reflect both uterine blood flow and placental metabolic competence. The reduction in MCR_{DS} following thiazide therapy may well represent decreased placental perfusion, although direct inhibition of enzymes important in DS metabolism is also possible. The knowledge that blood volume is decreased in preeclamptic patients coupled with the results of Gant's study constitutes a powerful argument for not using diuretic agents routinely in patients with PIH.

Thiazide therapy should never be initiated in obstetrical patients during a hypertensive crisis because in those rare situations where a diuretic is indicated a more rapidly acting parenteral agent should be used. Nevertheless, some pregnant women may be taking thiazides when a hypertensive crisis ensues and so the physician should be aware of the potential problems which may occur when these drugs are used. Complications of thiazide therapy during pregnancy include significant maternal electrolyte imbalances with severe hypokalemia and metabolic alkalosis[76,94] maternal hemorrhagic pancreatitis[58] thrombocytopenia,[101] hyperglycemia,[37] and hyperuricemia,[19] as well as neonatal hyponatremia[2] and thrombocytopenia.[90]

Furosemide. Furosemide is a potent diuretic which blocks the active reabsorption of chloride along with passive sodium reabsorption in the ascending loop of Henle. It can function even in the presence of significant renal insufficiency or volume depletion and is capable of causing severe electrolyte imbalance.[7,102]

Some authors have recommended the use of furosemide as part of the therapy of severe PIH.[12,20] Kelly,[45] however, lists specific indications for its use in the pregnant patient. These include:

1. Pulmonary edema with congestive heart failure in PIH, where severe vasoconstriction causes cardiac decompensation secondary to myocardial ischemia.
2. Pulmonary edema secondary to iatrogenic fluid overload.
3. Adjunctively with the administration of diazoxide, whose sodium-retaining and vasodilatory properties may cause oliguria.

It should be mentioned that Morris et al.[59] used diazoxide in the therapy of 12 patients with severe PIH and did not administer furosemide. The protocol in that series, however, limited the investigators to a maximum of three 300-mg boluses of diazoxide in a 24-h period. Furthermore, all pregnancies were terminated within 24 h of the initial administration of the drug. With this protocol it was not found necessary to treat any patient with furosemide.

No abnormalities have been reported in the fetuses of mothers who were given furosemide, but Gant's work suggests that it may decrease uterine blood flow.[29] Since it is such a potent diuretic, furosemide must be used with extreme caution in preeclamptic patients because of their contracted intravascular volume. It should rarely be necessary to use this drug except in patients with pulmonary edema. When diuretic therapy is indicated in women with severe PIH, however, flurosemide is the drug of choice.

Drugs Affecting the Sympathetic Nervous System

General Considerations. Adrenergic neural impulses initiate from various brain centers and pass through complex integrative areas of the brain stem via preganglionic neurons. They then pass down the spinal cord to the paravertebral ganglia, where they are propagated across the synapse via acetylcholine released from preganglionic terminal nerve fibers. Postganglionic fibers conduct the impulses to their respective nerve endings within the vascular wall or myocardium, where the stored neurohumoral substance norepinephrine is released. The liberated catecholamine stimulates alpha- and beta-receptor sites in the vascular smooth muscle or myocardial cell membrane. Alpha stimulation causes vasoconstriction, while beta-stimulation results in vasodilation. Alpha stimulation has little if any effect on the myocardium but beta stimulation increases heart rate, contractility, and conduction velocity, while decreasing the refractory period at the atrioventricular node. Alpha- and beta-receptor sites are also present in cell membranes of specific neurons in the hypothalamus and other brain centers. In the brain in contrast to the periphery, alpha stimulation reduces BP while beta stimulation increases it.

Increased adrenergic outflow from the brain causes increased renin release, which in turn results in increased angiotensin and aldosterone production. A rise in the latter results in sodium retention, and this in turn increases the effectiveness of the action of catecholamines on vessels and the heart. A decrease in adrenergic activity, on the other hand, causes an increase in plasma volume because the reduced hydrostatic pressure resulting from diminished vascular resistance permits influx of water from the extravascular compartment into the intravascular space. The only two types of antihypertensive agents that do not produce a retention of sodium and water are diuretics and beta-adrenergic blockers.[102] Intravascular volume depletion will augment the antihypertensive action of any drug that inhibits sympathetic activity.[26]

Sympathetic blockers cause a decrease in heart rate (HR), vascular resistance, and blood pressure. This is most pronounced when the patient is in the upright position because pooling of blood in dependent areas results in a diminished venous return and a subsequent decrease in cardiac output. The normal reflex response would be to increase HR and arteriolar constriction, but this is prevented by the sympathetic blockade. The result is orthostatic hypotension and syncope in severe cases. This sequence of events does not occur with agents which selectively block beta activity while leaving the alpha system intact.

Ganglionic blockers exert their action in paravertebral autonomic ganglia and prevent the attachment of released acetylcholine to postganglionic fibers. This results in the inhibition of all autonomic impulses, both sympathetic and parasympathetic.

The Beta-Adrenergic Antagonists. Five beta-blocking agents have currently been approved by the FDA for the treatment of hypertension. These drugs lower blood pressure by several mechanisms:

1. They decrease $beta_1$ stimulation of the heart, which results in a reduction in HR, myocardial contractility, and CO.
2. They act directly on the central nervous system to decrease BP by unopposed alpha stimulation.
3. They decrease renin secretion by the kidneys.[41]

The recent proliferation of these agents has been increased by the development of drugs possessing some selectivity for $beta_1$-adrenoceptors in the heart, as opposed to $beta_2$-receptors in the peripheral circulation and bronchi. Atenolol, like metoprolol is a $beta_1$-selective adrenergic blocker but has a longer plasma half-life, which allows for administration of single daily doses.[25] Propranolol, timolol, and nadolol, on the other hand, are nonselective beta-adrenergic blockers. All these drugs can be effective in the treatment of hypertension, but one may be better than another in decreasing side effects in specific clinical situations. Generally, if one agent in adequate doses does not work, neither will another, and the effect of these drugs is not additive.[24] There are theoretical advantages in using selective β_1 blockers, but the practical benefits seem to be limited to very specific cases. Propranolol is the agent in this group which has been most widely used in pregnant patients to date. While atenolol,[103] metoprolol,[93] and oxyprenolol[27,54] (not yet FDA-approved) have been used in some studies in obstetrical patients, no remarkable differences from propranolol have thus far been demonstrated.

Intravenous administration of propranolol results in a rapid decrease in HR and CO by direct inhibition of the rate and force of contractility. An initial increase in peripheral resistance secondary to generalized inhibition of beta-mediated vasodilation is reversed within a few hours by the drug's central action and by decreased renin production by the kidneys.

Since this drug does not block alpha-receptor stimulation, it leaves sympathetically mediated vasoconstrictor reflexes intact and causes neither orthostatic hypotension nor disturbances of sexual function. It has little effect on plasma volume but occasionally can precipitate cardiac failure. Most of the significant cardiovascular problems caused by this drug have been noted with low doses early in therapy and seem to occur primarily in those patients who depend on beta stimulation to maintain cardiac function.[7]

Additional side effect include bronchospasm, which occurs in 2 to 10 percent of patients with no history of asthma. Because of the increase in peripheral vascular resistance which may result from unopposed alpha vasoconstriction, this drug is contraindicated in patients with compromised peripheral vasculature or Raynaud's phenomenon. During acute stress, diabetics on propranolol may become more susceptible to hyperglycemia because of suppression of insulin release by beta blockade. On the other hand, acutely stressed insulin-dependent diabetics can become hypoglycemic because of the blockage of counterregulatory beta-mediated glycogenolysis. It is possible that selective $beta_1$-blockers will be shown to be safe for use as antihypertensive agents in some women with asthma, hypoglycemia, or peripheral vascular disease. Central nervous system effects of propranolol include insomnia, nightmares, hallucinations, depressions, paresthesias, ataxia, and dizziness.[41] Finally, acute hypertensive episodes have been reported when this drug was given in conjunction with methyldopa. Nies and Shand[64] have hypothesized that this is due to propranolol's potentiation of the pressor response to α-methylnorepinephrine, a metabolite of methyldopa.

Although there do not seem to be any maternal problems peculiar to the obstetrical patient taking propranolol, a number of fetal side effects have been noted. The drug easily crosses the placenta and is also secreted in breast milk. Experiments in pregnant sheep demonstrated a significant reduction in umbilical blood flow when propranolol was given intravenously to the mother.[66] In these studies no significant change in uterine blood flow was observed. Chronic administration has been associated with growth retardation,[77] neonatal hypoglycemia, and bradycardia which persists during the first day of extrauterine life.[31,85] Tunstall[104] has reported difficulty in establishing spontaneous respiratory activity at birth in neonates whose mothers had been given intravenous propranolol immediately prior to elective cesarean section. He hypothesizes that this is caused by beta-adrenergic blockade of the cervical sympathetic discharge which follows cord clamping.

In a retrospective study, Lieberman et al.[52] found that the fetal outcome was worse in nine pregnancies in which maternal hypertension was treated with propranolol than in 15 similar cases in which other antihypertensive agents were used. Rubin[92] however, in a review of the literature cites three prospective studies which found that treatment of hypertension with propranolol during pregnancy seemed to benefit the fetus. After including studies involving other beta-blockers in his analysis and criticizing methodologic flaws in the series with adverse results, Rubin concludes that when these agents are used to treat maternal hypertension, the likelihood that the fetus will be normal is improved. He states, however, that it is still not clear whether therapy with beta-blockers specifically improves the outcome in patients with PIH. Obviously, this issue has not yet been resolved. Additional large prospective trials with well-matched controls are necessary before it is clear that these agents offer advantages over other antihypertensive drugs for obstetric patients.

Methyldopa. The antihypertensive action of this drug is secondary to a reduction in peripheral arteriolar resistance. There is little or no effect on heart rate and cardiac output. The drug acts by:

1. Stimulation of alpha-adrenergic receptor sites in the hypothalamus and other portions of the central nervous system.
2. Inhibition of dopa decarboxylase, which results in decreased production of norepinephrine in the postganglionic nerve endings.
3. False neurohumoral transmission. α-Methyldopa is converted to α-methylnorepinephrine, which displaces norepinephrine from its vascular smooth muscle alpha-adrenergic receptor sites. This metabolite causes less vasoconstriction than norepinephrine.
4. Possibly suppression of the release of renal renin.[26]

Methyldopa is maximally effective when patients are standing, but postural variation of blood pressure is much less marked than with guanethidine. Orthostatic hypotension is uncommon. When methyldopa is administered chronically without the addition of a diuretic, plasma and extracellular fluid volumes are expanded. This reduces the drug's antihypertensive effectiveness.[46] Glomerular filtration rate and renal plasma flow are maintained in the presence of its hypotensive action, which makes methyldopa a good agent to use in patients with renal functional impairment.

Side effects include drowsiness, depression, sodium retention, and constipation. A positive Coombs test develops in 20 percent of nonpregnant patients within the first 12 months of therapy, but this rarely occurs with less than 6 months of use. Infrequently, the positive Coombs test is accompanied by a hemolytic anemia.[26] Very rarely, a flulike illness with high fever occurs, and a hepatitis syndrome has been described. Lactation, accompanied by high prolactin levels, has been reported in both males and females taking this drug.[63]

In many ways methyldopa is an ideal antihypertensive agent for long-term use during pregnancy. It has little or no effect on cardiac output, and regional blood flow to the kidneys and uterus seems to be unimpaired.[109] In a study by Redman's group published in 1976,[84] the outcome of 117 cases in which methyldopa was administered throughout pregnancy was studied. The authors concluded that the use of this medication for chronic maternal hypertension is safe for both mothers and their fetuses. A follow-up study[13] performed at the age of 7 1/2 showed the only significant difference between children of treated women and those of untreated controls was smaller head size in the sons of women who began taking methyldopa between 16 and 20 weeks gestation. No difference in mean intelligence quotient was evident. The authors therefore maintain their conviction that methyldopa is safe to use in pregnancy, but caution that, whenever possible, treatment with this agent should not be initiated between 16 and 20 weeks gestation.

While methyldopa is considered by many authorities to be the drug of choice for long-term antihypertensive therapy during pregnancy, it has not proved useful during the management of hypertensive crises. The onset of action is 4 to 6 h, even when given intravenously. This obviously is too long to wait when trying to lower blood pressures which have risen to dangerous levels. Furthermore, the intense vasospasm experienced by women with severe PIH is more effectively treated with primary vasodilators than with agents which act through the sympathetic nervous system.

Rauwolfia Alkaloids. Reserpine is one of approximately 20 related agents which comprise the family of *Rauwolfia* alkaloids. They act by depleting the natural stores of biogenic amines in the brain, myocardium, adrenal medulla, and postganglionic nerve endings. The transport of norepinephrine into its storage granules is blocked and the reuptake of released catecholamines by the nerve endings is inhibited.[26]

The hypotensive action of these drugs is due to a reduction in sympathetic stimulation of the blood vessels and heart and is associated with bradycardia as well as decrease in vascular resistance. The immediate result of the administration of an intravenous dose of reserpine is the release of pressor substances, which may cause a transient increase in BP. The usual oral dose is only sufficient to cause a modest decline in blood pressure, but this may be augmented significantly by diuretics. Reserpine, like the other sympathetic depressants, can decrease plasma renin activity.[46]

Side effects include postural and exercise hypotension, although these are uncommon when the drug is taken orally in effective amounts. Unopposed parasympathetic stimulation may cause an increase in gastric acid secretion, peptic ulceration, frequent bowel movements or diarrhea, prolonged atrioventricular conduction, and enhanced second-degree heart block. Nasal arteriolar dilatation may result in nasal stuffiness. Brain amine and serotonin depletion can cause depression and behavioral changes, and these serve as limiting factors in the long-term administration of high enough doses to cause major sympathoplegia.[46]

Reserpine crosses the placenta, and the major fetal complication is neonatal respiratory difficulties secondary to nasal congestion.[45,109]

Although some authors[21,109] have recommended reserpine as an alternative drug in the therapy of chronic hypertension in pregnancy, the large number of maternal side effects make this a less attractive choice than other agents which are currently available.

Clonidine. Clonidine is a sympathetic depressant. Its mechanism of action is stimulation of alpha-adrenergic receptor sites in the hypothalamus and other vasomotor centers of the central nervous system. It has no direct peripheral vasodilating effect and does not act on peripheral alpha-adrenergic receptors.[26] The renal release of renin, however, is suppressed.

Side effects include postural hypotension, sodium and fluid retention, bowel disturbances, drowsiness, and, rarely, a weakly positive Coombs test. Occasionally, following prolonged therapy a symptomatic hypertensive crisis occurs upon abrupt withdrawal of the drug.[26] This is accompanied by restlessness, tremor, headaches, and other symptoms suggestive of catecholamine release. A case has been published[111] of a woman with PIH who was given clonidine on the fifth postpartum day for control of her hypertension. The medication was inadvertently stopped after 2 days and she developed palpitations and tremor in association with a dramatic rise in BP to 250/190 mmHg. After unsuccessful attempts to adequately reduce the hypertension, clonidine was restarted in 3 days. Her BP then fell to 150/100 mmHg with relief of her symptoms, and gradual reduction in the dose of clonidine was achieved without further hypertensive overshoot.

No series have been published implicating clonidine as a teratogen, but a case report has described a child born with Robert's syndrome (tetraphocomelia, cleft lip and palate, and failure to thrive) to a woman who took this drug throughout her pregnancy.[99] Despite one report of its successful use in five Australian obstetrical patients[42] clonidine has been insufficiently evaluated to recommend its use in the pregnant patient. Other agents currently available can achieve the same objectives and have been more thoroughly studied.

Ganglionic Blockers. The ganglionic blocking agents have multiple maternal side effects. In addition they have been reported to cause meconium ileus in the fetus and newborn.[38] The intravenous administration of the extremely short-acting ganglionic blocker trimethaphan (Arfonad) has been used to produce controlled hypotension for neurosurgical procedures during pregnancy[1,57,71,108] This drug causes histamine release, however, and must be used with extreme caution in patients with a history of allergy.[34] Furthermore, interaction with succinylcholine may result in prolonged apnea.[72] Other antihypertensive agents are available for intravenous administration which are safer and more reliable than trimethaphan. The ganglionic blockers, therefore, currently have no role in the treatment of hypertension in pregnancy.

Vasodilators

General Considerations. Vasodilating agents which have been used in the therapy of hypertension during pregnancy include hydralazine, diazoxide, nitroprusside, prazosin, and nitroglycerin. Although they vary in their maximal vasodilatory action, even the least effective of these drugs can decrease total peripheral resistance by more than 50 percent.[47] Aside from prazosin, which has a different mechanism of action than the others, the long-term effectiveness of this group of antihypertensive agents is limited by:

1. Reflex increase in sympathetic activity, which causes an increase in HR and CO. This can diminish the hypotensive effect by 50 to 75 percent, and the increase in cardiac work may be poorly tolerated by patients with limited cardiac reserve.

2. Increase in plasma renin activity secondary to an increase in sympathetic discharge to the kidney.

3. Retention of sodium and water with expansion of extracellular fluid and plasma volume.[47]

The first two of these side effects can be prevented by beta-blockers, which isolate the heart from excessive sympathetic stimulation and decrease the renal release of renin. The third can be averted by the concomitant administration of a diuretic. Severe chronic hypertension may therefore require therapy with a drug from each of these three categories. The combination of a diuretic, beta-blocker, and vasodilator will control most degrees of hypertension and leave intact the vasoconstrictor reflexes required for cardiovascular homeostasis. In addition, this regimen is free from the other side effects of generalized sympathoplegia. In managing the acute hypertensive crisis of a woman with PIH, however, vasodilator therapy alone is often all that is required. This is because delivery following stabilization of the BP frequently causes a resolution of the hypertension, and long-term therapy with a vasodilator does not become necessary. Even when hypertension persists several days after delivery, it is often possible to control it with other agents.

Hydralazine. The mechanism of action of this drug is to decrease vascular resistance secondary to direct relaxation of arteriolar smoother muscle. Hydralazine primarily acts on the precapillary resistance vessels. Peripheral vasodilation is not uniform, and resistance in the coronary, cerebral, splanchnic, and renal circulations is reduced more than that in skin and muscle. There is no direct action on the heart, and the autonomic nervous system is not affected. Orthostatic hypotension consequently does not occur. The decreased BP which accompanies peripheral vasodilation activates baroreceptors, which stimulate an increased sympathetic discharge. This results in an increase in HR, left ventricular ejection velocity, stroke volume (SV) and CO.

Hydralazine causes increased sodium and water retention, expansion of plasma and extracellular fluid volumes, weight gain, and edema formation. These are not a result of decreases in renal blood flow or glomerular filtration rate, both of which are either increased or unchanged. They are due to the reduction in arterial pressure caused by hydralazine and may be mediated by both the renin-angiotensin-aldosterone system and by a direct renal mechanism.[49]

The major pathway of biotransformation is acteylation in the liver. The rate of this metabolic conversion is genetically determined by the activity of hepatic N-acetyltransferase. Consequently, when treated with a given dose of hydralazine, slow acetylators will have higher serum concentrations than fast acetylators.

The drug can be administered orally, intramuscularly, or intravenously. The latter route has been employed for the treatment of hypertensive crisis. The initial intravenous dose should never exceed 20 mg, and its onset of action is approximately 15 to 20 min. The dose and frequency of administration required for satisfactory blood pressure control are variable. Pritchard[73] has recommended that in order to avoid the creation of hypotension in women with PIH, the initial intravenous dose should be 5 mg, with additional 5 to 10 mg boluses being given every 20 min as needed. While 20-mg boluses may sometimes be necessary to maintain diastolic pressures between 90 and 110 mmHg, it is important to start with a low dose in order to avoid hypotensive overshoots in women who respond dramatically to the use of this drug.

Side effects include flushing, nasal congestion, headaches, dizziness, palpitations, anginal attacks, and EKG changes of myocardial ischemia. These are related to either direct or reflex-mediated hemodynamic actions of the drug. In doses exceeding 200 mg/day a syndrome similar to lupus erythematosis has developed in people who are slow acetylators. Very rarely drug fever, rash, peripheral neuropathy, and blood dyscrasias may develop.[49]

The literature contains conflicting reports of the effect of hydralazine on the uteroplacental circulation. Ladner et al.,[50] in a study of instrumented normotensive pregnant sheep, observed decreased uterine blood flow with a secondary decline in fetal pO_2 in response to hydralazine administration. No change was noted in fetal pH or cardiovascular parameters. The decrease in uterine blood flow was proportional to the reduction in maternal blood pressure. Gant and colleagues[29] reported a decrease in the MCR_{DS} by 6 to 59 percent in chronic hypertensive patients following the intravenous administration of hydralazine. Vink et al.[105] gave 12.5 mg dihydralazine intravenously over 4 min to 33 women with diastolic blood pressures of 110 mmHg or greater. Nineteen of these patients developed fetal heart rate (FHR) decelerations in association with drops in diastolic BP to 70 to 90 mmHg. Of the group with FHR decelerations, 68 percent (13/19) delivered growth-retarded babies, as opposed to 7 percent (1/14) of the group without decelerations.

Woods and Brinkman,[109] on the other hand, cite Page as showing that hydralazine increases uterine blood flow, and they state that propranolol effectively prevents this increase. Ring et al.[87] demonstrated a statistically significant increase in uterine blood flow when hydralazine was given to pregnant sheep made hypertensive with intravenously administered phenylephrine. No significant acid-base changes were noted in either the mother or fetus during these experiments. The authors also cite Brinkman and Assali as showing that hydralazine increases uterine blood flow in renal hypertensive pregnant sheep.

By virtue of its proven efficacy and safety, most authorities feel that hydralazine given intravenously is the antihypertensive drug of choice in the management of a hypertensive crisis in pregnancy. Its use in literally thousands of cases of PIH has demonstrated that it will adequately reduce the BP to acceptable limits in the overwhelming majority of cases and is well tolerated by the fetus in the absence of iatrogenically created hypotension. The latter can be avoided by administering the drug wisely and by careful attention to the appropriate infusion of fluids.

Diazoxide. Diazoxide is a benzothiadiazine derivative which is closely related chemically to the thiazide diuretics. It is a potent and rapidly acting antihypertensive agent and is marketed for the intravenous therapy of hypertensive emergencies. Its mechanism of action is a reduction in vascular resistance as a result of direct relaxation of arteriolar smooth muscle in all circulatory beds. Its use in the pregnant patient is controversial.

This drug has very little effect on capacitance vessels and no direct action on the heart. Like hydralazine, when diazoxide reduces arterial pressure, baroreceptors are activated which cause a reflex increase in HR, SV, and CO. Since cardiovascular reflexes in the sympathetic nervous system function normally, diazoxide rarely causes postural hypotension. This complication can occur, however, whenever the plasma and extracellular volumes have been markedly reduced. Sodium and water retention, expansion of plasma volume, and edema formation frequently occur with diazoxide therapy because of the drug's direct tubular antinaturetic action. Renal plasma flow and glomerular filtration rate may fall for a few hours after administration of this drug but thereafter are usually either unchanged or increased.[48]

Side effects include hyperglycemia, which is primarily caused by a reduction in insulin secretion by the pancreatic beta cells. There may also be a direct effect on the liver to increase its rate of glucose release. A mild hyperuricemia is caused by an inhibition of the tubular excretion of uric acid. Diuretics can potentiate both of these effects of diazoxide.[48] Displacement of coumarin anticoagulants from serum albumin can occur, and their dosage may therefore have to be reduced. Occasionally cardiac arrhythmias, palpitations, angina, headaches, and flushing occur. These are associated with the sympathetic reflex response to the diazoxide-induced vasodilation and can usually be controlled with propranolol. Finally, by direct action on uterine musculature, contractions may be abolished. These, however, can easily be reestablished by the intravenous administration of oxytocin.

Nuwayhid et al.[65] administered diazoxide to instrumented normotensive pregnant sheep and noted little change in uterine blood flow in association with moderate maternal hypotension. When, however, maternal systemic arterial pressure fell to a critical closing pressure level, there was a significant decrease in uterine blood flow. Diazoxide crossed the placenta, but fetal levels of the drug were always lower than those of the mother because of rapid loss of the drug by the fetus. Direct injection of the drug into the fetus resulted in minimal changes in its circulatory activity. Following maternal administration of diazoxide, moderate maternal and fetal hyperglycemia ensued.

Maximum duration and intensity of the drug is achieved when it is administered as an intravenous bolus which is injected within 10 to 30 s. The dependence of its effect on the injection rate is due to the rapidity with which the drug is bound by serum albumin when introduced more slowly. A drop in arterial pressure should be noted within 1 min, with maximal results being achieved in 2 to 5 min. Thereafter blood pressure increases gradually, returning to pretreatment levels within 3 to 15 h. If the initial response is unsatisfactory, a second dose may be given in 30 min. It is recommended that the second dose be given more rapidly than the first.[48]

The most serious potential side effect following the intravenous administration of a bolus of diazoxide to a toxemic patient is significant hypotension. Several series have shown some diastolic pressure drops to levels below 60 mmHg in severe preeclamptic patients with initial readings of 110 mmHg or higher.[56,59,62,69] A number of these patients have also demonstrated concomitant fetal bradycardia.[56,59,62] The standard dose of diazoxide employed in bolus injections has been 300 mg. Ram and Kaplan[81] have demonstrated, however, that in a group of 20 nonpregnant patients with diastolic pressures of 125 mmHg or greater, bolus injections of diazoxide 150 mg every 5 min as needed up to a maximum of 600 mg was successful in reducing the diastolic pressure to 110 mmHg or less. Six of these patients required only one injection, and none of them experienced hypotension.

Severe hypotensive responses have been specifically related to the potentiating effects of other antihypertensive drugs when given either prior or subsequent to administration of diazoxide.[39] These include vasodilating agents such as hydralazine and catecholamine-depleting drugs such as methyldopa or reserpine.

Because sodium and water are retained when diazoxide is used, the concomitant use of furosemide has been advised for the nonpregnant patient who is given this drug.[48] Finnerty[21] has recommended this combination of agents for treating the acutely hypertensive pregnant patient. The use of potent diuretics, however, may well be ill-advised in toxemic patients with significant hypovolemia.[70]

As has been mentioned, diazoxide routinely abolishes spontaneous uterine contractions. Termination of pregnancy is an integral part of the management of severely hypertensive toxemic patients. Should diazoxide be used to manage an acute hypertensive crisis in a toxemic patient, intravenous oxytocin must be administered if vaginal delivery is to be accomplished.

Sodium Nitroprusside. Sodium nitroprusside (SNP) is the most potent and predictably effective agent available for the treatment of hypertensive emergencies. It is uniquely specific for vascular receptors and dilates both resistance and capacitance blood vessels. As with hydralazine and diazoxide, there is no demonstrable effect on the autonomic or central nervous system. Changes in cardiac output and heart rate are variable and seem to be related to the preexisting state of cardiac performance.[67]

Since its action is virtually immediate and very evanescent, nitroprusside must be given by carefully monitored constant infusion. The average adult dose is 3 μg/kg/min and the maximum dose should not exceed 800 μg/min.[35]

Patients receiving this drug are usually asymptomatic if not made hypotensive by excessive infusion. However, prolonged adminsitration can cause cyanide toxicity. Cyanide is liberated by the direct combination of nitroprusside with sulfhydryl groups in red blood cells and tissue. In the liver, circulating cyanide is converted to thiocyanate.

Animal experiments have shown that the placenta is readily permeable to SNP. Naulty et al.[61] found that five out of eight normotensive pregnant sheep required a steadily increasing dose of this agent in order to maintain a reduction in blood pressure of 20 percent for 1 h. A marked accumulation of maternal and fetal cyanide was observed, with fetal blood levels being higher than those in the mother. All the fetuses in this group died. The authors comment that the significant buildup of cyanide could be due either to rapid formation within the fetus or to a slower rate of detoxification and/or excretion. In the remaining three sheep in this study, the therapeutic objective was obtained with a low rate of nitroprusside infusion. All the fetuses in the latter group survived and had low umbilical artery cyanide levels. No significant change in uterine blood flow was detected in either group. Ellis et al.[17] infused sufficient amounts of SNP into pregnant sheep with norepinephrine-induced hypertension to return the BP to control levels and found that neither maternal nor fetal blood samples contained more than 50 μg/L of cyanide. In their series the amount of drug necessary to achieve the therapeutic objective was quite low, and no fetal or maternal deaths occurred in association with this therapy.

Reports of the effects of SNP on uterine blood flow are conflicting. Ring et al.[87] found that SNP infusion did not change the reduction in uterine blood flow caused by phenylephrine-induced hypertension in pregnant ewes. Lieb et al.[51] administered nitroprusside to both normotensive ewes and those with one-kidney hypertension. They noted a progressive decrease in uterine blood flow in both groups, averaging 35 and 25 percent, respectively at the highest infusion rates. Ellis and colleagues[17] on the other hand, found that the administration of SNP to norepinephrine-induced hypertensive pregnant ewes caused a progressive increase in uterine blood flow.

In a small number of women, SNP has been successfully used to create controlled hypertension for intracranial surgery during pregnancy[16,86] and to stabilize the BP and reduce afterload prior to delivery in severe preeclampsia.[68] It has not been studied enough in pregnant patients, however, to adequately define its safety for the human fetus. Some of the animal data cited are worrisome in that they suggest that cyanide toxicity could occur in the fetus while the mother is asymptomatic. Furthermore, infusion of this drug may cause a significant reduction in uterine blood flow. At the current time, therefore, the use of SNP during hypertensive crises in pregnancy should be confined to those patients who are unresponsive to intravenous hydralazine or diazoxide. In that circumstance SNP should only be used to control the acute crisis, and delivery should be performed as quickly as possible thereafter.

Prazosin. Prazosin is a peripheral vasodilator which was released for clinical use in the United States in 1976.[36] Animal studies suggest that it works by relaxing peripheral arterioles secondary to blockade of postsynaptic alpha-receptors.[10] In humans, the drug causes decreased total peripheral resistance but, unlike hydralazine, rarely produces tachycardia.[9,36] It has been recommended that this drug should always be used in combination with a diuretic, because when used alone it is not as good as thiazides in lowering blood pressure.[8] Pretreatment with maximal doses of prazosin has not been shown to affect the hypotensive potency of hydralazine or diazoxide.[98] The antihypertensive effect of prazosin with either of these agents should be additive. Furthermore, Stokes and Oates[98] have speculated that this drug could prove useful in neutralizing the unwanted peripheral alpha-agonist effect of clonidine or those which may accompany sympathetic neuronal blockade.

Prazosin is said to be as effective as hydralazine with fewer adverse sequelae. Its most important side effect is the "first-dose phenomenon," which is a syndrome of severe dizziness and occasional syncope following the first dose. This is probably due to drug-induced hypotension without a compensatory reflex tachycardia to maintain CO. The effect can reportedly be minimized by beginning therapy with a low dose, which is increased gradually.[9,36]

Two sets of investigators[15,54] have studied the combination of prazosin and oxyprenolol in hypertensive obstetrical patients. Both found this combination to be safe for use in pregnancy and effective in the management of essential hypertension. Neither group, however, had impressive results in women with PIH. Davey and Dommisse[15] found that 18 of 50 multigravid women with severe hypertension prior to 36 weeks developed proteinuria while on a regimen of prazosin, oxyprenolol, and hydralazine. In this series 5 infants were stillborn, 4 died neonatally, and 19 were growth-retarded. Lubbe and Hodge[54] treated 17 pregnant women with hypertension, proteinuria, and edema with the combination of prazosin and oxyprenolol. Pregnancy had to be terminated because of inadequate control of BP in 13 of these patients, 11 of whom also required treatment with hydralazine. There were three stillbirths and one neonatal death in this small series. At the present time there is no direct evidence to suggest that prazosin has a role in the management of hypertensive crises during pregnancy.

Nitroglycerin. Nitroglycerin induces hypotension by a direct effect of the drug on vascular smooth muscle. Both resistance and capacitance vessels are dilated, but the effect on the latter is predominant. Fahmy[18] has suggested that it may have a more beneficial effect than SNP on the preservation of adequate myocardial profusion during hypotension induced by these agents. When administered intravenously, nitroglycerin acts rapidly and has a brief duration of action because of prompt hepatic metabolism.

Wheeler et al.[107] found that nitroglycerin caused a reduction in uterine blood flow when given to normotensive pregnant ewes. However, when it was given to either prevent or treat hypertension induced by norepinephrine in these animals, it antagonized the deleterious effect on uterine blood flow which otherwise occurred. Snyder et al.[96] reported the use of this agent in six severely hypertensive women given general anesthesia for cesarean section. The drug was successful in rapidly providing control of the hypertension and blunting the response to endotracheal intubation. No adverse effects on the neonates were detected. Writer et al.,[110] however, demonstrated that nitroglycerin infusion diminishes autoregulation of cerebral blood flow in hypertensive dogs, with an increase in blood flow to the brain occurring despite a reduction in mean arterial pressure (MAP). They caution that any further increase in MAP, such as occurs during endotracheal intubation, could significantly increase intracranial pressure. Since the intracranial dynamics of women with severe PIH may already be disturbed, a sudden increase in MAP could potentially have drastic consequences if nitroglycerin were being used. This issue should be further investigated before the use of nitroglycerin can be recommended for the treatment of hypertensive crises in women with PIH.

HEMODYNAMICS IN PATIENTS WITH SEVERE PIH DURING LABOR AND DELIVERY

Clinical investigations of the cardiopulmonary hemodynamics in severe PIH are difficult to perform because of the large number of important variables which must be kept constant. These include comparable patient populations (e.g., "pure" PIH versus chronic hypertension with superimposed hypertensive crisis in patients with no underlying cardiac disorders), fluid infusion rates, types of fluids infused (e.g., crystalloid versus colloid), medications administered, anesthetic regimen utilized, and type of delivery. Despite the limitations imposed by this problem, studies utilizing flow-directed pulmonary artery (Swan-Ganz) monitoring have provided considerable insight into the effect of severe PIH on the heart and lungs during parturition. This in turn has permitted the establishment of principles which serve as the core for an approach to the management of these critically ill patients.

Severe Toxemia without Pulmonary Edema

Benedetti et al.[5] studied 10 women who satisfied at least one of the American College of Obstetrics and Gynecology criteria for severe preeclampsia. Their MAPs varied between 100 and 153 mmHg and they all had 3 to 4+ proteinuria. All the patients were in early labor at the time of the insertion of a Swan-Ganz catheter. Six of these women delivered vaginally and the other four had cesarean sections under general anesthesia. In the entire group an increase in cardiac output, heart rate, and stroke volume over values in normotensive third-trimester patients was detected during early labor. There were no significant increases in mean pulmonary artery pressure (PAP) or pulmonary capillary wedge pressure (PCWP) when compared with normal, exercising third-trimester patients but there was an increase in systemic vascular resistance (SVR). No significant changes in any of the hemodynamic parameters studied were noted when early labor was compared with the early puerperium. Three patients in this series had central venous pressures (CVP) that did not reflect parallel changes in the PCWP. Finally, when left ventricular function was studied by plotting left ventricular stroke work index (LVSWI) against PCWP on a graph designating various levels of cardiac competence, all the patients had values above the lower limit for normal, and eight of them were in the hyperdynamic range.

Rafferty and Berkowitz[79] have published hemodynamic data from three previously normotensive women who presented in the third trimester with blood pressures of 170/120 mmHg or higher and 3 to 4+ proteinuria. All these women were delivered by cesarean section under general anesthesia although two had received oxytocin stimulation of labor for 4 to 6 h. The patients were all treated with intravenous $MgSO_4$ and had received or were receiving hydralazine during the period studied. The pulmonary arteriolar resistance (PAR) in these women were consistantly found to be within or below the normal nonpregnant range and the pulmonary artery diastolic pressure (PADP)–PCWP gradient did not exceed 7 mmHg in any patient. Normal PAR values for pregnancy are not known. The PCWP values were in the normal range during the antepartum period but rose significantly during delivery and remained elevated in the postpartum period. The cardiac index (CI) and LVSWI were noted to increase at the time of delivery and return to antepartum levels during the postpartum period. Total peripheral resistance (TPR) did not change at the time of delivery but fell postpartum. Finally, all the patients had left ventricular function which was in the normal or hyperdynamic range (Fig. 11-1).

When unpublished data from two additional patients were analyzed, the relationships described above were again observed. One of these patients was a primigravida with a BP of 170/120 mmHg on admission at 33 weeks, and the other was a

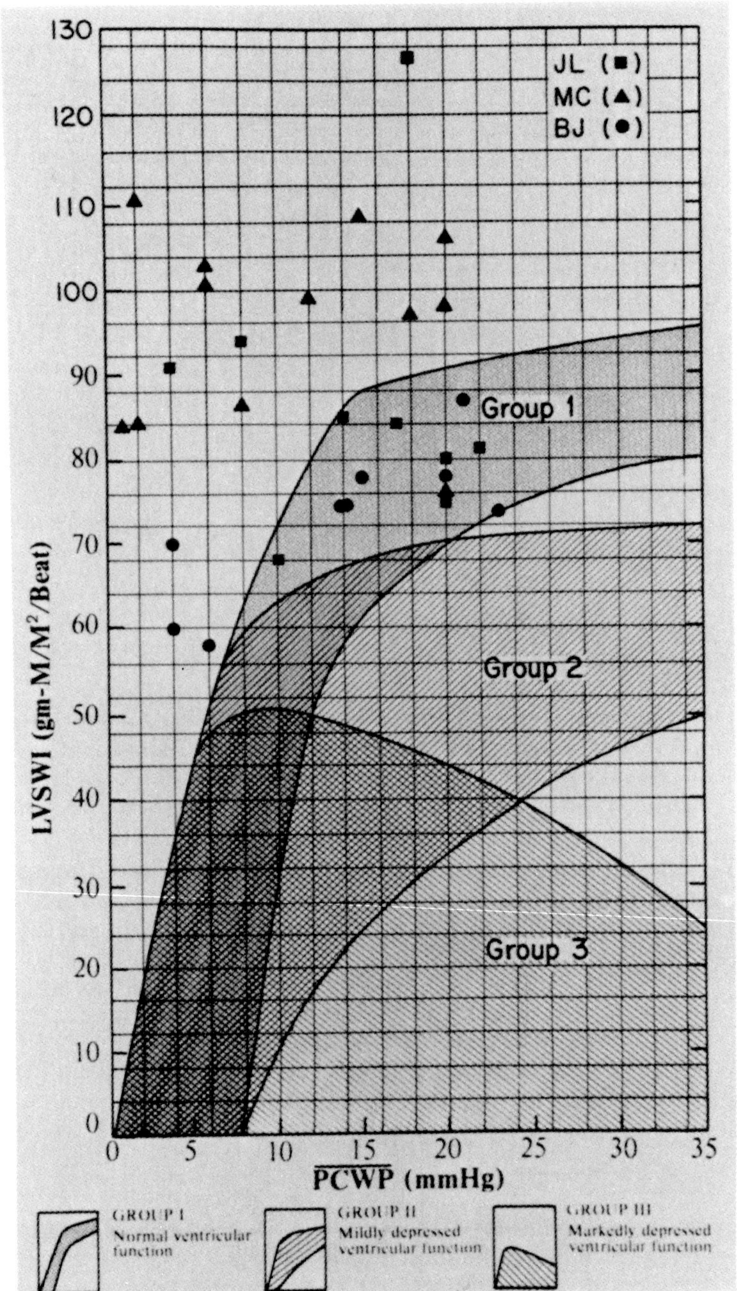

Fig. 11-1 This graph displays the ventricular function of three women with severe PIH during labor, delivery, and the postpartum period. The graph distinguishes among three levels of ventricular competence. Each of the patients demonstrated excellent ventricular function by these criteria, even in the presence of markedly elevated PCWP values. (From Rafferty, T.R. and Berkowitz, R.L.: Hemodynamics in patients with severe toxemia during labor and delivery. Am. J. Obstet. Gynecol., 138:263, 1980.)

chronically hypertensive grand multipara who presented at 24 weeks with a blood pressure of 170/130 mmHg. Both were delivered by cesarean section under general anesthesia. Mean values from these five patients are presented in Table 11-1.

Before considering the implications of these studies, it is important to point out that all these women were receiving drug and fluid therapy while the data were being collected. The data do not, therefore, necessarily provide insight into the natural history of severe hypertension at the time of delivery and must be interpreted with this in mind.

None of the patients studied by Benedetti et al. or by our group showed evidence of left ventricular failure as determined by analysis of their ventricular function curves. Furthermore, none of them had pulmonary hypertension, which suggests that their pulmonary vasculature was not involved in a primary vasospastic process. Because of the wide range of body surface areas (BSA) in our patients we expressed their COs and related variables as indices. Owing to the lack of normative data in obstetrical patients expressed in these terms, it was not possible to make direct comparisons with normotensive women during labor and delivery. Nevertheless, the data obtained from all the patients studied above suggest that their hearts are working hard to overcome significant systemic vascular resistance.

In nonpregnant patients the normal range of PCWP is 7 to 15 mmHg. In our series of five patients the highest PCWP value obtained immediately following the insertion of the Swan-Ganz catheter in the antepartum period was 5 mmHg, and one woman had an initial value of 2 mmHg. the antepartum PCWP values all rose into the normal range when hydration was coupled with antihypertensive therapy. Chesley[11] has stated that in severe toxemia the plasma volume can be decreased by as much as 30 to 40 percent. A decrease in PCWP below the limits of normal may reflect diminished cardiac preload, and in our patients this explanation for the low values is consistent with Chesley's assertion.

Dramatic increases were noted in systemic and pulmonary blood pressures as well as PCWP and CI values in our patients at the time of their delivery by cesarean section. This was undoubtedly due in part to extrusion of blood from the uteroplacental bed into the central circulation, resulting in increased cardiac preload. The rapid induction-intubation sequence associated with the light general anesthesia used in these patients may have compounded the situation.[78] Benedetti et al. did not publish hemodynamic data obtained at the time of delivery.

Table 11-1. Mean Hemodynamic Values from Five Severely Hypertensive Women during Labor and Delivery

	AP	Delivery	PP
Initial PCWP (mmHg)	2–5		
PCWP (mmHg)	7.5 ± 3.6	12.4 ± 1.7*	14.7 ± 1.5*
CI (L/min/m²)	5.2 ± 0.2	6.1 ± 0.4*	5.4 ± 0.4 (N.S.)
LVSWI (g · m/m²)	84.2 ± 11.2	103.1 ± 6.4*	75.6 ± 9.8 (N.S.)
TPR (mmHg min L^{-1} m^2)	21.7 ± 0.9	20.3 ± 0.3 (N.S.)	18.7 ± 0.9 (N.S.)

AP, antepartum; PP, postpartum; PCWP, pulmonary capillary wedge pressure; CI, cardiac index; LVSWI, Left ventricular stroke work index; TPR, total peripheral resistance (indexed as HR units); *, stasticially significant change from AP values (at least $p > 0.05$); N.S., not significantly different from AP values (From Rafferty, T.R. and Berkowitz, R.L.: unpublished data).

Table 11-2. High Output State 7 to 9 Hours Following Delivery

	7 h PP		8 h PP		9 h PP
Measured Values					
CO (L/min)	8.8		9.0		6.7
P (beats/min)	113		112		105
BP (mmHg)	160/90		154/90		116/90
PCWP (mmHg)	23		20		4
Derived Values					
CI (L/min/m²)	6.8		6.9		5.1
SVI (ml/beat/m²)	60.5	HYDRALAZINE 25 mg IV	62.2	FUROSEMIDE 20 mg IV	50.9
LVSWI (g · m/m²)	73.8		77.9		69.9
TPR (mm Hg min L⁻¹ m²)	15.5		15.1		18.8

Following cesarean section under general anesthesia, the only medication this patient had received was a continuous infusion of $MgSO_4$ (1 g/h) and one injection of morphine sulfate (10 mg IM) for pain. She had received 2,400 ml of crystalloid solution over the previous 7 h and had put out 485 ml of urine. The estimated blood loss was 600 ml at the time of delivery. Her urinary output increased to 350 ml in the hour following administration of the furosemide indicated above.

CO, cardiac output; P, pulse; BP, blood pressure; SVI, stroke volume index; for the remaining abbreviations see footnote to Table 11-1. (From Rafferty, T.R. and Berkowitz, R.L.: Hemodynamics in patients with severe toxemia during labor and delivery. Am. J. Obstet. Gynecol., *138*:263, 1980.)

All the patients in the studies being discussed continued to demonstrate excellent left ventricular function in the postpartum period. The patients in our series had all received hydralazine and the cardiovascular effects of this agent include decreased vascular resistance and increased HR, SV, and CI.[48] While hydralazine may have assisted the ventricular performance, it is unlikely to have played a major role because of the inconstancy of its administration and the small doses employed. Despite the excellence of their ventricular function two of our patients required postpartum diuretic therapy because of elevated indices of left-heart filling pressure in the face of fluid restriction. Therapy was directed towards a high output state characterized by hypertension, elevated CI and LVSWI, and PCWP values in excess of 20 mmHg. Illustrative data from one of these patients are shown in Table 11-2.

Severe Toxemia Complicated by Pulmonary Edema

Cardiogenic pulmonary edema is caused by an increase in hydrostatic pressure within pulmonary capillaries, while noncardiogenic pulmonary edema results from an increase in capillary wall permeability. Hydrostatic and colloid osmotic pressures, both within the capillary lumen and in the surrounding interstitium, determine the movement of fluid across capillary walls according to a relationship originally described by Starling. These pressures cannot easily be measured in interstitial fluid, but PCWP reflects intravascular hydrostatic pressure, and plasma colloid osmotic pressure (COP) can be measured directly with a commercially available oncometer. Within a capillary, hydrostatic pressure tends to move fluid from the lumen into the intravascular space while COP pulls fluid from the interstitium into the vessel lumen. Some authors feel that a clinically useful estimate of the net intravascular fluid filtration pressure can be obtained by simply subtracting the PCWP from the plasma COP. In normal supine nonpregnant individuals the COP-PCWP gradient ranges from 9 to 17 mmHg, and some reports have suggested that a reduction in this gradient may be associated with the development of pulmonary edema even at relatively low PCWP values.[14,97] Other authors have not found the COP-PCWP gradient to be a useful parameter to follow in patients at risk to develop pulmonary edema.[80,106] This subject is covered in more detail in Chapters 1 and 3 but it is mentioned here because of its potential relevance in understanding the etiology of pulmonary edema in women with severe PIH.

Normal pregnant women have been shown to have a decline in COP from prepregnant values of 27.6 ± 2.3 mmHg to 22.4 ± 1.9 mmHg at term.[89] Benedetti and Carlson[4] measured COP in normal ambulatory women when they presented in labor at term and from these same patients in the supine position 6 and 24 h postpartum. Mean values were 22.0 ± 0.5 mmHg prior to delivery and 18.2 ± 0.5 mmHg postpartum. They also found that a group of women with PIH had values which were significantly lower than these. This is not surprising, since a fall in COP might be expected in patients with significant proteinuria. One hypertensive patient in their series developed pulmonary edema with a moderately elevated PCWP of 18 mmHg. That woman's COP was 13 mmHg and therefore her COP-PCWP gradient was −5 mmHg. This patient was simply treated with fluid restriction and the pulmonary edema resolved within 24 h of delivery. Is this case representative of women with PIH who develop pulmonary edema, and what role should COP determinations play in the evaluation of that condition?

In 1977 Freund et al.[23] published a case report of a 22-year-old primagravida who presented at 34 weeks gestation with a BP of 180/140 mmHg. At the time of cesarean section she was found to have a placental abruption, and 3,500 ml of ascites was present in her peritoneal cavity. Postoperatively, she had x-ray evidence of pulmonary edema, and a Swan-Ganz catheter was inserted. Data obtained 12 h postpartum revealed an elevated PCWP (24 mmHg), a decreased plasma volume index (23.7 ml/kg), a decreased plasma COP (12 mmHg) and a markedly decreased CI (2.8 L/min/m^2). Details of therapy are not given, but it included infusions of colloidal fluids and injections of furosemide. The only other central data presented are a set of values obtained 36 h after delivery. These reveal a reduction of PCWP (12 mmHg), an increase in plasma volume index (30.7 ml/kg), no change in COP, and a further reduction in CI (2.4 L/min/m^2). Pulse rates of 120 and 132 per minute at 12 and 36 h postpartum were recorded. The patient steadily improved and recovered completely. The data presented in this report suggest that there was significant compromise in cardiac function. The patient's LVSWI and PCWP values demonstrated moderately depressed ventricular function and the reduced COP may have aggravated the potential for pulmonary edema to occur. The COP-PCWP gradient was −12 and 0 mmHg 12 and 36 h postpartum.

Strauss et al.[100] have provided central hemodynamic data from three severely toxemic women who developed cardiogenic pulmonary edema. Their case histories are as follows.

1. A 25-year-old secundigravida was diagnosed as being hypertensive at 32 weeks and started on phenobarbital and methyldopa. One week later she presented in pulmonary edema with a BP of 190/140 mmHg. Treatment with furosemide, hydralazine, digoxin, and morphine reduced the BP to 160/100 mmHg with little symptomatic improvement. The PCWP was 33 mmHg, CVP 8 mmHg, and CO 5 L/min. Treatment with sodium nitroprusside infusion reduced the BP to 175/90 mmHg and CO increased to 9.5 L/min. With continued infusion of SNP, the PCWP fell to 20 mmHg and a cesarean section was performed 30 min after infusion of that drug had been started. Postpartum the SNP was increased until MAP fell to 80 mmHg and PCWP to 11 mmHg. The cardiac silhouette narrowed but pulmonary edema persisted and the patient was hypoxemic on 40 percent oxygen. Constant positive airway pressure (CPAP) was administered by face mask and the PO_2 increased from 54 to 131 mmHg. Digoxin and methyldopa therapy were resumed, the patient was weaned from SNP and CPAP over 48 h, and the x-ray evidence of pulmonary edema resolved entirely by the fifth postoperative day. Improvement continued, and 4 months after discharge the patient was normotensive and asymptomatic on no medications.

2. A 35-year-old secundigravida with no history of hypertension or heart disease presented at 37 weeks with severe toxemia and pulmonary edema. After receiving hydralazine and furosemide, she was transferred to the authors' hospital and her BP was 170/125 mmHg on admission. Her PCWP and CVP were initially 23 and 10 mmHg, respectively, and her CO was 4.7 L/min. Following continuous hydralazine infusion, the MAP and PCWP fell to 110 and 20 mmHg, respectively, and the CO increased to 6 L/min. Cesarean section was performed uneventfully, and postoperatively she was controlled with methyldopa, digoxin, and intermittent hydralazine. Hypoxemia was treated with CPAP. Her CO ranged from 6 to 8 L/min and the pulmonary edema had cleared by 72 h after surgery. She was discharged on methyldopa.

3. A 25-year-old multipara who had been hypertensive during her first pregnancy presented at 34 weeks with a BP of 190/110 mmHg and a normal cardiopulmonary examination. Cesarean section under general anesthesia was performed and postoperatively her BP rose to 190/135 mmHg despite repeated doses of hydralazine and morphine. Three hours after surgery she developed respiratory distress, and a chest x-ray demonstrated pulmonary edema and cardiomegaly. Eight hours later her MAP was 120 mmHg, her PCWP was 22 mmHg, her CVP was 18 mmHg, and her CO was 4.6 L/min. Sodium nitroprusside was started. It initially lowered the MAP to 115 mmHg, with a concomitant increase in CO to 8.84 L/min and fall in PCWP and CVP to 16 and 9 mmHg, respectively. Further reduction in the MAP to 85 to 90 mmHg resulted in stabilization of the PCWP (11 to 14 mmHg), CVP (6 to 11 mmHg), and CO (7.5 to 10.4 L/min). The SNP was slowly tapered over 36 h and the patient gradually improved. She was discharged on no medications.

These three women with no evidence of preexisting heart disease or fluid overload developed acute pulmonary edema in association with severe PIH. The first two cases showed evidence of dissociation between left and right ventricular function since their initial PCWP values were elevated (33 and 23 mmHg) in the face of normal CVPs (8 and 10 mmHg). The third case presented with elevations of both the PCWP and CVP (33 and 23 mmHg). All these patients showed an immediate and dramatic improvement following reductions in afterload with effective arteriolar vasodilation. The initial effect of fairly low-dose therapy was a near doubling of CO without significant changes in BP or pulse. It was necessary to produce relatively hypotensive arterial pressures in some of these cases in order to achieve optimal cardiopulmonary function, but this was done in the postpartum period. Interestingly, two of these patients required the use of SNP after hydralazine had failed to adequately lower BP. Unfortunately, it was not possible to plot the relationship of LVSWI to PCWP in these patients because of insufficient data in the case reports. However, the dramatic increase in CO following the reduction in afterload and continued improvement thereafter suggest that the cardiogenic pulmonary edema was not due to an inherent problem in myocardial contractility. Plasma COP values were not reported for these patients. It is certainly possible that abnormally low COP-PCWP gradients were present and aggravated the pulmonary edema, but the elevated hydrostatic pressures were significant in and of themselves in these cases.

ANESTHESIA FOR THE PATIENT WITH SEVERE PIH

Epidural anesthesia is a potentially useful adjunct to the management of obstetrical patients with hypertensive crises. The lumbar sympathetic blockade it causes results in generalized vasodilation in the pelvis and lower extremities with subsequent venous pooling of blood. The major reason usually given for avoiding the use of epidural anesthesia in women with PIH is that their decreased intravascular volume puts them at increased risk for a dramatic hypotensive response to the sympathetic blockade.[73] It has been demonstrated, however, that epidural analgesia and/or anesthesia can be safely and effectively used if appropriate volume replacement with either crystalloid[43] or colloid[44] solutions is administered prior to performing the chemical sympathectomy.

Effective lumbar epidural analgesia eliminates the necessity of administering narcotics and sedatives and reduces the maternal production of endogenous catecholamines. When used as anesthesia for cesarean section in women with severe PIH, the dangerous hemodynamic changes which may accompany endotracheal intubation can be avoided. Hodgkinson et al.[40] studied 20 severely preeclamptic patients receiving either epidural or general anesthesia for cesarean section. The MAP, PAP, and PCWP were recorded every 5 min for 60 min prior to surgery and every 2 min during anesthesia. The 10 patients receiving general anesthesia had these pressures recorded every minute during intubation and extubation. The latter group showed highly significant mean increases in MAP, PAP, and PCWP during intubation and extubation. One patient's BP increased from 200/90 mmHg to 360/150 mmHg during suction and extubation. On the other hand, the 10 women receiving epidural anesthesia showed a slight decrease in MAP with no significant change in PAP and PCWP. The authors conclude that tracheal intubation of patients with severe gestational hypertension may initiate hemodynamic responses which lead to an increased risk of cerebral hemorrhage. Occasionally, however, epidural anesthesia is contraindicated in women with severe PIH. These situations include the need to perform an emergency cesarean section for fetal distress, when the time necessary to achieve a satisfactory anesthetic level or adequately prehydrate the patient would further compromise the fetus, and a coagulopathy, in which the risk of an intraspinal hematoma is increased.

These issues are all discussed in more detail in Chapter 5, along with guidelines for administering lumbar epidural anesthesia to severely hypertensive patients and an approach to the therapy of postblockade hypotension, should it occur.

MAGNESIUM SULFATE AND THE PREVENTION OF CONVULSIONS

Debate rages over the effectiveness of $MgSO_4$ in preventing eclamptic convulsions, with obstetricians usually claiming that it does and neurologists and internists insisting that it does not. The major argument given by the former group is that it is almost universally used in the management of severe preeclampsia in the United States and that when it is used in appropriate doses, the incidence of seizures is extremely low. The latter group argues that since $MgSO_4$ in therapeutic doses does not cross the blood-brain barrier, it has no central effect and consequently its curariform action on motor end plates only blocks the peripheral response to eclampsia-induced cortical dysfunction. It is also argued that while the peripheral action of $MgSO_4$ may diminish the hyperreflexia elicited by a reflex hammer, it is the concomitant use of antihypertensive agents which truly prevents most preeclamptic patients from seizure.

$MgSO_4$ is not an effective antihypertensive agent and its use in the management of women with severe PIH is confined specifically to its purported antiseizure activity. The drug is an integral part of Pritchard's management of preeclampsia, and his group has published extraordinarily good results with their therapeutic approach to this disease.[75] It is true, however, that some women have had seizures with blood levels of Mg^{2+} documented to be in the therapeutic range.[95] A more detailed analysis of the argument for and against the effectiveness of this drug in preventing eclamptic seizures is beyond the scope of this chapter. The interested reader is referred to an article by Pritchard[74] defending the use of this agent and Chapter 13 in this book for the opposing view.

RECOMMENDATIONS

On Admission

All patients with the acute onset of severe hypertension in pregnancy should be admitted to the delivery floor for evaluation and stabilization. Since termination of the pregnancy is the most important part of the definitive management of PIH, the overwhelming majority of these patients should be delivered after being stabilized. Very occasionally, however, a rapid response to minimal therapy in a woman with a pulmonically immature fetus permits continued observation in the hospital in an attempt to allow the fetus to mature further in utero.

The initial approach to a severely hypertensive obstetrical patient includes taking a history for seizures, abdominal pain, episodes of bleeding, recent urinary output, current medications, the presence of contractions, and the status of the membranes. The physical examination should focus on the state of consciousness, focal neurological abnormalities, vascular changes in the eye grounds, auscultatory evidence of pulmonary edema or cardiac abnormalities, signs of right ventricular failure, upper abdominal or uterine tenderness, the presence of fetal heart tones, the status of the reflexes, the degree of edema, and the presence of bleeding sites or petichiae. A pelvic examination should be performed to evaluate the dilatation and effacement of the cervix. Vital signs must be taken at least every 5 min until they are stable and an external fetal heart rate monitor must be applied to the maternal abdomen for continuous monitoring. An intravenous infusion should be started with a crystalloid solution delivered through an 18-gauge catheter. A Foley catheter should be inserted and hourly input and output determinations charted. Blood should be sent for a complete blood count, platelet count, type and crossmatch, blood urea nitrogen, creatinine, uric acid, serum glutamic oxylacetic transferase, and albumin/globulin ratio. A hematocrit determination should be performed on the delivery floor, along wth a peripheral smear to look for evidence of microangiopathic hemolytic anemia (the presence of schistocytes) and significant platelet depletion. A specimen of 5 ml of whole blood is placed in a plain glass test tube, which is inverted every 30 s, and the time necessary for clotting to occur is recorded. A complete urine analysis should be performed by the laboratory, but the protein content should be assessed by dipstick analysis on the delivery floor.

If abnormal neurologic signs are found, a neurologist should be urgently consulted in order to assist with the diagnosis and management of cerebral edema or an intracranial hemorrhage (see Ch. 13). If an overt coagulopathy is evident, the patient should be treated for disseminated intravascular coagulopathy, as described in Chapter 9. In this setting the possibility of a placental abruption is very high and must be ruled out.

These initial steps are not controversial and should be part of the management of all women with acutely severe hypertension. From this point on, however, management approaches may vary considerably. I will describe the approach I use and try to point out where facts end and opinions begin.

General Approach When Pulmonary Edema Is Not Present

Many investigators have shown that women with PIH are intravascularly depleted. The severity of the circulating volume reduction seems to be proportional to the degree of hypertension.[43,44] This is consistent with the very low initial PCWP values found in our series of centrally monitored severely hypertensive women. If the generalized vasospasm of PIH is rapidly reversed without concomitant replacement of a significant intravascular deficit, the potential exists for diminished perfusion of the maternal brain, kidneys, and uteroplacental circulation. In our series it was possible to raise the PCWP into the normal range by infusing crystalloid solution while concomitantly reducing systemic blood pressure with hydralazine. Cardiac output increased significantly at the time of delivery in our patients but returned to antepartum values shortly thereafter. The PCWP remained elevated, however, and some of our patients developed a hyperdynamic state which was consistent with intravascular volume overload. This may have been due to overvigorous hydration or to the mobilization of extravascular fluid in the postpartum period in association with suboptimal renal function. Conclusions reached from this interpretation of our data have resulted in the set of simple management principles described below.

Acutely hypertensive women are significantly volume-depleted and should be treated with a limited fluid challenge over a period of 1 to 2 h. Response to this therapy should be followed with hourly urinary outputs and serial hematocrit determinations. Concurrently, BP should be lowered to the range of 140 to 160/100 to 110 mmHg with a rapidly acting arteriolar dilator. I think that diuretics are contraindicated at this time because of their potential for reducing flow to the uteroplacental unit. After a urinary output of 30 ml/h or greater has been established, the fluid infusion should be cut back to a relatively low maintenance rate in order to prevent overexpansion of the intravascular space and reduce the potential for cardiac overload or cerebral edema.[6] I favor the cautious administration of epidural anesthesia after the BP has been stabilized and satisfactory urinary output has been demonstrated in patients who have no evidence of fetal distress. This frequently allows one to control the BP with lower doses of antihypertensive agents. Postpartum infusion of crystalloid solutions should be reduced even further because of the increased risk of volume overload. Diminished urinary output at this time should be treated either with the infusion of colloid solutions or the administration of a parenteral diuretic. Finally, although I admit that questions about $MgSO_4$ remain unresolved, I continue to use it. I am impressed with its safety when used appropriately and have personally rarely seen a patient have a seizure when being treated with it. If a woman does have a convulsion while $MgSO_4$ is being administered, however, a Mg^{2+} blood level should be sent to the laboratory and the hourly intravenous dose increased. If she has another seizure pending the laboratory results or if the Mg^{2+} is found to be in the therapeutic range at the time of the convulsion, I would switch to an infusion of intravenous Dilantin for continued antiseizure prophylaxis.

Specific Recommendations for Therapy

Fluids Administration. I administer a crystalloid solution (D5W/0.45 percent saline) in doses of 500 ml every half hour up to a total of 2,000 ml. The therapeutic objective at this point is to maintain a urinary output of 30 ml/h or greater. No advantage is obtained by increasing the urinary output to more than 30 ml/h and therefore when this rate has been achieved, the rate of fluid infusion should be cut back to 125 ml/h. If the initial fluid challenge does not produce the appropriate renal response, central monitoring is instituted in order to safely push more fluids. A Swan-Ganz catheter is preferable to a CVP line because of the discrepancies which have been shown to exist between PCWP and CVP values in some patients with severe PIH.[5] It should be stressed, however, that most patients will respond to the initial fluid challenge with an appropriate diuresis and consequently will not need central monitoring. Rolbin et al.[91] have presented four cases of patients with severe PIH who had central monitoring and advocate that "all patients with severe preeclampsia should have cardiac filling pressures monitored." I do not agree with this statement and feel that most, if not all, of the cases in their small series could have been managed safely and effectively without Swan-Ganz catheters.

Joyce and Loon[44] have shown that albumin infused in 25-g increments over 30 min in association with Ringer's lactate solution delivered at a rate of 75 ml/h is capable of achieving a rise in CVP of 6 to 8 mmHg in patients with severe PIH. Furthermore, this regimen may cause less of an elevation in the postpartum PCWP than the infusion of larger amounts of crystalloid solution during the antepartum period. There is a 20- to 30-min lag in increased urinary output following the albumin infusion, however, and therefore the physician must either exercise greater patience in evaluating the effectiveness of the infusion or use central monitoring to be sure that the patient's intravascular space is not being overexpanded.

Postpartum, the infusion of crystalloid solution should be slowed to a rate of 75 ml/h and the patient checked frequently for the development of tachypnea, tachycardia, cyanosis, or auscultatory evidence of pulmonary edema. Again, a urinary output of 30 ml/h is completely satisfactory and therapy is not necessary to increase it above this level. If the urinary output falls below 30 ml/h for 2 h, 20 to 40 mg furosemide can be administered intravenously or, alternatively, 25 g albumin infused over half an hour.

Drugs. Hydralazine is the antihypertensive drug of choice for the treatment of severe PIH because of its proven effectiveness in reversing the vasoconstriction which is the hallmark of that condition. Despite recommendations to the contrary,[12,20] I feel that the concomitant use of furosemide is contraindicated unless cardiogenic pulmonary edema is evident. The objective of antihypertensive therapy in these patients should be to relieve vascular spasm while at the same time repleting their diminished intravascular volume. Reduction in BP for maternal indications should not compromise the fetus by diminishing flow to the uteroplacental unit. The use of a potent diuretic is counterproductive because it aggravates the depletion of intravascular volume and increases the difficulty of maintaining an adequate circulating blood volume after vasodilation has been accomplished.

The initial dose of hydralazine should be 5 mg given intravenously, since some patients respond dramatically to small doses of this drug. Thereafter the drug can be administered in 5- to 20-mg intravenous boluses every 20 to 30 min until the BP is brought into the range of 140 to 160/100 to 110 mmHg. Once this has been achieved, intermittent bolus therapy or administration of a continuous hydralazine drip is usually quite effective in maintaining reasonable pressures until the delivery has been accomplished.

If sustained maternal tachycardia in excess of 140 beats per minute occurs in response to hydralazine therapy and delivery is not imminent, intravenous propranolol may be cautiously administered to nonasthmatic patients. Women with healthy hearts who do not depend on sympathetic stimulation to maintain effective cardiac output should not be compromised by the use of this drug. Short-term exposure to propranolol has not been shown to adversely affect the fetus except for causing some difficulty in initiating spontaneous respiration at birth. This, of course, should be anticipated and neonatologists must be present at the time of delivery to provide respiratory support to the infant if this is necessary. Propranolol is administered intravenously by slowly injecting 1 mg every 5 min up to a maximum of 5 mg until the desired reduction in heart rate has been achieved. Continuous maternal EKG monitoring is mandatory during this period. Serial blood sugars must be followed closely in diabetic women who have been given propranolol.

Despite the successful use of diazoxide in toxemic patients, the reports of profound hypotensive responses to the rapid bolus administration of 300 mg of this drug are a matter for concern. Perhaps this will prove to be less of a problem if the drug is administered in 150-mg boluses, but that has not yet been demonstrated to be true in obstetrical patients. Furthermore, diazoxide must never be administered in conjunction with either hydralazine or methyldopa, as these combinations have been reported to result in BP dropping to levels as low as 60/0 mmHg. Since a reduction in diastolic pressure below 90 mmHg may significantly reduce uterine perfusion, diazoxide is not an optimal drug for the management of women with severe PIH. If it is used at all to treat an obstetric patient having an acute hypertensive episode, it should probably be administered in 150-mg boluses. It must also be the *first* antihypertensive agent employed, and after its use hydralazine should not be administered for a minimum of 4 h. Ideally, any woman with PIH who is treated with diazoxide should have been given sufficient intravenous fluid prior to its use to raise her CVP to 6 to 8 mmHg. If a hypotensive episode occurs following its administration, the initial therapy should be the rapid infusion of 1 L of crystalloid solution. The use of sympathomimetic agents such as norepinephrine to restore BP should be avoided unless there is no response to the infusion of fluids, and this will almost never be the case. Maternal blood sugars should be monitored regularly and a cord blood glucose obtained from the neonate. Oxytocin administration may be necessary in order to reinstitute uterine contractions which are routinely abolished by the diazoxide.

In those rare situations in which hydralazine is unsuccessful in lowering the BP of a severely hypertensive obstetrical patient or when an emergency cesarean section must be performed under general anesthesia in a woman whose BP has not yet been stabilized, I recommend the use of sodium nitroprusside. Despite theoretical considerations about dangers to the fetus, SNP has been used successfully in a small number of selected cases. The action of the drug is very rapid and of short duration. The solution must be prepared freshly for each use, wrapped in foil to protect it from light, and delivered by infusion pump. The infusion should be started at a rate of 0.5 μg/kg/min and steadily increased in small increments until the therapeutic objectives have been achieved.

The principal concern regarding the use of SNP is based on animal studies which suggest that the fetus might be particularly vulnerable to cyanide toxicity. Maternal hepatic function is often compromised in severe PIH, and since the liver is intimately involved in cyanide metabolism, the potential for toxicity may be increased in this setting. Because of this concern the pregnancy should obviously be terminated as rapidly as possible after the SNP has stabilized the maternal BP. Until more human data exist, it is probably wise to follow the advice of Strauss et al.[100] and to limit fetal exposure to this drug to 30 min or less.

If an epidural anesthetic has been administered prior to giving the SNP, it will complement the action of that drug. Furthermore, if a sympathetic blockade above the level of T4 has been achieved, there will be a reduction in maternal heart rate secondary to the decrease in sympathetic cardiac stimulation. However, it frequently takes 15 to 20 min following administration of an epidural blockade to achieve sufficient sensory anesthesia to perform a cesarean section. As this necessary delay will prolong the fetal exposure to maternal SNP, it is not worth postponing the delivery in order to avoid the use of general anesthesia in this setting. This is particularly true when SNP is being administered because the proper use of this agent can effectively control the dramatic swings in BP accompanying intubation and extubation, which are the greatest concerns about the use of general anesthesia in women with severe PIH.

$MgSO_4$ may be administered either intravenously or intramuscularly. I prefer the former route because it is far less painful and provides more predictable blood levels. A loading dose of 4 g is infused over 20 min and then a maintenance dose of 1 to 2 g/h delivered. Reflexes should be checked every half hour and the maintenance dose adjusted accordingly. This drug is generally quite safe to administer as long as maternal urinary output is satisfactory and attention is paid to these basic guidelines. I usually continue infusing $MgSO_4$ for 24 h following delivery in cases of severe PIH but will prolong this period for an additional 12 to 24 h if significant hyperreflexia or clonus persists.

After delivery has been accomplished, the physician has much more latitude in treating maternal hypertension because fetal well-being is no longer a consideration. In the immediate postpartum period the agent which has successfully controlled the BP prior to delivery should be continued. This usually will mean that intermittent bolus therapy with hydralazine will be all that is necessary. If SNP has been used, this infusion should be continued until it can be safely tapered. It should be remembered that many of these women will have been delivered by cesarean section and often will have BP elevations secondary to the release of catecholamines associated with pain. The treatment of choice in this setting is obviously the provision of effective analgesia, usually with intravenous morphine or meperidine.

If therapy is necessary for more than 48 h following delivery, oral medication should be started. A thiazide diuretic alone or in combination with methyldopa or propranolol is the regimen I employ. The parenteral antihypertensive agent being administered should be continued as indicated during the first 24 to 36 h of oral therapy.

Delivery. Delivery is the ultimate key to the management of PIH. Whatever it is that sets this process in motion is effectively reversed when the patient is no longer pregnant. On rare occasions, women with the acute onset of severe hypertension dramatically respond to bed rest and minimal antihypertensive therapy. In those situations in which the fetus is very immature, there is an irresistible temptation to leave the patient undelivered and hope for further development in utero to occur. These patients, however, are often extremely labile and may suddenly worsen at any time. They must therefore be carefully watched in the hospital and delivered quickly if their condition, or that of the fetus, deteriorates. In the vast majority of cases, however, delivery should be accomplished as part of the therapy of the acute hypertensive crisis.

In the absence of fetal distress or a life-threatening maternal complication of PIH, it is not necessary to perform a cesarean section soon after admission. The fetus must be monitored and the maternal BP stabilized, but in the absence of obstetrical contraindications there is time in most cases to attempt a vaginal delivery. This will be better for the mother because it avoids the risks of a major anesthetic, abdominal surgery with its attendant problems of blood loss, and implications for future deliveries if a cesarean section is performed. Regardless of the initial Bishop score it is often possible to successfully induce labor in women with severe PIH.[75] The membranes should be artificially ruptured as soon as possible and an oxytocin infusion started when the BP has been stabilized. If after 6 to 8 h there has been no appreciable progress toward delivery, I feel that a cesarean section should be performed unless the patient has been so easy to control that further efforts at a vaginal delivery seem warranted. In most cases she will either be well into the active stage at this point or will have proved herself to be extremely labile, and the decision as to the route of delivery will be fairly straightforward.

Pulmonary Edema

When pulmonary edema is present in an undelivered woman with severe PIH, the physician is faced with an extremely difficult situation because inappropriate therapy for the maternal problem may adversely affect the fetus. It is therefore essential to evaluate the central hemodynamics in this situation in order to more rationally evolve a treatment plan.

If the patient is suffering from respiratory distress, she must be offered symptomatic relief as quickly as possible. Oxygen should be delivered by face mask and intravenous morphine and a single dose of 20 mg furosemide administered. As soon as the patient is comfortable, a Swan-Ganz catheter (or as a poor second choice a CVP line) and an arterial line should be introduced. Blood gases, PAP, PCWP, and if possible the COP should be determined. It is also extremely helpful to calculate the LVSWI so that a hemodynamic tracking profile can be constructed (see Ch. 1). If the PCWP is high and ventricular function is suboptimal, therapy consists of relief of vasospasm with hydralazine or SNP, cardiac support with digoxin, and reduction of intravascular volume with the judicious use of furosemide. If the PCWP is low and left ventricular function is normal, however, the pulmonary edema is noncardiogenic in origin and treatment should consist of positive airway pressure and volume expansion as necessary (see Ch. 20). Unless there are clinical or historical clues to suggest the presence of noncardiogenic pulmonary edema, cardiogenic origin is more likely and therefore I feel the empirical administration of a single dose of furosemide is warranted prior to obtaining objective confirmation of an elevated PCWP. When elevated hydrostatic pressures are present, the COP may shed light on the role of hypoproteinemia in aggravating the situation. If the COP-PCWP gradient is abnormally low and the PCWP is high, the cautious use of solutions containing albumin may accelerate the reversal of the pulmonary edema while helping to maintain an intravascular volume which is adequate to prevent significant reductions in uteroplacental flow following vasodilatory therapy. Obviously, the maternal PCWP must be carefully followed when colloidal solutions are infused in this situation. It must also be remembered that the pulmonary edema may be significantly worsened by the infusion of albumin if capillary permeability in the lungs has been altered to the point that this material can gain access to the interstitial fluid.

Once stabilized, women with pulmonary edema and severe PIH should be delivered as rapidly as possible and then cared for in an intensive care setting in cooperation with appropriate consultants. Their management in the postpartum period consists of following the same principles utilized prior to delivery, but again this is easier because fetal well-being is no longer a consideration. The report of Strauss et al.[100] suggests that these women recover fairly rapidly after delivering if they have been managed aggressively during the antepartum period and do not suffer from underlying cardiac disease. For a discussion of the management of congestive failure in obstetrical patients with heart disease, the reader is referred to Chapter 19.

REFERENCES

1. Aitken, R.R. and Drake, C.G.: A technique of anesthesia with induced hypotension for surgical correction of intracranial aneurysms. Clin. Neurosurg., *21*:107, 1974.
2. Altstatt, L.B.: Transplacental hyponatremia in the newborn infant. J. Pediatr., *66*:985, 1965.
3. Assali, N.S. and Vaughn, D.L.: Blood volume in pre-eclampsia: fantasy and reality. Am. J. Obstet. Gynecol., *129*:355, 1977.
4. Benedetti, T.J. and Carlson, R.W.: Studies of colloid osmotic pressure in pregnancy-induced hypertension. Am. J. Obstet. Gynecol., *135*:308, 1979.
5. Benedetti, T.J., Cotton, D.B., Read, J.C., and Miller, F.C.: Hemodynamic observations in severe preeclampsia with a flow-directed pulmonary artery catheter. Am. J. Obstet. Gynecol., *136*:465, 1980.
6. Benedetti, T.J. and Quilligan, E.J.: Cerebral edema in severe pregnancy-induced hypertension. Am. J. Obstet. Gynecol., *137*:860, 1980.
7. Black, H.R.: Management of hypertension. Primary Care, *4*:13, 1977.
8. Black, H.R.: Prazosin. Drugs in Patient Care, Yale-New Haven Hospital 6(10), 1978.
9. Brogden, R.N., Heel, R.C., Speight, T.M., and Avery, G.S.: Prazosin: a review of its pharmacological properties and therapeutic efficacy in hypertension. Drugs, *14*:163, 1977.
10. Cambridge, D., Davey, M.J., and Massingham, R.: The pharmacology of antihypertensive drugs with special reference to vasodilators, α-andrenergic blocking agents and prazosin. Med. J. Aust., spec. supp. 2,2, 1977.
11. Chesley, L.C.: Hypertensive Disorders in Pregnancies. p. 203. Appleton-Century-Crofts, Norwalk, Conn., 1978.
12. Clark, A.D., Sevitt, L.H., and Hawkins, D.F.: Use of furosemide in severe toxaemia of pregnancy. Lancet, *1*:35, 1972.

13. Cockburn, J., Ounsted, M., Moar, V.A., and Redman, C.W.G.: Final report of study on hypertension during pregnancy: The effects of specific treatment on the growth and development of the children. Lancet, *1*:647, 1982.
14. daLuz, P.L., Shubin, H., Weil, M.H. et al.: Pulmonary edema related to changes in colloid osmotic and pulmonary artery wedge pressure in patients after acute myocardial infarction. Circulation, *51*:350, 1975.
15. Davey, D.A. and Dommisse, J.: The management of hypertension in pregnancy. Response to Letter to the Editor by Lubbe, W.F. S. Afr. Med. J., 59:320, 1981.
16. Donchin, Y., Amirav, B., Sahar, A., and Yarkoni, S.: Sodium nitroprusside for aneurysm surgery in pregnancy. Br. J. Anaesth., *50*:849, 1978.
17. Ellis, S.C., Wheeler, A.S., James, F.M. et al.: Fetal and maternal effects of sodium nitroprusside used to counteract hypertension in gravid ewes. Am. J. Obstet. Gynecol., *143*:766, 1982.
18. Fahmy, N.R.: Nitroglycerin as a hypotensive drug during general anesthesia. Anethesiology, *49*:17, 1978.
19. Feitelson, P.J. and Lindheimer, M.D.: Management of hypertensive gravidas. J. Reprod. Med., *8*:111, 1972.
20. Ferris, T.F. Toxemia and hypertension. In Burrow, G.N., and Ferris, T.F. Eds.: Medical Complications during Pregnancy, 2nd Ed. W.B. Saunders, 1982.
21. Finnerty, F.A., Jr.: Hypertension in pregnancy. Clin. Obstet. Gynecol., *18*:145, 1975.
22. Fisher, K.A., Luger, A., Spargo, B.H., and Lindheimer, M.D.: Hypertension in pregnancy: clinical-pathological correlations and remote prognosis. Medicine, *60*:267, 1981.
23. Freund, U., French, W., Carlson, R.W. et al.: Hemodynamic and metabolic studies of a case of toxemia of pregnancy. Am. J. Gynecol., *127*:206, 1977.
24. Frishman, W.H.: β-Adrenoceptor antagonists: new drugs and new indications. N. Engl. J. Med., *305*:500, 1981.
25. Frishman, W.H.: Atenolol and Timolol, two new systemic β-adrenoceptor antagonists. N. Engl. J. Med., *306*:1456, 1982.
26. Frohlich, E.D.: The sympathetic depressant antihypertensives. Drug Therapy, May/June, 1975, p. 24.
27. Gallery, E.D.M., Saunders, D.M., Hunyor, S.H., and Gyory, A.Z.: Randomised comparison of methyldopa and oxprenolol for treatment of hypertension in pregnancy. Br. Med. J., *1*:1591, 1979.
28. Gant, N.F., Madden, J.D., Siiteri, P.K., and MacDonald, P.C.: The metabolic clearance rate of dehydroisoandrosterone sulfate. III. The effect of thiazide diuretics in normal and future pre-eclamptic pregnancies. Am. J. Obstet. Gynecol., *123*:159, 1975.
29. Gant, N.F., Madden, J.D., Siiteri, P.K., and MacDonald, P.C.: The metabolic clearance rate of dehydroisoandrosterone sulfate. IV. Acute effects of induced hypertension, hypotension, and naturesis in normal and hypertensive pregnancies. Am. J. Obstet. Gynecol., *124*:143, 1976.
30. Gibbs, C.E. and Locke, W.E.: Maternal deaths in Texas, 1969–1973: A report of 501 consecutive deaths from the Texas Medical Association's Committee on Maternal Health. Am. J. Obstet. Gynecol., *126*:687, 1976.
31. Gladstone, G.R., Hordof, A., and Gersony, W.M.: Propranolol administration during pregnancy: effects on the fetus. J. Pediatr., *86*:962, 1975.
32. Goldby, F.S. and Beilin, L.J.: Relationship between arterial pressure and the permeability of arterioles to carbon particles in acute hypertension in the rat. Cardiovasc. Res., *6*:384, 1972.
33. Goodlin, R.C.: Beware the great imitator—severe preeclampsia. Contemp. Obstet. Gynecol., *20*:215, 1982.

34. Goodman, L.S. and Gilman, A.: p. 573. In: The Pharmacological Basis of Therapeutics. 5th Ed., Macmillan, New York, 1975.
35. Goodman, L.S. and Gilman, A.: p. 715. In: The Pharmacological Basis of Therapeutics. 5th Ed., MacMillan, New York, 1975.
36. Graham, R.M. and Pettinger, W.A.: Prazosin. N. Engl. J. Med., *300*:232, 1979.
37. Gray, M.J.: Use and abuse of thiazides in pregnancy. Clin. Obstet. Gynecol., *11*:568, 1968.
38. Hallum, J.L. and Hatchuel, W.L.F.: Congenital paralytic ileus in a premature baby as a complication of hexamethonium therapy for toxemia of pregnancy. Arch. Dis. Child., *29*:354, 1974.
39. Henrich, W.L., Cronin, R., Miller, P.D., and Anderson, R.J.: Hypotensive sequelae of diazoxide and hydralazine therapy. JAMA, *237*:264, 1977.
40. Hodgkinson, R., Husain, F.J., and Hayashi, R.H.: Systemic and pulmonary blood pressure during caesarean section in parturients with gestational hypertension. Can. Anaesth. Soc. J., *27*:389, 1980.
41. Holland, O.B. and Kaplan, N.M.: Propranolol in the treatment of hypertension. N. Engl. J. Med., *294*:930, 1976.
42. Johnston, C.I. and Aickin, D.R.: The control of high blood pressure during labor with clonidine ("Catapres"): Med. J. Aust. *2*:132, 1971.
43. Joyce, T.H. III, Debnath, K.S., and Baker, E.A.: Preeclampsia—relationship of CVP and epidural analgesia. Anesthesiology, *51*:S297, 1979.
44. Joyce, T.H. III and Loon, M.: Pre-eclampsia: Effect of albumin 25% infusion. Anesthesiology, *55*:A313, 1981.
45. Kelly, J.V.: Drugs used in the management of toxemia of pregnancy. Clin. Obstet. Gynecol., *20*:395, 1977.
46. Koch-Weser, J.: Correlation of pathophysiology and pharmacotherapy in primary hypertension. Am. J. Cardiol., *32*:499, 1973.
47. Koch-Weser, J.: The vasodilator antihypertensives. Drug Therapy, May/June 1975, p. 17.
48. Koch-Weser, J.: Diazoxide. N. Engl. J. Med., *294*:1271, 1976.
49. Koch-Weser, J.: Hydralazine. N. Engl. J. Med., *295*:320, 1976.
50. Ladner, C.N., Weston, P.V., Brinkman, C.R., and Assali, N.S.: Effects of hydralazine on uteroplacental and fetal circulations. Am. J. Obstet. Gynecol., *108*:375, 1970.
51. Lieb, S.M., Zugaib, M., Nuwayhid, B. et al.: Nitroprusside-induced hemodynamic alteration in normotensive and hypertensive pregnant sheep. Am. J. Obstet. Gynecol., *139*:925, 1981.
52. Lieberman, B.A., Stirrat, G.M., Cohen, S.L. et al.: The possible adverse effect of propranolol on the fetus in pregnancies complicated by severe hypertension. Br. J. Obstet. Gynaecol., *85*:678, 1978.
53. Lindheimer, M.D. and Katz, A.I.: Sodium and diuretics in pregnancy. N. Engl. J. Med., *288*:891, 1973.
54. Lubbe, W.F. and Hodge, J.V.: Combined α- and β-adrenoceptor antagonism with prazosin and oxprenolol in control of severe hypertension in pregnancy. NZ Med. J., *94*:169, 1981.
55. Lubbe, W.F., Hodge, J.V., and Kellaway, G.S.M.: Antihypertensive treatment and fetal welfare in essential hypertension in pregnancy: A retrospective survey of experience with various regimes at National Women's Hospital, Auckland, 1970–80. NZ Med. J., 95:1, 1982.
56. Michael, C.A.: Intravenous diazoxide in the treatment of severe pre-eclampsia, toxaemia and eclampsia. Aust. NZ. J. Obstet. Gynaecol., *13*:143, 1973.
57. Minielly, R., Yuzpe, A.A., and Drake, C.G.: Subarachnoid hemorrhage secondary to ruptured cerebral aneurysm in pregnancy. Obstet. Gynecol., *53*:64, 1979.

58. Minkowitz, S., Soloway, H.B., Hall, J.E., and Yermakov, V.: Fatal hemorrhagic pancreatitis following chlorothiazide administration in pregnancy. Obstet. Gynecol., *24:*337, 1964.
59. Morris, J.A., Arce, J.J., Hamilton, C.J. et al.: The management of severe preeclampsia and eclampsia with intravenous diazoxide. Obstet. Gynecol., *49:*675, 1977.
60. Naeye, R.L. and Friedman, E.A.: Causes of perinatal death associated with gestational hypertension and proteinuria. Am. J. Obstet. Gynecol., *133:*8, 1979.
61. Naulty, J., Cefalo, R.C., and Lewis, P.E.: Fetal toxicity of nitroprusside in the pregnant ewe. Am. J. Obstet. Gynecol., *139:*708, 1981.
62. Neuman, J., Weiss, B., Rabello, Y. et al.: Diazoxide for the acute control of severe hypertension complicating pregnancy: a pilot study. Obstet. Gynecol., 53 suppl., 50S, 1979.
63. Nies, A.S.: Adverse reactions and interactions limiting the use of antihypertensive drugs. Am. J. Med., *58:*495, 1975.
64. Nies, A.S. and Shand, D.G.: Hypertensive response to propranolol in a patient treated with methyldopa—a proposed mechanism. Clin. Pharmacol. Ther., *14:*823, 1973.
65. Nuwayhid, B., Brinkman, C.R., III, Katchen, B., and Symchowicz, S.: Maternal and fetal hemodynamic effects of diazoxide. Obstet. Gynecol., *46:*197, 1975.
66. Oakes, G.K., Walker, A.M., Ehrenkranz, R.A., and Chez, R.A.: Effect of propranolol infusion on the umbilical and uterine circulations of pregnant sheep. Am. J. Obstet. Gynecol., *126:*1038, 1976.
67. Palmer, R.F. and Lasseter, K.C.: Sodium nitroprusside. N. Engl. J. Med., *292:*294, 1975.
68. Paull, J.: Clinical report of the use of sodium nitroprusside in severe pre-eclampsia. Anaesth. Intensive Care, *3:*72, 1975.
69. Pennington, J.C. and Picker, R.H.: Diazoxide and the treatment of the acute hypertensive emergency in obstetrics. Med. J. Aust. *2:*1051, 1972.
70. Perkins, R.P.: Diazoxide in treatment of severe pre-eclampsia and hypertensive encephalopathy. Am. J. Obstet. Gynecol., *126:*296, 1976.
71. Pevehouse, B.C. and Boldrey, E.: Hypothermia and hypotension for intracranial surgery during pregnancy. Am. J. Surg. *100:*633, 1960.
72. Poulton, T.J., James, F.M., III, and Lockridge, O.: Prolonged apnea following trimethaphan and succinylcholine. Anesthesiology, *50:*54, 1979.
73. Pritchard, J.A. and McDonald, P.C. Eds. p. 219 in: Williams Obstetrics. 15th Ed., Appleton-Century-Crofts, Norwalk, Conn., 1976.
74. Pritchard, J.A.: Management of preeclampsia and eclampsia. Kidney Int., *18:*259, 1980.
75. Pritchard, J.A. and Pritchard, S.A.: Standardized treatment of 154 consecutive cases of eclampsia. Am. J. Obstet. Gynecol., *123:*543, 1975.
76. Pritchard, J.A. and Walley, P.J.: Severe hypokalemia due to prolonged administration of chlorothiazide during pregnancy. Am. J. Obstet. Gynecol., *81:*1241, 1961.
77. Pruyn, S.C., Phelan, J.P., and Buchanan, G.C.: Long-term propranolol therapy in pregnancy: Maternal and fetal outcome. Am. J. Obstet. Gynecol., *135:*485, 1979.
78. Prys-Roberts, L.T., Meloche, G.R., and Foex, P.: Studies of anesthesia in relation to hypertension. II. Haemodynamic consequences of induction and endotracheal intubation. Br. J. Anaesth., *43:*531, 1971.
79. Rafferty, T.D. and Berkowitz, R.L.: Hemodynamics in patients with severe toxemia during labor and delivery. Am. J. Obstet. Gynecol., *138:*263, 1980.
80. Rafferty, T.D., Ljungquist, R., Firestone, L. et al.: The plasma colloid oncotic pressure–pulmonary artery occlusion pressure gradient—a poor predictor of pulmonary edema in surgical intensive care unit patients. Arch. Surg. (in press).
81. Ram, C.V.S. and Kaplan, N.M.: Individual titration of diazoxide dosage in the treatment of severe hypertension. Am. J. Cardiol., *43:*627, 1979.

82. Redman, C.W.G.: Treatment of hypertension in pregnancy. Kidney Int., *18:*267, 1980.
83. Redman, C.W.G., Beilin, L.J., and Bonnar, J.: Treatment of hypertension in pregnancy with methylalopa: blood pressure control and side effects. Br. J. Obstet. Gynecol., *84:*419, 1977.
84. Redman, C.W.G., Beilin, L.J., Bonnar, J., and Ounsted, M.K.: Fetal outcome in trial of antihypertensive treatment in pregnancy. Lancet, *2:*753, 1976.
85. Reed, R.L., Cheney, C.B., Fearon, R.E. et al.: Propranolol therapy throughout pregnancy: a case report. Anesth. Analg. (Cleve) *53:*214, 1974.
86. Rigg, D. and McDonogh, A.: Use of sodium nitroprusside for deliberate hypotension during pregnancy. Br. J. Anaesth., *53:*985, 1981.
87. Ring, G., Krames, E., Shnider, S.M. et al.: Comparison of nitroprusside and hydralazine in hypertensive pregnant ewes. Obstet. Gynecol., *50:*598, 1977.
88. Roberts, J.M. and Perloff, D.L.: Hypertension and the obstetrician-gynecologist. Am. J. Obstet. Gynecol., *127:*316, 1977.
89. Robertson, E.G. and Cheyne, G.A.: Plasma biochemistry in relation to oedema of pregnancy. J. Obstet. Gynecol. Br. Commonw., *79:*769, 1972.
90. Rodriguez, S.U., Leikin, S.L., and Hiller, M.C.: Neonatal thrombocytopenia associated with antepartum administration of thiazide drugs. N. Engl. J. Med., *270:*881, 1964.
91. Rolbin, S.H., Cole, A.F.D., and Hew, E.M.: Haemodynamic monitoring in the management of severe pre-eclampsia and eclampsia. Can. Anaesth. Soc. J., *28:*363, 1981.
92. Rubin, P.C.: Beta-blockers in pregnancy. N. Engl. J. Med., *305:*1323, 1981.
93. Sandstrom, B.: Antihypertensive treatment with the adrenergic beta-receptor blocker metoprolol during pregnancy. Gynecol. Obstet. Invest., *9:*195, 1978.
94. Schifrin, B.S., Spellacy, W.N., and Little, W.A.: Maternal death associated with excessive ingestion of a chlorothiazide diuretic. Obstet. Gynecol., *34:*215, 1969.
95. Sibai, B.M., Lipshitz, J., Anderson, G.D., and Dilts, P.V.: Reassessment of intravenous $MgSO_4$ therapy in preeclampsia-eclampsia. Obstet. Gynecol., *57:*199, 1981.
96. Snyder, S.W., Wheeler, A.S., and James, F.M.: The use of nitroglycerin to control severe hypertension of pregnancy during cesarean section. Anesthesiology, *51:*563, 1979.
97. Stein, L., Beraud, J.J., Morissette, M. et al.: Pulmonary edema during volume infusion. Circulation, *52:*483, 1975.
98. Stokes, G.S. and Oates, H.F.: Comparative and interaction studies with peripherally acting hypotensive agents. Med. J. Aust., specl suppl., *2:*9, 1977.
99. Stoll, C., Levy, J.M., and Beshara, D.: Robert's syndrome and clonidine. J. Med. Genet., *16:*486, 1979.
100. Strauss, R.G., Keefer, R., Burke, T., and Civetta, J.M.: Hemodynamic monitoring of cardiogenic pulmonary edema complicating toxemia of pregnancy. Obstet. Gynecol., *55:*170, 1980.
101. Sullivan, J.M.: Blood pressure elevation in pregnancy. Prog. Cardiovasc. Dis., *16:*373, 1974.
102. Tarazi, R.C.: The diuretic antihypertensives. Drug Therapy, May/June 1975, p. 11.
103. Thorley, K.J., McAinsh, J., and Cruickshank, J.M.: Atenolol in the treatment of pregnancy-induced hypertension. Br. J. Clin. Pharmacol., *12:*725, 1981.
104. Tunstall, M.E.: The effect of propranolol on the onset of breathing at birth. Br. J. Anaesthesia *41:*792, 1969.
105. Vink, G.J., Moodley, J., and Philpott, R.H.: Effects of hydralazine on the fetus in the treatment of maternal hypertension. Obstet. Gynecol. *55:*519, 1980.
106. Virgilio, R.W., Smith, D.E., Rice, C.L. et al.: Effect of colloid osmotic pressure and pulmonary capillary wedge pressure in intrapulmonary shunt. Surg. Forum, *27:*168, 1976.
107. Wheeler, A.S., James, F.M., Meis, P.J. et al.: Effects of nitroglycerin and nitroprusside on the uterine vasculature of gravid ewes. Anesthesiology, *52:*390, 1980.

108. Wilson, F. and Sedzimir, C.B.: Hypothermia and hypotension during craniotomy in a pregnant woman. Lancet, *2*:947, 1959.
109. Woods, J.R. and Brinkman, C.R.: The treatment of gestational hypertension. J. Reprod. Med., *15*:195, 1975.
110. Writer, W.D.R., James, F.M., Stullken, E.H., and Koontz, F.A.: Intracranial effects of nitroglycerin—an obstetrical hazard? Anesthesiology, *53*:S309, 1980.
111. Yudkin, J.S.: Withdrawal of clonidine. Lancet, *1*:546, 1977.

12

Asthma and Other Severe Respiratory Diseases during Pregnancy

Michael S. Niederman, M.D.
Richard A. Matthay, M.D.

The respiratory system adapts to the physiologic stress of pregnancy more easily than does the cardiovascular system; however, pulmonary disease frequently manifests itself during pregnancy and labor, imparting life-threatening risks to both mother and fetus.[18] Awareness of the physiologic changes affecting the lung during gestation will allow the physician not only to recognize and reassure the 60 to 76 percent of normal women who experience symptomatic dyspnea during pregnancy, but also to diagnose the early manifestations of severe respiratory illness in previously normal women. During pregnancy, this population can be affected by pulmonary infections, pulmonary embolus, or labor-associated aspiration pneumonitis. Although chronic respiratory illness in women of childbearing age is not common, conditions such as restrictive lung disease, asthma, cystic fibrosis, and other obstructive lung diseases do occur and must be properly evaluated and treated to avoid progression to life-threatening complications for mother and fetus.

In this chapter, we first review diagnostic techniques, including history and physical examination, pulmonary function tests, arterial blood gases, and radiographic tests. Then, we summarize the physiologic alterations of the respiratory system during pregnancy. Specific illnesses in women with chronic disease as well as those who were previously normal are discussed. Special attention is given to the following areas: (1) how women with chronic respiratory illness can be recognized, followed, and managed to prevent progression to extreme illness; (2) how pregnancy alters the course of chronic respiratory disease; (3) how disease can affect both maternal and fetal outcomes during pregnancy; and (4) how pharmacologic treatment of lung disease can be undertaken to minimize adverse affects to both mother and fetus.

Other chapters in this book deal with the topics of ventilator management, adult respiratory distress syndrome (ARDS), amniotic fluid embolization, and noncardiogenic pulmonary edema. These are not discussed further here. Pulmonary tuberculosis, rarely an advanced and life-threatening illness today, is discussed in detail elsewhere and is omitted in this discussion of severe respiratory illness during pregnancy.[75,85]

PULMONARY EVALUATION OF THE PREGNANT PATIENT

History and Physical Examination

An accurate history of the pregnant woman will help identify the patient with respiratory disease. Inquiry should focus on symptoms of shortness of breath, degree of exercise limitation, cough (which can be the sole manifestation of bronchial asthma), sputum production (a clue to the diagnosis of chronic bronchitis or bronchiectasis), wheezing and chest tightness, fever, chills, night sweats (a clue to the presence of active tuberculosis), and hemoptysis. History of heavy smoking or respiratory illness is particularly helpful in identifying potential high-risk patients. Physical examination can demonstrate the presence of wheezing, rales, rhonchi, expiratory prolongation, pleural rubs and effusions, lobar consolidation, or chest wall abnormalities.

The most common respiratory symptom that the physician must evaluate is dyspnea. As many as 60 to 76 percent of previously normal women note dyspnea at some time during pregnancy, usually beginning in the first or second trimester but being most prevalent at term.[16,28,56] This symptom often is not a sign of underlying heart or lung disease; features that help to distinguish physiologic from pathologic dyspnea are its improvement with exercise and with the progression of gestation.[16,28] There is no widely accepted explanation for this dyspnea, but some believe that it results from an awareness of the "new" sensation of hyperventilation accompanying pregnancy.[16] In support of this theory is the frequent improvement or stabilization of dyspnea as pregnancy progresses and the sensation of hyperventilation becomes less "new." In addition, women with chronic respiratory insufficiency are accustomed to a sensation of hyperventilation and rarely note subjective dyspnea at rest during pregnancy.[25] One study showed that maximum dyspnea correlated with the time of lowest arterial carbon dioxide tension, suggesting a role for hypocarbia in mediating this symptom.[28]

Arterial Blood Gases

Arterial blood sampling can give valuable data about maternal oxygenation and acid-base status. Proper evaluation of this information and its impact on fetal well-being are discussed below. Because of the well-documented risks of fetal hypoxia and the good response of umbilical-vein oxygen tension to maternal oxygen administration, arterial blood gas data should be obtained in the mother with any acute respiratory complaint. For maximal fetal safety, oxygen should be administered to keep maternal arterial oxygen tension greater than 70 mmHg, and blood gas determination should be used to properly titrate the pharmacologic effect of oxygen administration.

The adequacy of alveolar gas exchange can be assessed by calculating the alveolar-arterial oxygen tension gradient. If ideal alveolar oxygen tension ($P_{A}O_2$) greatly exceeds arterial oxygen tension (PaO_2), gas exchange is abnormal because of a mismatching of alveolar ventilation and perfusion or because of right-to-left shunting of unoxygenated blood. To assess the $(A - a)O_2$ gradient, arterial blood gas sampling is necessary to measure PaO_2. Ideal alveolar oxygen tension ($P_{A}O_2$) is calculated as follows:

$$P_{A}O_2 = F_{I}O_2 \times (P_{B} - 47) - PaCO_2/0.8$$

where $F_{I}O_2$ = fractional percent of inspired oxygen
P_{B} = barometric pressure
47 = water vapor pressure
$PaCO_2$ = arterial blood tension of carbon dioxide
0.8 = respiratory quotient

This equation states that ideal alveolar oxygen tension equals the tension of oxygen in inspired air minus the amount of oxygen taken up by the lung in exchange for carbon dioxide. This latter exchange relationship, the respiratory quotient, is equal to 0.8 volume of carbon dioxide released in exchange for every volume of oxygen delivered.

As an example, if arterial blood gas analysis showed pH = 7.40, $PaCO_2$ = 32 mmHg, and PaO_2 = 105 mmHg in a 30-year-old patient breathing room air (21 percent oxygen) at a barometric pressure of 760 mmHg, then:

$$\begin{aligned} P_{A}O_2 &= 0.21\,(760 - 47) - 32/0.8 \\ &= 110 \text{ mmHg} \end{aligned}$$

Since PaO_2 = 105 mmHg, the $(A - a)O_2$ gradient is equal to 110 minus 105 or 5 mmHg.

In the nonpregnant patient, $(A - a)O_2$ gradients vary with age.[7] While a prediction formula for the expected range of normal is useful in the nonpregnant patient, it is not applicable during pregnancy. In one study, the mean $(A - a)O_2$ gradient in normal pregnant women in the supine position during the third trimester was 20 mmHg. That mean was exceeded in 11 of 23 patients, and the highest value was 35 mmHg.[4] In the sitting position, the mean $(A - a)O_2$ gradient decreased to 14.3 mmHg. In another study of normal obstetric patients, arterial PO_2 increased by 13 mmHg in changing from supine to sitting, and arterial PCO_2 decreased by 2 mmHg, leading to a net decrease in $(A - a)O_2$ gradient of 10 mmHg.[2] Since most acute lung diseases are accompanied by an increased $(A - a)O_2$ gradient, we recommend that this be assessed with the pregnant patient in the upright position and be considered abnormal if it exceeds 25 mm Hg. It is important to emphasize that blood gas analysis should be accompanied by calculation of the gradient, because on casual observation, with the usual decreased PCO_2 of pregnancy, a "normal" PaO_2 can be seen even with an abnormally increased $(A - a)O_2$ gradient.

Pulmonary Function Testing

Basic pulmonary parameters are defined as follows (Fig. 12-1)[11]:

Total lung capacity (TLC): The volume of air in the lungs at maximal inspiration
Vital capacity (VC): The maximum amount of air that can be exhaled after a maximal inspiration to TLC
Residual volume (RV): The volume of air remaining in the lung after a vital capacity maneuver
Tidal volume (VT): The volume of air inhaled or exhaled with each breath
Functional residual capacity (FRC): The volume of air remaining in the lungs after an ordinary expiration
Forced vital capacity (FVC): The volume of air exhaled during a rapid forced expiration starting at full inspiration
Forced expiratory volume in 1 second ($FEV_{1.0}$): The volume of air expelled in 1 s during a forced expiration starting at full inspiration

Lung volumes can be calculated after a patient has breathed insoluble helium by measuring the extent of gas dilution. Clinical spirometry can be used to study airway function by measuring rates and volumes of air flow. Abnormal spirometry usually is classified as a pattern that is either obstructive or restrictive. Normal spirometric lung values are within 20 percent of a predicted normal, which is based on the patient's age, sex, height, and weight. A restrictive pattern is present when total lung capacity is below 80 percent of the predicted normal.[79] With restrictive disease, air flow rate, expressed by FEV_1 as a percent of FVC (FEV_1/FVC), is frequently greater than 85 percent. Restrictive ventilatory defects are caused by skeletal, neuromuscular, pleural, interstitial, and alveolar diseases that lead to a reduction in lung volume. Sarcoidosis and chest-wall deformity are the most common restrictive lung diseases seen in women of childbearing age.

An obstructive pattern is present when FEV_1/FVC is less than 75 percent and FEV_1 is less than 80 percent of predicted volume. Lung volumes may be normal or they may be increased if air is trapped as a result of early airway closure. Asthma is the most common obstructive airway disease encountered during pregnancy.

As can be seen in Figure 12-2, the spirogram can help the clinician determine whether a reduction in vital capacity is the result of a restrictive or obstructive

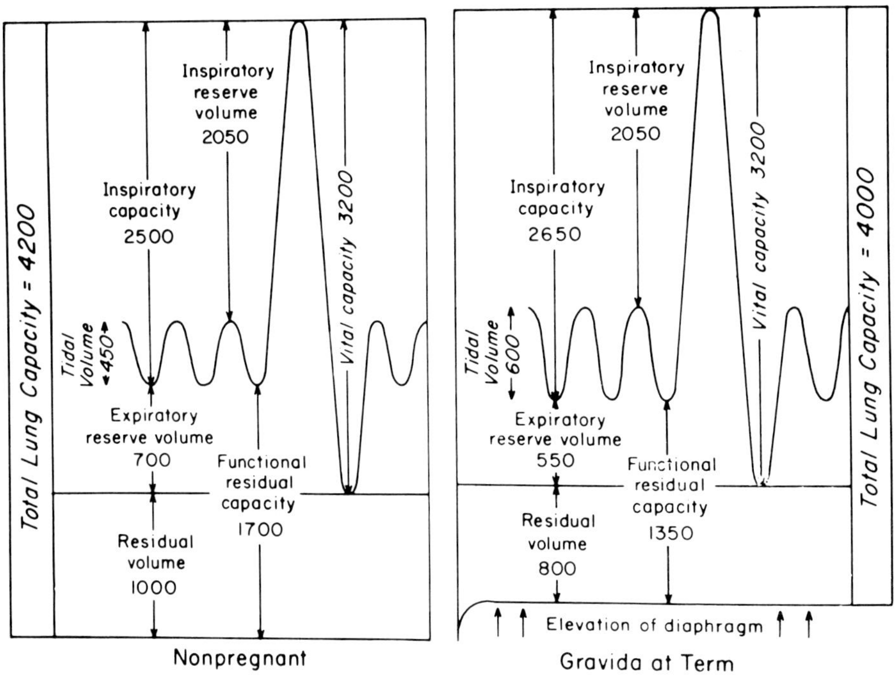

Fig. 12-1 Pulmonary volumes and capacities in the normal nonpregnant woman and the gravida at term. (Reproduced with permission from Leontic, E.A.: Respiratory disease in pregnancy. Med. Clin. North Am., *61*:111, 1977.)

disease. In the restrictive disease, FEV_1/FVC is normal or supranormal, while in the obstructive disease, this ratio is reduced.

When a patient with lung disease seeks advice about the risks of pregnancy, pulmonary function studies should be obtained. In addition to assessing the patient's current pulmonary status, data obtained from these studies will help classify her condition. This is important because there is good evidence that while patients with restrictive lung disease tolerate pregnancy well, those with obstructive disease vary widely in their tolerance of pregnancy.[25,85]

No strict guideline can be given as to the level of pulmonary function that will prohibit a safe pregnancy. As a rough rule of thumb, a patient with a vital capacity less than 1 L will have significant difficulties, although pregnancy has been tolerated well in a patient with a vital capacity of 800 ml.[44] If the FEV_1 exceeds 1 L, the maximal breathing capacity will be 35 to 40 times this, or 35 to 40 L/min. Since resting minute ventilation at term rarely exceeds 15 L/min, such a woman would be breathing at less than 50 percent of her maximum breathing capacity and thus not experience dyspnea at rest. As further protection for the patient with respiratory insufficiency, resting ventilation during pregnancy is increased less in this group than in normals.[25] Studies in patients with restrictive lung disease due to lung resection demonstrate a potential for normal pregnancy and fetal development.[50] Indeed, even intrapartum lung resection has been done when necessary without adverse outcome.[77] In view of these data, a woman with a respiratory disease that is unlikely to deteriorate during pregnancy (this is more likely for restrictive than obstructive dis-

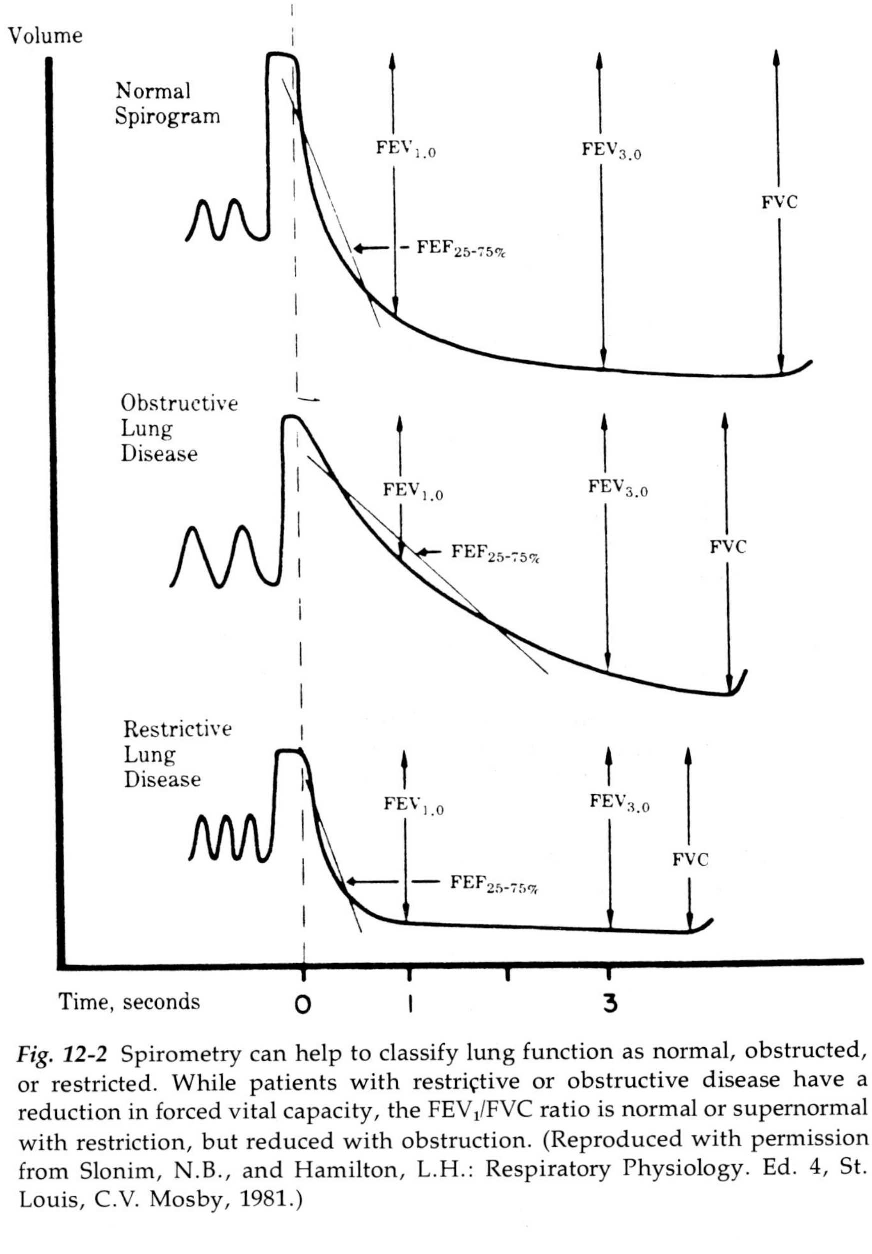

Fig. 12-2 Spirometry can help to classify lung function as normal, obstructed, or restricted. While patients with restrictive or obstructive disease have a reduction in forced vital capacity, the FEV_1/FVC ratio is normal or supernormal with restriction, but reduced with obstruction. (Reproduced with permission from Slonim, N.B., and Hamilton, L.H.: Respiratory Physiology. Ed. 4, St. Louis, C.V. Mosby, 1981.)

eases), an FEV_1 greater than 1 L, and no dyspnea at rest, can undertake pregnancy safely.

When a pregnant patient must undergo general anesthesia, either for cesarean section or for emergency surgery, pulmonary function should be assessed. Postoperative respiratory complications of atelectasis, inadequate secretion clearance, infection, or respiratory failure are more likely to occur when the FEV_1 is less than 2 L.[78] A higher FEV_1 is required to tolerate surgery than to tolerate pregnancy alone because of an expected reduction of lung function in the immediate postoperative period.

To assess the patient with respiratory complaints properly, pulmonary function data are useful, both in the evaluation of maternal risk during pregnancy and surgery and as an aid in the management of patients with obstructive airway disease. This is particularly true in the asthmatic woman, in whom baseline and serial FEV_1 and FEV_1/FVC measurements should be obtained to follow disease status and to assess the severity of exacerbations.

Radiographic Testing

Excessive radiation during pregnancy is undesirable because it exposes the fetus to risks of congenital anomaly, increased frequency of cancer, and spontaneous genetic mutation. While any radiation in the first trimester is theoretically dangerous, the risk of congenital anomaly is increased by 1 to 3 percent if a woman receives more than 5 rads to the pelvis in the first trimester.[76] A posteroanterior chest radiograph, however, should never be omitted if indicated by history or physical examination, since it exposes the fetus to only 36 mrads.[76] Thus, if chest radiography is inadvertently performed on a pregnant patient, the fetal risk is minimal. If, however, radiography must be done in a woman who is known to be pregnant, this minimal risk can be reduced further by shielding the abdomen with a lead apron so that the fetus receives virtually no radiation.[10] A semielective radiograph is best delayed until the second trimester. It is our belief that routine chest radiographs are unnecessary during pregnancy and that they should be performed only in patients with clinical signs or symptoms suggesting lung disease. When this approach is followed, significant disease is not overlooked.[10]

When chest radiographs are performed in the pregnant patient, one should be aware of normal findings that differ from those seen in nonpregnant women of childbearing age.[51] Specifically, the diaphragm may be elevated 4 cm at term but there will be a compensatory increase in anteroposterior diameter. Also, lung markings may be increased, giving a false impression of mild congestive heart failure.

PHYSIOLOGY OF THE RESPIRATORY SYSTEM DURING PREGNANCY

Changes in Pulmonary Mechanics and Ventilation

Serial studies of pulmonary volumes and ventilation in normal women during pregnancy have been performed by many investigators, but one of the earliest comprehensive studies was made by Cugell et al. in 1953.[16,51] These authors observed an increase in pulmonary ventilation at rest that exceeded the increased oxygen consumption associated with pregnancy and thus resulted in hyperventilation as early as the first trimester. At term, ventilation was 48 percent above normal, while oxygen consumption was only increased 21 percent[63] (Fig. 12-3). Because of the early onset of this change, they suspected that hormonal, not mechanical, factors were mediating this increased ventilation. Indeed, others have shown that progesterone probably leads to increased ventilation by increasing the respiratory center's sensitivity to CO_2.[58] Cugell and colleagues found that in normal pregnant women, even as the uterus enlarged, the diaphragm continued to move normally and the increase in minute ventilation was achieved by an increase in tidal volume and not by an increase in respiratory rate. As tidal volume increased, the dead space-to-tidal volume ratio decreased, explaining the hypocarbia and chronic compensated respiratory alkalosis seen during pregnancy. Other observations in this study included preservation of vital capacity as inspiratory capacity increased and expiratory reserve volume decreased. The second half of pregnancy saw a slight reduction in FRC (18 percent), RV, and TLC caused by compression of the resting lung by elevated intra-abdominal pressure secondary to uterine enlargement (Fig. 12-1).

These changes in respiratory function were not observed in pregnant patients with restrictive lung disease resulting from previous removal of functioning lung tissue. In these patients, ventilation changed inversely with the degree of baseline respiratory insufficiency.[25] Thus, the patients with the most severe baseline deficits had the smallest increase in ventilation during pregnancy. Also, the increase in ventilation that did occur was achieved by an increased respiratory rate, not by an increased tidal volume, which was already stressed to full capacity in these patients.

Airway function studies in normal pregnant women have shown no change in airway conductance or FEV_1.[58,85] No change has been seen in studies of small airway function (airways < 2 mm diameter) during pregnancy, except for closing volume. Closing volume is the lung volume at which the small airways in the dependent lung zones begin to collapse. During tidal breathing, in normals, end tidal volume (or FRC) exceeds closing volume. However, in pregnancy, closing volume can exceed

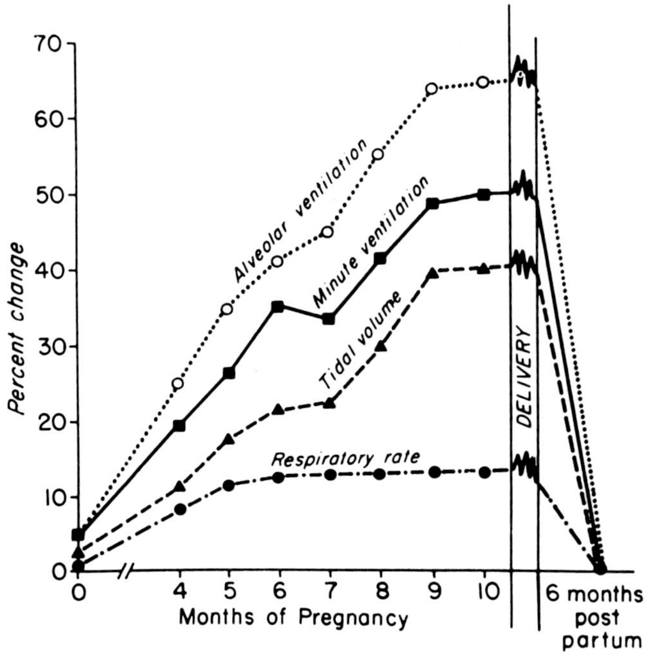

Fig. 12-3 Changes in respiratory function during pregnancy. (Reproduced from Leontic, E.A.: Respiratory disease in pregnancy. Med. Clin. North Am., *61*:111, 1977.)

FRC owing to an increase in VC and a decrease in FRC.[26,58] This finding means that during pregnancy, dependent lung zones may collapse during normal ventilation.[4] Airway closure above FRC is particularly marked in the supine position.[2,4] Although many authors have shown that closing volume can exceed FRC because the latter is reduced, only one study has shown an actual increase in closing volume.[26] The explanation for this observation is not known, and the observation itself has been questioned by others.[58]

Studies of diffusing capacity have shown a slight increase during the first trimester, a slow decrease until a plateau level at 27 weeks, and then a slow return to normal postpartum.[58] Some authors have suggested that the fall in diffusion is caused by an estrogen-medicated increase in acid mucopolysaccharides in the alveolar capillary membrane, but this has not been proved.[58,85]

In summary, pulmonary function testing in the normal pregnant patient shows an increased minute ventilation due to an increased tidal volume, with no change in respiratory rate. In the second half of pregnancy, FRC and TLC are reduced, but vital capacity does not change in spite of an elevation of the diaphragm. Air flow rates do not change in normals, but closing volume may be increased above FRC. Diffusing capacity will show a slight decline after the first trimester.

Arterial Blood Gases and Acid-Base Status

As mentioned, pregnancy is accompanied by a hormonally mediated increase in ventilation, leading to hypocarbia and chronic respiratory alkalosis. Arterial carbon dioxide tensions range from 27 to 32 mmHg (normal 38 to 45 mmHg) while pH remains in the range of 7.40 to 7.45 because of compensatory renal bicarbonate loss to a serum level of 18 to 21 mEq/L (normal 24 to 30 mEq/L).[85] Appreciation of the primary respiratory and secondary metabolic basis of these changes has led to abolishing the previously held concept of "acidosis of pregnancy."[63]

For reasons that are not entirely clear, the alveolar-arterial oxygen gradient is increased in pregnancy. This is probably due in part to the relationship of closing volume to FRC mentioned earlier. As noted, this change is most marked in the supine position, but can be as high as 25 mmHg in the sitting position.[2,4]

Hormonal Changes in Pregnancy and Their Relation to Respiratory Function

The increase in progesterone throughout pregnancy leads to hyperventilation secondary to increased CO_2 sensitivity. Progesterone also decreases smooth muscle tone and can lead to bronchial dilation, a theoretical effect which is not seen in pregnancy.[58,81]

Estrogen levels are increased during pregnancy and may contribute to the drop in diffusing capacity seen after the first trimester.[58]

Increased transcortin levels lead to an increased total plasma cortisol level, but decreased cortisol clearance also leads to a two- to threefold elevation of free cortisol. Theoretically this could lead to improvement in corticosteroid responsive lung disease (e.g., asthma) during pregnancy.[81,85]

Prostaglandin F is increased during all trimesters, prostaglandin E during the third trimester, and PG $F_{2\alpha}$ during labor.[85] $PGF_{2\alpha}$ is a bronchoconstrictor and PGE_1 and E_2 are bronchodilators when given as aerosols; however, both $PGF_{2\alpha}$ and PGE_2 cause airway obstruction when given intravenously.[73] This does not become clinically relevant during normal labor, but may be important when $PGF_{2\alpha}$ is given by the intra-amniotic route. A greater than 50 percent decrease in small airway flow occurred in two patients with a family history of asthma who were given intra-amniotic $PGF_{2\alpha}$ for second-trimester therapeutic abortion.[48]

Maternal-Fetal Oxygen Exchange

While available evidence shows prolonged hypoxia has a deleterious fetal effect, the level of reduction in oxygenation that can be tolerated is not well defined. In one study of healthy human neonates at birth, the normal fetal umbilical vein PO_2 was 32 mmHg, while in another it was 28.5 mmHg, demonstrating the large maternal-fetal oxygen gradient that is normally present.[55,81] However, with reductions in human maternal PaO_2 to levels as low as 47 mmHg, placental oxygen extraction increased and maintained the umbilical vein PO_2 at 27 mmHg.[81] Although the fetus can maintain oxygenation in the face of moderate maternal hypoxia, it does benefit directly from oxygen administration to the mother. In one study, maternal oxygen administration led to an increase in fetal PO_2 after at least 10 min of oxygen delivery.[55] In experimental models, chronic hypoxia of maternal animals can lead to fetal pulmonary artery thickening, a complication that is avoided by normal or hyperoxic conditions.[30]

Fetal oxygenation can be affected by maternal acid-base status. Several studies in humans and animals have shown that hyperventilation and the alkalosis that results can decrease uterine blood flow.[53,81] This becomes further compounded by the fact that maternal alkalosis shifts the hemoglobin-oxygen dissociation curve to the left, reducing the amount of oxygen released to the fetus at the placental exchange site.

ASTHMA

Definition

Bronchial asthma is the most common obstructive lung disease in women of childbearing age, encountered in 0.4 to 1.3 percent of all pregnancies.[85,86] By definition, asthma is a condition of hyperreactivity of small and large airways to a variety of stimuli (allergens, infectious agents, cold air, exercise, and others) which results in reversible bronchoconstriction.[75] Along with bronchial smooth muscle contraction, asthma is accompanied by excessive mucus production; both factors lead to plugging of small airways and narrowing of larger airways. In its usual form the condition is manifested by wheezing as a result of airway narrowing. Cough, especially at night, also can be a manifestation of asthma.[69]

Airway narrowing is the central physiologic defect of asthma. In mild asthma, small airways (less than 2 mm) are narrowed, and since they make up only 10 to 30 percent of airway resistance, their obstruction is detected by sensitive small airways tests.[69] Such a test would be the air flow rate between 25 and 75 percent of the forced expiratory flow (FEF_{25-75}) (Fig. 12-2). Only with progressive bronchospasm do larger airways become obstructed and cause a fall in the FEV_1.

Classically, asthmatics have been divided into two clinical groups, extrinsic and intrinsic.[69] Those with extrinsic asthma are younger and have had the disease since childhood. Their attacks are often seasonal, precipitated by well-defined allergens, and accompanied by a history of hayfever or atopic dermatitis. Blood and sputum eosinophilia are common. Intrinsic asthma is an adult-onset illness without a preceding atopic history, usually requiring long-term treatment rather than short-term therapy limited to acute attacks. The intrinsic asthmatic is sensitive to environmental irritants, and acute exacerbations are often precipitated by viral respiratory illness. Blood eosinophilia is unusual in this group of patients.

Effects of Pregnancy on Asthma

An overall pattern emerges from studies of the effect of pregnancy on the course of asthma. Although serial pulmonary function tests show no change in FEV_1/FVC during an asthmatic's pregnancy, clinical studies suggest that approximately one-third improve during pregnancy, one-third show no change, and one-third deteriorate.[72,86] Improvement in asthma may result from the net effect of several hormonal changes during pregnancy: bronchial dilatation by progesterone, increased serum-free cortisol levels, increased maternal histaminase, and increased serum cyclic adenosine 3′,5′-monophosphate (cAMP) levels.[86] However, offsetting these beneficial effects are alterations that can worsen asthma: antigenicity of the fetus, increased mouth breathing due to nasal congestion, increased susceptibility to viral infections, and hyperventilation.[29] Although it is impossible to predict accurately how a specific patient's asthma will act during pregnancy, most exacerbations occur in the second half of pregnancy, and women with a history of prior pregnancy-induced exacerbations are likely to repeat this pattern.[29,86] Serum IgE levels may help predict exacerbations, with an increase during pregnancy identifying a group of patients likely to deteriorate.[29] The degree of deterioration of asthma during pregnancy is variable but can be severe, and a case of status asthmaticus relieved only by abortion has been reported.[80]

Effects of Asthma on Pregnancy

The presence of asthma can affect the course and outcome of pregnancy for both mother and fetus. In one study of 277 asthmatics during pregnancy, perinatal mortality was 5.9 percent.[32] However, one-quarter of all infant deaths came from a small group of mothers with severe asthma. This maternal subgroup may not have been managed optimally, since it had a 25 percent mortality rate. Contrast this data with a series of 55 corticosteroid-treated asthmatics under close medical supervision for asthma throughout pregnancy. In this group, maternal and fetal mortality was not increased above a control population and there was only a slight increase in the incidence of premature births.[68] Taken together, these studies show that asthma is a potentially serious illness during pregnancy and if managed improperly, can lead to increased maternal and fetal mortality. However, it appears that these life-threatening risks can be avoided by careful medical attention and control of symptoms with corticosteroids, if necessary.[81]

Agents for Therapy of Asthma

Because asthma is a disease of variable severity, therapy must be individualized. In the woman who is only symptomatic during an acute exacerbation from a clearly defined precipitant, therapy is only necessary during the attack itself and may not be necessary at all if the precipitant can be avoided. Other patients may have a chronic baseline wheeze that worsens during an acute attack. These women will need both chronic and more intensive therapy for acute exacerbations. It is this latter group that should be followed closely and treated for exacerbations as soon as possible to avoid progression to status asthmaticus.

An in-depth discussion of the pathophysiology of asthma is beyond the scope of this chapter. However, a basic understanding is necessary to develop a rational approach to pharmacologic management of the disease.[84] The normal bronchial smooth muscle cell has adrenergic receptors. $Beta_2$-receptors cause bronchodilation, while alpha-receptors cause bronchoconstriction. $Beta_1$-receptors are present in the cardiovascular system, and their stimulation by nonselective betamimetic agents leads to the cardiac side effects (especially tachycardia) of these drugs. $Beta_2$-receptor stimulation leads to intracellular bronchial smooth muscle cell conversion of adenosine triphosphate (ATP) to cyclic AMP (cAMP) via adenylcyclase (Fig. 12-4). The cAMP acts as a "second messenger" to reduce bronchial smooth muscle tone. It is broken down by a cytoplasmic enzyme, phosphodiesterase, which can be inhibited by methylxanthines such as theophylline. Cyclic guanosine monophosphate (cGMP) is a "second messenger" under parasympathetic control, which leads to bronchoconstriction. The hyperreactivity of the asthmatic's airways results from an imbalance in these smooth muscle control systems, possibly from an excess of cGMP or a lack of cAMP. Partial blockade of the $beta_2$-receptor also may play a role.[84]

Stimuli that precipitate asthma can lead to bronchoconstriction by causing release of chemical mediators. Extrinsic asthmatics have allergen-specific IgE anti-

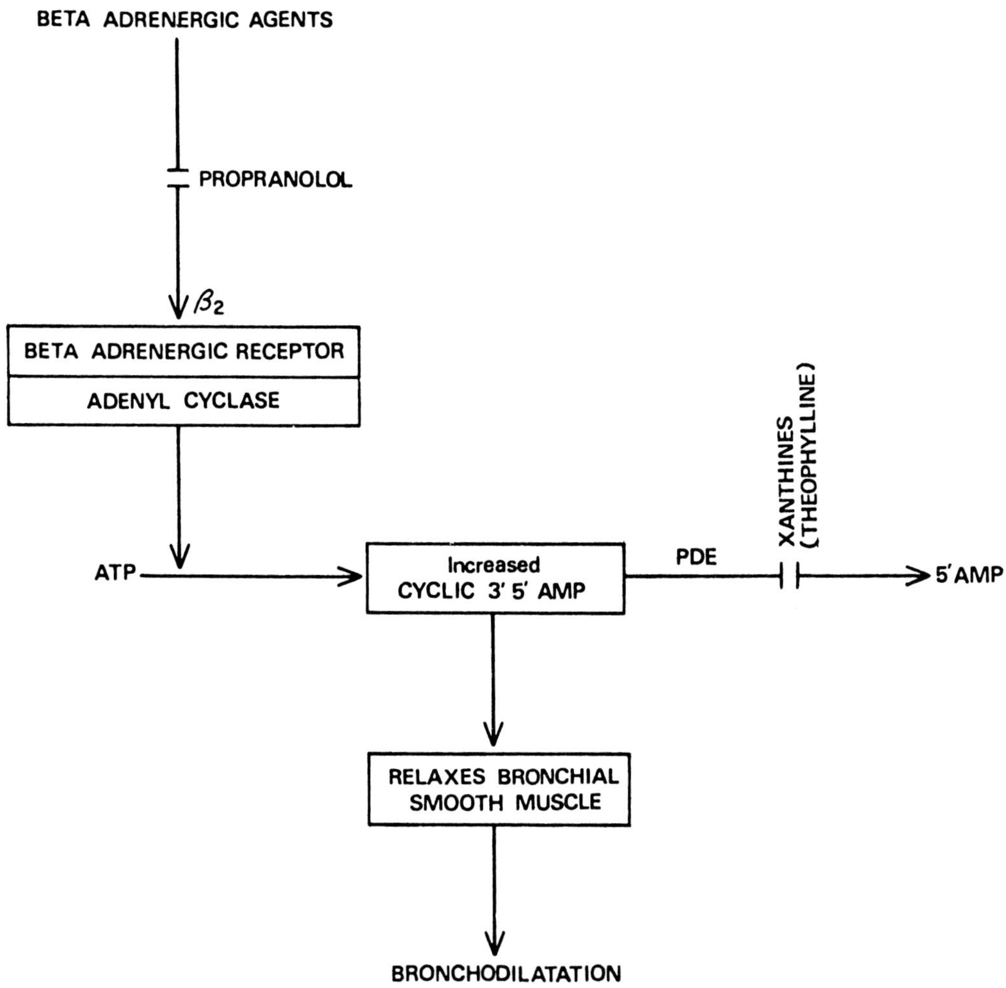

Fig. 12-4 Beta-adrenergic pathways in bronchial smooth muscle. Stimulation of beta$_2$-receptors or inhibition of phosphodiesterase breakdown (PDE) of cyclic AMP leads to bronchodilation. Reprinted, by permission of the New England Journal of Medicine, from Webb-Johnson, D.C., and Andrews, J.L.: Bronchodilator therapy. N. Engl. J. Med., 297:476, 758, 1977.

bodies on the surface of the mast cells lining their tracheobronchial tree. When an allergen molecule bridges two adjacent IgE molecules, the mast cell is activated and a variety of mediators are released, which can initiate bronchospasm. Beta$_2$-receptor stimulation can block the action of these mediators on bronchial smooth muscle sites. Furthermore, mast cells have beta-adrenergic receptors on their surface and when these are stimulated, mediator release is blocked. Intrinsic asthma is not caused by IgE-mediated mechanisms, but beta$_2$ stimulation will also block the bronchoconstriction found in this disease.

Agents that selectively stimulate $beta_2$-receptors include isoetharine, albuterol, metaproterenol, and terbutaline, all of which are available in aerosol form. Metaproterenol and terbutaline are available in oral preparations and terbutaline also can be administered subcutaneously. Less selective sympathomimetic agents include epinephrine and ephedrine, with both alpha- and beta-stimulating effects, and isoproterenol with similar $beta_1$ and $beta_2$ effects but no alpha effects. Epinephrine is available in subcutaneous form or as an aerosol, isoproterenol as an aerosol, and ephedrine as an oral medication. Theophylline, a nonsympathomimetic bronchodilator, is available in oral and intravenous forms.[69,84]

For severe asthma, corticosteroids are important pharmacologic agents that act through different mechanisms than the bronchodilators. Their actions are multiple and include vasoconstriction of the bronchial vasculature, with reduction in edema formation and dilation of bronchial smooth muscle.[84] They inhibit antibody formation and penetration of antigen through the bronchial mucosa. In addition, they block the formation and action of many inflammatory mediators. Corticosteroids are useful in conjunction with sympathomimetic agents because they can restore adrenergic responsiveness to the asthmatic.[84]

Before outlining a specific treatment protocol for an exacerbation of asthma, we will briefly review data regarding the use of antiasthmatic agents during pregnancy. More comprehensive reviews of this topic appear elsewhere.[81,85,86]

Theophylline. Theophylline preparations appear to be safe during pregnancy and pose no teratogenic risk to the fetus. One study even showed that intramuscular theophylline can reduce perinatal mortality and the frequency of respiratory distress syndrome in premature infants.[36] However, theophylline does cross the placenta and if given in excessive doses can lead to both maternal and neonatal toxicity. Neonatal toxic reactions include jitteriness, tachycardia, gagging, vomiting, and opisthotonus, all of which can occur at neonatal theophylline blood levels which are therapeutic for the adult (10 to 20 μg/ml).[3] Adult reactions can include seizures as well as the above findings. One study showed that fetal toxicity can occur in the absence of maternal toxicity owing to increased fetal sensitivity to and slower elimination of the drug.[3] Another study showed that although the fetus may have higher heelstick theophylline levels than maternal blood levels, side effects that frequently occur are minor and transient, making maternal theophylline use safe for the fetus at term.[49] To avoid toxic complications theophylline, in the form of intravenous aminophylline, should be used in lower doses than the usually recommended 5.6 mg/kg loading dose followed by 0.9 mg/kg/h.[40] Use of 0.5 mg/kg/h, or less than 1 g aminophylline per 24 h, will reduce the potential for toxicity while still providing adequate bronchodilation.[82] Calculations are based on lean body weight. Higher doses can be used if serum levels are followed, but we recommend maintaining serum theophylline levels no higher than 14 μg/ml in the pregnant patient, realizing that bronchodilation has been seen with levels as low as 5 μg/ml.[82] Patients with congestive heart failure, liver dysfunction, or coincident cimetidine therapy should receive no more than 0.3 mg/kg/h. Smokers and patients younger than age 20 can be given 0.7 mg/kg/h. The loading dose of 5.6 mg/kg is still appropriate for the patient not currently receiving theophylline, but no more than a 400-mg loading dose should be administered.

Theophylline blood levels should be measured 10 h after therapy is begun and at least daily after that in the acutely ill patient. For chronic outpatient therapy, oral theophylline can be administered in two or three daily doses of any of the currently available long-acting, slow-release preparations. Blood theophylline levels are monitored 6 h after an oral dose is given.

Beta-Adrenergic Agents. Beta-stimulating drugs such as metaproterenol, terbutaline, and albuterol have been used during pregnancy but their safety has not yet been established. These drugs inhibit uterine activity and delay the onset of labor. If beta-stimulating drugs are needed to control asthma, we believe they should be given, but it is probably wise to discontinue their use, if possible, near term. A case report of postpartum uterine atony and hemorrhage from albuterol used during labor points to one potential problem with these agents.[83] Also, there are reports of betamimetic therapy, with or without glucocorticoids, precipitating high-output congestive heart failure at term.[46,47]

Unless needed for life-threatening anaphylaxis, epinephrine, especially the sustained-release preparations, should be avoided because of an increased incidence of fetal malformations after use during the first 4 months of pregnancy.[81] To allow individualized therapy of asthma, fixed drug combinations of theophylline and ephedrine are best avoided.

Corticosteroids. Corticosteroid therapy with prednisone is safe during pregnancy and, if used to control asthma promptly, it can prevent excess maternal and fetal mortality.[81] Human studies have not confirmed the increased risk of cleft palate seen in offspring of corticosteroid-treated animals. Neonatal adrenal suppression has been seen only rarely. This is probably because of rapid conversion of prednisone to its active form, prednisolone, in the mother and poor placental passage of prednisolone.[8] Additionally, the fetus may not be able to convert prednisone, which can cross the placenta, to prednisolone.[85] Although not specifically studied, inhaled corticosteroid preparations probably are also safe for the fetus. Thus, if asthma is severe during pregnancy, corticosteroid therapy is far preferable to and of lower risk than poorly controlled asthma. The use of unconventional corticosteroid doses (gram quantities) in status asthmaticus is of unproven safety.

Other Agents. Atropine by inhalation and disodium cromoglycate have been used safely during pregnancy, but because their safety is not officially established, they should be avoided if possible. Drugs to be avoided specifically in the pregnant asthmatic are the antihistamines brompheniramine (fetal malformations); hydroxyzine and cyproheptadine (insufficient data); tetracycline (damage to fetal teeth, bone, and liver); iodide expectorants (life-threatening fetal goiter); amobarbital, an agent in some combination medications (cardiovascular malformations); and aspirin or tartrazine dye in sensitive patients (precipitates asthma).[33] Immunotherapy appears to be safe during pregnancy but increases in dosage should be avoided to prevent the possibility of life-threatening anaphylaxis.[81]

Management of Acute Asthma Exacerbations during Pregnancy

Acute asthmatic exacerbations (Fig. 12-5) can occur in response to viral or bacterial respiratory infections, exposure to noxious stimuli or allergens, exposure to aspirin or tartrazine dyes in sensitive patients (often with a history of nasal polyposis), after exercise or cold-air exposure.[69] The patient presents with shortness of breath, chest tightness, and wheezing and also may report symptoms of respiratory infection with a change in sputum characteristics, fever, and chills. A quick search for a precipitating event and questioning about prior and current corticosteroid use are part of the initial history. Then examination should include measurement of pulse, blood pressure, respiratory rate, pulsus paradox, and FEV_1. A pulse >120/min, respiratory rate >30/min, FEV_1 <1 L, pulsus paradox >18 mmHg, moderate to severe dyspnea, accessory muscle use, and severe wheezing at the time of initial evaluation are all signs of life-threatening disease and may well be predictive of need for hospitalization.[23] In assessing the degree of wheezing present, the combination of inspiratory and expiratory wheezes signifies more obstruction than if expiratory wheezes alone are present. In the most severe cases of asthma, relatively few wheezes are heard because very little air is moved through the markedly narrowed airways.

It is probably safest to obtain an arterial blood gas sample on all pregnant women with an acute asthmatic exacerbation so that hypoxemia can be rapidly identified and treated to avoid fetal embarrassment. Also, blood gas analysis can identify acute respiratory alkalosis, which, as stated, can impair delivery of oxygen to the fetus. In mild asthma, arterial carbon dioxide tension is normal or slightly reduced. In the more severe stages of asthma, normocarbia or hypercarbia develops while arterial hypoxemia becomes more marked.[24] Administration of oxygen will alleviate both hypoxemia and respiratory alkalosis. Chest radiography is probably necessary only in patients with clinical signs of pneumonia or pneumothorax accompanying asthma. A recent study in acute asthma patients found that chest radiography does not reveal pathology unsuspected by an adequate history and physical examination.[21] Bedside spirometry with measurement of FEV_1/FVC and peak expiratory flow rate are also useful, especially when compared with previous values and when followed serially through an attack.

In the pregnant patient, treatment is begun with an inhaled bronchodilator such as isoetharine, 0.5 ml of a 1 percent solution in 1.5 ml of saline given by nebulizer. This can be repeated every 1 to 2 h if needed. Intravenous aminophylline also is begun. If the patient already is taking a theophylline preparation, no loading dose is necessary; if not, aminophylline, 5.6 mg/kg, is given intravenously over 30 min. As stated, no more than 400 mg should be given as a loading dose. If it appears that the patient has been taking too little theophylline, a partial loading dose can be given. After this, a continuous aminophylline infusion is given at 0.5 mg/kg/h, preferably via an infusion pump. After 10 to 12 h, a theophylline blood level is obtained to confirm that the concentration is in the safe, effective range of 10 to 14 μg/ml. Supportive management includes intravenous hydration with 100 to 125 ml/h of 0.5 N saline and administration of oxygen. In the usual patient, oxygen is given by nasal cannula at a rate of 2 to 3 L/min. If the patient has CO_2 retention ($PaCO_2$ >45 mmHg), oxygen

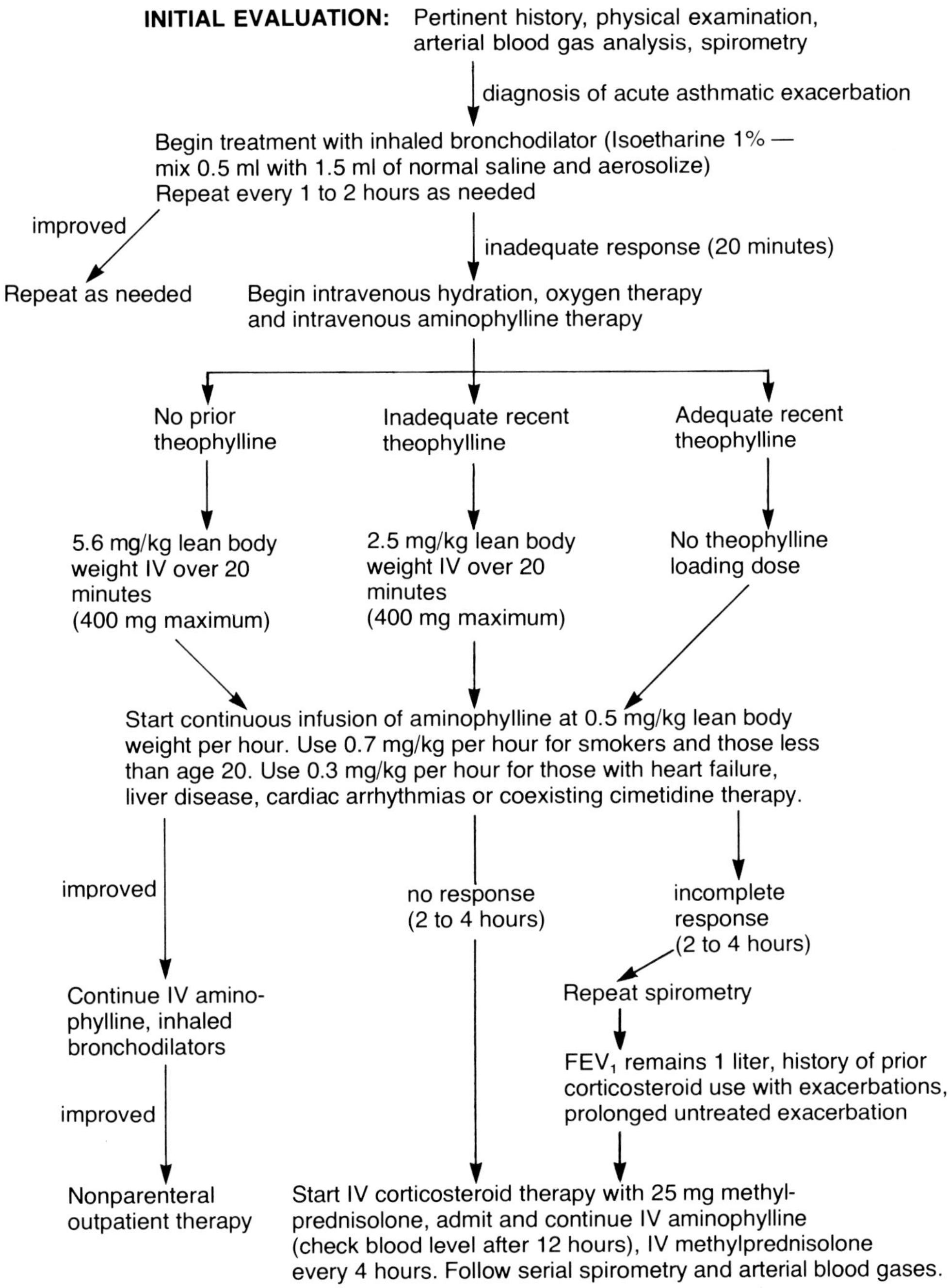

Fig. 12-5 Management of severe asthma during pregnancy.

must be titrated more carefully and a Venturi mask (either 24, 28, or 31 percent oxygen) used to deliver as much oxygen as can be given without causing further CO_2 retention. If oxygen is administered, an arterial $PO_2 \geq 70$ mmHg should be achieved.

If clinical examination and spirometry (FEV_1 remains less than 1 L) show that the patient is not responding to therapy after 2 to 4 h, if the patient has a long history of corticosteroid use for prior acute exacerbations, if the attack has been present for several days before the patient seeks help, or if the patient already is taking corticosteroids, then corticosteroid therapy is indicated. For an acute attack, 25 mg of methylprednisolone is given intravenously every 4 h. If corticosteroids are used, the patient is admitted to the hospital and this regimen is continued until the attack is resolved. Corticosteroids are then continued orally at a starting dose of 60 mg of prednisone daily. If the patient is free of wheezing, this dose is reduced by 20 mg at 4-day intervals until a daily dose of 20 mg is reached. From this point, the dose is tapered weekly by 5 mg until corticosteroids are stopped or the lowest dose that keeps the patient free of wheezes is reached. If corticosteroids cannot be tapered completely, an alternate-day regimen is preferable to a daily regimen. Inhaled corticosteroids can sometimes help to facilitate oral corticosteroid tapering. However, they should not be added until wheezing is controlled, since during an attack they will not be able to penetrate the airways effectively. Because adequate control of asthma is essential for optimizing fetal and maternal outcome, there should be no hesitation to continue corticosteroids indefinitely, if needed, to control the asthma.

Antibiotics also are used in an acute asthma attack if pneumonia is present or if bacterial respiratory infection appears to have precipitated the attack. For therapy of an infectious bronchitis, oral ampicillin or an oral cephalosporin is used until the results of a sputum culture are available to allow a more specific antibiotic choice. A 10-day course of therapy is given. Antibiotic therapy of bacterial penumonia is discussed later.

As the acute attack begins to resolve and oral corticosteroids are started, an outpatient bronchochilator program is also initiated. An oral form of theophylline replaces intravenous aminophylline. In making this transition, the 24-h intravenous aminophylline dose is recorded. Since 85 percent of aminophylline is theophylline, a 24-h theophylline dose can be calculated. This dose can be divided conveniently into two or three daily doses of a long-acting theophylline preparation, which is begun while the intravenous infusion is continued for an additional 3 to 4 h. An oral betamimetic agent such as terbutaline can be added to theophylline, if needed, in a dose of 2.5 to 5 mg 3 times per day, as there is good evidence of synergy between these two agents for the asthmatic patient. To complement this regimen of oral agents, an inhaled bronchodilator such as metaproterenol, two puffs 4 times daily, may be helpful. When betamimetic agents are used, caution should be exercised as the delivery date approaches so that the complications of high-output congestive failure and postpartum uterine atony can be avoided.

Although this treatment program will manage most episodes of acute asthma, there is a small subgroup of patients who remain refractory to therapy. As stated, documentation of a normal or elevated arterial PCO_2 during an asthma attack, rather than the expected hypocarbia, identifies the patient with severe, life-threatening asthma.[24] If the previously outlined therapy does not rapidly reverse this degree of airway obstruction carbon dioxide retention, respiratory acidoses and obtundation will ensue, and endotracheal intubation and mechanical ventilation are indicated. Although mechanical ventilation is an important resource for the severe asthmatic, it is associated with a high incidence of complications and a 38 percent mortality in one series.[71] This difficulty arises because the severely obstructed asthmatic requires high airway pressures to achieve an adequate tidal volume, and barotrauma frequently follows. To reduce complications of mechanical ventilation in the asthmatic, Scoggin and colleagues suggest: (1) use the largest endotracheal tube possible, at least 8 mm diameter, to reduce expiratory air flow resistance; (2) deliver constant volumes with a volume ventilator; (3) humidify the air delivered; (4) allow adequate expiratory time by using the lowest rate that allows carbon dioxide elimination; and (5) suppress agitation and ventilatory drive with sedatives and paralysis. Paralysis can be achieved with pancuronium bromide, which does not cross the placental barrier well and is safe for short-term use in pregnancy.[66] Paralysis must be accompanied with sedation but histamine-releasing drugs such as morphine and meperidine should be avoided. Valium should also be avoided, whenever possible, during pregnancy. If labor occurs during pancuronium bromide therapy, the fetus should be carefully observed for flaccidity and respiratory depression.

The elevated airway pressures of an acute asthmatic attack in a spontaneously breathing or mechanically ventilated patient can lead to mediastinal emphysema. This complication is uncommon but can occur if the increased airway pressures in asthma lead to rupture of an alveolus and air leakage along the vascular sheaths to the hilum and mediastinum.[37] Mediastinal emphysema can occur not only with asthma but also during the second stage of labor, with hyperemesis of early pregnancy, or after a bout of coughing.[37] Clinically, the patient presents with sharp retrosternal pain, which can radiate to the shoulders and arms. On examination, subcutaneous emphysema is present and a crunching noise, Hamman's sign, can be heard with each heartbeat at the left sternal edge. Pneumothorax, often on the left, is associated in some cases. Treatment involves analgesia and oxygen, drainage by chest tube of an associated pneumothorax, and careful observation. If tension builds in the mediastinum leading to cardiovascular compromise, release of air is achieved by incisions over sites of subcutaneous air accumulation.[37]

When the asthmatic enters labor, several precautionary measures are warranted. As mentioned, betamimetic agents should be discontinued if possible and if the patient is not allowed to take anything by mouth, her antiasthmatic medications should be administered intravenously. The corticosteroid-dependent asthmatic should be regarded as adrenally suppressed and given additional "stress" doses of glucocorticoids to avoid an Addisonian crisis. An appropriate regimen consists of 100 mg of hydrocortisone intramuscularly on admission to the labor room, followed by 100 mg of hydrocortisone intramuscularly every 8 h for 24 h; the patient then returns to her previous oral steroid regimen.[81] If general anesthesia is necessary for delivery, halogenated gases are broncholytic and are preferable to nonhalogenated agents.

OTHER OBSTRUCTIVE LUNG DISEASES

Severe emphysema due to alpha$_1$-antitrypsin deficiency and cystic fibrosis (CF) can occur in the woman of childbearing age. Care for these patients is primarily supportive, with attention to the physiologic parameters of lung function and oxygenation that we have discussed. As noted, the effect of pregnancy on these diseases and the effect of these diseases on fetal outcome are more variable than with restrictive lung disorders. This is primarily because pulmonary function can deteriorate rapidly as a result of the respiratory infections which frequently complicate these diseases.

A National Institute of Health study followed 129 pregnancies in CF patients. These pregnancies produced only 86 viable infants, leading the investigators to conclude that CF patients have greatly increased fetal wastage.[13] In the study, there were 6 spontaneous abortions, 25 therapeutic abortions, and 11 perinatal deaths. Ten of the perinatal deaths occurred in infants born at less than 37 weeks gestation. Premature labor occurred in 26 of the 129 pregnancies. The maternal mortality was 18 percent within 24 months of delivery. The authors recommended that pregnancy be avoided unless the potential mother with CF is clinically healthy. This study and others strongly recommend that any CF patient with cor pulmonale and pulmonary hypertension not undertake pregnancy because of her inability to tolerate the increased cardiac load and circulating blood volume. A reasonable set of guidelines is to advise against pregnancy in any CF patient with a VC <50 percent of that predicted, hypoxemia, cor pulmonale, or pancreatic insufficiency. The absence of pancreatic insufficiency may identify a subgroup more able to tolerate pregnancy.[15]

Since respiratory infections may be responsible for the increased fetal and maternal mortality during a CF pregnancy, these infections should be treated vigorously. This entails chest physiotherapy, nebulized bronchodilators, and use of antibiotics. Although no data exist to support the use of continuous antibiotic therapy in these patients, therapy for acute exacerbations accompanied by a change in sputum character is effective.[45] Therapy often is given intravenously with antibiotics directed at *Pseudomonas aeruginos* and *Staphylococcus aureus*, which commonly infect CF patients. However, to guide therapy baseline sputum cultures should be obtained in these patients and when exacerbations occur. Penicillins (carbenicillin, oxacillin) are preferable to potentially fetal-toxic aminoglycosides.[13] In the penicillin-allergic CF patient, cephalosporins and aerosolized aminoglycosides can be used.

If the patient with obstructive lung disease has no exertional dyspnea, is clinically stable, and has an FEV_1 greater than 1 L, pregnancy can be attempted. Such a woman must certainly be regarded as a high-risk patient and serial spirometry and blood gas analyses are indicated. The expectant mother should be urged not to smoke cigarettes and should be treated aggressively for any respiratory infection. These usually present initially as a change in sputum quantity and nature. Using this program, a woman with $alpha_1$-antitrypsin deficiency and an FEV_1 of 1.07 L was successfully managed and gave birth to a healthy child.[27]

Bronchiectasis, which may be associated with frequent infections and airway obstruction, also can be successfully managed during pregnancy if attention is given to the basics of care outlined.[42]

RESPIRATORY INFECTIONS

Influenza and bacterial pneumonias can affect any pregnant patient, and morbidity can be lowered by attempts to prevent illness and efforts at early diagnosis and treatment. Aspiration pneumonitis, a complication of labor and anesthesia, is discussed in another part of this chapter.

Influenza is associated with a higher fatality rate in pregnant women than in the nonpregnant.[70] Although the magnitude of increased maternal fatality from influenza is not known, some data are available. During the 1918 influenza epidemic, maternal mortality with the illness was 27 percent. In one study of the 1957 epidemic, pregnancy increased mortality ninefold in the 20 to 29 year age group.[54] In a review of all deaths due to influenza in 1957through 1960, 1 to 11 percent occurred in pregnant patients.[20] These deaths were concentrated in the late third trimester and early puerperium and were more likely to occur with increased maternal age. The disease can progress rapidly to fulminant cardiopulmonary failure after several days of preceding malaise, fever, cough, and myalgia. The physician cannot effectively treat the viral infection with antimicrobial drugs but should be vigilant for secondary bacterial infection caused by pneumococcus, staphylococcus, *Hemophilus influenza*, or streptococcus, which require antibiotic treatment. While these secondary infections can occur in any severe case, pregnant patients seem more susceptible than nonpregnant individuals to progressive, fatal primary influenza pneumonia.[60]

Influenza and other viral pneumonias may progress rapidly to respiratory failure and ARDS.[22] This complication is heralded by dyspnea and can occur 24 to 36 h after the start of the illness. Findings include profound tachypnea, arterial hypoxemia that responds minimally to oxygen, bilateral diffuse interstitial infiltrates or alveolar filling patterns on chest radiograph, and sputum showing few white cells and normal bacterial flora. ARDS is caused by capillary leaking of fluid into the alveolar spaces, with subsequent alveolar closure and arterial hypoxemia due to intrapulmonary shunting of unoxygenated blood. This nonspecific response to viral infection requires aggressive supportive treatment. Intubation and mechanical ventilation are begun immediately. Positive end-expiratory pressure (PEEP) frequently is used to correct hypoxemia refractory to high concentrations of oxygen. PEEP increases FRC and prevents airway closure, which results in better ventilation and perfusion relationships.[22] The concentration of supplemental oxygen can be reduced by the use of PEEP at levels of 10 to 15 cmH_2O. However, the risk of oxygen toxicity persists if oxygen concentrations greater than 50 percent are required for more than 3 to 4 days.

When PEEP is used, a Swan-Ganz catheter should be inserted. This will allow direct measurements of cardiac output and mixed venous oxygen tension (a measure of tissue oxygen delivery) in response to changes in PEEP. Also, it allows the physician to keep the patient's intravascular volume at the lowest level that maintains adequate cardiac and renal function. With PEEP therapy, arterial oxygen tension should be kept above 65 mmHg. ARDS is accompanied by stiff, noncompliant lungs, and high airway pressures may develop during mechanical ventilation. For this reason, constant vigilance for barotrauma is necessary.

In one study, the survival rate of influenza patients with ARDS was 45 percent.[87] Survivors were ventilated earlier than those who died. Ventilator support was required for at least 14 days in survivors and definite radiographic improvement preceded successful weaning from the respirator. The chest radiograph was only 50 percent improved after 3 weeks. There is controversy about whether corticosteroid therapy hastens improvement, but our recommendation is not to use corticosteroids because there is no proof of their benefit.[60]

Although influenza virus can cross the placenta, the infection does not appear to cause congenital defects except for those related to maternal drug treatment.[70,85] Congenital anomalies attributed to influenza include circulatory defects, central nervous system malformations, cleft lip, and childhood cancer. But a review of this subject concluded that no definite influenza-induced congenital syndrome exists.[54] In support of this is a case report of transplacental viral passage without fetal tissue infection.[89] Although influenza vaccination is available, it is of unproven safety and is recommended only during an anticipated pandemic. Since increased mortality from infections occurs late in pregnancy, vaccination can be delayed until the middle of the second trimester.[70]

Other life-threatening viral pneumonias can develop in the pregnant patient. Varicella pneumonia can accompany chickenpox and can range from a mild to a rapidly fatal illness. In pregnancy, varicella is rare, but if pneumonia develops, mortality is high.[19] Pneumonia is accompanied by dyspnea, pleuritic chest pain, and infiltrates on chest radiograph, which are worst when the skin eruption is maximal. In its more severe forms, varicella pneumonia requires the same supportive care outlined for influenza pneumonia. Maternal varicella infection in any trimester of pregnancy can be associated with infrequent, but possibly lethal, congenital anomalies. If maternal infection occurs within 5 days of delivery, the infant is at risk of a fatal disseminated infection. Some authors have recommended administration of varicella-zoster immune globulin, if available, to both mother and fetus exposed to peripartum varicella.[17]

Pneumonia of all etiologies is the second most common cause of nonobstetric maternal mortality. It occurs in 0.1 to 0.84 percent of all pregnancies, with a mortality of 3.5 to 8.6 percent.[41] The two most common infectious agents are *Streptococcus pneumoniae* and *Mycoplasma pneumoniae*. Pneumococcal pneumonia classically begins with a shaking chill, pleuritic chest pain, fever, cough, and shortness of breath. Physical signs and chest radiographic evidence of lobar consolidation in a toxic patient help to distinguish this disease from pulmonary infarction. Procaine penicillin G in a dose of 1.2 million units/day in divided doses is the treatment of choice and will lead to defervescence within 24 h in half of the patients and within 3 to 4 days in the rest.[70] Erythromycin is used for the penicillin-allergic patient. Good medical management also requires that the physician monitor arterial blood gases, deliver oxygen as needed, and provide chest physiotherapy to help drain secretions. If the pneumonia becomes progressive or if it is not treated until a late stage, mechanical ventilation may become necessary. Indications for this intervention are progressive retention of carbon dioxide with uncompensated respiratory acidosis, inadequate oxygenation (PaO_2 <60 mmHg) on greater than 50 percent FIO_2, impaired mental status leading to inability to protect the airway from aspiration and obstruction, and inability to clear respiratory secretions.

Mycoplasma pneumonia produces symptoms similar to those of a viral infection, with a flulike syndrome and interstitial infiltrates and alveolar filling. Small pleural effusions are common, and 10 percent of infected patients have cold agglutinins in their serum. Because tetracycline is contraindicated in pregnancy, erythromycin is the drug of choice.

Different antibiotics may be indicated for the other bacterial pneumonias and a brief summary of their safety in pregnancy is presented here.[52] All penicillins are safe in the nonallergic patient, pass through the placenta, and thus potentially can treat fetal infections. Semisynthetic antistaphylococcal penicillins, while safe, have variable placental transfer, with methicillin being similar to penicillin G. The older cephalosporins are safe, although specific inquiry should be made before using one of the newer agents. Tetracyclines are unsafe because of fetal tooth and bone abnormalities and third-trimester maternal hepatitis.[52] Sulfonamides are safe for the fetus but should be discontinued before delivery owing to fetal inability to conjugate the drug. This may result in neonatal kernicterus due to competition with bilirubin for metabolism.[52] Sulfa-trimethoprim combinations are unproven in pregnancy. Chloramphenicol must be used cautiously to avoid bone marrow toxicity and "gray baby syndrome" due to inadequate fetal metabolism.[52] Aminoglycosides are needed for life-threatening infection but can cause fetal ototoxicity and nephrotoxicity.[52] Erythromycin is safe but penetrates the placenta poorly. Clindamycin appears to be safe during pregnancy.

One other respiratory infection to be aware of in the postpartum period is a solitary lung abscess. This has been described in one case report as the presenting sign of septic pelvic thrombophlebitis.[31] Recognition of this association will lead to prompt therapy, which requires heparin in addition to antibiotics.

PULMONARY THROMBOEMBOLISM

Venous thrombosis, especially in the thigh, is the source of blood clots which can dislodge and migrate to the lung, resulting in the pulmonary embolism syndrome. More than 95 percent of thrombi that result in pulmonary embolism are from the legs, and the majority come from sites above the knee.[61] However, in the postpartum patient the pelvic veins can be the source of pulmonary emboli. Postpartum pelvic thrombophlebitis is usually suppurative and associated with a septic postpartum course with signs of pelvic infection. Mycotic emboli can travel to the lung and lead to infarction or abscess. Unlike bland pulmonary emboli, these emboli require antibiotics along with anticoagulants.[34] If this therapy is ineffective, ligation of the vena cava and pelvic veins may be necessary.[14]

Available evidence shows an increased risk of venous thrombosis and thrombophlebitis in the immediate postpartum period. In the first postpartum month, this risk is 49 times that in the nonpregnant woman.[39] In one series, the incidence of deep venous thrombosis was 1.5 per 1,000 pregnancies, and that of pulmonary embolism was 0.4 per 1,000 pregnancies.[1,85] Factors that may lead to this increased risk in the pregnant patient include an increase in clotting factors VII, VIII, and X, along with increased fibrinogen level and decreased fibrinolytic activity.[85] The venous stasis of pregnancy and the postpartum use of estrogen to suppress lactation also may add to this risk.

When pulmonary embolism occurs, it is almost always manifested by the nonspecific finding of tachypnea, with a respiratory rate above 16.[61] Depending on the size and location of the embolus, several different clinical pictures can result. A small peripheral embolus can lead to pulmonary hemorrhage or infarction and present with shortness of breath, pleuritic chest pain, hemoptysis, low-grade fever, pleural effusion, and hypoxemia. A large central embolus can present as syncope and cardiovascular collapse. Multiple small emboli can present as unexplained dyspnea. In any of these instances, clinical signs of thrombophlebitis may be present, but frequently this is not the case. Other physical findings that may be present in the patient with pulmonary embolism include wheezing, pleural friction rub, and an accentuated second heart sound. Ominous findings, suggesting severe pulmonary hypertension, are a wide and fixed split of the second heart sound, a pulmonary vascular flow murmur, and massive jugular venous A waves. Laboratory evaluation always shows an increased $(A - a)O_2$ difference. The EKG can show tachycardia, right-axis deviation, and acute cor pulmonale findings of an S wave in lead 1 and Q wave and T wave inversion in lead 3 (S_1, Q_3, T_3 pattern). The chest radiograph may be normal or it may show atelectasis, vascular oligemia, or an infiltrate and effusion.

Pulmonary embolism must be diagnosed with certainty, particularly in the pregnant or postpartum patient. If this disease is not diagnosed and treated, it can result in repeated episodes of embolism and maternal mortality as high as 28 percent.[39] If, however, pulmonary embolism is treated without proper diagnostic documentation, the mother and fetus may be exposed to anticoagulants and possibly hemorrhage without adequate justification. Additionally, anticoagulant treatment with either heparin or warfarin can result in adverse outcome for the fetus.

To diagnose this disease, attempts are made to document thrombophlebitis by the noninvasive methods of Doppler ultrasound and impedance plethysmography, which may be difficult to interpret during pregnancy.[85] If phlebitis without embolism is suspected, venography with pelvic shielding is done. If pulmonary embolism is suspected, a lung perfusion scan with radioactive technetium and a ventilation scan with radioactive xenon are performed. Using values obtained from the *Physicians Desk Reference for Radiology and Nuclear Medicine* and assuming an equivalent total body dose for mother and fetus, this technique will deliver approximately 50 mrad of radiation to the fetus. In later gestation, as the larger fetus is closer to the maternal lung, a fetal body part nearest to the lung might receive 500 mrad of radiation. These figures are only rough estimates but they lead us to conclude that lung scans should be done, if indicated, in the pregnant patient. If the lung scan is totally normal, pulmonary embolism is virtually ruled out.[65] If the perfusion lung scan shows multiple segmental defects in areas with normal ventilation and no abnormality on plain radiograph, pulmonary embolism is likely. If a patient has a convincing clinical history and a high probability of pulmonary embolism by lung scanning, treatment can be started without a pulmonary angiogram. However, in many instances, perfusion scan results are indeterminate and definitive documentation by pulmonary angiogram is necessary. This clearly exposes the fetus to radiation, but the dose can be minimized by pelvic shielding and by attempts at selective angiography directed at areas that are abnormal with perfusion scanning.

Once pulmonary embolism is documented, the patient is treated with anticoagulants. Initial therapy consists of a bolus of 5,000 to 10,000 units of heparin intravenously. This is followed by a continuous infusion of heparin,[61] which during the acute period causes less hemorrhagic morbidity than intermittent administration.[67] The infusion can be begun at 1,000 units/h and the partial thromboplastin time (PTT) is measured after 3 hr of therapy. The infusion rate is then adjusted to maintain the PTT at 1½ to 2 times the control value. If the infusion rate must be increased, a partial heparin bolus (1,000 units) is sometimes helpful. During therapy, stool and urine must be observed for evidence of hemorrhage and serial hematocrits followed. Arterial hypoxemia is treated with oxygen, and deep vein thrombosis is treated with bed rest, leg elevation, and local application of heat.

In the presence of hypotension, vasopressors may be required. Patients with massive pulmonary emboli and pulmonary hypertension are at risk from further large emboli, and it may be necessary to supplement anticoagulation therapy with vena cava interruption.[61] This intervention should also be considered if the patient sustains recurrent pulmonary emboli during adequate therapy or has an absolute contraindication to anticoagulant use (e.g., an active bleeding site elsewhere). Vena caval interruption is achieved either by surgical plication or by insertion of an umbrella filter. Ligation of the vena cava has been performed in eight pregnant women via a transabdominal approach. Two had the procedure in the first trimester, four in midtrimester, and two near term. All eight patients went to term and had normal, uncomplicated deliveries.[14] The umbrella filter, recently developed by Mobin-Uddin and colleagues, also can provide successful vena caval interruption.[59] The device is inserted transvenously under local anesthesia into the internal jugular vein and then advanced into the inferior vena cava. Although this procedure avoids the need for major surgery during pregnancy, abdominal radiography is required for proper filter placement. In hemodynamically unstable patients with acute cor pulmonale, effective caval interruption by the umbrella filter will avoid the major risk of general anesthesia. Either interruptive procedure is associated with a risk of continued small emboli through collateral venous channels, but, by preventing immediate large emboli, the procedures can be life-saving. There is limited experience with the use of thrombolytic therapy in the pregnant patient and no specific recommendation can be given.[85]

Once continuous heparin therapy is started, it is continued, following the PTT determination, for 7 to 10 days. Then, the patient is switched to an outpatient subcutaneous heparin regimen, which is continued through the remainder of gestation. This consists of a heparin injection every 6 to 12 h, adjusted to give a dose that prolongs the midinterval PTT 1½ times the control value. One recent study used such a regimen with heparin every 12 h to successfully manage deep vein thrombosis in a nonpregnant population.[43] Heparin needs may increase as pregnancy progresses, and dosage should be reevaluated every 1 to 2 weeks. Long-term heparin use can lead to osteoporosis. Thrombocytopenia may also result, making it mandatory to follow platelet counts.[12]

If pulmonary embolism occurs postpartum, the patient is treated with oral warfarin after the initial 7 to 10 days of continuous intravenous heparin therapy. Warfarin therapy is continued for 6 weeks postpartum.

Anticoagulant therapy poses the problem not only of hemorrhage but also of teratogenicity. Warfarin, an oral anticoagulant ideal for chronic therapy, crosses the placenta and can result in a specific embryopathy and central nervous system abnormalities.[38] Heparin, which does not cross the placenta, has been reported to cause a higher incidence of maternal bleeding than warfarin and an increased incidence of perinatal mortality, fetal prematurity, and stillbirths.[38] Hall et al.[38] have estimated that only two-thirds of pregnancies in which either warfarin or heparin is used will result in a normal outcome. For patients already taking anticoagulants they recommend avoidance of pregnancy; or for women who must begin taking these drugs during pregnancy, they suggest therapeutic abortion. Given these data and recommendations, anticoagulation must not be taken lightly in the pregnant patient. However, in discussing the possibility of abortion with the pregnant patient treated with anticoagulants, the physician should have a good knowledge of both risks and alternative approaches.

Warfarin embryopathy occurs in 4 percent of the exposed offspring and is characterized by nasal hypoplasia and stippled bony epiphyses.[38] In addition, 3 percent of exposed offspring can develop unrelated central nervous system abnormalities. While the central nervous system abnormalities can occur after warfarin exposure any time in pregnancy, the embryopathy syndrome only occurs after warfarin exposure during weeks 6 to 9 of gestation.[38] Also, although exposure to warfarin leads to persistent fetal sequelae in 10.4 percent of pregnancies, heparin exposure causes persistent sequelae in only 0.7 percent of fetuses.[38] Keeping these data in mind, one can understand the use of a combination anticoagulant regimen in the pregnant patient, which some authors have reported is safe. This regimen, studied only in small series, consists of: (1) initial therapy with heparin intravenously, then subcutaneously throughout the first trimester; (2) maintenance therapy with oral warfarin after the first trimester; (3) discontinuation of warfarin at 37 weeks by use of 5 mg of vitamin K and institution of intravenous heparin therapy; (4) induction of labor 7 to 10 days later with heparin discontinued through labor and the subsequent 6 h; and (5) institution of warfarin postpartum and discontinuation of heparin after warfarin begins to act.[57,62,85]

Our recommendation for anticoagulation of the pregnant patient is to use intravenous and subcutaneous heparin in the regimen outlined earlier. Such an approach avoids two potential problems that exist when using a combination heparin-warfarin program. First, with heparin but not warfarin, the fetus is not anticoagulated and is not susceptible to hemorrhage from minor maternal trauma. Second, if premature labor begins, heparin can be stopped but warfarin is not easy to reverse and warfarin therapy makes peripartum maternal and fetal hemorrhage possible. When heparin is used in the management of antepartum pulmonary embolism, the patient is admitted to the hospital just prior to term and labor is induced. Heparin is stopped through labor and the subsequent 6 h. Then, a continuous intravenous infusion is begun and continued until warfarin, which is begun postpartum, begins to act. Warfarin is used for at least 6 weeks postpartum.

The above regimen can also be used in the anticoagulated patient who chooses to become pregnant after learning the risks involved and after she is switched to subcutaneous heparin during the period of conception. Outpatient use of heparin can be achieved with good patient acceptance and outcome.[74] Low-dose subcutaneous heparin, 5,000 units every 12 h, also can be used prophylactically throughout pregnancy in patients at increased risk of thromboembolic events.[85] High-risk patients include those with previous thrombophlebitis or pulmonary embolism during pregnancy or in the postpartum period. Such patients also have been successfully managed with the previously outlined heparin-warfarin combination regimen.[62]

ASPIRATION OF STOMACH CONTENTS

Mendelson's syndrome, the aspiration of low-pH liquid stomach contents into the tracheobronchial tree, with subsequent chemical pneumonitis, was first described in women undergoing labor and delivery.[88] This syndrome is most likely to develop if aspirated material has a pH less than 2.5. Other syndromes which can result from aspiration are bronchial obstruction by an aspirated foreign body and bacterial pneumonia from aspiration of oropharyngeal bacteria.

Foreign-body aspiration is managed by bronchoscopic removal. Aspiration bacterial pneumonia is treated with antibiotics, which are chosen on the basis of whether the event occurred out of the hospital or shortly after admission, or if it occurred during a prolonged hospital stay.[6]

In the pregnant patient, the acid aspiration syndrome is more frequently encountered and can lead to maternal mortality.[5] The pregnant woman is vulnerable to this problem because the gravid uterus can compress the stomach and elevate intragastric pressure, while progesterone relaxes the gastroesophageal sphincter. Labor itself delays gastric emptying, and in one study 55 percent of intrapartum patients had greater than 40 ml of liquid gastric juice and 42 percent had a pH less than 2.5.[5] Alcohol, which is rarely used today as a tocolytic agent, can stimulate gastric acid secretion and lead to obtundation, thus facilitating aspiration.[35] Forceful abdominal manipulation and obtundation during anesthesia also add to the risk of aspiration.

When acid aspiration occurs, clinical illness may become apparent immediately if the aspiration is massive, but in some cases there is a delay of 6 to 8 h. The illness is characterized by bronchospasm, tachycardia, hypotension, tachypnea, cyanosis, and then frothy pink sputum production. The latter finding appears if noncardiogenic pulmonary edema and capillary leak develop. Diagnosis is facilitated by having a high index of suspicion in the postpartum patient with respiratory distress.

Treatment of acid aspiration is supportive with oxygen and mechanical ventilation with PEEP, if needed. If aspiration is observed, endotracheal suctioning should be performed, but saline lavage is not indicated and may even serve to spread the acid to uninvolved areas.[35,88] Bronchodilators may control bronchospasm. Fluid therapy is directed at keeping intravascular volume as low as possible while still preserving cardiac output, a goal which may require monitoring of pulmonary capillary wedge pressure because of rapid volume loss across the injured pulmonary capillary. Corticosteroid treatment is of unproven benefit but can be justified if given immediately after a witnessed aspiration in which gastric fluid, obtained simultaneously by nasogastric tube, has a pH less than 2.5.[5,64,88] The dose used by some authors is 1 g hydrocortisone every 6 h for 1 to 2 days, followed by 1 to 2 days of 1 g daily.[5] Others have used one-time methylpredinisolone therapy in a dose of 30 mg/kg. Antibiotic treatment is best withheld until the patient develops signs of infection; therapy is then directed at the organisms found on sputum gram stain and culture.[88]

Prophylaxis of aspiration should always be attempted.[5,64] All patients in labor should be assumed to have a full stomach and should be given nothing by mouth except medication. If gross stomach distension is present, nasogastric evacuation can be performed. Regional anesthesia should be used instead of general whenever possible. When general anesthesia is administered, the patient should be intubated with a cuffed endotracheal tube. The optimal intubation position is not established but cricoid pressure during intubation can reduce aspiration risk.

Antacids should be given routinely during labor. One study found that 25 percent of patients in labor had more than 25 ml of gastric fluid with a pH less than 2.5 and were thus at risk for aspiration pneumonia. This risk was reduced to less than 3 percent by administration of 30 ml of antacid every 3 h after the onset of labor.[64] Still, aspiration pneumonitis with subsequent pulmonary edema has been described in an antacid-treated patient with a gastric pH of 6.4.[9]

In summary, the acid and nonacid aspiration syndromes are common complications of labor and delivery, and every effort must be made to prevent these illnesses and to diagnose them early when prevention has failed.

RESTRICTIVE LUNG DISEASES

Restrictive lung diseases have been mentioned earlier and generally are better tolerated by the mother than obstructive diseases. This stems from the basic nature of the physiologic defect and also from the fact that some of the steroid-responsive restrictive diseases, such as sarcoidosis, may improve in pregnancy.[85] In managing the patient with restrictive disease, pulmonary function evaluation and application of the guidelines discussed is appropriate, in addition to the usual supportive measures used in other lung diseases.

REFERENCES

1. Aaro, L.A. and Juergens, J.L.: Thrombophlebitis associated with pregnancy. Am. J. Obstet. Gynecol., *109:*1128, 1971.
2. Ang, C.K., Tan, T.H., Walters, W.A.W., and Wood, C.: Postural influence on maternal capillary oxygen and carbon dioxide tension. Br. Med. J., *4:*201, 1969.
3. Arwood, L.L., Dasta, J.F., and Friedman, C.: Placental transfer of theophylline: two case reports. Pediatrics, *63:*844, 1979.
4. Awe, R.J., Nicotra, M.B., Newsom, T.D., and Viles, R.: Arterial oxygenation and alveolar-arterial gradients in term pregnancy. Obstet. Gynecol., *53:*182, 1979.
5. Baggish, M.S. and Hopper, S.: Aspiration as a cause of maternal death. Obstet. Gynecol., *43:*327, 1974.
6. Bartlett, J.G. and Borbach, S.L.: The triple threat of aspiration pneumonia. Chest, *68:*560, 1975.
7. Bates, D.V., Macklem, P.T., and Christie R.V.: Respiratory Function in Disease. 2nd Ed. W.B. Saunders, Philadelphia, 1971.
8. Beitins, J.Z., Bayard, F., Ances, I.G. et al.: The transplacental passage of prednisone and prednisolone in pregnancy near term. J. Pediatr., *81:*936, 1972.
9. Bond, V.K., Stoelting, R.K., and Gupta, C.O.: Pulmonary aspiration syndrome after inhalation of gastric fluid containing antacid. Anesthesiology, *51:*452, 1979.

10. Bonebrake, C.R., Noller, K.L., Loehnen, C.P. et al.: Routine chest roentgenography in pregnancy. JAMA, *240:*2747, 1978.
11. Cherniak, R.M.: Pulmonary function testing. W.B. Saunders, Philadelphia, 1977.
12. Cines, D.B., Kaywin, P., Bina, M. et al.: Heparin-associated thrombocytopenia. N. Engl. J. Med., *303:*788, 1980.
13. Cohen, L.F., DiSanti' Agnese, P.A., and Friedlander, J.: Cystic fibrosis and pregnancy. A national survey. Lancet, *2:*842, 1980.
14. Collins, C.G.: Suppurative pelvic thrombophlebitis. Am. J. Obstet. Gynecol., *108:*681, 1970.
15. Corkey, C.W.B., Newth, C.J.L., Corey, M., and Levison, H.: Pregnancy in cystic fibrosis: a better prognosis in patients with pancreatic function. Am. J. Obstet. Gynecol., *140:*737, 1981.
16. Cugell, D.W., Frank, N.R., Gaensler, E.A. et al.: Pulmonary function in pregnancy. I. Serial observations in normal women. Am. Rev. Tuberc., *67:*568, 1953.
17. DeNicola, L.K. and Hanshaw, J.B.: Congenital an neonatal varicella. J. Pediatr., *94:*175, 1979.
18. De Swiet, M.: Respiratory disease in pregnancy. Postgrad. Med. J., *55:*325, 1979.
19. Duong, C.M. and Munns, R.E.: Varicella pneumonia during pregnancy. J. Fam. Pract., *8:*277, 1979.
20. Eickhoff, T.C., Sherman, I.L., and Serling, R.E., Observations on excesss mortality associated with epidemic influenza. JAMA, *176:*776, 1961.
21. Findley, L.J. and Sahn, S.A.: The value of chest roentgenograms in acute asthma in adults. Chest, *80:*535, 1981.
22. Ferstenfeld, J.E., Schlueter, D.P., Rytel, M.W., and Molloy, R.P.: Recognition and treatment of adult respiratory distress syndrome secondary to viral interstitial pneumonia. Am. J. Med., *58:*709, 1975.
23. Fischl, M.A., Pitchenik, A., and Gardner, L.B.: An index predicting relapse and need for hospitalization in patients with acute bronchial asthma. N. Engl. J. Med., *305:*789, 1981.
24. Franklin, W.: Treatment of severe asthma. N. Engl. J. Med., *290:*1469, 1974.
25. Gaensler, E.A., Patton, W.E., Verstraeten, J.M. et al.: Pulmonary function in pregnancy. III. Serial observations in patients with pulmonary insufficiency. Am. Rev. Tuberc., *67:*779, 1953.
26. Garrard, G.S., Littler, W.A., and Redman, C.W.G.: Closing volume during normal pregnancy. Thorax, *33:*488, 1978.
27. Giesler, C.F., Buehler, J.H., and Depp, R.: Alpha-1-antitrypsin deficiency. Severe obstructive lung disease and pregnancy. Obstet. Gynecol., *49:*31, 1977.
28. Gilbert, R. and Auchincloss, J.H., Jr.: Dyspnea of pregnancy: clinical and physiological observations. Am. J. Med. Sci., *252:*270, 1966.
29. Gluck, J.C. and Gluck, P.A.: The effects of pregnancy on asthma: a prospective study. Ann. Allergy, *37:*164, 1976.
30. Goldberg, S.J., Levy, R.A., Siassi, B., and Betten, J.: The effects of maternal hypoxia and hyperoxia upon the neonatal pulmonary vasculature. Pediatrics, *48:*528, 1971.
31. Good, J.T. and Waite, D.: Postpartum solitary lung abcess. Am. J. Obstet. Gynecol., *132:*338, 1978.
32. Gordon, M., Niswander, K.R., Berendes, H., and Kantor, A.G.: Fetal morbidity following potentially anoxygenic obstetric conditions. VII. Bronchial asthma. Am. J. Obstet. Gynecol., *106:*421, 1970.
33. Greenberger, P. and Patterson, R.: Safety of therapy for allergic symptoms during pregnancy. Ann. Intern. Med., *89:*234, 1978.
34. Greenhill, J.P. and Friedman, E.A.: Biological Principles and Modern Practice of Obstetrics. W.B. Saunders, Philadelphia, 1974.

35. Greenhouse, B.S., Hook, R., and Hehre, F.W.: Aspiration pneumonia following intravenous administration of alcohol during labor. JAMA, *210*:2393, 1969.
36. Hadjigeoriou, E., Kitsiou, S., Psarondakis, A. et al.: Antepartum aminophylline treatment for prevention of the respiratory distress syndrome in premature infants. Am. J. Obstet. Gynecol., *135*:257, 1979.
37. Hague, W.M.: Mediastinal and subcutaneous emphysema in a pregnant patient with asthma. Br. J. Obstet. Gynaecol., *87*:440, 1980.
38. Hall, J.G., Pauli, R.M., and Wilson, K.M.: Maternal and fetal sequelae of anticoagulation during pregnancy. Am. J. Med., *68*:122, 1980.
39. Handin, R.I.: Thromboembolic complications of pregnancy and oral contraceptives. Prog. Cardiovasc. Dis., *16*:395, 1974.
40. Hernandez, E., Angell, C.S., and Johnson, J.W.C.: Asthma in pregnancy: current concepts. Obstet. Gynecol., *55*:739, 1980.
41. Hopwood, H.G.: Pneumonia in pregnancy. Obstet. Gynecol., *25*:875, 1965.
42. Howie, A.D. and Milne, J.A.: Pregnancy in patients with bronchiectasis. Br. J. Obstet. Gynaecol., *85*:197, 1978
43. Hull, R., Delmore, T., Carter, C. et al.: Adjusted subcutaneous heparin versus warfarin sodium in the long-term treatment of venous thrombosis. N. Engl. J. Med., *306*:189, 1982.
44. Hung, C.T., Pelosi, M., Langer, A., and Harrigan, J.T.: Blood gas measurements in the kyphoscoliotic gravida and her fetus: report of a case. Am. J. Obstet. Gynecol., *121*:287, 1975.
45. Hyatt, A.C., Chipps, B.E., Kumor, K.M. et al.: A double-blind controlled trial of anti-*Pseudomonas* chemotherapy for acute respiratory exacerbations in patients with cystic fibrosis. Pediatrics, *99*:307, 1981.
46. Jacobs, M.M., Knight, A.B., and Arias, F.: Maternal pulmonary edema resulting from betamimetic and glucocorticoid therapy. Obstet. Gynecol., *56*:56, 1980.
47. Katz, M., Robertson, P.A., and Creasy, R.K.: Cardiovascular complications associated with terbutaline treatment for preterm labor. Am. J. Obstet. Gynecol., *139*:605, 1981.
48. Kreisman, H., Van de Wiel, W., and Mitchell, C.A.: Respiratory function during prostaglandin-induced labor. Am. Rev. Respir. Dis., *111*:564, 1975.
49. Labovitz, E. and Spector, S.: Placental theophylline transfer in pregnant asthmatics. JAMA, *247*:786, 1982.
50. Laros, K.D.: The postpneumonectomy mother. Respiration, *39*:185, 1980.
51. Leontic, E.A.: Respiratory disease in pregnancy. Med. Clin. North Am., *61*:111, 1977.
52. Levin, S. and Jupa, J.E.: Principles of antibiotic use in obstetrics and gynecology. Obstet. Gynecol. Annu., *5*:293, 1976.
53. Levinson, G., Shnider, S.M., deLorimier, A.A., and Steffenson, J.L.: Effects of maternal hyperventilation on uterine blood flow and fetal oxygenation and acid-base status. Anesthesiology, *40*:340, 1974.
54. MacKenzie, J.S. and Houghton, M.: Influenza infections during pregnancy: association with congenital malformations and with subsequent neoplasms in children and potential hazards of live virus vaccines. Bacteriol. Rev., *38*:356, 1974.
55. McClure, J.H. and James, J.M.: Oxygen administration to the mother and its relation to blood oxygen in the newborn infant. Am. J. Obstet. Gynecol., *80*:554, 1960.
56. Milne, J.A., Howie, A.D., Pack, A.I.: Dyspnea during normal pregnancy. Br. J. Obstet. Gynaecol., *85*:260, 1978.
57. Merril, L.K. and VerBurg, D.J.: The choice of long-term anticoagulants for the pregnant patient. Obstet. Gynecol., *47*:711, 1976.
58. Milne, J.A.: The respiratory response to pregnancy. Postgrad. Med. J., *55*:318, 1979.

59. Mobin-Uddin, K., Collard, G.M., Bolooki, H. et al.: Transvenous caval interruption with umbrella filter. N. Engl. J. Med., *286:*55, 1972.
60. Monif, G.R.G., Sowards, D.L., and Eitzman, D.V.: Serologic and immunologic evaluation of neonates following maternal influenza infection during the second and third trimesters of gestation. Am. J. Obstet. Gynecol., *114:*239, 1972.
61. Moser, K.M.: Pulmonary embolism. Am. Rev. Respir. Dis., *115:*829, 1977.
62. Pridmore, B.R., Murray, K.H., and McAllen, P.M.: The management of anticoagulant therapy during and after pregnancy. Br. J. Obstet. Gynaecol., *82:*740, 1975.
63. Prowse, C.M. and Gaensler, E.A.: Respiratory and acid-base changes during pregnancy. Anesthesiology, *26:*381, 1965.
64. Roberts, R.B. and Shirley, M.A.: The obstetrician's role in reducing the risk of aspiration pneumonitis, with particular reference to the use of oral antacids. Am. J. Obstet. Gynecol., *124:*611, 1976.
65. Robin, E.D.: Overdiagnosis and overtreatment of pulmonary embolism: the emperor may have no clothes. Ann. Intern. Med., *87:*775, 1977.
66. Roizen, M.F. and Feeley, T.W.: Pancuronium bromide. Ann. Intern. Med., *88:*64, 1978.
67. Salzman, E.W., Deykin, D., Shapiro, R.M., and Rosenberg, R.: Management of heparin therapy. N. Engl. J. Med., *292:*1046, 1975.
68. Schatz, M., Patterson, R., Zeitz, S. et al.: Corticosteroid therapy for the pregnant asthmatic patient. JAMA, *233:*804, 1975.
69. Scherter, C.B., Polnitsky, C.A., and Matthay, R.A.: Chronic obstructive pulmonary diseases (asthma, bronchitis, emphysema, bronchiectasis and cystic fibrosis). In George, R., Light, R., and Matthay, R., Eds.: Pulmonary Diseases. Churchill Livingstone, New York, 1982.
70. Schoenbaum, S.C. and Weinstein, L.: Respiratory infections in pregnancy. Clin Obstet. Gynecol., 22:293, 1979.
71. Scoggin, C.H., Sahn, S.A., and Petty, T.L.: Status asthmaticus: a nine-year experience. JAMA, *238:*1158, 1977.
72. Sims, C.D., Chamberlain, G.V.P., and DeSwiet, M.: Lung function tests in bronchial asthma during and after pregnancy. Br. J. Obstet. Gynaecol., *83:*434, 1976.
73. Smith, A.P.: The effects of intravenous infusion of graded doses of prostaglandins F2α and E2 on lung resistance in patients undergoing termination of pregnancy. Clin. Sci. Mol. Med., *44:*17, 1973.
74. Spearing, G., Fraser, I., Turner, G., and Dixon, G.: Long-term self-administered subcutaneous heparin in pregnancy. Br. Med. J., *1:*1457, 1978.
75. Sulavik, S.B.: Pulmonary disease. p. 549. In Burrow, G.N., Ferris, T.F., Eds.: Medical Complications During Pregnancy. W.B. Saunders, Philadelphia, 1975.
76. Swartz, H.M. and Reichling, B.A.: Hazards of radiation exposure for pregnant women. JAMA, *239:*1907, 1978.
77. Tarnoff, J., Lees, W.M., and Fox, R.T.: Major thoracic surgery during pregnancy. Am. Rev. Respir. Dis., *96:*1169, 1967.
78. Tisi, G.M.: Preoperative evaluation of pulmonary function. Am. Rev. Respir. Dis., *119:*293, 1979.
79. Tisi, G.M.: Pulmonary Physiology in Clinical Medicine. Williams and Wilkins, Baltimore, 1980.
80. Topilsky, M., Levo, Y., Spitzer, S.A. et al.: Status asthmaticus in pregnancy: a case report. Ann. Allergy, 32:151, 1974.
81. Turner, E.S., Greenberger, P.A., and Patterson, R.: Management of the pregnant asthmatic patient. Ann. Intern. Med., *93:*905, 1980.
82. Van Dellen, R.G.: Intravenous aminophylline. Chest, *76:*2, 1979.

83. Vinall, P.S. and Jenkins, D.M.: Salbutamol and haemorrhage at spontaneous abortion: Lancet, *2:*1355, 1977.
84. Webb-Johnson, D.C. and Andrews, J.L.: Bronchodilator therapy, N. Engl. J. Med., *297:*476, 758, 1977.
85. Weinberger, S.E., Weiss, S.T., Cohen, W.R. et al.: Pregnancy and the lung. Am. Rev. Respir. Dis., *121:*559, 1980.
86. Weinstein, A.M., Dubin, B.D., Podleski, W.K. et al.: Asthma and pregnancy. JAMA, *241:*1161, 1979.
87. Winterbauer, R.H., Ludwig, W.R., and Hanmar, S.P.: Clinical course, management, and long term sequelae of respiratory failure due to influenza viral pneumonia. Johns Hopkins Med. J., *141:*148, 1977.
88. Wynne, J.W. and Modell, J.H.: Respiratory aspiration of stomach contents. Ann. Intern. Med., *87:*466, 1977.
89. Yawn, D.H., Pyeatta, J.C., Joseph, J.M. et al., Transplacental transfer of influenza virus. JAMA, *216:*1022, 1971.

13

Neurologic Emergencies during Pregnancy

James O. Donaldson, M.D.

INTRODUCTION

Neurologic emergencies during pregnancy are unusual but account for a large share of maternal mortality. This chapter is devoted to the management of these crises in obstetrical patients. Other sources with extensive bibliographies deal with the broad range of nonemergent neurologic problems coexistent with pregnancy.[3,19]

STATUS EPILEPTICUS

Status epilepticus is the state wherein a patient has seizures and does not fully recover between them or has one seizure lasting more than 30 min. Generalized tonic-clonic (grand mal) status epilepticus is the most frequent and dangerous type; however, status epilepticus also occurs with petit mal (spike-wave stupor) and focal seizures of the temporal lobe and motor cortex (epilepsia partialis continua). The convulsions themselves, regardless of cause, result in a 2.5 percent mortality rate and a 12.5 percent morbidity rate.[4] Status epilepticus in a pregnant woman, especially one not known to be an epileptic, should be considered symptomatic of another disorder such as eclampsia, encephalitis, meningitis, frontal lobe tumor, drug withdrawal, and a variety of toxic and metablic conditions until proven otherwise.[4,45]

Inadvertent intravenous injection of local anesthetics intended for a paracervical block may cause continuous seizures for 10 to 20 min.[2,8,56] If hypoxia is prevented, the electroencephalogram may be normal in these patients within 1 h after the seizure.

"Status hystericus," i.e., continuous pseudoseizures, will be misdiagnosed and mistreated unless a "seizure" is critically observed. During pseudoseizures pupillary light reactions are characteristically present; opisthotonus, pelvic thrusting, and to-and-fro head thrashing are common; and the patient may respond to or remember what is said. During true generalized convulsions, the pupillary light responses are absent and the tonic phase usually is either stiffening of the body or bilateral flexion of hips and knees, followed by clonic movements which are bilaterally synchronous jerks. Pupillary light responses are the most reliable signs. The diagnosis of status epilepticus should not be made until a physician has critically witnessed one convulsion.

Before effective anticonvulsants became available, status epilepticus during pregnancy was always fatal to both mother and fetus.[30] Termination of pregnancy did not stop noneclamptic status epilepticus. The effect of isolated maternal seizures and status epilepticus upon fetal physiology, organogenesis, and growth has not been established, except that fetal bradycardia has been noted to occur during a convulsion.[60] It is reasonable to believe, however, that maternal seizures are potentially harmful to the fetus. Nevertheless, healthy, normal infants have been born to mothers who had status epilepticus during pregnancy.[30]

Status epilepticus in a pregnant epileptic usually occurs in the second half of pregnancy and is frequently associated with subtherapeutic blood levels of anticonvulsant drugs.[39,50] Anticonvulsant blood levels should be followed once a month throughout pregnancy if epilepsy is controlled, and more frequently if it is not. It is common for the oral daily dosage of phenytoin to double or triple during pregnancy because drug absorption in the gut is decreased and metabolism is increased. Also, the patient may not strictly adhere to the prescribed drug regimen. Table 13-1 lists the range of therapeutic blood levels for several different anticonvulsants.

The complex physiologic changes which occur during seizures must be understood in order to properly treat status epilepticus and to prevent its complications. The hypertension, tachycardia, hypoxia, and lactic acidosis which inevitably occur during an isolated seizure lasting less than 3 min do not have a chance to resolve spontaneously in status epilepticus. As a consequence, cerebral blood flow and cerebral utilization of oxygen and glucose increase severalfold.[35] Hypotension and hypoglycemia may ensue. Prolonged muscular contractions may cause rhabdomyolysis, hyperthermia, and myoglobinuric acute renal tubular necrosis.

Adults with status epilepticus lasting more than 2 h may develop permanent neurologic dysfunction due to neuronal loss similar to that caused by hypoxic encephalopathy. Some patients, however, may seize for much longer times without demonstrable impairment.[3,45] When damage occurs, it can be attributed both to the

Table 13-1. Therapeutic Concentrations of Anticonvulsants

Phenytoin	10–20 mg/L
Phenobarbital	15–40 mg/L
Carbamazepine	4–12 mg/L
Primidone	5–12 mg/L
Ethosuximide	40–100 mg/L

continuous firing of neurons and to hypoxemia because status epilepticus in paralyzed, well-ventilated animals causes similar pathologic changes.[35]

The therapeutic goal is to control status epilepticus within 30 min while maintaining ventilation and preventing injury.[12] Do not jam a wooden tongue blade or a spoon between clenched teeth because it only causes trauma. Give all medications intravenously. Monitoring of the maternal EKG and the fetal heart rate is recommended, especially during infusions of drugs; however the dosages and infusion rates recommended herein are usually safe for both mother and fetus.

Diazepam is an excellent drug to break status epilepticus. Adults are given 10 mg intravenously over 2 min and thereafter 2 mg/min IV until the convulsion stops. Usually, less than 20 mg will be needed to give a seizure-free interval long enough to catheterize a large vein and to insert a soft plastic oral airway. If an oral airway can not be introduced, intubate without hesitation.

Yeh et al. reported that maternal and fetal heart rates increased transiently after the IV administration of 5 to 10 mg diazepam to women in labor and had no adverse effect upon maternal, fetal, or neonatal pH, pO_2, or pCO_2.[67] The intrapartum IV administration of up to 20 mg diazepam did not increase the incidence of neonatal hypotonia and respiratory depression. Larger total doses of diazepam, however, can depress both mother and fetus.

After blood has been drawn for the determination of concentrations of glucose, electrolytes, and calcium, the following should be administered IV: 50 ml of a 50 percent dextrose solution, a loading dose of a long-acting anticonvulsant (phenytoin or phenobarbital), and, if there is any possibility of alcoholism, thiamine hydrochloride, 100 mg. Phenytoin is the first choice because, unlike phenobarbital, it does not depress either respiration or level of consciousness.

The loading dose of phenytoin sodium is usually 1 g (approximately 14 to 18 mg/kg), diluted in normal saline and infused at a rate of 50 mg/min.[16,65] Peak brain levels may not occur for 1 h. Seizures in the interim can be treated with additional diazepam. The loading dose of phenytoin should be followed with 100 mg every 6 h to ensure consistently high therapeutic concentrations of this drug.

Status epilepticus which is intractable to this regimen is usually caused by an acute, active brain disorder such as encephalitis or tumor. When seizure activity persists, the next steps are endotracheal intubation, if that has not already been done, and the IV administration of phenobarbital at 60 mg/min until convulsions cease or until a total dose of 20 mg/kg has been administered.[12] The total daily maintenance dose, 1.5 to 2.0 mg/kg, can be adjusted according to phenobarbital blood levels.

If this fails, general anesthesia will be required. Hyperthermia and rhabdomyolysis are treated by a cooling blanket and curare. Paralyzed patients need electroencephalographic monitoring to guide anticonvulsant therapy.[64]

ACUTE INTERMITTENT PORPHYRIA

Acute intermittent porphyria (AIP) is an inborn error of heme synthesis in which a deficiency of uroporphyrinogen I synthase prevents sufficient negative

Table 13-2. Precipitants of Porphyric Crises

Fasting	Anticonvulsants:
Sulfonamides	Barbiturates
Griseofulvin	Phenytoin
Estrogens	Mephenytoin
Chlordiazepoxide	Methsuximide
Meprobamate	Phensuximide
Methyprylon	Carbamazepine
Glutethimide	Valproic acid
Isopropylmeprobamate	Clonazepam (high dose)
Dicloralphenazone	
Ergot	

From Tschudy, D.P., Valsamis, M., and Magnussen, C.R.: Acute intermittent porphyria: clinical and selected research aspects. Ann. Intern. Med., 83:851, 1975.

feedback regulation of porphyrin synthesis. A variety of substances and situations which stimulate aminolevulinic acid (ALA) synthase and porphyrin synthesis can provoke a crisis (Table 13-2). Crises are clinically manifested by abdominal pain and mental aberrations, followed several days later by an acute areflexic polyneuropathy. The greatest risk to a pregnant woman occurs when the existence of porphyria is unknown.[19] Then the hypertension, tachycardia, and seizures which accompany a crisis may lead to the mistaken diagnosis of eclampsia. Postpartum crisis with paralysis is often induced by intrapartum administration of barbiturates and other drugs, surgery, or the fasting state.

The initial treatment of a porphyric crisis consists of discontinuation of barbiturates and other offending drugs and maintenance of a high carbohydrate intake (300 to 800 g/day PO and IV).[31] Resolution of hypertension and tachycardia is an excellent measure of therapeutic success unless propranolol, administered to treat an arrhythmia, masks these responses.

If this approach is not successful within 3 days, an IV infusion of hematin (3 mg/kg/day) should be administered. Hematin is a powder of crystallized heme prepared from human red cells, which effectively decreases porphyrin synthesis by inhibiting ALA synthase.[31] Hematin infusions will not reverse neuropathic weakness. Fetal effects of this therapy are unknown, as to date there have been no reports of the use of hematin during pregnancy.

Unless convulsions abate with these measures, seizure management is a serious problem because all anticonvulsants except bromide salts induce ALA synthase and may exacerbate acute prophyria. Patients whose seizures are unresponsive to clonazepam in low doses (1 to 3 mg/day) may respond to bromide at blood levels of 15 mEq/L (about 90 mg/dl).[10,32] The usual dosage of triple bromide solution is 3 ml twice daily by mouth. Higher maternal doses may cause neonatal bromism, as manifested by hypotonia, hyporeflexia, lethargy, and irritability.

ECLAMPSIA

The neurologic manifestations of eclampsia are convulsions, coma, and, rarely, cortical blindness. The convulsions may be focal, generalized, or generalized with focal features such as adversive eye movements. Sudden coma with or without convulsions can occur as a result of a large intracerebral hematoma. In most instances the patient progresses through the stages of impaired consciousness to stupor and coma. Headache and brisk reflexes are common.

Cerebral pathology causes at least 30 percent of deaths due to eclampsia. Modern neurologic tools, including electroencephalography and computerized tomography (CT) are rarely used, although they may prove to make valuable contributions to the management of eclampsia. The entity of "late postpartum eclampsia" usually proves to be a cerebral venous thrombosis.[55]

The gross neuropathologic hallmarks of eclampsia are clusters of small hemorrhages and intermixed microinfarctions which occur in the border zones between the the major cerebral arteries, in the terminal distribution of small arterioles supplying the deep cerebral nuclei and corona radiata, and in the pons.[55] Closely packed petechiae may be difficult to distinguish from one large hematoma on CT scan. There is special predilection for involvement of the occipital lobes, and the rest of the brain may be normal. The classic microscopic lesion is a ring hemorrhage surrounding a thrombosed precapillary.[55]

Eclamptic convulsions can be attributed to the cortical lesions. Individual lesions in the visual cortex or retina may cause the flashes of light which eclamptic women often experience and for which eclampsia was named. Multiple lesions in the occipital cortex can cause cortical blindness. Hyperreflexia may not be caused by any cerebral lesion; it may be due to high catecholamine levels.

Conventional wisdom has maintained that these lesions are caused by cerebral vasospasm.[48] Research in the past decade, however, indicates that the ring hemorrhages result from the failure of cerebral vasoconstriction to reduce blood flow to the capillary bed and to limit the pressure exerted upon thin-walled capillaries.[59] These forces rupture small vessels, with exudation of plasma and diapedesis of erythrocytes. This damage coexists with and may initiate the deposition of fibrinoid material within both the lumen and media of arterioles (Fig. 13-1).

In physiologic terms the upper limit of the autoregulation of cerebral perfusion has been breached.[59] In experimental animals the greatest change in arteriolar diameter and the earliest rupture of vessels occur in the anastomotic arterioles be-

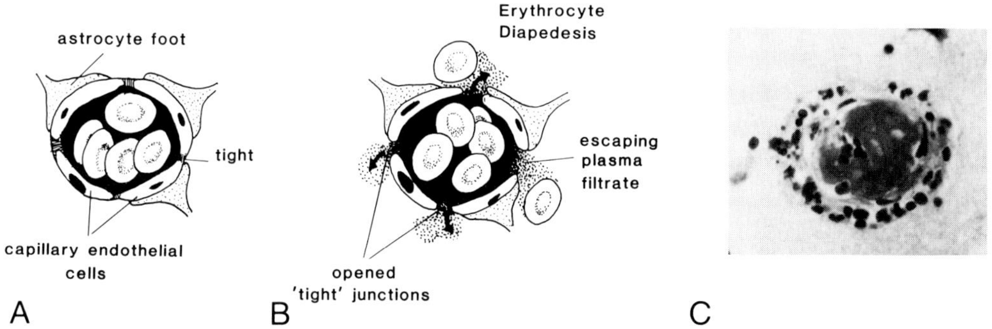

Fig. 13-1 Pathogenesis of ring hemorrhages in eclamptic hypertensive encephalopathy. (A) Intact cerebral capillary. (B) Ruptured capillary junctions with leakage of red cells and plasma. (C) A thrombosed cerebral precapillary surrounded by hemorrhage.

tween major watersheds. These areas act as safety valves through which blood flow may increase two- or threefold without the remaining 90 percent of brain being affected. At higher pressures the entire cortex is affected similarly.

The upper limit of the range of blood pressures throughout which cerebral perfusion is held constant is dependent upon an individual patient's usual blood pressure. A pregnant teenager who previously had a blood pressure of 95/60 mmHg may convulse at a sustained blood pressure of 140/90 mmHg, well below most arbitrary thresholds for the diagnosis of severe preeclampsia. Thus, each patient must be considered individually.

Control of hypertension is fundamental to the prevention of the cerebral manifestations of eclampsia.[19] The antihypertensive drug chosen should decrease vascular resistance in the rest of the body and not directly affect cerebral vasconstriction. Lowering of peripheral resistance and blood pressure is followed automatically by relaxation of cerebral vasoconstriction; in experimental animals a lag of 1 to 2 min exists. If a drug directly relaxes cerebral vasoconstriction but does not significantly lower blood pressure at the same time, cerebral damage could worsen. Hypercarbia, which lowers the upper limit of cerebral perfusion autoregulation in this manner, must be avoided. Similarly, nitroglycerin is potentially dangerous. The antihypertensive drugs which meet these specifications are hydralazine, nitroprusside, and diazoxide.

Anticonvulsant Therapy. The best anticonvulsant treatment is effective antihypertensive therapy. Individual seizures can be stopped with diazepam, and thereafter a loading dose of phenytoin should be administered intravenously as prophylaxis against additional seizures. In Europe intravenous chlormethiazole is often used instead of phenytoin. Women who have received magnesium sulfate should be treated similarly although respiratory depression is more likely to occur during an infusion of diazepam. Unless hypertension is treated commitantly, new cerebral lesions could develop without convulsions to alert the clinician.

Magnesium "Therapy". Each year in the United States tons of magnesium sulfate are administered to women with preeclampsia and eclampsia.[48] Magnesium sulfate is infrequently used in Britain and Scandinavia. Its use is empiric.[38] Most regimens include both magnesium sulfate and an effective antihypertensive drug such as hydralazine.[48] Magnesium sulfate is a poor anticonvulsant and a poor antihypertensive agent, and its risks to mother and fetus are significant.

Hypermagnesemia depresses neuromuscular transmission by inhibiting the presynaptic release of acetylcholine in response to a nerve action potential. Its effects upon skeletal and cardiac muscle are dependent upon blood magnesium concentrations.[38] Hypotension may occur during intravenous infusions of magnesium solutions. The fetal level reaches 90 percent of the maternal level within 3 h, and manifestations of neonatal hypermagnesemia are more common than usually are appreciated.[51]

If the blood-brain barrier is intact, as it is in preeclampsia, acute hypermagnesemia does not affect either the function of the central nervous system or the magnesium concentrations in cerebropsinal fluid (CSF).[44,57] Intracerebral, intraventricular, and intrathecal instillation of magnesium ions can profoundly depress central nervous system activity.[11] Seizure foci induced by experimental methods which disrupt the blood-brain barrier are depressed but not abolished by intravenous magnesium sulfate infusions with an efficacy proportional to blood magnesium concentrations.[11] It could be argued that an eclamptic seizure focus from a patch of ring hemorrhages could be damped by magnesium sulfate because the blood-brain capillary barrier is broken, but this hypothesis has never been tested by electroencephalographic monitoring of an eclamptic seizure treated in this fashion. It is unlikely that hypermagnesemia would stop generalized seizures triggered by the focus because the blood-brain barrier would be intact in the remainder of the brain. High levels of magnesium, on the other hand, could block the motor response to cortical seizures. Chesley[15] has documented eclamptic seizures in spite of magnesium levels of 6.3 mEq/L.

ISCHEMIC STROKE

Ischemic strokes present as the sudden onset of deficits in central nervous system function, such as hemiplegia, hemianopsia, aphasia, and apraxia. Headache and seizures occur but less frequently than with intracerebral hemorrhage or cerebral venous disease. Ischemic strokes in young adults, especially pregnant or puerperal women, must be thoroughly investigated in order to discover treatable conditions, to prevent additional strokes, and to properly counsel the patients.

Some of the conditions which may cause strokes in pregnant women are listed in Table 13-3. A medical history and physical examination done with the differential diagnosis in mind is the critical first step in evaluating the patient. Optic fundi must be inspected for emboli, Roth's spots, and signs of arteriolar sclerosis and hypertension. Blood pressures must be determined in both arms. Ocular, cervical, and subclavian bruits must be listened for. A careful cardiac examination is manditory. Phlebitis, ecchymoses, and splinter subungual hemorrhages are important physical findings.

Most relevant laboratory studies, including routine hemogram, platelet count, erythrocyte sedimentation rate, chest x-ray, electrocardiography, two-dimensional echocardiography, and computed tomography are noninvasive. Oculoplatysmography and oculodynamometry supply clues to the etiology of the stroke but are

Table 13-3. Diseases Causing Stroke during Pregnancy

Heart Disease
Rheumatic heart disease
Atrial fibrillation
Peripartum cardiomyopathy
Infective endocarditis
Mitral valve prolapse
Paradoxical embolism
Sickle hemoglobinopathy
Arteritis
Thrombotic thrombocytopenic purpura
Metastatic choriocarcinoma

accurately interpreted only in retrospect after an angiogram. A CT scan will clearly show intracerebral hemorrhage in addition to mass effects and edema. If an obvious source for emboli or a systemic disease is not found, cerebral angiography is recommended. Percutaneous transfemoral angiography can be done with abdominal shielding so that fetal exposure is limited to little more than right-angle scatter.

Strokes symptomatic of heart disease and other systemic disorders more commonly cause maternal and fetal mortality than ischemic stroke due to premature atheroma.[17,20] Pregnant patients with stroke due to atrial fibrillation and peripartum cardiomyopathy need immediate anticoagulation with heparin unless intracerebral hemorrhage is present.[66] Subacute bacterial endocarditis, sickle hemoglobinopathy, metastatic choriocarcinoma, thrombotic thrombocytopenic purpura, and arteritis must be appropriately managed.

Paradoxical cerebral embolism usually coexists with pulmonary emboli from puerperal pelvic phlebitis.[18] Often other major arteries are occluded, and this combination of problems can be devastating. In one case, however, a puerperal paradoxical embolus was removed from the carotid bifurcation with subsequent complete recovery from hemiplegia.[41] Emergency carotid thromboendarterectomy must be done within 4 h after the onset of stroke and only after the diagnosis has been established with arteriography. Rarely can this logistic feat be accomplished.

Unless cardiac or other systemic disease dictates otherwise, women who have had a stroke during pregnancy may be delivered vaginally and they may be allowed to push. If delivery occurs within 6 weeks of the stroke and thus before the infarcted area has healed, hypotension and systemic hypertension must be avoided in order to prevent either extension of the infarction or hemorrhage into the softened brain. The Valsalva maneuver may be permitted during this period.

PUERPERAL CEREBRAL PHLEBOTHROMBOSIS

Aseptic cerebral venous thrombosis usually presents 3 days to 4 weeks postpartum as a syndrome of increasingly severe headaches culminating in generalized and focal convulsions, which are followed by weakness, aphasia, and other deficits in cerebral cortical function.[14,20] Recurrence of seizures implies spread of the clot. Intracranial hypertension can be caused by obstruction of CSF absorption by clot in the superior sagittal sinus and by the mass effect of venous infarctions with hemorrhage. A rapid progression of symptoms is a poor prognostic sign because it implies extension of the thrombus with less time for anastomotic veins to enlarge. The long-term prognosis is good if the patient survives the initial insult.

The diagnosis may be established by cerebral angiography if enough films are taken during the venous phase. Computed tomography will determine the extent of hemorrhagic cerebral infarction and may suggest a thrombosis of some major sinuses.[63] Aseptic cerebral venous thrombosis may occur with hyperviscosity syndromes, during sickle-cell crises, and after minor head trauma.

The treatment of puerperal cerebral venous thromboses with heparin was first suggested in 1942 and has been controversial ever since.[6,24,58] Heparin would prevent propagation of the clot into unaffected brain; however, it could increase hemorrhage into those venous infarctions already present. Also, it would treat concomitant phlebitis in the pelvis and legs but increase the risk of uterine hemorrhage.[14] The controversy may be resolved by the CT scan's unique ability to determine the presence and extent of intracerebral bleeding. Perhaps those patients without intracerebral hemorrhage should be treated with heparin. Seizures should be treated with anticonvulsants.

SUBARACHNOID HEMORRHAGE

Spontaneous subarachnoid hemorrhage due to ruptured berry aneurysms and arteriovenous malformations causes approximately 5 to 10 percent of maternal deaths. Patients complain of the sudden onset of the worst headache of their lives, followed by nausea and retching, diaphoresis, and neck stiffness; some lapse into coma. Patients often have hypertension and a wide variety of electrocardiographic abnormalities. Patients who are awake and have a normal neurologic examination after their initial hemorrhage still have a 15 percent chance of death due to rebleeding. The more stuporous the patient is and the more abnormal the neurologic examination, the greater the mortality rate.

The diagnosis is confirmed by finding grossly bloody CSF on lumbar puncture. The CSF will have a xanthrochromic supernatant after contrifugation if more than 6 h have passed from the time of the subarachnoid bleed. A CT scan will demonstrate intracerebral hematomas and often blood in the subarachnoid space. After exclusion of hematologic disorders and systemic diseases, (including bacterial endocarditis, sickle hemoglobinopathy, and metastatic choriocarcinoma) which may cause subarachnoid hemorrhage, angiography of all four major intracranial arteries will be needed for a definitive diagnosis and detection of multiple aneurysms.

Unless the patient is in active labor, neurologic evaluation and treatment take precedence over fetal concerns. Subarachnoid hemorrhage due to aneurysms occurs most commonly during pregnancy in the third trimester, and, if it occurs near term, may initiate labor.[27,52,53] Subarachnoid hemorrhage frequently occurs during labor, probably in part because of the hemodynamic changes resulting from the Valsalva maneuver, which almost irresistibly accompanies the second stage of labor. If the patient is in labor, bearing down must be prevented and the pregnancy should be terminated with urgency in order to prevent rebleeding and to maximize fetal survival.

The initial step in management of a mild subarachnoid hemorrhage is the administration of enough sedative to relieve anxiety and to allow toleration of bed rest in a quite room. During pregnancy phenobarbital is recommended for sedation instead of diazepam because chronic maternal use of diazepam causes fetal depression due to fetal retention of the drug and its active metabolites. Cigarette smoking is not permitted, and smoker's cough is suppressed. Constipation is prevented by stool softeners. Hypertension must be controlled.

Antifibrinolytic therapy with ϵ-aminocaproic acid or tranexamic acid does not alter the natural history of ruptured aneurysms although some experimental evidence supports its current widespread use.[49] It can not be recommended for pregnant patients.

Curative surgery before childbirth is the treatment of choice in the nonlaboring patient.[37]

Hypothermia. In experienced hands, hypothermia and controlled hypotension have been used extensively during intracranial operations performed on pregnant women with demonstrated safety for both mother and fetus.[26,29,37] Hypothermia reduces cerebral oxygen requirements and cerebral edema. Uterine blood flow and fetal metabolic requirements decrease. The uterus contracts and becomes firm but labor does not ensue. Fetal hypoxia does not occur if maternal ventilation is adequate.

Hypotension. Intraoperative controlled hypotension decreases rebleeding from an aneurysm during surgery.[1] This technique has been used safely during pregnancy with continuous monitoring of fetal heart rate; fetal bradycardia occurs if maternal blood pressure is too low.[1,37] The limit of tolerable hypotension varies with each person. Nitroprusside is the drug of choice because its effect can be titrated and quickly reversed. The effect of ganglionic blocking agents cannot be strictly controlled. This probably accounts for the unfavorable early reports on the use of hypotension during intracranial surgery upon pregnant women. Also, ganglionic blocking agents can cause meconium ileus in the fetus.

If the ruptured aneurysm is clipped or the arteriovenous malformation can be excised, vaginal delivery can be permitted thereafter without concern. Patients with inoperable lesions are usually delivered by elective cesarean section at 38 weeks gestation although some physicians have permitted a multiparous women to deliver vaginally with lumbar epidural anesthesia or continuous caudal anesthesia.[27,34] Panting during contractions early in labor will help to prevent Valsalva's maneuver.

CHOREA GRAVIDARUM

Chorea gravidarum is chorea or hemichorea acquired during pregnancy. These jerky movements and associated limb hypotonia usually begin sometime after the first trimester and cease after 2 or 3 months or following childbirth. Chorea gravidarum caused by rheumatic heart disease or systemic lupus erythematosus has a high morbidity due to the underlying disease. Unrelenting, severe chorea per se is dangerous because it can cause rhabdomyolysis, myoglobinuria, and hyperthermia.[28,34]

At one time treatment consisted of quiet isolation and sedation with barbiturates because chorea stops during sleep. Chorea is now effectively treated by competitively blocking dopamine receptors and thereby correcting a relative preponderance of dopaminergic activity within the corpus striatum. Phenothiazines and butyrophenones are both effective classes of domamine antagonists. Haloperidol, however, is the recommended drug because it is both potent and acceptably safe for use during pregnancy. The incidence of birth defects is not increased among infants born to women who took haloperidol for control of hyperemesis gravidarum.[21]

Moderate chorea gravidarum will usually respond to haloperidol 1 to 6 mg/day in divided doses.[21] More severe cases may require initial dosages in excess of 20 mg/day to control the chorea.

MYASTHENIC CRISIS

Myasthenia gravis is an autoimmune disease of the motor end plates of striated muscles which is clinically manifested by fluctuating fatigability of the muscles. Antibodies against nicotinic acetylcholine receptors block neuromuscular transmission and also accelerate the turnover of receptors, which can lead to irreversible deformation of the postsynaptic membrane. The immunogenesis of the disease is altered by thymectomy and corticosteroid therapy. Remissions may also occur spontaneously. Symptomatic treatment with the cholinesterase inhibitors neostigmine and pyridostigmine stimulates both muscarinic and nicotinic acetylcholine receptors. I arbitrarily advise young women with generalized myasthenia gravis to have a thymectomy and then to wait at least 1 year or until their disease stabilizes before attempting to become pregnant.

Myasthenic women usually have uncomplicated childbirth. Smooth muscles and myometrium are unaffected by myasthenia gravis. Furthermore, myasthenia may improve during pregnancy because α-fetoprotein blocks the interaction of anti-acetylcholine receptor antibody with its antigen. Maternal exhaustion must be avoided during labor. Serial determinations of vital capacity will detect respiratory fatigue at an early stage. Magnesium sulfate is contraindicated in myasthenia gravis because it will precipitate a myasthenic crisis.

Regional anesthesia with lidocaine is recommended during vaginal delivery.[54] Administration of procaine, 2-chloroprocaine, or other ester-type local anesthetics may be toxic if their hydrolysis by plasma cholinesterase is inhibited by neostigmine or pyridostigmine. Lidocaine and other aminoacyl amide drugs, on the other hand, are inactivated in the liver. If general anesthesia is required, a nitrous oxide–oxygen mixture and halothane are recommended. Ether should be avoided because it can block neuromuscular transmission.

After labor begins, cholinesterase inhibitors are given intravenously to ensure absorption. The intravenous dosage of neostigmine and pyridostigmine is one-thirtieth of the oral dose. Any IV administration of these drugs must be preceded by an injection of atropine, 0.4 to 1.0 mg or more, to prevent muscarinic side effects, especially bronchorrhea.

Patients with myasthenia gravis may develop rapidly progressive weakness and respiratory failure caused either by worsening of their myasthenia or by overdosage with the acetylcholinesterase inhibitors pyridostigmine and neostigmine (cholinergic crisis).

A myasthenic crisis may be caused by infection or by unusually strenuous physical exertion such as prolonged labor.[47] Neuromuscular transmission may be blocked by curare, aminoglycoside antibiotics, quinine, quinidine, and magnesium.[54] Respiratory drive may be depressed by narcotic analgesics. Hyperthyroidism and potassium depletion may contribute to muscle weakness.

The weakness of a cholinergic crisis is caused by continuous depolarization of the sarcoplasmic membrane due to persistent stimulation of nicotinic acetylcholine receptors. This is usually accompanied by overstimulation of muscarinic acetylcholine receptors, which produces diarrhea, belching, vomiting, sweating, hypersalivation, fasciculations, and pallor. Pupils measuring less than 2 mm in diameter in normal room lighting are often a harbinger of bradycardia and hypotension. Atropine sulfate, 2 mg IV, is an effective antidote, which may be repeated every hour as needed.

The distinction between myasthenic and cholinergic crises is important but can be difficult to make because the same patient's limb muscles may have myasthenic weakness and her diaphragm cholinergic weakness. In both cases the patient should be immediately intubated and her ventilation assisted. An edrophonium (Tensilon) test should not be part of the initial management of a crisis. Although the effect of edrophonium may last only 5 min, its additional cholinergic effect in a cholinergic crisis may be enough to cause fatal cardiorespiratory collapse. Patients with myasthenic weakness will usually strengthen after the intravenous injection of edrophonium; however, ventilation may be further compromised by increased pulmonary secretions. Furthermore, patients slipping into a myasthenic crisis may have gobbled extra acetylcholinesterase inhibitors in the false hope of increasing their strength.

When a crisis occurs, all medication should be discontinued for at least 24 h. If the patient's vital capacity is below 1.2 L or she tires when ventilation is not assisted, it is unlikely that antiacetylcholinesterase drugs will increase her strength enough to permit extubation with safety. If the patient is no stronger the following day, plasmapheresis will be needed. Most nonpregnant patients respond to three to five 2-L exchanges.

WERNICKE'S ENCEPHALOPATHY

Wernicke's encephalopathy is clinically characterized by the acute onset of global confusion, ataxia, gaze paresis, and nystagmus and is caused by thiamine deficiency. The neuritic symptoms of chronic thiamine deprivation need not be present. Even previously well-nourished women can develop thiamine deficiency after 3 to 6 weeks of intractable vomiting.[9] Vomiting ceases with the presentation of neurologic symptoms. The diagnosis can be verified by measuring erythrocyte transketolase activity and sometimes by the clinical response to the IV administration of 100 mg thiamine. A gaze palsy may disappear within minutes following thiamine administration. These patients should be treated with an adequate diet, correction of any electrolyte imbalances caused by the pernicious vomiting, and large doses of thiamine and other vitamins. Parenteral administration of thiamine, 100 mg twice daily, for at least 1 week is recommended because malabsorption can occur, especially in alcoholics.

AUTONOMIC HYPERREFLEXIA

Patients with high spinal cord transections (i.e., above T_{5-6}) often develop autonomic hyperreflexia, a syndrome of paroxysmal hypertension, cardiac arrhythmias, throbbing headaches, facial flushing, and sweating due to the sudden release of catecholamines.[25,42] Some pregnant paraplegics are able to time their contractions without feeling any pain by monitoring these paroxysms. In these patients the splanchnic sympathetic bed, uninhibited by higher centers, is overstimulated by many stimuli, including bladder distension, fecal impaction, and uterine contractions. These same stimuli may also increase somatic hyperreflexia and thereby produce flexor or extensor spasms and sustained clonus, which may make delivery difficult.

Autonomic hyperreflexia and its cardiac arrhythmias may be treated with a β-adrenergic blocking agent such as propranolol, 1 mg IV, repeated as necessary every 5 min up to a total of 8 to 10 mg. Both somatic and autonomic hyperreflexia will be prevented by a peridural or spinal anesthetic to the T_{10} level.

LUMBAR DISK DISEASE

Low back pain is a common complaint during pregnancy. Fortunately, radicular pain and weakness due to acute protrusions of lumbar intervertebral disks are infrequent. Myelography and emergency surgery are indicated if bladder and bowel sphincter control are lost. Otherwise patients should be treated with analgesics and enforced bed rest for at least 2 weeks.[46] Those who do not improve should be considered for myelography and lumbar laminectomy with extraction of disk material. Laminectomies have been performed during pregnancy without incident. Thereafter normal vaginal delivery is possible. If surgery is not done, labor may cause insufferable radicular pain and necessitate the additional risk of cesarean section.

Whenever a spinal cord tumor is suspected, myelography is indicated.

BRAIN TUMORS

The size of brain tumors increases during the second half of pregnancy and, at least temporarily, remits after childbirth. In most cases brain tumors do not cause emergencies during pregnancy. Their neurosurgical treatment is frequently postponed until several weeks postpartum, by which time the tumor is less vascular. Exceptions include metastatic choriocarcinoma, which may cause hemorrhage into an intracranial compartment;[57] tumors which cause intractable seizures, acoustic neuromas, which compress the brain stem; and pituitary tumors, which cause sudden visual failure.

Pregnancy accelerates the growth of pituitary adenomas[22,40,43] and it is not possible to predict which women will become symptomatic. Most women with prolactin-secreting pituitary adenomas are infertile until treated with human gonadotropin or bromocriptine in order to induce ovulation. Women known to have large pituitary adenomas who wish to become pregnant should have their tumors treated before any attempt is made to induce ovulation.

Treatment with bromocriptine is usually stopped once pregnancy has been achieved. During pregnancy, visual fields and visual acuity should be determined at least monthly, and more frequently if any visual failure is detected. Early visual failure with gradual progression may be carefully observed. Alternatively, bromocriptine therapy may be reinstituted, although experience with the latter approach during pregnancy is in an evolutionary phase. If visual acuity decreases to less than 20/50 or if bitemporal hemianopia encroaches upon the nasal sectors, treatment is mandatory. Therapeutic choices include bromocriptine, hypophysectomy, and delivery. Patients with sudden visual loss or pituitary apoplexy are candidates for emergency neurosurgery. Transsphenoidal hypophysectomy is the procedure of choice in most instances.

CEREBRAL EDEMA

The medical management of cerebral edema is usually the responsibility of a neurosurgeon or neurologist, for whom this section is intended as a guide to special concerns during pregnancy. Electronic fetal heart rate monitoring is helpful in following the status of the fetus in these circumstances. Hypothermia has already been discussed in the section on subarachnoid hemorrhage.

Hyperventilation. Hyperventilation safely reduces cerebral blood flow and decreases intracranial hypertension during pregnancy.[36]

Corticosteroid Therapy. High-dose corticosteroid therapy (dexamethasone, 4 to 6 mg every 6 h) is widely used in the treatment of cerebral edema of any cause. Its efficacy is debated except in cases of tumors metastatic to the brain, where it is clearly effective. Glucocorticoid steroids can affect division, differentiation, and myelination of developing animal brain cells.[62] The effect of high-dose corticosteroid therapy upon the human fetus at different stages in gestation is unknown. Neonates with respiratory distress syndrome who were treated with glucocorticosteroids have been reported to grow and develop normally, at least for the first year of life.[23] Whatever fetal risk may exist owing to the administration of high-dose corticosteroids to a seriously ill pregnant woman should be considered acceptable given currently available information.

Hyperosmolar Mannitol. Hyperosmolar mannitol therapy produces acute cerebral dehydration and decreased brain volume if the blood-brain barrier is intact. It is often effective in providing more space for an intracranial mass such as a hematoma and is used in the treatment of cerebral edema. A 10 percent increase in plasma osmolarity as produced by a bolus of 100 g mannitol (12.5 g/ampule) is the therapeutic goal although some patients may respond to less.

Hypertonic expansion of the maternal extracellular space with mannitol produces osmotic forces that result in a flow of water from the fetus and amniotic fluid into the maternal circulation. In a study by Battaglia et al.,[7] a 10 percent increase in the plasma osmolarity of three healthy women infused with 1 L of 20 percent mannitol during the hour before childbirth was associated with a similar increase in umbilical cord blood. The condition of the neonates in this study was not mentioned nor were fetal heart rates monitored. Bruns et al.[13] reported that a 25 percent increase in plasma osmolarity in pregnant rabbits was associated with fetal bradycardia, cyanosis, and a 50 percent reduction in fetal blood volume.

Hypertonic mannitol therapy should be used with caution during pregnancy. It is contraindicated for eclamptic hypertensive encephalopathy because of the widespread disruption of cerebral capillaries in that condition. Furthermore, mannitol administered to an eclamptic woman may trigger or worsen pulmonary edema.

REFERENCES

1. Aitken, R.R. and Drake, C.G.: A technique of anesthesia with induced hypotension for surgical correction of intracranial aneurysms. Clin. Neurosurg., *21:*107, 1974.
2. Alper, M.H.: Toxicity of local anesthetics. N. Engl. J. Med., 295:1432, 1976.
3. Aminoff, M.J.: Neurological disorders and pregnancy. Am. J. Obstet. Gynecol., *132:*325, 1978.
4. Aminoff, M.J. and Simon, R.P.: Status epilepticus. Am. J. Med., *69:*657, 1980.
5. Assali, N.S. and Westin, B.: Effects of hypothermia on uterine circulation and on the fetus. Proc. Soc. Exp. Biol. Med., *109:*485, 1962.
6. Averback, P.: Primary cerebral venous thrombosis in young adults: the diverse manifestations of an underrecognized disease. Ann. Neurol., 3:81, 1978.
7. Battaglia, F., Prystowsky, H., Smisson, C. et al.: Fetal blood studies. XIII. The effect of the administration of fluids intravenously to mothers upon the concentrations of water and electrolytes in plasma of human fetuses. Pediatrics, *25:*2, 1960.
8. Berger, G.S., Tyler, C.W., and Harrod, E.K.: Maternal deaths associated with paracervical block anesthesia. Am. J. Obstet. Gynecol., *118:*1142, 1974.
9. Berkwitz, N.J. and Lufkin, N.H.: Toxic neuronitis of pregnancy. Surg. Gynecol. Obstet., *54:*743, 1932.
10. Bonkowsky, H. L., Sinclair, P. R., Emery, S., and Sinclair, J.F.: Seizure management in acute hepatic porphyria: risks of valproate and clonazepam. Neurology (New York), *30:*588, 1980.
11. Borges, L.F. and Gücer, G.: Effect of magnesium on epileptic foci. Epilepsia, *19:*81, 1978.
12. Browne, T.R.: Drug therapy reviews: drug therapy of status epilepticus. Am. J. Hosp. Pharm., *35:*915, 1978.
13. Bruns, P.D., Linder, R.O., Drose, V.E., and Battaglia, F.: The placental transfer of water from fetus to mother following the intravenous infusion of hypertonic mannitol to the maternal rabbit. Am. J. Obstet. Gynecol., *86:*160, 1963.
14. Carroll, J.D., Leak, D., and Lee, H.A.: Cerebral thrombophlebitis in pregnancy and the puerperium. Q. J. Med., *35:*347, 1966.
15. Chesley, L.C. and Tepper, I.: Plasma levels of magnesium attained in magnesium sulfate therapy for preeclampsia and eclampsia. Surg. Clin. North Am., *37:*353, 1957.
16. Cranford, R.E., Leppik, I.E., Patrick, B. et al.: Intravenous phenytoin: clinical and pharmacokinetic aspects. Neurology, *28:*874, 1978.

17. Cross, J.N., Castro, P.O., and Jennett, W.B.: Cerebral strokes associated with pregnancy and the puerperium. Br. Med. J., *3:*214, 1968.
18. De Swiet, J. and Lond, M.D.: Puerperal paradoxical embolism. Lancet, *2:*1197, 1962.
19. Donaldson, J.O.: Neurology of Pregnancy. W.B. Saunders, Philadelphia, 1978.
20. Donaldson, J.O.: Stroke. Clin. Obstet. Gynecol., *24:*825, 1981.
21. Donaldson, J.O.: Control of chorea gravidarum with haloperidol. Obstet. Gynecol., *59:*381, 1982.
22. Falconer, M.A. and Stafford-Bell, M.A.: Visual failure from pituitary and parasellar tumours occurring with favourable outcome in pregnant women. J. Neurol. Neurosurg. Psychiatry, *38:*919, 1975.
23. Fitzhardinge, P.M., Eisen, A., Lejtenyl, C. et al.: Sequelae of early steroid administration to the newborn infant. Pediatrics, *53:*877, 1974.
24. Gettelfinger, D.M. and Kokmen, E.: Superior sagittal sinus thrombosis. Arch. Neurol., *34:*2, 1977.
25. Guttmann, L., Frankel, H.L., and Paeslak, V.: Cardiac irregularities during labour in paraplegic women. Paraplegia, *3:*144, 1965.
26. Hehre, F.W.: Hypothermia for operations during pregnancy. Anesth. Analg. (Cleve), *44:*424, 1965.
27. Hunt, H.B., Schifrin, B.S., and Suzuki, K.: Ruptured berry aneurysms and pregnancy. Obstet. Gynecol., *43:*827, 1974.
28. Ichikawa, K., Kim, R.C., Givelber, H., and Collins, G.H.: Chorea gravidarum. Report of a fatal case with neuropathological observations. Arch. Neurol., *37:*429, 1980.
29. Kamrin, R.P. and Masland, W.: Intracranial surgery under hypothermia during pregnancy. Arch. Neurol., *13:*70, 1965.
30. Knight, A.H. and Rhind, E.G.: Epilepsy and pregnancy: a study of 153 pregnancies in 59 patients. Epilepsia, *16:*99, 1975.
31. Lamon, J.M., Frykholm, B.C., Hess, R.A., and Tschudy, D.P.: Hematin therapy for acute porphyria. Medicine (Baltimore), *58:*252, 1979.
32. Larson, A.W., Wasserstrom, W.R., Felsher, B.F., and Shih, J.C.: Posttraumatic epilepsy and acute intermittent porphyria: effects of phenytoin, carbamazepine, and clonazepam. Neurology (Minneap.), *28:*824, 1978.
33. Laubstein, M.B., Kotz, H.L., and Hehre, F.W.: Obstetric and anesthetic management following spontaneous subarachnoid hemorrhage. Obstet. Gynecol., *20:*661, 1962.
34. Lewis, B.V. and Parsons, M.: Chorea gravidarum. Lancet, *1:*284, 1966.
35. Meldrum, B.S. and Nilsson, B.: Cerebral blood flow and metabolic rate early and late in prolonged epileptic seizures induced in rats by bicuculline. Brain, *99:*523, 1976.
36. Miller, F.C., Petrie, R.H., Arce, J.J. et al.: Hyperventilation during labor. Am. J. Obstet. Gynecol., *120:*489, 1974.
37. Minielly, R., Yuzpe, A.A., and Drake, C.G.: Subarachnoid hemorrhage secondary to ruptured cerebral aneurysm in pregnancy. Obstet. Gynecol., *53:*64, 1979.
38. Mordes, J.P. and Wacker, W.C.: Excess magnesium. Pharmocol. Rev., *29:*273, 1978.
39. Mygind, K.I., Dam, M., and Christiansen, J.: Phenytoin and phenobarbitone plasma clearance during pregnancy. Acta Neurol. Scand., *54:*160, 1976.
40. Nagulesparan, M. and Roper, J.: Haemorrhage into the anterior pituitary during pregnancy after induction of ovulation with clomiphene. Br. J. Obstet. Gynaecol., *85:*153, 1978.
41. Najafi, H., Javid, H., Dye, W.S. et al.: Emergency carotid thromboendarterectomy. Arch. Surg., *103:*610, 1971.
42. Nath, M., Vivian, J.M., and Chernny, W.B.: Autonomic hyperreflexia in pregnancy and labor: a case report. Am. J. Obstet. Gynecol., *134:*390, 1979.
43. Nelson, P.B., Robinson, A.G., Archer, D.F., and Maroon, J.C.: Symptomatic pituitary tumor enlargement after induced pregnancy. J. Neurosurg., *49:*283, 1978.

44. Oppelt, W.W., MacIntyre, I., and Rall, D.P.: Magnesium exchange between blood and cerebrospinal fluid. Am. J. Physiol., *205*:959, 1963.
45. Oxbury, J.M. and Whitty, C.W.M.: Causes and consequences of status epilepticus in adults. Brain, *94*:733, 1971.
46. Pearce, J. and Moll, J.M.H.: Conservative treatment and natural history of acute lumbar disc lesions. J. Neurol. Neurosurg. Psychiatry, *30*:13, 1967.
47. Plauché, W.C.: Myasthenia gravis in pregnancy: an update. Am. J. Obstet. Gynecol., *135*:691, 1979.
48. Pritchard, J.A.: Management of preeclampsia and eclampsia. Kidney Int., *18*:259, 1980.
49. Ramirez-Lassepas, M.: Antifibrinolytic therapy in subarachnoid hemorrhage caused by ruptured intracranial aneurysm. Neurology (New York), *31*:316, 1981.
50. Ramsay, R.E., Strauss, R.G., Wilder, B.J., and Willmore, L.J.: Status epilepticus in pregnancy: effect of phenytoin malabsorption on seizure control. Neurology (Minneap.), *28*:85, 1978.
51. Rasch, D.K., Huber, P.A., Richardson, C.J. et al.: Neurobehavioral effects of neonatal hypermagnesemia. J. Pediatr., *100*:272, 1982.
52. Robinson, J.L., Hall, C.J., and Sedzimir, C.B.: Subarachnoid hemorrhage in pregnancy. J. Neurosurg., *36*:27, 1972.
53. Robinson, J.L., Hall, C.S., and Sedzimir, C.B.: Arteriovenous malformations, aneurysms, and pregnancy. J. Neurosurg., *41*:63, 1974.
54. Rolbin, S.H., Levinson, G., Shnider, S.M., and Wright, R.G.: Anesthetic considerations for myasthenia gravis and pregnancy. Anesth. Analg. (Cleve), *57*:441, 1978.
55. Sheehan, H.L., Lynch, J.B.: Pathology of Toxaemia of Pregnancy. Churchill Livingstone, Edinburgh, 1973.
56. Smith, B.E., Hehre, F.W., and Hess, O.W.: Convulsions associated with anesthetic agents during labor and delivery. Anesth. Analg. (Cleve), *43*:476, 1964.
57. Somjen, G., Hilmy, M., and Stephen, C.R.: Failure to anesthetize human subjects by intravenous administration of magnesium sulfate. J. Pharm. Exp. Ther., *154*:652, 1966.
58. Stansfield, F.R.: Puerperal cerebral thrombophlebitis treated by heparin. Br. Med. J., *1*:436, 1942.
59. Strandgaard, S.: Autoregulation of cerebral circulation in hypertension. Acta. Neurol. Scand., *57*:suppl. 66, 1, 1978.
60. Teramo, K., Hiilesmaa, V., Bardy, A., and Saarikoski, S.: Fetal heart rate during a maternal grand mal epileptic seizure. J. Perinat. Med., *7*:3, 1979.
61. Weed, J.C. and Hammond, C.B.: Cerebral metastatic choriocarcinoma: intensive therapy and prognosis. Obstet. Gynecol., *55*:89, 1980.
62. Weichsel, Jr., M.E.: The therapeutic use of glucocorticoid hormones in the perinatal period: potential neurological hazards. Ann. Neurol., *2*:364, 1977.
63. Wendling, L.R.: Intracranial venous sinus thrombosis: diagnosis suggested by computer tomography. Am. J. Roentgenol., *130*:978, 1978.
64. Whitty, C.W.M. and James, J.L.: The electroencephalogram as a monitor of status epilepticus suppressed peripherally by curarisation. Lancet, *2*:239, 1961.
65. Wilder, B.J., Ramsay, R.E., Willmore, L.J. et al.: Efficacy of intravenous phenytoin in the treatment of status epilepticus: kinetics of central nervous system penetration. Ann. Neurol., *1*:511, 1977.
66. Yatsu, F.M. and Mohr, J.P.: Anticoagulation therapy for cardiogenic emboli to brain. Neurology (New York), *32*:274, 1982.
67. Yeh, S.Y., Paul, R.H., Cordero, L., and Hon, E.H.: A study of diazepam during labor. Obstet. Gynecol., *43*:363, 1974.

14

Endocrine Emergencies during Pregnancy

Alan H. DeCherney, M.D.
Alexander M. Dlugi, M.D.
Burton V. Caldwell, M.D.

INTRODUCTION

Although endocrine emergencies in pregnancies are uncommon, their occurrence presents both a diagnostic and a therapeutic challenge. Ranging from the most commonly seen thyroid disorders to rare aberrations in adrenal or pituitary function, all endocrinopathies occurring throughout gestation are difficult to evaluate and manage, yet accurate diagnosis and rapid and appropriate therapy are essential. This chapter will emphasize the special problems that confront the physician faced with treating the mother while protecting the fetus from the possible adverse effects of the pharmaceutical agents used.

THYROID DISEASE

With the exception of diabetes mellitus (see Ch. 15), thyroid disease is the most common endocrine disorder in women in the reproductive age group and also the most common cause of endocrine crisis in pregnancy.

Thyrotoxicosis

The mere nomenclature of the most severe stage of the disorder, "thyroid storm," indicates its life-threatening potential. An infrequent medical emergency, it is even more infrequent in pregnancy but warrants prompt attention when present. Death from left ventricular failure may ensue secondary to cardiac arrhythmias, shock, coma, hyperpyrexia, and pulmonary edema. In addition, marked pregnancy wastage is seen in inadequately managed patients.

This entity usually occurs in cases of known diffuse toxic goiter (Graves' disease), but can occur *de novo* in previously undiagnosed patients in response to a variety of stresses, including pregnancy. Although hyperthyroid patients generally require less suppression when pregnant, occasionally there is "escape" and an acute exacerbation of a previously well-controlled state.[9] The manifestations of this disorder are due in part to increased catecholamine release and action.[3] There is no evidence that the serum levels of thyroid hormones are any higher during thyroid storm than in the previous few days before the onset of crisis. Earlier diagnosis of hyperthyroidism and careful treatment and monitoring have contributed to the relative rarity of this endocrine crisis during pregnancy (Table 14-1).

Diagnosis. The hallmark of thyrotoxicosis is marked hypermetabolism and fever (100 to 106°F) due to the intracellular effects of thyroxine (T_4), tri-iodothyronine (T_3), and catecholamines. Sinus tachycardia and atrial fibrillation may lead to acute pulmonary edema; congestive heart failure, however, is more likely to occur in patients with preexisting cardiac disease. Other signs and symptoms that are frequently encountered are diarrhea and vomiting, leading to hypovolemia, hypokalemia, dehydration, and eventually shock. Neurologic deterioration may progress from restlessness to delirium and result in a state of stupor and coma.[13]

Physical examination generally reveals thyroid enlargement with bruits, systolic hypertension with a wide pulse pressure, and ophthalmoplegia, which may coexist with preexisting exophthalmus. Jaundice from hepatocellular damage can ensue. Some patients may present with acute psychosis.

Laboratory Findings. The thyroid gland mainly secretes T_4 and about 15 percent of the T_3 found in the circulation. The T_4 is converted to the more active T_3 in peripheral tissues by monodeiodination. Over 99 percent of both these compounds are bound to thyroid-binding globulin (TBG), a liver protein which increases greatly during pregnancy as a result of estrogen stimulation. The free hormone, which is the sole metabolically active form, remains within the normal range in pregnancy despite the near doubling of total thyroxine produced by the thyroid. There has been no direct correlation between the severity of thyroid storm and the level of free T_4 and T_3, but both are elevated during crisis and appropriate laboratory tests will confirm the presence of hyperthyroidism.[46] Rarely, a patient will present with T_3-toxicosis in which the T_3 is elevated in association with a normal free T_4. Other laboratory tests such as a decrease in serum cholesterol and an increase in urea nitrogen secondary to increased catabolism of protein may be helpful in diagnosing

Table 14-1. Hyperthyroidism: Manifestations

	History	Physical Examination
General	Weight loss with good appetite Heat intolerance	
Skin		Warm, moist, smooth Onycholysis Pretibial myxedema (Graves' disease)
Eyes	Burning Tearing Diplopia	Lid lag, stare Exophthalmos, soft-tissue swelling, extraocular muscle paresis, corneal involvement (Graves' disease)
Neck	Enlargement	Goiter Diffuse Nodular
Respiratory	Dyspnea	
Cardiovascular	Palpitations Angina pectoris	Sinus tachycardia Atrial fibrillation Increased systolic blood pressure Decreased diastolic blood pressure Scratchy systolic ejection murmur Congestive heart failure, right-side more severe than left-sided
Gastrointestinal	Diarrhea	
Genitourinary	Nocturia Hypomenorrhea	Gynecomastia
Neuromuscular	Tremor Weakness	Peripheral and bulbar myopathy Brisk deep tendon reflexes
Psychiatric	Emotional instability Hyperkinesia Insomnia Anxiety	

From Bacchus, H: Metabolic and Endocrine Emergencies: Recognition and Management. University Park Press, Baltimore, 1977.

these unusual cases. The definitive laboratory test is the radioimmunoassay of free T_4 level.

Differential Diagnosis. In pregnancy, thyroid storm can be confused with infection because of the hyperpyrexia and associated tachycardia; an elevated white blood cell count, however, is not often encountered in thyrotoxicosis. Nausea, vomiting, and diarrhea might suggest hyperemesis gravidarum.[24] There may be difficulty in distinguishing the increase in blood pressure from pregnancy-induced hypertension or a pheochromocytoma, although systolic hypertension is the hallmark of thyroid hormone excess. The presence of a palpable thyroid gland is helpful in these particular situations. The characteristic ophthalmological findings in hyperthyroidism also provide a helpful clinical clue in this differential diagnosis. Hyperreflexia, weakness, and tremor are always seen in thyroid storm.[3]

Psychiatric and neurologic disease frequently can be confused with hyperthyroidism both in the pregnant and in the nonpregnant state. Amphetamine abuse can also mimic this condition.[13]

The etiology of thyrotoxicosis in pregnancy is difficult to establish since the techniques usually used for differentiating Graves' disease from acute viral thyroiditis should not be performed. A radioactive thyroxine uptake and scan would, however, show markedly increased uptake in Graves' disease while demonstrating decreased localization of radioactive iodine in the thyroid of patients with viral-induced release of hormone. In the near future it will be possible to measure the level of thyroid-stimulating circulating immunoglobulins (TSIGs) present only in Graves' disease both as a means of diagnosis and a guide to management. Although the treatment for these two conditions is the same, the clinical response is different, since viral thyroiditis is a self-limiting entity responding best to beta-blockade and anti-inflammatory drugs while Graves' disease responds mainly to inhibitors of thyroid hormone synthesis (Table 14-2) (see below).

Therapy. Bacchus[3] lists four specific principles in the management of thyroid storm: (1) to halt increased synthesis and secretion of T_4 and T_3; (2) to suppress iodothyronine-catecholamine synergism in target cells; (3) to treat the precipitating illness (not always applicable if pregnancy is the only etiologic association that can be found after all other possibilities, especially infection, have been excluded); and (4) to support body defense mechanisms.

General measures include treating the hyperpyrexia with acetaminophen or cooling blankets. Infection must be ruled out at this juncture, with urinary tract infection and amnionitis requiring particular attention in the pregnant patient. The patient must be adequately hydrated and electrolytes replaced when diarrhea and vomiting occur.

Thyroid hormone synthesis is most effectively blocked by the use of propylthiouracil (PTU). Methimazole (Tapazole) can also be used and has a longer half-

Table 14-2. Causes of Hyperthyroidism

1. Graves' disease (diffuse toxic goiter)
2. Toxic multinodular goiter (Plummer disease)
3. Toxic uninodular goiter (toxic adenoma)
4. Hyperthyroidism associated with thyroiditis
    a. Subacute thyroiditis
    b. Hashimoto's thyroiditis (Hashitoxicosis)
    c. Silent thyroiditis
    d. Radiation thyroiditis (rare)
5. Hyperthyroidism due to exogenous iodide (Job-Basedow effect)
6. Exogenous thyroid hormone
    a. Thyrotoxicosis factitia
    b. Overenthusiastic therapy for hypothyroidism
    c. T_3 suppression test
7. Malignancies with circulating thyroid stimulators
    a. Choriocarcinoma and hydatidiform mole
    b. Embryonal carcinoma of the testis
    c. Other malignancies
8. Struma ovarii with hyperthyroidism
9. Albright syndrome (polyostotic fibrous dysplasia)
10. Metastatic thyroid carcinoma
11. TSH-producing tumor (pituitary or ectopic)
12. Pituitary resistance to thyroid hormone

Lang, R.: Special issue on thyroid disorders. Contemp Ob/Gyn. *19*, 1982.

life than PTU[21]; however, it is relatively contraindicated in pregnancy because of the potential for fetal scalp abnormalities.[9,11] Also, only PTU decreases peripheral T_4-to-T_3 conversion. Recommended doses of PTU for the treatment of thyroid storm are 1,200 to 1,500 mg daily (in three individual doses), given by mouth or crushed and administered by nasogastric tube.[10]

Lugol's iodine, 30 drops per day orally, can be given in order to retard the release of stored T_4 and T_3 from the thyroid gland; however transplacental passage will occur and may also block the fetal thyroid. Iodine should only be used late in pregnancy because escape from the block usually occurs in 2 to 4 weeks. Blockade of thyroxine production can be achieved in hours but clinical manifestations might take weeks to resolve entirely. The serum half-life of T_4 is approximately 7 days and that of T_3 is 1 day[46]; however, the apparent biological half-life is at least 2 to 3 times as long.

Since there is no known antidote to thyroid hormone, the only effective way to interfere with the peripheral effects of thyroid storm is by beta-adrenergic blockade. This is best accomplished by the use of propanolol hydrochloride given intravenously (1 mg starting dose, with increases dependent upon responses).[3,13] Propranolol and other beta blockers also decrease T_4-T_3 conversion.[8] Concomitant EKG monitoring is mandatory. Guanethidine and reserpine have been used effectively in thyroid storm, but these drugs are not recommended for use in pregnancy because other antihypertensive agents are equally effective and have fewer adverse side effects.[5]

In the presence of congestive heart failure, propanolol should be administered with extreme caution and with continuous central monitoring.[46] Propanolol may have adverse effects in pregnancy, such as growth retardation of the fetus, neonatal hypoglycemia, and bradycardia persisting through the first day of life. These are usually associated with long-term administration but the benefits of propanolol therapy during thyroid storm outweigh any risk of these occurrences.[5]

Other adjunctive therapy such as digitalis and diuretics may be necessary in the management of some women with thyroid storm, especially when congestive heart failure develops.[2] Also, immunosuppressive doses of glucocorticoids may be needed (Solumedrol 100 mg every 12 h with tapering over 4 to 5 days) to decrease T_4-to-T_3 conversion and also to inhibit the production of TSIGs.

Hypothyroidism

Myxedema coma is an extreme form of hypothyroidism that warrants immediate recognition and intervention. While a history of indolent thyroid disease is helpful in the diagnosis, it is not a prerequisite. It has been predicted that myxedema coma will become more common in the general population because of the increasing use of surgery and radioactive iodine to treat thyroid disease.[13,35] This does not seem to have occurred in obstetric patients since profound disease of this nature is almost incompatible with conception.

Patients usually present in winter months[2,45] with clinical manifestations which include hypothermia and hypoventilation with concomitant respiratory acidosis. This may progress to lethargy, stupor, and eventual coma as a result of the severe metabolic changes induced by the low output of thyroid hormone. Carbon dioxide narcosis is a serious complication of myxedema. This is occasionally caused by a large tongue leading to upper airway obstruction, but may be due to chest wall infiltration with mucopolysaccharide deposition, pleural effusion, and ascites and to direct suppression of the respiratory center in the medulla.[3,13] Patients may present with severe dehydration and cachexia from vomiting. Profound hypoglycemia may also occur. In pregnancy, this disease entity can most commonly be confused with neuropsychiatric disease or a nutritional deprivation state. Edema and obesity are inconsistent and relatively rare findings in myxedema crisis unless a long-standing hypothyroid state has preceded the acute event.

It should be stressed that women with myxedema crises are acutely as well as chronically ill. Of these patients, 95 percent will have primary hypothyroidism on the basis of Hashimoto's thyroiditis, automimmune thyroiditis, radioactive iodine therapy, or thyroid surgery.[13,45] Chronic manifestations of the disease include decreased pubic and axillary hair, diminished libido, and hyporeflexia. In the postpartum period, this disease must be differentiated from Sheehan's syndrome. Acute pituitary apoplexy due to infarction or hemorrhage is extremely rare, and multiple hormonal deficiencies will be present in that condition (see section on pituitary crisis). See also Table 14-3.

Laboratory Diagnosis. Primary hypothyroidism is associated with an elevated thyroid-stimulating hormone (TSH) level and low T_3 and T_4 levels. Secondary hypothyroidism, however, has diminished TSH levels as well as decreased T_3 and T_4 levels, since this entity is based on failure of the pituitary rather than on failure of the thyroid gland itself. Just as in thyroid storm there is little correlation between the actual thyroid hormone level, or the free thyroxine concentration, and the severity of the myxedema crisis.[44] In fact, many patients with profound hypothyroidism have associated low protein production, which raises the circulating free thyroxine. In addition to the above, other supportive laboratory tests, which are essential more for management than for diagnosis, are arterial blood gases to determine the severity of the respiratory acidosis, plasma glucose levels, and electrolytes. An EKG will generally reveal sinus bradycardia and low voltage with widespread T-wave changes.[3] A chest x-ray frequently indicates the presence of pleural or pleuropericardial effusions. Muscle creatine phosphokinase (CPK) and cholesterol levels are usually elevated. Panhypopituitarism or adrenal cortical failure must be ruled out by appropriate hormone measurements. The definitive diagnosis is made by documenting depressed free T_4 levels associated with elevated TSH. Early in pregnancy, high levels of human chorionic gonadotropin may falsely elevate TSH levels because of cross reaction in some radioimmunoassays. Antithyroid antibodies are not helpful Table 14-4).

Treatment. Specific goals have been outlined in the general schema of treating patients with myxedema coma.[3,13] They include replacing the patient's extrathyroidal hormone pool, treating the precipitating factor, and assisting ventilation. An endotracheal tube or even tracheostomy might be necessary in these patients. Depressant drugs should be avoided. The hypometabolism and hypotension should be corrected.

Table 14-3. Hypothyroidism: Manifestations

	History	Physical Examination	Laboratory Findings
General	Intolerance to cold Weight gain with decreased appetite Obesity (rare) Radioactive iodine therapy Thyroidectomy	Hypothermia	Decreased thyroxine, T_3 resin Increased TSH (primary hypothyroidism) Elevated cholesterol, triglycerides, sedimentation rate, CPK, cerebrospinal fluid protein
Cardiovascular		Sinus bradycardia Increased diastolic blood pressure Cardiomegaly Distant heart sounds	
Skin		Dry, cool, coarse, thickened Carotenodermia Patchy alopecia Periorbital edema	
Mouth		Enlarged tongue	
Neck		Goiter Surgical scar	
Gastrointestinal	Constipation	Ileus	
Genitourinary	Menorrhagia (primary hypothyroidism) Amenorrhea (secondary hypothyroidism)		
Neurologic	Muscle cramps Parathesias Unsteadiness	Ataxic gait Delay in relaxation of deep tendon reflexes Obtundation	
Psychiatric	Lethary Depression Mental slowing	Apathy Psychosis Myxedema "wit"	

From Bacchus, H: Metabolic and Endocrine Emergencies: Recognition and Management. University Park Press, Baltimore, 1977.

Thyroid replacement should be in the form of levothyroxine sodium in a dose of 25 to 100 μg IV daily.[9,13] When the patient is stable, she should be placed on maintenance oral doses of levothyroxine (100 to 200 μg/day) and followed with free thyroxin determinations as well as periodic TSH levels.[9,13] The latter may take 4 to 6 weeks to fall. Electrolyte imbalance and hypoglycemia should be corrected with appropriate IV solutions. Rapid external warming should be avoided. Because of the hypometabolic state, decreased drug metabolism may occur. Therefore, any supportive drugs given these patients, such as sedatives and narcotics, must be cautiously administered. Pressor agents for the treatment of hypotension are not effective unless there is adequate replacement of thyroid hormone. Some authors recommend the use of a corticosteroid as secondary treatment in patients with severe primary hypothyroidism since they may present with relative adrenal insufficiency. This is due to suppression of the conversion of cortisol to cortisone, since the 11-β-dehydrogenase reaction is partially dependent on thyroid hormone.[3]

Table 14-4. Causes of Hypothyroidism

I. Reduced function of thyroid tissue
  A. Hereditary defects in hormonogenesis
  B. Inhibition of hormone synthesis
    1. Iodine deficiency
    2. Antithyroid drugs (iodine, perchlorate, lithium, etc.)
  C. Decreased TSH stimulation
    1. Hypothalamic hypothyroidism or decreased TRH
    2. Hypopituitarism with decreased TSH
    3. Antibodies to thyroid cellular products (Hashimoto thyroiditis)
  D. Transient inflammation
    1. Subacute thyroiditis
    2. Silent thyroiditis
II. Reduced mass of thyroid tissues
  A. Postthyroidectomy
  B. Postradioactive iodine treatment
  C. Postroentgen therapy (e.g., Hodgkins disease)
  D. Autoimmune destruction (Hashimoto thyroiditis)
  E. Replacement by metastatic cancer
  F. Destruction from infection

Lang, R.: Special issue on thyroid disorders. Contemp Ob/Gyn. *19*, 1982.

Special Considerations in the Pregnant Patient. Hypothyroidism is extremely uncommon in pregnancy,[9] in part because of the difficulty that these women have in conceiving. It is also primarily a disease of older women. For prophylaxis against thyroid instability, replacement therapy during known hypothyroid pregnancies should be increased, since increased TBG production binds the thyroxine given orally. Levels of TSH and of free T_4 should be measured every 6 to 8 weeks.[11]

Therapy consists of thyroid replacement, respiratory support, and correction of electrolyte and metabolic imbalances. Improvement should be seen within the first day of therapy. Continuous electronic fetal monitoring should be utilized until the patient is stabilized and on maintenance therapy. Probably the only special consideration is that pregnant patients who have hypothyroidism should be given other medications with caution because of the altered metabolic clearance rate associated with this disorder.

The IgG antibodies present in the maternal circulation in autoimmune hypothyroidism do not cause hypothyroidism in the newborn. Hypothyroidism results from destruction of intracellular structures, and the fetal thyroid remains intact and does not permit the antibodies to enter and destroy thyroxine-producing enzymes.

ADRENAL DISEASE

Excess cortisol production (Cushing's disease) occurs rarely and creates a relatively mild emergent situation. Acute adrenal cortical insufficiency (Addison's disease), however, is life-threatening. The manifestations of the latter are due primarily to a deficiency in the production of cortisol and aldosterone, the primary glucocorticoid and mineralocorticoid, respectively.

Addison's Disease

Destruction of the adrenal gland with concomitant adrenal insufficiency may be an indolent process (e.g., secondary to tuberculosis or autoimmune disease) or it may present as a catastrophic acute situation (e.g., adrenal hemorrhage secondary to infection). A more important consideration is that 5 million people in the United States are receiving steroids in doses great enough to suppress the pituitary-adrenal axis.[3] Doses equivalent to 50 mg of cortisone acetate daily for as little as 10 days are capable of causing mild suppression[13]; but suppression is more common in patients on high doses of corticosteroids for longer than 2 to 3 months. If these drugs are discontinued suddenly or tapered too rapidly, acute adrenal insufficiency may occur. Therefore special consideration should be given to pregnant patients being treated with steroids for acute inflammatory conditions or severe asthmatic attacks unresponsive to other therapy, since it is possible for an Addisonian crisis to occur if a stressful situation intervenes even though the patient might be on steroids for relatively brief periods of time.

Symptoms. Symptoms include nausea and vomiting with severe epigastric pain. Weakness and lassitude are often quite profound, as are hypotension and hypothermia. Evidence of overwhelming infection might be present, and in this setting consideration should be given to adrenal hemorrhage as an etiology of the adrenal crisis. It should be remembered that acute steroid administration will increase white blood cell count to 15,000/mm^3 or more. Eventually unconsciousness, shock, and death will occur if an Addisonian crisis remains untreated.

The concomitant aldosterone deficiency and its associated salt loss lead to extracellular fluid volume depletion. This disease presents most commonly in the summer months because of the stress of additional salt loss,[3,13] and acute dehydration must be included in the differential diagnosis. Hypotension, azotemia, and hyperkalemia are usually present. The complete absence of cortisol production leads to a decrease in gluconeogenesis, with symptomatic hypoglycemia. Often, these patients will be hyperpigmented because of increased melanocyte-stimulating hormone (MSH) and ACTH production due to lack of negative feedback by cortisol on pituitary β-lipotropin production.

Diagnosis. Diagnosis is based on a specific constellation of symptoms, clinically evident signs, and characteristic laboratory findings. Hyperpigmentation may represent a long-standing underlying problem or be caused by an immediately overwhelmingly stressful situation. Plasma cortisol levels should be drawn, preferably in the morning. Normal a.m. nonpregnant limits are between 7 and 18 μg/100 ml. In pregnancy normal values are slightly elevated because of increased cortisol-binding globulin (CBG).[11] Levels below 7 μg/ml are suggestive of Addison's disease.[46] A total eosinophil count may also prove to be helpful. In Addisonian crisis the total eosinophil count is often greater than 300/mm^3 whereas in shock of any other etiology it is usually markedly decreased and may be zero.[13] Serum electrolytes must be determined. A sodium/potassium ratio of less than 30 reflects the hyperkalemia and normal or decreased sodium values in the emergent state.

When possible, ACTH diagnostic testing should be employed utilizing Cortrosyn, 250 units IV, with cortisol levels measured at baseline and 1 h after injection. Occasionally it is necessary to prolong the test, i.e., 250 units in 500 ml of 5 percent dextrose solution over a course of 8 h on three consecutive days. This is safe in pregnancy since little ACTH crosses the placenta. In normal women the plasma cortisol level will increase to more than 20 μg/ml. ACTH levels may also aid in the diagnosis and differentiate Addison's disease from panhypopituitarism.[46]

Treatment. Treatment consists of immediate steroid replacement and supportive therapy to counteract dehydration and the metabolic effects of adrenal depletion.

To treat the concomitant hypotension and shock, appropriate amounts of 5 percent glucose in saline should be administered with monitoring of the central venous pressure with a central line or Swan-Ganz catheter. It might be necessary to replace as much as 20 percent of lost extracellular fluid, as deficits of 3 L or more are not uncommon.[46] The response to saline administration is often dramatic. This sometimes contributes to the late recognition of adrenal crisis since the infusion of saline alone will temporarily improve the patient's clinical condition. Potassium, 20 to 40 mEq/day, should be given after 24 to 48 h to replace total body depletion of this electrolyte. Urine output and other parameters of clinical responsiveness should be continuously assessed. Initially, vasopressors might have to be employed, such as phenylephrine (Neo-Synephrine) in doses of 0.25 to 0.5 mg as an IV bolus.

Glucocorticoid Replacement. Intravenous hydrocortisone sodium succinate should be administered as a stat dose of 100 mg IV followed by cortisone acetate 75 mg IM every 6 h. After a few days the dosage can be cut by 50 percent until maintenance requirements are established.[3,13] The repeated dosage is based on the short biological half-life of *d*-glucocorticoids.[9]

Mineralocorticoids. These may be given to prevent the loss of sodium but the large doses of glucocorticoids administered will have a significant mineralocorticoid effect, especially when IV saline is infused.[46] The use of mineralocorticoids should be given serious consideration, however, if the blood pressure remains low despite adequate saline infusion, if hyperkalemia persists, or if synthetic glucocorticoids such as prednisolone with little mineralocorticoid activity are used. Similarly, when the dose of cortisone is being tapered, mineralocorticoids might be added to the regimen. Desoxycorticosterone acetate (DOCA), 5 mg IM b.i.d., or fluorohydrocortisone acetate (Flurinef), 0.05 to 0.1 mg per day orally, is recommended.[13] Careful observation for signs of edema is recommended.

Special Considerations in Pregnancy. In 1948 Brent[7] reviewed the 39 cases of Addison's disease occurring during pregnancy in the literature at that time. Eighteen of these patients died during pregnancy. Postmorten studies demonstrated primary tuberculosis to be the most common cause of the adrenal insufficiency. With the improved treatment of tuberculosis, Addison's disease has become uncommon and it is now rarely seen in obstetric patients. Brent found no symptoms in this group of patients with Addisonian crisis which were peculiar to pregnancy. She also reported that Addison's disease did not influence labor. She did report, however, that the patients were extremely sensitive to other medications such as barbiturates and morphine because of their decreased metabolic clearance rates. Thus, it is suggested that sedation of these patients should be kept at a minimum.

Fetal outcome was good in all but two of these patients—one in which the infant died in the neonatal period of "gastrointestinal disturbances" and one stillbirth. Brent found that latent Addison's disease presented as crisis most frequently in the first trimester or in the puerperium. Based on one maternal death after cesarean section, she cautions against operative intervention in obstetrical patients with inadequately treated Addisonian crisis.

A potential concern in adrenal cortical steroid depletion in pregnancy are the ramifications of administering replacement medications. Berkowitz et al.[5] state that prolonged high-dose glucocorticoid ingestion in the first trimester may be associated with an increased incidence of cleft palate. Animal studies have suggested an effect on neurologic and pulmonary development, primarily with chronic use. Large doses of corticosteroids may suppress fetal adrenal production and give falsely lowered estriol readings. These are minor considerations, however, since glucocorticoid therapy is life-sustaining in patients with adrenal insufficiency. It should also be pointed out that replacement therapy following recovery from an Addisonian crisis involves the use of much lower doses of steroids than are administered for therapeutic purposes. No data are available on the acute use of mineralocorticoids during early or late pregnancy.

Cushing's Syndrome

In 1978 Blumsohn[6] reviewed the world literature and reported on 25 patients who had Cushing's syndrome in pregnancy. Only one of these patients presented in critical condition during pregnancy; the rest had a more indolent form of the disease.[14] Perhaps this is due to the fact that these patients are usually anovulatory and consequently infertile. According to Grimes et al.,[20] the etiology of hypercoritsonism in pregnancy is usually adrenal hyperplasia, accounting for 50 to 70 percent of the cases. Other potential etiologic factors include carcinoma, primary pituitary disease, and ectopic production of corticosteroids.[20]

Signs and Symptoms. A great deal of difficulty arises in diagnosing Cushing's syndrome in obstetric patients since many of the symptoms of pregnancy itself mimic the clinical findings associated with this disorder.[10] These include obesity, glucose intolerance, easy bruisability, emotional disturbances, hypertension, weight gain, stria, edema, and increased pigmentation. There is no evidence that pregnancy clinically exacerbates Cushing's syndrome; however, there are reported cases in the literature of amelioration of Cushing's syndrome in association with pregnancy termination.[11,29,31,45]

The physiologic changes in glucocorticosteroid metabolism in pregnancy mimic Cushing's syndrome and include up to a seven-fold increase in 17-hydroxycorticosteroids and cortisol; these levels return to normal by the sixth postpartum day.[6,12] Exaggerated ACTH response has also been reported by Burrows. Grimes[20] has summarized the glucocorticoid and related changes associated with pregnancy as: (1) increased unconjugated cortisol and rising plasma globulins; (2) decreased rate of glucuronide conjugation of cortisol metabolites; (3) increased levels of transcortin; (4) elevated 17-hydroxycorticosteroids, with no change in urinary excretion of these products; (5) decreased peripheral metabolism of cortisol; (6) maintenance of normal hypothalamic pituitary control, i.e., diurnal variation; and (7) increased levels of bound and free cortisol. The diagnosis of hypercortisolism is made with 24-h urinary free cortisol levels in excess of 150 μg/24 h.

The etiology of Cushing's syndrome in pregnancy can be determined by suppression tests. If cortisol levels decrease by 100 percent after 8 mg of dexamethasone is administered daily for 4 days (2 mg every 6 h), adrenal hyperplasia or pituitary adenoma is responsible for the hypercorticosteroidism and an adrenal adenoma or carcinoma can usually be ruled out.[20,21]

Effects on the Fetus. Effects on the fetus remain theoretical, with virilization and cleft palate being the primary concerns.[20,47] Neonatal adrenal insufficiency in cases of Cushing syndrome has been reported and is of real concern. This is caused by maternal cortisol crossing the placenta and supressing fetal ACTH production.[29]

Burrow[10] reports that Cushing's syndrome is extremely unusual but is associated with poor fetal outcome. Of 16 cases reported, 4 had abortions, 4 ended in stillbirth, and the remaining 8 presented with premature labor.

Treatment. Treatment consists of surgical removal of the source of increased cortisol production or source of ACTH. Either unilateral or bilateral adrenalectomy or if appropriate, transsphenoidal pituitary resection may be performed. Medical management with blockers of glucocorticoid synthesis should not be undertaken because of potential side effects on the fetus. The critical problem associated with Cushing's syndrome in pregnancy lies not in the increased production of steroids but in the postoperative Addisonian crisis that can occur if appropriate replacement therapy is not immediately provided. Grimes[20] recommends 5 to 10 times maintenance requirements for 48 h, after which the patient may be tapered to maintenance levels.

Pheochromocytoma

Pheochromocytoma can present as a real crisis in pregnancy as well as in the nonpregnant state. It is due to an overproduction of catecholamines by chromaffin tissue from either the adrenal medulla or ectopic neural crest tissues.

In a review of the literature, Durham[16] reported 111 cases of pheochromocytomas associated with pregnancy, with a maternal mortality of 48 percent and a fetal loss of 58 percent. Most of the maternal deaths occurred from pulmonary edema or cerebral vascular accidents. Of these patients, 58 percent died before the diagnosis was made.

Signs and Symptoms. Serious problems caused by this disorder are primarily cardiovascular in nature, hypertensive crisis, cerebral vascular hemorrhage, and congestive heart failure being the most prevalent. Signs and symptoms include sustained or paroxysmal hypertension, headache, epigastric pain, chest pain, palpitations, perspiration, pallor, flushing, feeling of warmth, feeling of numbness, dizziness, and fainting. Postural hypotension is seen in 60 percent of cases.[3] Cardiac hypertrophy, cardiomyopathy, sinus arrhythmias, and hypertensive encephalopathy may also occur. In pregnant patients, the major symptom seems to be severe headache.[20,41] Pheochromocytomas may be associated with neuromas or neurofibromas; in these cases café au lait spots are often present.

Laboratory Findings. Laboratory findings include hyperglycemia in 60 percent of patients,[3] increased hematocrit, decreased plasma volume, and increased serum free fatty acids secondary to alterations in catecholamine metabolism. Definitive diagnosis depends on the demonstration of increased catecholamines, metanephrine, and vanillylmandelic acid (VMA) in the urine or increased catecholamines in the blood. The urinary assays are more reliable since blood cathecholamines may be elevated in other causes of hypertension.

Differential Diagnosis. Any hypertensive cardiovascular catastrophe may mimic a pheochromocytoma. The diagnosis of this condition may be made on the basis of tertiary alpha-adrenergic blockade; however, urine and blood assays for catecholamines and catecholamine metabolites are preferable. Hypertensive disease of pregnancy and toxemia should be differentiated from pheochromocytoma. Other diseases not necessarily associated with pregnancy may also mimic this entity. The hypertension of thyrotoxicosis is caused by catecholamine synergism with increased circulating thyroid hormones, although the systolic hypertension is not of the same magnitude as in pheochromocytoma. Ingestion of excess monoamine oxidase inhibitor drugs may increase the tissue levels of norepinephrine by blocking intraneuronal metabolism,[3] with subsequent hypertension and epilepsy and an acute abdomen.

A hypertensive crisis can be acutely precipitated under various circumstances such as local pressure over the tumor (perhaps by the gravid uterus), micturition if the tumor is located near the bladder, palpation of the tumor, or ingestion of food with increased tyramine levels.

Stimulation and Suppression Testing. Along with the direct evidence provided by measuring blood and urine for catecholamine excess, stimulation and suppression tests have also been advocated to aid in the definitive diagnosis of pheochromocytoma. The phentolamine (Regitine) test utilizes an alpha-adrenergic blocker in a dose range of 1 to 5 mg IV. A fall in blood pressure of 35 systolic/25 diastolic lasting for 4 min is a positive test and will successfully identify 45 percent of patients with pheochromocytoma.[11]

The histamine-provocative test is utilized in patients who are normotensive but suspected of having a pheochromocytoma based on history. This is a somewhat dangerous test and if it is employed, an alpha-adrenergic blocker should be readily available. Thus, 25 to 50 mg of histamine is injected IV, with a positive test yielding marked elevation in blood pressure in 1 to 2 min.[3,13,46] The potential danger of profound hypertension from an overly effective response or of induced hypotension in treating the elevated blood pressure makes this test contraindicated in pregnancy.

Management of Pheochromocytoma. There are two distinct problems in the management of pheochromocytoma. The first is that of the acute management of malignant hypertension. This entails lowering the blood pressure, managing fluid volumes, and preventing cardiac decompensation. The definitive management of this disorder, however, is surgical removal of the tumor, which involves the second problem—preparing the patient for surgery.

Control of Blood Pressure. All patients should be confined to strict bed rest. Control of blood pressures can be accomplished with phentolamine hydrochloride, an alpha-adrenergic blocking agent injected intravenously, 2 to 5 mg every 5 min until the blood pressure stabilizes.[3] Phenoxybenzamine hydrochloride (Dibenzyline) can also be used in this fashion, but phentolamine has a shorter half-life and permits minute-to-minute control of blood pressure. Phenoxybenzamine has the advantage that it can be given in oral doses varying from 4 to 100 mg every 12 h without the gastric side effects associated with phentolamine.[13] Maintenance therapy is not the rule and treatment is primarily aimed at stabilization in preparation for surgical removal of the tumor.

The beta-adrenergic blocking agents are helpful in patients with associated cardiac arrhythmias from catecholamine excess which are not responsive to the alpha-adrenergic blockers. Routine use of these agents in the management of pheochromocytoma has not been advocated and they should only be administered after adequate alpha blockade has been achieved.[40]

Sodium restriction is not a therapeutic requirement since these patients may have markedly decreased intravascular volumes. If that is the case, volume expanders such as whole blood, serum albumin, or saline should be administered. If intravascular volume depletion is profound, a central line should be employed during the period of hydration. Most authors recommend a period of 7 to 10 days of stabilization prior to surgery.[3,39]

Ross[39] quotes an operative mortality rate of up to 25 percent; in patients with undiagnosed cases who inadvertently undergo surgery, the mortality rate can be as high as 50 percent. The continued use of alpha- and beta-adrenergic blockers throughout the surgical procedure and in the immediate postoperative period is mandatory.

Anesthetic Considerations. The safe anesthetic management of the patient with pheochromocytoma begins with and is predicated upon preoperative "normalization" of blood pressure and intravascular blood volume with alpha-adrenergic blockade (phenoxybenzamine) and control of tachyarrhythmias and ventricular ectopy with beta-adrenergic blockade (propranolol). Preoperative cardiovascular stability helps to ensure intraoperative hemodynamic control and to limit volatile responses to circulating catecholamines.

Many anesthetic techniques and agents have been safely used to anesthetize these patients. Halothane sensitizes the myocardium to catecholamines and is best avoided. Enflurane, isoflurane, balanced nitrous oxide and narcotics, and regional anesthesia have all been used successfully.

The patient with a pheochromocytoma will require careful intra- and postoperative cardiovascular monitoring. This is best accomplished with intra-arterial and pulmonary artery catheters. Because the patient may display hemodynamic instability following tumor excision as a result of changing levels of plasma catecholamines and altered vascular resistance and capacitance, she should be admitted to an intensive care unit following surgery, where monitoring can be continued and rapid therapeutic interventions can be made.

Special Considerations during Pregnancy. Schenker and Chowers,[41] in a survey of 89 cases, reported a 58 percent maternal mortality rate when the diagnosis was not made until delivery or the postpartum period. If the diagnosis was made prior to delivery, the mortality rate was 17.3 percent. A major problem with pheochromocytoma during pregnancy is the increased vascularity of the tumor compared with the nonpregnant state. Furthermore, drastic swings in blood pressure may lead to placental abruption. These tumors should be operated upon in obstetrical patients whenever they are detected. A transverse upper abdominal incision is recommended. Schenker and Chowers state that if the tumor is detected at term, "labor and vaginal delivery should be avoided. Cesarean section, and removal of the tumor are recommended at the same time."[41] They also found that only 10 percent of pheochromocytomas in pregnancy were of nonadrenal origin. In the nonpregnant state localization of the tumor is by selective radiologic catheterization or computerized axial tomography (CAT) scan; in pregnancy only CAT scans are employed because of the large dose of radiation exposure which accompanies selective angiography.

Unlike the mother, the fetus has a 56 percent mortality rate regardless of when this disorder becomes manifest in pregnancy.[41] The level of catecholamines has been shown to be lower in cord blood than that of the mother. This difference is explained by enzymatic degradation by the placenta. Catechol methyltransferase, which methylates the epinephrine to an inactive metabolite, has been isolated from the placenta. However, Schenker[41] hypothesizes that even these small levels are quite detrimental to fetal homeostasis.

Drug Considerations. Berkowitz et al.[5] recommend that phenoxybenzamine (Dibenzyline) only be used in obstetric patients for maintenance of blood pressure control in women with pheochromocytoma, and not for management of an acute hypertensive crisis associated with that disorder. Side effects include postural hypertension, reflex tachycardia, and sedation. In patients who are hypovolemic, catastrophic drops in blood pressure might be noted.

Phentolamine (Regitine) "should be limited to the treatment of acute hypertensive episodes, in patients with pheochromocytoma."[5] It is not recommended as a diagnostic agent for pheochromocytoma during pregnancy because it may cause a rapid drop in maternal blood pressure with an associated decrease in uterine blood flow and subsequent fetal anoxia. Therefore, the diagnosis of pheochromocytoma in pregnancy should be based on blood and urine testing alone. Propranolol can be used to control cardiovascular arrhyhthmias but should not be used alone in the treatment of pheochromocytoma since an acute hypertensive episode can result.

PARATHYROID DISEASE

Burrow[10] has described a physiologic hyperparathyroidism associated with pregnancy with elevation of parathyroid hormone and calcium levels. Also, according to Shangold,[42] there is a sudden increase in serum calcium immediately postpartum. This is due to: (1) "removal of the transplacental calcium shunted from the mother to the fetus by active transport"; and (2) "markedly elevated maternal serum levels of 1,25-dihydroxy Vitamin D at term, which causes both increased intestinal absorption of calcium and enhanced action of parathyroid hormone on bone resorption."

Hypocalcemia

The manifestations of hypocalcemia arise primarily from the increased need for and decreased availability of calcium ion; this can be due to acute hypoparathyroidism. Another etiology of hypocalcemia is acute pancreatitis, the pathogenesis of which is a direct inhibitory effect on bone resorption by glucagon release, as well as the stimulation of calcitonin by glucagon. Calcium binding by saponification of fats is also contributory. Hypocalcemia can also be seen in phenothiazine drug reactions, epilepsy, brain tumors, and, most commonly, in surgical removal of the thyroid gland with inadvertent interruption of parathyroid function.[3] Other entities to rule out in the differential diagnosis of hypocalcemia include acute renal failure, decompensated alcoholic liver, and rare malabsorption syndromes.[46]

The diagnosis of hypocalcemia is based primarily on laboratory results rather than on physical findings. Clinical signs, however, may include tetany, which ranges in a continuum from elicited tetancy (Chvostek's sign) to frank seizure activity. Other signs and symptoms include papilledema, hallucinations, and, in the chronic state, cataracts and characteristic coarse skin changes.

The laboratory diagnosis is based on low serum calcium levels (<8 mg/100 ml), and usually an elevation in serum phosphate. The latter finding is unpredictable, however, since the phosphate level is usually proportional to the serum calcium. Prolongation of the QT wave is a frequent EKG change. Care must be taken to correct the calcium level for the albumin concentration. When the serum albumin concentration is abnormally low multiply it by 0.8 and add the value to the serum calcium. (For example, if serum calcium is 7.4 and serum albumin is 2, then the true serum calcium is $0.8 \times 2 + 7.4 = 9$ mg/100 ml. This value is normal.) In the future the use of "ionized" calcium levels may prove to be more reliable; however, insufficient data are available to recommend this approach at present.

Hypocalcemia when associated with pancreatitis can be accompanied by acute hypoglycemia, with resulting respiratory acidosis. The fall in pH will rapidly increase the protein binding of ionized calcium and this aggravates the problem.[3]

Management consists of rapidly administering an ampule of 10 percent Ca gluconate and then slowly infusing 1 g of calcium gluconate over a 6- to 8-h period, or 15 mg of calcium per kilogram body weight every 4 to 6 h.[3] It is very important to monitor serum calcium levels dynamically during the acute phase of treatment. Vitamin D may be started at 50,000 units/day if hypocalcemia persists.

Special Considerations in Pregnancy. The most common cause of hypoparathyroidism in pregnancy is previous removal of the thyroid gland for treatment of hyperthyroidism. Hypoparathyroidism in pregnancy theoretically can affect the fetus, but Burrow[10] reports no adverse effects either in the mother or fetus other than anecdotal reports of symptoms that are not related to the hypoparathyroidism. Neonatal hypocalcemia may occur, especially in infants born to mothers with hyperparathyroidism.[3]

Hypercalcemia

Serum calcium levels in excess of 12 to 13 mg/100 ml are associated with specific clinical findings, including anorexia, nausea, vomiting, weakness, fatigue, and severe abdominal pain. This is characteristic of hyperparathyroidism and associated hypercalcemia. These patients may also have polyuria and associated nephrolithiasis. Neuropsychiatric manifestations such as hallucinations and delusions have also been reported. Frequently patients will have hypertension in the acute state. These patients often present in a stupor and coma and the diagnosis must be made without the benefit of a history. A serum calcium greater than 16 mg/100 ml is an ominous sign, with death being attributable to intractable nausea and vomiting, polyuria, myocardial necrosis, circulatory collapse, and cerebral thrombosis.

The elevated serum calcium level leads to polyuria by its effect on the basement membrane of the renal tubular cell, causing an impairment of concentration of the urine. Calcium phosphate crystals may then precipitate in small vessels throughout the body, producing pancreatitis, pulmonary thrombosis, and even focal neurologic abnormalities[13] (Table 14-5).

Differential Diagnosis. Hypercalcemias can be divided into two specific types with different etiologies: those with increased parathyroid hormone (PTH) levels and those with normal or low PTH levels. Patients with elevated PTH levels have parathyroid adenomas, parathyroid hyperplasia, or ectopic production of PTH by a malignancy.[3] The PTH increases serum calcium by stimulating resorption of bone, inhibiting renal phosphate absorption, and increasing absorption from the gastrointestinal tract.[10] Those cases with normal PTH levels are usually attributable to malignancies with bony metastases, the use of thiazide diuretics, adrenal corticol insufficiency, milk alkali syndrome, physical immobilization, or hypo- or hyperthyroidism. The severity of the disease is much more profound in those cases with elevated PTH levels. Other conditions to consider in the differential diagnosis of hypercalcemia include hypervitaminosis D and A, sarcoidosis, thyrotoxicosis, and Paget's disease.

Laboratory Findings. Characteristic laboratory values include elevated serum calcium levels, low or low normal serum phosphate levels, chloride levels above 104

Table 14-5. Manifestations of Primary Hyperparathyroidism

1. Hypercalcemia
   a. Neuropsychiatric, e.g., lassitude, decreased recent memory, irritability, depression, and personality changes
   b. Peptic ulcer symptoms
2. Abnormal deposition of calcium in the tissues
   a. Renal calculi and nephrocalcinosis
   b. Band keratopathy
   c. Calcifications in capsules around joints and in tendons
   d. Chondrocalcinosis
   e. Pancreatitis
3. Skeletal findings
   a. Osteitis fibrosa cystica
   b. Osteoporosis
   c. Osteomalacia
   d. Osteosclerosis
   e. Subperiosteal erosions
   f. Bone cysts

From Bacchus, H: Metabolic and Endocrine Emergencies: Recognition and Management. University Park Press, Baltimore, 1977.

mEq/L, and an EKG with a shortened QT interval. According to Bacchus, serum calcium values greater than 10.5 mg/100 ml are considered elevated but hypercalcemic crisis rarely occurs with serum calcium levels less than 15 mg/100 ml.[3] Again, correction to normal albumin levels should be made, subtracting the factor 0.8 × albumin concentration from the serum calcium level. Serum PTH levels are usually inappropriately elevated in primary hyperparathyroidism, but the most useful diagnostic test is the measurement of nephrogenic cyclic AMP levels in a 24-h urine collection.

Management. In the chronic state, hypercalcemia is treated by preventing of calcium absorption from the GI tract, increasing urinary calcium excretion, decreasing bone resorption, or increasing bone formation. In the acute stage, in which vigorous and quick treatment is necessary, available modalities include: (1) infusion of large volumes of isotonic saline for dilutional effects; (2) administration of furosemide, 20 to 40 mg every 4 to 6 h, to increase the renal clearance of calcium (it should be noted that the calcium-lowering effect of furosemide may be transient); and (3) subcutaneous or intramuscular calcitonin, which is a safe and reliable new form of therapy for nonpregnant patients although its safety in pregnancy has not been totally established. Clearly the first order of treatment is adequate hydration and the establishment of a brisk diuresis. Since a vigorous natriuresis ensues, continuous monitoring of potassium levels and the EKG is crucial. In occasional severe cases, hemodialysis has been employed to treat these patients.[13] Some cases of hypercalcemia secondary to hyperparathyroidism and unresponsive to medical therapy may require rapid surgical intervention (Table 14-6).

Special Considerations in Pregnancy. Maternal calcium absorption increases from approximately 150 to 400 mg/day at 20 weeks, at which point it stabilizes.[1] The placenta allows the fetus to concentrate calcium, fetal serum calcium

Table 14-6. Treatment of Hypercalcemic Crisis

Hydration and natriuresis
1. Normal saline solution 3 L, if cardiorenal function permits, alternating with 5% D/W, 1 L. Infusion rate is determined by urinary flow rate.
2. Potassium replacement as determined by urinary K^+ measurements and EKG monitoring
3. Furosemide, 40 to 100 mg IV every 4 to 6 h
Phosphate (Inphos), 0.5 to 1.0 g PO every 6 h, or 50 to 100 mmol IV over 8 to 12 h
Mithramycin, 25 μg/kg body weight IV over 10 min; may be repeated in 24 to 48 h
Hemodialysis
Calcitonin

From Bacchus, H: Metabolic and Endocrine Emergencies: Recognition and Management. University Park Press, Baltimore, 1977.

levels being greater than those of the mother. This tends to promote hypercalcemia in the fetus of a mother with hyperparathyroidism.

In a review of the world literature, Shangold[42] reported 63 women with primary hyperparathyroidism associated with pregnancy. Ten patients were asymptomatic while the remainder had mild or nonspecific symptoms. A 50 percent complication rate has been reported in pregnancies associated with hyperparathyroidism, neonatal death and stillbirth being the most commonly reported problems.[27,32]

The actual effect of pregnancy on hyperparathyroidism is unknown but when these pregnancies were interrupted, there was a remission in some patients.[42]

PITUITARY DISEASE

Prolactin-Producing Adenomas

The true incidence of pituitary adenomas in the general population is unknown. This probably reflects the fact that these tumors are small and generally asymptomatic. Autopsy series place the incidence anywhere from 13 to 25 percent.[14,28] More recently, Coulam et al.[15] reported the incidence of pituitary tumors presenting clinically in women of reproductive age to be 7.1 per 100,000. Although this population of women tends to have a lower fertility rate, early diagnosis and modern therapeutic techniques have enabled many of them to achieve a successful pregnancy. Most often the pregnancy will be carried to term uneventfully with delivery of a normal, healthy infant. However, in 1 to 5 percent of these patients, complications may arise that are directly attributable to the pituitary lesion.[18,23,34]

Signs and Symptoms. Gemzell et al. reported the risk of developing complications during pregnancy to be 5.5 percent for women with untreated microadenomas, 35.7 percent for women with untreated macroadenomas, and 7.1 percent for women with treated adenomas of any size.[18] The most common tumor-related symptoms are headache and visual disturbances. Headache may be attributed to expansion of the adenoma, with resultant stretching of the diaphragmatic sella or adjacent dura mater. In Magyar's[33] series of 91 pregnancies in 73 patients, 23 percent developed headache. Of these, 66 percent developed symptoms in the first trimester, 24 percent in the second trimester, and 10 percent in the third trimester.

The progressive development of visual disturbances tends to follow the onset of headaches by at least 4 weeks.[34] The visual or optic changes that occur may be as subtle as pallor of the optic disk but can also include diplopia and eventually the more serious occurrence of bitemporal hemianopia due to impingement of the optic chiasma by the expanding pituitary adenoma. In Magyar's[33] study, 25 percent of patients with large untreated pituitary tumors developed visual disturbances. The onset of visual changes does not appear to differ significantly from one trimester to the next; the median time of onset was at 14 weeks.

Although most authors tend not to differentiate between micro- and macroadenomas, Gemzell's[18] review of the subject in 1979 suggests that patients with untreated macroadenomas had a significantly higher risk of developing complications during pregnancy. Those patients with macroadenomas which were excised prior to pregnancy appeared to do as well as women with microadenomas.

Diagnosis. The suspicion of a pituitary tumor complicating pregnancy should be aroused in any patient presenting with severe headaches with or without visual changes. This is particularly true in a patient with a previous history of oligo- or anovulation in whom prolactin levels may have been elevated prior to conception. The diagnosis in pregnancy is primarily a radiologic one since plasma prolactin concentrations may normally be elevated to levels as high as or higher than 400 ng/ml in normal obstetrical patients. Although coned-down views of the sella turcica are useful to detect large tumors, these radiologic procedures are being replaced by third-generation computer tomography. At the present time pneumoencephalography and arteriography are rarely indicated.

Other disorders that may result in headache and/or visual disturbance during pregnancy and must therefore be included in the differential diagnosis include tension headache, migraine headache, other vascular headaches such as temporal arteritis, and of course preeclampsia. The disorders can generally be excluded by accurate history and physical examination.

Management. In the past, most authors decided that patients with macroadenomas should be treated by surgical removal before ovulation was induced and pregnancy attempted. Recently, however, it has become clearly preferable to pursue noninvasive methods of therapy if an operative procedure can be avoided and favorable results obtained. Thus, modern therapeutic measures have tended to move away from surgical or radiation therapy with their potential for complications of infection, diabetes insipidus, anosmia, visual-field defects, and hypopituitarism to more conservative medical management. Jewelewicz et al.[26] reported a case in 1977, before adequate nonsurgical treatment was available in the United States, of a patient who at 22 weeks gestation noted the onset of blurred vision. She subsequently went on to develop abnormal visual fields and an enlarged sella turcica on x-ray by 30 weeks gestation. This patient was treated with dexamethasone 12 mg/day in divided doses and managed conservatively until 36 weeks, when she underwent cesarean section for obstetric indications. Since then, Bergh et al.,[4] Jewelewicz and Vande Wiele,[15] and McGregor et al.[35] have reported the use of bromocriptine to markedly reduce the size of prolactin-secreting adenomas. The dosage of bromocriptine used ranged from 5 to 20 mg/day, and this is now the treatment of choice for pituitary adenomas that become symptomatic. Those that are not symptomatic should be followed by visual fields and prolactin levels each trimester.

The onset of visual symptomatology appears to correlate most closely with the need for therapeutic intervention in pregnancy. In Magyar's series,[33] therapy was required by 53 percent of patients with headaches, 61 percent of those with visual changes, and 79 percent of those with a combination of headache and visual disturbances ($p < 0.05$). Furthermore, once visual symptoms develop, the likelihood that the patients will receive therapy during pregnancy appears to be influenced by gestational age. Thus, in Magyar's study treatment was given to 78 percent of the patients developing symptoms in the first trimester, 83 percent of those in the second trimester, but only 25 percent of those in the third trimester ($p < 0.5$). Finally, it is important to note that 96 percent of patients with untreated asymptomatic tumors have no permanent sequelae.

Special Considerations in Pregnancy. In normal pregnancy the pituitary gland increases in size and weight. In 1934 Rasmussen[38] reported a mean increase of hypophyseal weight of 102 mg in pregnant women. At present, it is impossible to predict which patients with pituitary tumors will undergo sufficient enlargement of the tumor to cause symptomatology. All patients should have a baseline neurologic examination and then be followed with ophthalmologic consultation to assess visual fields and acuity every 3 months. Once symptomatology, particularly visual disturbances, occurs, radiologic reevaluation is necessary. If the findings suggest that treatment is necessary, therapy must be individualized. If the fetus is not mature, control of tumor growth may be accomplished by conservative medical management with bromocriptine. If fetal lung maturity can be documented, induction of labor and delivery of the infant may prove beneficial. In most cases, vaginal delivery should be attempted, with cesarean section being reserved for true obstetric indications.

Pregnancy outcome does not appear to be markedly affected by the presence of a pituitary tumor. Gemzell and Wang[18] reported a fetal wastage rate of 15.4 percent in patients with previously untreated microadenomas. Perinatal mortality is similarly not increased over that in the general population. Prematurity, however, appears to be increased in patients who undergo treatment during preganancy. This has been ascribed to premature induction of labor and preterm cesarean section and not to the spontaneous onset of labor.[33] The long-term effects of medication such as bromocriptine on the fetus have not as yet been determined although the preliminary data are reassuring.

The pregnant patient with a pituitary adenoma should not be neglected once delivery has been effected. Follow-up radiographic examination should be performed from 4 to 6 months after delivery. Finally, the recommendations to a patient who desires further pregnancies must follow complete reevaluation. Gemzell[17] and Gemzell and Wang[18] in 1975 studied women with untreated pituitary adenomas who had more than one pregnancy. The frequency with which symptoms occurred in the second pregnancy did not appear to be statistically different from that in the first pregnancy.

DIABETES INSIPIDUS

Diabetes insipidus is a rare disease with a slightly greater incidence in young adults and in males. A recent review of the subject reported the incidence in the general population to be anywhere from 1 in 16,000 to 1 in 82,000.[22] The disease is due to a lack or extremely low levels of vasopressin (antidiuretic hormone) production. This results in large volume losses via the kidney. Central diabetes insipidus appears to be caused as a result of a disruption of the normal functional integrity of either the supraoptic and paraventricular nuclei, the supraoptic hypophyseal tract, or the posterior lobe of the hypophysis. The full-blown disease occurs only when the tract is interrupted close enough to the hypothalamus to cause a degeneration of at least a majority of the supraoptic and paraventricular neurons.

Signs and Symptoms. The chief symptoms of diabetes insipidus are those of polyurea and polydipsia. The urine tends to be dilute, with specific gravities less than 1.005. As much as 15 to 30 L may be lost per day. This results in dehydration, with its related signs and symptoms of dry skin, constipation, and intense thirst.

Diagrosis and Differential Diagnosis. Diagnosis is suggested by the symptoms, plus the large urine volumes with specific gravities below 1.010. In addition, the urine osmolality is less than that of plasma. The diagnosis is confirmed by a water deprivation test wherein the patient remains polyuric with little increase in urine osmolality despite significant water restriction. The subsequent IM injection of vasopressin will result in an antidiuretic response reflected in a substantial increase in urine osmolality and decrease in free-water clearance.

Central diabetes insipidus must be differentiated from nephrogenic diabetes insipidus, wherein there is refractoriness of the renal tubules to vasopressin. The latter condition can be ruled out by giving vasopressin as a test substance. Other conditions causing polyuria must also be excluded: these include acute and chronic renal disease, diabetes mellitus, the hypercalcemia of hyperparathyroidism, vitamin D intoxication, primary aldosteronism, hypochloremic alkalosis, and psychogenic polydipsia. These disorders can be ruled out by appropriate laboratory studies.

Therapy. Therapy is geared towards replacement of antidiuretic hormone activity. At the present time this is best accomplished by intransasal administration of L-diamino-8-*d*-arginine vasopressin (DDAVP). Dosages in the order of 0.1 ml nasally are administered up to 3 times daily. Response is virtually immediate. Vasopressin in oil (10 IU IM) can be given and is usually effective up to 48 h.

Special Considerations in Pregnancy. The course of diabetes insipidus in pregnancy is variable and unpredictable. In a review of the literature, Hime and Richardson[22] reported that the majority of patients had a worsening of the condition in pregnancy, while a smaller percentage showed either improvement or no change in the condition. Of 67 cases reviewed, a majority were labeled idiopathic, 4 were secondary to head injury, 1 was ascribed to hypophysectomy and 4 to metastatic breast carcinoma, 1 was secondary to encephalitis, and 1 was thought to be due to tuberculosis.

The suggestion that inadequate labor occurs in diabetes insipidus has not been substantiated by the reports of Gordon[19] and Pico.[37] Indeed, labor and delivery appear to progress normally. In the absence of underlying pathology such as chronic renal disease or diabetes mellitus, the outcome for the fetus should be expected to be excellent. The long-term effect of DDAVP administration on the fetus, however, is not known at the present time and therefore use of this treatment during pregnancy is not recommended. Vasopressin in oil is therefore the therapy of choice. The appearance of diabetes insipidus in pregnancy requires a CAT scan to rule out pituitary or hypothalamic lesions.

SHEEHAN'S SYNDROME

In 1914 Simmonds described a syndrome of pituitary apoplexy as a result of a destructive lesion of the anterior pituitary. Twenty-five years later, Sheehan[43] called attention to some cases of Simmonds' disease that he felt were due to postpartum necrosis of the anterior pituitary. At that time, Sheehan estimated the incidence of the syndrome that would subsequently bear his name was somewhere in the order of 9 per 10,000 term pregnancies.

Sheehan's syndrome occurs in patients with severe postpartum hemorrhage, particularly when accompanied by hypotension. The exact etiology is unknown; however, contributing factors may include the presence of a small sella, swelling of the pituitary during pregnancy owing to increased size and number of lactotropes, hemorrhage and hypotension, and fibrosis of the remaining pituitary. Sheehan[43] noted that a loss of 50 percent of the pituitary gland produced no clinical evidence of hypopituitarism. With 75 percent loss of the gland, moderate hypopituitarism was noted, and it was only when 90 to 98 percent of the gland was affected that severe symptoms of hypopituitarism were demonstrated. Thus, varying gradations of the severity of this syndrome may be seen clinically.

Diagnosis and Differential Diagnosis. The diagnosis of Sheehan's syndrome is based primarily on a very characteristic clinical picture, particularly when there is history of antecedent intra- or postpartum hemorrhage accompanied by shock. Interestingly, the full-blown picture may take years to become manifest. The earliest sign of the disease appears in the puerpurium: the patient fails to lactate. The breasts atrophy rapidly and remain dry. In patients whose subsequent symptoms of hypopituitarism are only moderate, the failure of lactation occurs in only about half the cases. Hypoglycemia secondary to growth hormone deficiency was also reported by Sheehan[43] in the puerperal period, with blood sugars remaining at levels of approximately 50 mg/100 ml. Deficiency of luteinizing hormone (LH) and follicle-stimulating hormone (FSH) lead to atrophy of the ovaries, with complete loss of ovarian function. This results in amenorrhea, with attendant infertility, decreased libido, and urinary and genital atrophy. The uterus may undergo suprainvolution. The vagina loses its glycogen and takes on a characteristic senile appearance. Less severe cases of Sheehan's syndrome generally tend to demonstrate amenorrhea but not the complete genital atrophy. In still less severe cases there may, with time, be a return to menstruation. In addition to the specific symptoms, more general symptoms of lethargy and apathy may become evident during the puerpurium.

The later signs and symptoms of Sheehan's syndrome, like the early ones, vary in intensity based on the degree of anterior pituitary necrosis. In addition, the signs and symptoms may appear in any combination. Loss of body hair, particularly axillary and pubic hair, signs and symptoms of hypothyroidism, pallor secondary to decreased ACTH and MSH, signs and symptoms of adrenal insufficiency, and hyperchromic anemia were all described in Sheehan's original paper. Although weight loss may occur, a severely emaciated patient as described by Simmonds is rarely seen in Sheehan's syndrome.

The differential diagnosis of Sheehan's syndrome include all those conditions which may result in anterior pituitary deficiency. Common causes include pituitary tumors; tumors of the hypothalamus or pituitary stalk; granulomatous disease, particularly tuberculosis; and other causes of pituitary infarction—namely, idiopathic infarction and, more rarely, the infarction seen in association with either diabetes mellitus or sickle-cell disease. Surgical hypophysectomy, irradiation of the pituitary, head trauma, congenital malformations of the hypothalamus, and hemachromatosis must all be included in the differential diagnosis. More rarely, para-, supra-, or intrasellar tumors, metastatic cancer, lymphoma, aneurysms of the internal carotid artery, abscess formation, cavernous sinus thrombosis, or congenital defects may be encountered.

Laboratory Diagnosis. The laboratory diagnosis of Sheehan's syndrome rests on the demonstration of deficient anterior pituitary function. Growth hormone deficiency may be demonstrated with either an L-dopa test, an arginine infusion test, or insulin-induced hypoglycemia. Prolactin deficiency and TSH deficiency may both be demonstrated with a TRH (thyrotropin releasing hormone) stimulation test. Similarly, LH deficiency may be demonstrated through the use of an LRH (luteinizing hormone releasing hormone) stimulation test. ACTH deficiency may be inferred when lower than normal serum corticosteroid levels respond appropriately to ACTH infusion. A discussion of these tests is beyond the scope of this chapter. The interested reader is referred to some articles in the reference list for detailed descriptions of how to perform and interpret these studies.[3,10,13,46]

Treatment. The treatment of Sheehan's syndrome consists primarily in replacing those anterior pituitary hormones that are essential for maintaining homeostasis and responding to stress. Thus, thyroid hormone and corticosteroid replacement are essential when these hormones are deficient. Thyroid replacement may be given in the form of L-thyroxine in a dosage of 0.1 to 0.2 μg PO daily. Corticosteroids should be replaced in those individuals in whom adrenal insufficiency has been proved. Cortisone acetate in a dose of 25 to 37.5 mg daily may be used. Replacement of LH and FSH would be required only in those instances in which ovulation is induced for purposes of achieving pregnancy. In those individuals with urogenital atrophy, estrogen replacement (0.625 mg/day) would prove beneficial. Growth hormone replacement is not necessary in adults.

REFERENCES

1. Aurbach, G., Marx, S., and Spoegel, A.: Parathyroid hormone, calcitonin, and the calciferols. In Williams, R.: Textbook of Endocrinology. W.B. Saunders, Philadelphia, 1981.
2. Ayromlooi, J., Zervoudakis, I.A., and Sadaghat, A.: Thyrotoxicosis in pregnancy. Am. J. Obstet. Gynecol., *117*:818, 1973.
3. Bacchus, H.: Metabolic and Endocrine Emergencies: Recognition and Management. University Park Press, Baltimore, 1977.
4. Bergh, T., Nillius, S.J., and Wide, L.: Clinical course and outcome of pregnancies in amenorrhoeic women with hyperprolactinaemia and pituitary tumours. Br. Med. J., *1*:875, 1978.
5. Berkowitz, R.L., Coustan, D.R., and Mochizuki, T.K.: Handbook for Prescribing Medications during Pregnancy. Little, Brown, Boston, 1981.
6. Blumsohn, D., Munyadziwa, E.H., Dajie, S.K. et al.: Cushing's syndrome and pregnancy: a case report. S. Afr. Med. J., *53*:338, 1978.
7. Brent, F.: Addison's disease and pregnancy. Am. J. Surg., 645, 1950.
8. Bullock, J.L., Harris, R.E., and Young, R.: Treatment of thyrotoxicosis during pregnancy with propranolol. Am. J. Obstet. Gynecol., *121*:242, 1975.
9. Burrow, G.N.: Hyperthyroidism during pregnancy. N. Engl. J. Med., *298*:150, 1978.
10. Burrow, G.N. and Ferris, T.F.: Medical Complications During Pregnancy. W.B. Saunders, Philadelphia, 1975.
11. Calodney, N., Eaton, R.P., Black, W., and Cohn, F.: Exacerbation of Cushing's syndrome during pregnancy: report of a case: J. Clin. Endocrinol. Metab., *36*:81, 1973.
12. Carr, B.R., Parker, C.R., Jr., Madden, J.D., and MacDonald, P.C.: Maternal plasma adrenocorticotropin and cortisol relationships throughout human pregnancy. Am. J. Obstet. Gynecol., *139*:416, 1981.
13. Cohen, A.S., Freidin, R.B., and Samuels, M.A.: Medical Emergencies: Diagnostic and Management Procedures from Boston City Hospital. Little, Brown, Boston, 1977.
14. Costello, R.T.: Subclinical adenoma of the pituitary gland. Am. J. Pathol., *12*:205, 1936.
15. Coulam, C.B., Annergers, J.F., Abboud, C.F. et al.: Pituitary adenoma and oral contraceptives: a case-control study. Fertil. Steril., *31*:25, 1979.
16. Durham, J.A.: A noradrenaline pheochromocytoma complicating pregnancy. Aust. NZ. J. Obstet. Gynaecol., *17*:53, 1977.
17. Gemzell, C.: Induction of ovulation in infertile women with pituitary tumors. Am. J. Obstet. Gynecol., *121*:311, 1975.
18. Gemzell, C. and Wang, C.F.: Outcome of pregnancy in women with pituitary adenoma. Fertil. Steril., *31*:363, 1979.
19. Gordon, G. and Bradford, W.: Pregnancy in a patient with diabetes insipidus following induction of ovulation with clomiphene. J. Obstet. Gynaecol. Br. Commonw., *77*:467, 1970.
20. Grimes, E.M., Fayez, J.A., and Miller, G.L.: Cushing's syndrome and pregnancy. Obstet. Gynecol., *42*:550, 1973.
21. Hawe, P.: The management of thyrotoxicosis during pregnancy. Br. J. Surg., *52*:731, 1965.
22. Hime, M.C. and Richardson, J.: Diabetes insipidus and pregnancy: case report, incidence, and review of literature. Obstet. Gynecol. Surv., *33*:375, 1978.

23. Husami, N., Jewelewicz, R., and Vande Wiele, R.L.: Pregnancy in patients with pituitary tumors. Fertil. Steril., *28:*920, 1977.
24. Innerfield, R. and Hollander, C.S.: Thyroidal complications of pregnancy. Med. Clin. North Am., *61:*67, 1977.
25. Jewelewicz, R. and Vande Wiele, R.L.: Clinical course and outcome of pregnancy in twenty-five patients with pituitary microadenomas. Am. J. Obstet. Gynecol., *136:*339, 1980.
26. Jewelewicz, R., Zimmerman, E.A., and Carmel, P.W.: Conservative management of a pituitary tumor during pregnancy following induction of ovulation with gonadotropins. Fertil. Steril., *28:*35, 1977.
27. Johnstone, R.E., II, Kreindler, T., Johnstone, R.E.: Hyperparathyroidism during pregnancy. Obstet. Gynecol., *40:*580, 1972.
28. Kraus, J.: Neoplastic diseases of the human hypophysis. Arch. Pathol., *39:*343, 1945.
29. Krienes, K. and DeVaux, W.D.: Neonatal adrenal insufficiency associated with maternal Cushing's syndrome. Pediatrics, *47:*516, 1971.
30. Leak, D., Carroll, J.J., Robinson, D.C., and Ashworth, E.J.: Management of pheochromocytoma during pregnancy. Can. Med. Assoc. J. *116:*371, 1977.
31. Lee, R. and Rapoport, A.: Cushing's syndrome with amelioration during pregnancy. JAMA, *221:*392, 1972.
32. Ludwig, G.D.: Hyperparathyroidism in relation to pregnancy. N. Engl. J. Med., *267:*637, 1962.
33. Magyar, D.M. and Marshall, J.R.: Pituitary tumors and pregnancy. Am. J. Obstet. Gynecol., *132:*739, 1978.
34. Magyar, D.M. and Marshall, J.R.: When your pregnant patient has a pituitary adenoma. Contemp. Obstet. Gynecol., *17:*121, 1981.
35. McGregor, A., Scanlon, M., Hall, K. et al.: Reduction in size of a pituitary tumor by bromocriptine therapy. N. Engl. J. Med., *300:*291, 1979.
36. Menendez, C.E. and Rivlin, R.S.: Thyrotoxic crisis and myxedema coma. Med. Clin. North Am., *57:*1463, 1973.
37. Pico, I. and Greenblatt, R.: Diabetes insipidus and pregnancy. Fertil. Steril., *20:*384, 1969.
38. Rasmussen, A.T.: The weight of the principal components of the normal hypophysis cerebri of the adult human female. Am. J. Anat., *55:*253, 1934.
39. Ross, E.J., Prichard, B.N.C., Kaufman, L. et al.: Preoperative and operative management of patients with phaeochromocytoma. Br. Med. J., *1:*191, 1967.
40. Rubin, P.C.: Beta-blockers in pregnancy. N. Engl. J. Med., *305:*1323, 1981.
41. Schenker, J.G. and Chowers, I.: Pheochromocytoma and pregnancy. Obstet. Gynecol. Surv., *26:*739, 1971.
42. Shangold, M.M., Dor, N., Welt, S.I. et al.: Hyperparathyroidism and pregnancy: a review. Obstet. Gynecol. Surv., *37:*217, 1982.
43. Sheehan, H.L.: Simmonds's disease due to post-partum necrosis of the anterior pituitary. Q. J. Med., *8:*277, 1939.
44. Urbanic, R.C. and Mazzaferri, E.L.: Thyrotoxic crisis and myxedema coma. Heart Lung, *7:*435, 1978.
45. Wieland, R.G., Shaffer, M.B., and Glove, R.P.: Cushing's syndrome complicating pregnancy: a case report. Obstet. Gynecol., *38:*841, 1971.
46. Wilkins, E.W., Dineen, J., Moncure, A.C., and Fitzgerald, C.P.: MGH Textbook of Emergency Medicine. Williams & Wilkins, Baltimore, 1978.
47. Yackel, D.B., Kempers, R.D., and McConahey, W.M.: Adrenocorticosteroid therapy in pregnancy. Am. J. Obstet. Gynecol., *96:*985, 1966.

15

Diabetic Ketoacidosis

Donald R. Coustan, M.D.

INTRODUCTION

In the nonpregnant patient, diabetic ketoacidosis (DKA) carries a 5 to 15 percent mortality rate,[10] with death most often due to some serious intercurrent event (sepsis, pancreatitis, myocardial infarction). In pregnancy, DKA is an even more serious occurrence, since estimates of the incidence of fetal death run from 50 to 90 percent![9,31] Indeed, DKA is one of Pedersen's "prognostically bad signs in pregnancy"[22] and is clearly the most ominous. With modern approaches to the medical management of diabetes in pregnancy, DKA should be an exceedingly rare complication. Nevertheless, it does happen. It is thus important for the perinatologist to be able to recognize DKA and to treat this problem rapidly and appropriately. In this chapter I shall review the pathophysiology of DKA,[10,19] outline the differential diagnosis, and suggest a plan of management.

PATHOPHYSIOLOGY

Diabetic ketoacidosis is characterized by a state of hyperglycemia and accelerated ketogenesis. Both these problems are related to an absolute or relative lack of insulin and to an excess of glucagon. This may be thought of as a decrease in the insulin/glucagon ratio. The signs and symptoms of DKA all follow from hyperglycemia and acclerated ketogenesis.

Hyperglycemia

The plasma glucose level is dependent upon a number of factors: (1) ingested carbohydrate and amino acids; (2) peripheral glucose utilization; and (3) hepatic storage and release, i.e., glycogen production and breakdown, and gluconeogenesis. Although tissue glucose utilization is diminished in DKA, the main problem is increased hepatic gluconeogenesis from endogenous precursors. While normal postabsorptive subjects release 150 to 200 mg of glucose per minute from their livers, diabetics in DKA have been demonstrated to increase hepatic glucose release to 400 to 600 mg/min. This explains the occurrence of severe hyperglycemia in ketoacidotic patients who have not eaten for as long as 24 h.

When glucose enters the liver, it is phosphorylated to glucose 6-phosphate. This activated glucose may go down a number of possible pathways (Fig. 15-1). One possibility is storage in the form of glycogen. It is not completely clear what factors are most important in activating this pathway. They may include high hepatic glucose levels, insulin and/or other regulatory hormones. There is clearly an inverse relationship between glycogen synthetase activity and intracellular cyclic AMP levels, but this probably represents an intermediate regulatory step.

Glycolysis (the Embden-Meyerhof pathway) is another direction in which hepatic glucose 6-phosphate may travel (Fig. 15-2). The end product is pyruvate, which may then enter the Krebs cycle to be metabolized to CO_2 and water, with concomitant production of energy. Under anaerobic conditions, lactate is produced from pyruvate. The first *committed* step in glycolysis, and the most important regulatory

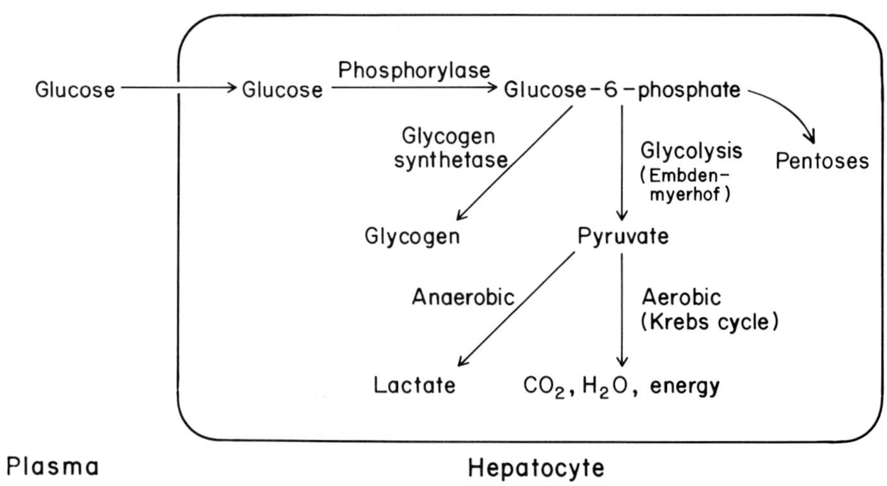

Fig. 15-1 Hepatic fate of glucose.

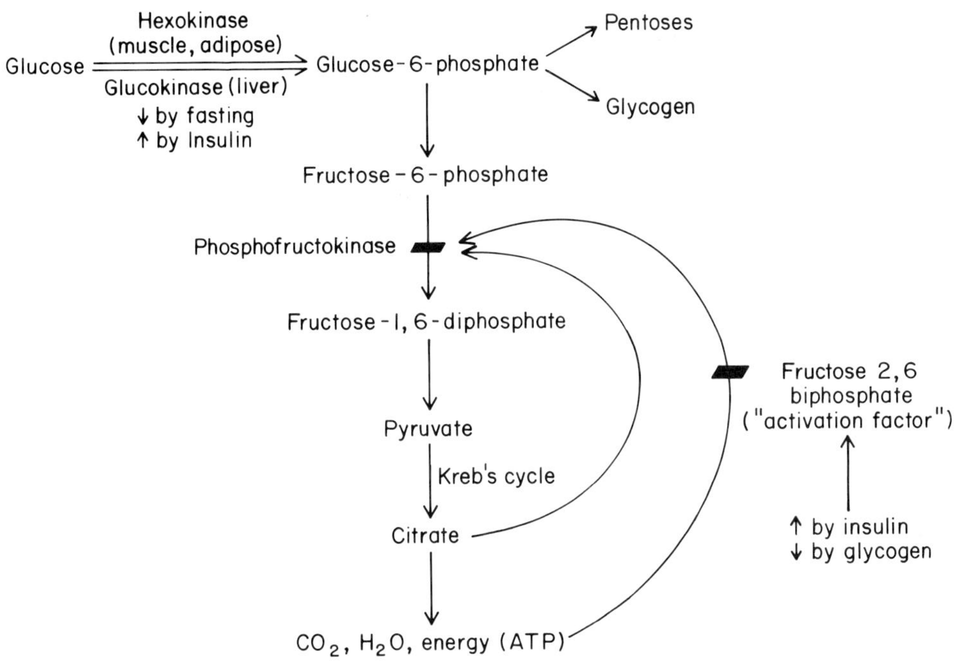

Fig. 15-2 Glycolysis.

step, is the conversion of fructose 6-phosphate to fructose 1,6-diphosphate. This step is irreversible and is catalyzed by the enzyme phosphofructokinase. This enzyme is inhibited by the presence of large amounts of ATP and citrate (important end products of glycolysis) in a negative feedback manner. Of interest is the fact that fructose 2,6-biphosphate is an "activation factor" which protects phosphofructokinase against inhibition by ATP. This activation factor is increased by insulin and decreased by glucagon. Thus, we see that diminished insulin and/or increased glucagon can block glycolysis, preventing the normal utilization of glucose for energy production.

The reverse of glycolysis, the formation of glucose from noncarbohydrate sources (lactate, pyruvate, amino acids, odd-chain fatty acids), is called gluconeogenesis. Key steps in gluconeogenesis are catalyzed by different enzymes from those involved in glycolysis and are irreversible. The liver is the major site of gluconeogenesis; muscle and heart do not contain the necessary enzymes. Gluconeogenesis is enhanced by glucagon and diminished by insulin. Thus it is apparent that hyperglycemia results from insulin lack and/or glucagon excess because of diminished glycolysis and enhanced gluconeogenesis in the liver.

Maternal Effects of Hyperglycemia. Maternal hyperglycemia, associated with a diminution in the insulin/glucagon ratio, is responsible for many of the clinical problems seen in DKA. In the first place, high glucose levels cause an osmotic diuresis, with the loss of large amounts of water and electrolytes. Dehydration and hyperosmolarity result. These problems are further magnified by the water and electrolyte loss due to vomiting which almost invariably accompanies acidosis. Dehydration is present in both intravascular and extravascular spaces. The hypovolemia may lead to hypotension, impaired renal function, diminished mentation, and ultimately shock.

Although during an osmotic diuresis, the urine is always hypotonic and hyponatremic relative to plasma, total body sodium depletion results. In addition, total body potassium is reduced, although serum potassium levels may be normal or even elevated secondary to insulin deficiency. Total body phosphate, chloride, bicarbonate, and magnesium are also depleted.

Fetal Effects of Hyperglycemia. When gluconeogenesis is enhanced and glycolysis is diminished, amino acids become the major precursors for glucose production. These amino acids are derived from body protein, so that gluconeogenesis brings about negative nitrogen balance. Since amino acids serve as a source of fuel and as building blocks for fetal development, there is a theoretical risk to fetal growth and metabolism when maternal gluconeogenesis is enhanced. Furthermore, elevated maternal glucose levels are translated directly into fetal hyperglycemia. According to the Pedersen hypothesis, fetal hyperglycemia is the ultimate cause of diabetic fetopathy. Fetal hyperglycemia is believed to cause fetal hyperinsulinemia, leading to excessive fetal growth, neonatal hypoglycemia, and possibly the observed delay in fetal pulmonary maturation.

The dehydration, hypovolemia, and electrolyte depletion brought about by hyperglycemia may themselves have detrimental effects upon the fetus. Profound intravascular depletion would be expected to lower uterine blood flow, with a possible consequence being acute hypoxia. Although one might hypothesize that chronic maternal hyperglycemia would lead to intrauterine growth retardation because of an associated chronic intravascular depletion, the opposite is true—maternal hyperglycemia is associated with fetal macrosomia. This is most likely due to the fact that maternal glucose easily crosses to the fetus by facilitated diffusion, evoking a fetal insulin response. High fetal insulin levels promote increased fetal growth. Macrosomia is the result.

Ketosis

The liver is the site of ketone body production. It is also the major site of synthesis of fatty acids. Combustion of fatty acids produces energy. This occurs in various tissues throughout the body, including heart, muscle, and liver. The liver may thus be thought of as a clearing house in fat metabolism. It produces fatty acids for the rest of the body to use or breaks them down when they are overly abundant or when other substrates are unavailable, as in starvation.

A relative or absolute lack of insulin has numerous consequences, many of which increase the level of ketone bodies in the circulation. The presence of insulin exerts a restraining influence on lipase, an enzyme in adipose tissue which brings about lipolysis (Fig. 15-3). If insulin is diminished, lipase activity is enhanced and free fatty acids (FFAs) are released in greater quantity. Additionally, if insulin is lacking, glucose transport into adipocytes is reduced. This lack of intracellular glucose decreases the availability of glycerol 3-phosphate, an essential precursor in the in situ reesterification of fatty acids. Thus, insulin deficiency acts peripherally to increase lipolysis and decrease reutilization of FFAs, thereby providing more substrate for hepatic ketogenesis.

In the liver, the normal state of events is fatty acid synthesis rather than breakdown. Glucose is oxidized via the Krebs cycle, citrate being an end product. If fatty acids are to be made, citrate is split into acetylcoenzyme A (acetyl-CoA) and oxaloacetate (Fig. 15-4). The acetyl-CoA can then be used to produce malonyl-CoA, the first committed intermediate in fatty acid synthesis. Malonyl-CoA is also the physiologic inhibitor of an enzyme, carnitine acyltransferase I (CAT I), which is responsible for allowing fatty acids to cross the mitochondrial membrane and enter the mitochondrion, where oxidation to ketone bodies occurs. Thus, in the fed state, fatty acid synthesis feeds back negatively on fatty acid breakdown and ketosis.

In order for fatty acids to be broken down to ketones, they must first be transported into the mitochondria of hepatic cells. Otherwise, they will be reesterified and used for the formation of very low density lipoproteins. When fatty acids reach the liver, they are immediately esterified to coenyzme A (CoA), forming fatty acyl-CoA (Fig. 15-4). In order to cross the mitochondrial membrane, they have to be transesterified with carnitine to form fatty acylcarnitine. This transesterification is accomplished by the enzyme CAT I, mentioned above. This is the rate-limiting step in the formation of ketones. Once fatty acylcarnitines are formed, they cross the mitochondrial membrane, are again transesterified to fatty acyl-CoA, and are then oxidized almost exclusively to ketone bodies. The presence of excess glucagon (i.e., a lower insulin/glucagon ratio) activates ketogenesis in two ways. First, the availability of carnitine to the liver is increased. Second, malonyl-CoA production is blocked, and the inhibition of CAT I is removed. The net result is the formation of acetoacetate and its partial conversion to β-hydroxybutyrate, the ketone bodies.

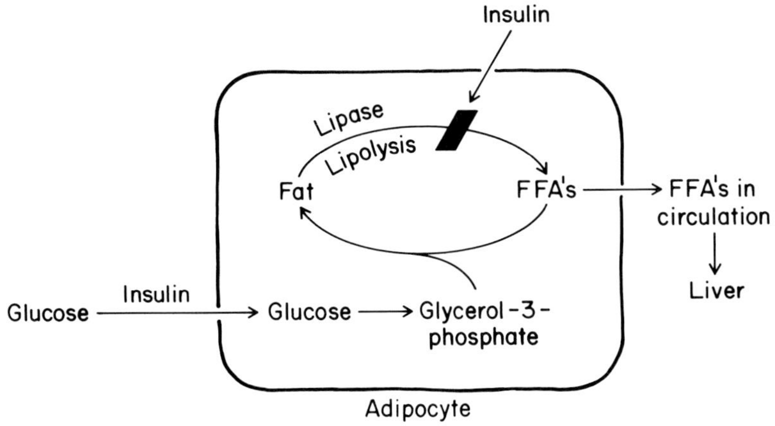

Fig. 15-3 Effects of insulin on adipose tissue.

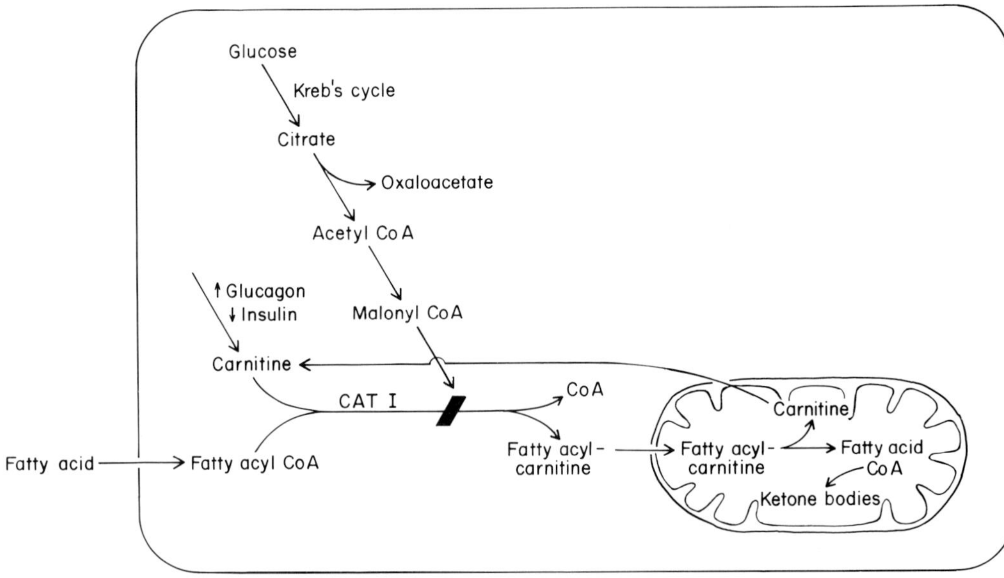

Fig. 15-4 Effects of insulin and glucagon on ketone production in hepatocytes.

The importance of increased glucagon in activating CAT I has been demonstrated by experiments in which glucagon was blocked with somatostatin in insulin-withdrawn diabetics.[11] In these circumstances ketosis was diminished. Additionally, individuals who have undergone pancreatectomy (and thus have neither insulin nor glucagon) are less ketosis-prone than diabetics.

Insulin deficiency decreases the ability of muscle to dispose of ketones. This is

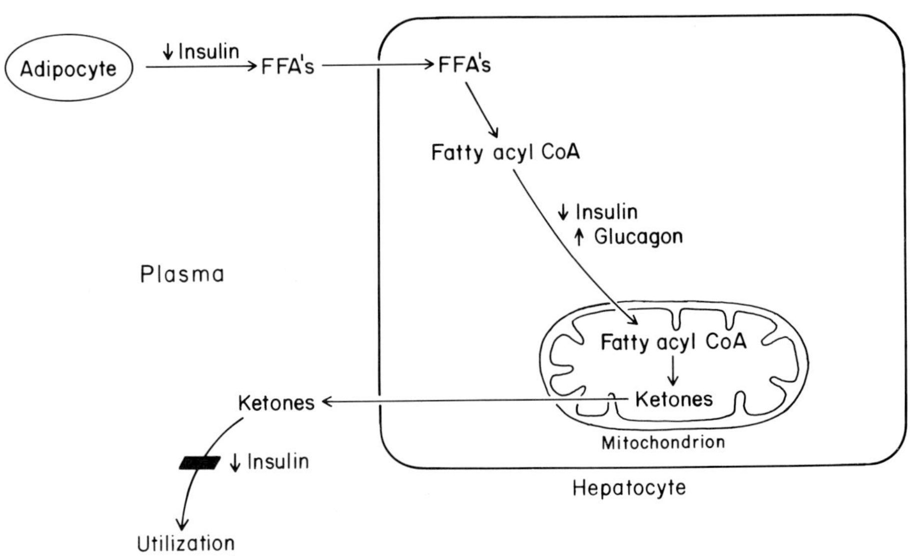

Fig. 15-5 Effects of lack of insulin on ketosis.

true even with mild degrees of insulin lack, and is a more sensitive index of insulin lack than is ketone overproduction.

Figure 15-5 summarizes the mechanisms involved in ketosis. Insulin lack causes increased peripheral release of FFAs, increasing hepatic substrate for fatty acid oxidation. Insulin lack and glucagon excess activate CAT I, allowing fatty acids to enter the mitochondria in liver cells, where they are oxidized to ketones. Peripheral ketone utilization is diminished by reduced insulin levels. The net effect is a buildup of ketones in the blood.

Maternal Effects of Ketoacidosis. Ketone bodies are moderately strong acids. In DKA, the concentration of hydrogen ions is increased in all body fluids (i.e., the pH decreases). The serum bicarbonate falls, and the anion gap is increased (i.e., the serum sodium minus the sum of bicarbonate and chloride is greater than the normal value of 10 to 15 mEq/L). The acidosis leads to increased respiratory rate and depth in an attempt to compensate by creating a respiratory alkalosis. This is the cause of Kussmaul's respiration. Nausea and vomiting are extremely common, and this increases the tendency toward dehydration and electrolyte depletion. Aberrations of mental function ranging from drowsiness to coma may occur.

Fetal Effects of Ketoacidosis. By a mechanism not as yet understood, DKA has been implicated in sudden intrauterine death, with fetal mortaility rates approaching 90 percent when diabetic coma occurred.[9,31] At least one case has been reported of an apparently normal fetus dying in utero during an episode of ketoacidosis induced by administration of ritodrine to a diabetic mother.[25] Unfortunately, the effects of maternal acidosis per se on fetal circulatory dynamics are poorly understood. The administration of ammonium chloride to humans has been shown to result in lower pH values in the cord bloods of their neonates.[12] Because CO_2 crosses the placenta freely, maternal respiratory acidosis or alkalosis is rapidly transmitted to the fetus. However, charged ions such as HCO_3^- cross much more slowly. Thus, in the situation of maternal metabolic acid-base imbalance, fetal changes will occur much more slowly. If the fetus becomes acidotic, it is not clear what effect this has upon circulatory dynamics in the absence of hypoxia.

At least two studies have linked maternal ketonuria in the third trimester with childhood intellectual deficits.[8,30] However, controversy exists as to the validity of these findings.[21] It is clear that ketone bodies freely cross the placenta and that the adult brain is capable of utilizing these substrates for energy. It is not known whether their use by the fetal brain is detrimental to normal development.

Myers has suggested that fetal brain damage due to hypoxia is enhanced by elevated lactate levels.[20] He has linked increases in fetal brain lactate to increased availability of glucose as a substrate. It may then be hypothesized that diabetic ketoacidosis may have adverse effects on the fetal brain in at least two ways: (1) If the patient has severe enough DKA to be hypovolemic, diminished placental perfusion may cause fetal hypoxia. In the presence of severe hyperglycemia, the fetal brain may be more susceptible to hypoxic insult. (2) If the mother is hypotensive, poor tissue perfusion will add lactic acidosis to her list of problems. High lactic acid levels in the fetal brain probably also predispose to hypoxic injury.

DIAGNOSIS OF DIABETIC KETOACIDOSIS

Because of the great risk to both mother and fetus, it is important that the diagnosis of DKA be made rapidly and reliably. This is most quickly done by measuring urinary glucose and ketones, arterial blood gases, and serum ketones. The diagnosis is established if the urine is 4+ for glucose with strong ketones, the arterial pH is below 7.3 and $PaCO_2$ not above 35 mmHg (normal for pregnancy is 30 to 35 mmHg), and undiluted serum is strongly positive for ketones. All these tests can be done rapidly. The problem, then, is in knowing when and on which patient to peform them.

The classic patient in DKA is drowsy or comatose, has rapid and shallow respirations, complains of nausea and/or vomiting, may have abdominal pain, and appears dehydrated. The pulse is rapid, and blood pressure is often low. The typical "fruity odor" of the breath is due to the presence of acetone. Acetone is formed by the spontaneous decarboxylation of acetoacetate and has a low vapor pressure. Because of this, it is excreted by the lungs and is detectable by smelling the patient's breath.

Because the specific tests for the measurement of acetoacetate and β-hydroxybutyrate are involved and expensive, the nitroprusside reaction (Acetest®) is generally used instead. In this test, a tablet containing nitroprusside reagent is crushed. One or two drops of undiluted serum or plasma are placed on the mound of powder, and the development of a purple color signifies the presence of ketone acids. The nitroprusside reaction measures acetoacetate and acetone but not β-hydroxybutyrate. In the typical DKA patient, β-hydroxybutyrate is present in 3 times the amount of acetoacetate. Thus, a strongly purple color in the nitroprusside test on the undiluted plasma or serum of a woman with DKA indicates the presence of at least 4 m*M*/L of ketone acids. In certain situations, however, the test may be misleading. For example, when DKA has been treated with insulin, β-hydroxybutyrate falls before acetoacetate starts to diminish. Thus the Acetest reaction may give a falsely high estimate of the total amount of ketone acids present. On the other hand, in situations such as alcoholic ketoacidosis or a combined DKA and lactic acidosis, in which acetoacetate accounts for less than 25 percent of the ketone acids present, the nitroprusside reaction may underestimate the degree of ketosis.

In the pregnant woman, DKA may occur at lower plasma glucose values than in the nonobstetric patient. This difference is presumably related to the relative insulin resistance of pregnancy, with a greater tendency toward ketosis. In pregnant women DKA has been observed at plasma glucose levels as low as 200 mg/dl.

Differential Diagnosis

1. Alcoholic ketoacidosis. This is seen in nondiabetic poorly nourished alcoholics with repeated vomiting. Ketone acids accumulate, but blood glucose is generally below 200 mg/dl and may in fact be much lower. The plasma ketone reaction (nitroprusside) is only moderately positive, because the ratio of β-hydroxybutyrate to acetoacetate is increased. A proposed mechanism[16] for alcoholic ketoacidosis is that the combination of prolonged excessive alcohol intake and food deprivation leads to extremely high serum FFA levels, perhaps because of a hormonal response with low insulin and high growth hormone, catecholamines, cortisol, and/or glucagon. These FFAs in the presence of low insulin levels may then act as a substrate for the production of large amounts of ketone bodies, with resultant ketoacidosis. Alcoholic ketoacidosis responds to empiric treatment with intravenous fluids containing glucose and if necessary, bicarbonate.

2. Acidosis of Uremia or Methanol Poisoning. Ketosis is not present.

3. Hypoglycemic Coma. Blood sugar is low. The onset is rapid and neither hyperventilation nor dehydration is present. If in doubt, draw a blood sugar and give 25 g of glucose intravenously.

4. Nonketotic Hyperosmolar Coma. This is severe hyperglycemia occurring in the absence of ketoacidosis. Seizures are common. The condition is often associated with the administration of hyperglycemia-producing drugs (diuretics, corticosteroids, etc.) and/or acute pancreatitis. Hyperglycemia is at least 600 mg/dl. Hyperosmolarity is at least 310 mosm/L (normal pregnant osmolarity is 280 mosm/L). Blood urea nitrogen is elevated to an average of 70 to 90 mg/dl. There is marked dehydration, and this is probably the main problem. Treatment consists of intravenous insulin by continuous infusion at a rate of 6 to 10 units/h, large amounts of hypotonic saline, and potassium replacement. If hypotension exists, isotonic saline should be used. If a patient with nonketotic hyperosmolar coma also has a low pH and increased anion gap but tests negative for ketone acids, lactic acidosis is probably present.

5. Lactic Acidosis. This is metabolic acidosis related to an excess of lactate in the body. This lactate accumulation is thought to be secondary to reduced tissue perfusion in hypotensive, hypovolemic states, resulting in increased peripheral lactate production and diminished hepatic uptake. The antidiabetic drug phenformin can cause the same phenomena to occur. Symptoms of lactic acidosis include Kussmaul's respiration, lethargy, dehydration, and abdominal pain, with coma sometimes occurring. The arterial pH is below 7.3 (with normal or low $PaCO_2$), HCO_3 is reduced, and the anion gap is increased, but serum ketone acids are absent or present in only trace amounts. A serum lactate in excess of 5 mM/L confirms the diagnosis. Treatment is with large volumes of saline and bicarbonate. If hyperglycemia accompanies the problem, as occurs with combined DKA and lactic acidosis or combined nonketotic hyperosmorality and lactic acidosis, insulin should, of course, be added.

TREATMENT OF DIABETIC KETOACIDOSIS

The treatment of DKA is directed towards reversing dehydration and electrolyte imbalance, normalizing metabolism, and identifying the underlying cause so as to prevent relapse.

Insulin

There is general agreement that only short-acting (regular) insulin should be used. Currently in this country the continuous intravenous or subcutaneous infusion of 5 to 10 units of insulin per hour is the most popular form of therapy. This is called *low-dose* insulin treatment, in contradistinction to *high dose* therapy, in which 50 to 100 units is given subcutaneously or as a combination of IV boluses and subcutaneous injections every 2 to 4 h. The major advantage of low-dose insulin administration is a reduction in the incidence of hypoglycemia and hypokalemia. The advantage of IV use is more rapid and predictable action, especially in the hypovolemic patient whose peripheral tissue perfusion may be marginal. Continuous low-dose IV insulin therapy is accomplished by adding 50 units of regular insulin to 500 ml of normal saline. This mixture then contains 1 unit of insulin per 10 ml of solution. It is usually infused by an infusion pump at a rate of 50 to 100 ml/h, yielding a dose of 5 to 10 units/h. This infusion can be conveniently "piggy-backed" into the main IV fluid line so that the insulin dose can be varied independently of fluid and electrolyte administration. If an infusion pump is not available, little is lost by using a "minidrip" chamber, although closer surveillance is necessary to make certain the infusion rate does not vary too widely.

Parameters used to monitor the response to treatment include blood glucose, pH, serum electrolytes, and serum and/or urine ketone bodies. These measurements should be made at 2-h intervals. If the blood glucose level does not fall by 30 percent (or more) in 2 h, the insulin dose should be doubled. This doubling should be repeated at 2-h intervals until the glucose level responds. For the nonpregnant individual, it is recommended that insulin infusion be discontinued when the blood glucose levels reach 250 mg/dl. This is intended to avoid hypoglycemia and possible cerebral edema. Because of the relative insulin resistance seen in late pregnancy, however, and because of the tremendous fetal risk of DKA, I recommend that the insulin infusion rate be cut in half when the blood glucose reaches 200 to 250 mg/dl, and that hourly blood glucose determinations be followed. When the blood glucose falls below 150 mg/dl, a second halving of the insulin dose should be made. If the blood glucose is below 150 mg/dl, the arterial pH is normal, and the urine or serum ketones are decreasing, then a basal insulin infusion rate of 1 to 2 units/h should suffice. In patients treated for DKA, the blood glucose starts to fall before the acidosis begins to clear. If the arterial pH remains below 7.3, and is not rising, insulin dosage should be increased despite a falling glucose level. In this situation, 5 percent glucose should be infused (200 ml/h) in order to avoid hypoglycemia and possibly cerebral edema. If the pH does not improve but ketones clear, consideration must be given to the possibility of a concomitant lactic acidosis and the possible need for bicarbonate.

Resumption of conventional subcutaneous insulin treatment should be undertaken when the patient has no detectable ketones in her urine, is symptom-free, and is able to tolerate oral food intake. If the woman was in good metabolic control prior to her episode of DKA and the cause of the DKA has been eliminated, the usual subcutaneous insulin dose may be reinstituted. If she has been on IV short-acting insulin exclusively for more than 18 to 24 h, it would not be unexpected to encounter some instability of control on the first day subcutaneous insulin is resumed. Presumably this is because there is no unabsorbed intermediate-acting insulin in the patient's previous subcutaneous injection sites, and a new steady state has to be established.

Fluids

Estimates of the average total fluid deficit in patients presenting with DKA range from 3 to 6 L, but occasionally exceed 10 L. With the osmotic diuresis induced by hyperglycemia, relatively more water is lost than salt. Thus 0.5 *N* (0.45 percent) or 1 *N* (0.9 percent) saline should be infused, with 1 L being given over the first hour and 300 to 500 ml/h thereafter. In the patient with severe enough hypovolemia to be hypotensive, it is most important to expand the intravascular volume. Thus, the best choice in this situation would be 1 *N* saline.

Once the blood glucose level has gone below 200 mg/dl in the pregnant patient with DKA, 5 percent glucose in water or 0.45 percent saline should be infused. It is important that glucose be administered, both to prevent hypoglycemia and to avoid the possible complication of cerebral edema, which may accompany rapid insulin-induced drops in blood glucose.

Total fluid replacement in the first 12 h should usually be about 5 L, but the patient's state of dehydration may require more or less than this amount. Because of the osmotic diuresis that accompanies hyperglycemia, copious urine output is not necessarily a sign of adequate intravascular volume. However, anuria or low urine output in the face of diabetic ketoacidosis is worrisome. If it does not respond to IV fluids over the first 1 or 2 h of treatment, consideration should be given to central monitoring and further assessment of renal function. Diminished urine output in this setting may be a reflection of hypovolemia, but alternatively could be due to severe renal failure. In the treated patient with a relatively normal blood glucose value and little or no glycosuria, a brisk ($\geq$50 ml/h) urine output with a low specific gravity is a sign that intravascular volume has been adequately replaced. When this occurs, the rate of IV fluid administration can be reduced to approximately 100 ml/h.

Bicarbonate

Bicarbonate should only be administered to patients with an arterial pH below 7.1 or serum HCO_3^- below 5 mEq/L and should be repeated only if the pH is still below 7.25 after 2 h. It should be given as 88 mEq sodium bicarbonate in 1 L of 0.45 percent saline to avoid giving a hypertonic solution and aggravating hyperosmolarity. When the pH is less than 7.0, 132 mEq should be administered. Rapid correction of acidosis in the pregnant diabetic in DKA is especially important because of the tremendous fetal risk. *Severe* acidosis should be treated with bicarbonate in order to avoid a potential worsening of central nervous system depression and detrimental effects on myocardial function. Nevertheless, in mild degrees of acidosis when the pH exceeds 7.1, bicarbonate should not be given for the following three reasons: (1) As ketone acids are oxidized, bicarbonate is produced, leading to a return of serum bicarbonate levels towards normal. This assumes, of course, that insulin therapy has prevented the continuing production of ketone acids. Thus, giving exogenous bicarbonate may eventually result in a mild metabolic alkalosis. (2) A rapid elevation in arterial pH may be accompanied by a fall in cerebrospinal fluid (CSF) pH, worsening neurologic symptoms. This phenomenon is explained by the fact that CO_2 diffuses quickly between blood and CSF, whereas bicarbonate moves much more slowly. If the pH is rapidly elevated, the acidotic respiratory drive is removed. As respiration rate and depth diminish, the PCO_2 rises. This CO_2 rapidly diffuses into the CSF where bicarbonate is still low despite more normal blood levels. As CO_2 combines with water, bicarbonate and hydrogen ions are released, making the CSF more acidotic. (3) Red-blood-cell 2,3-DPG is reduced in DKA. Alkalization will shift the oxygen dissociation curve to the left, limiting oxygen availability to tissues.

Potassium

The osmotic diuresis and vomiting of DKA bring about a deficit in total body potassium of 5 to 10 mEq/kg of body weight. However, acidosis is generally accompanied by a shift of potassium from intracellular to extracellular fluid. Thus, a normal or elevated serum potassium at the time DKA is diagnosed may mask the fact that the patient is depleted of potassium. Once the acidosis is corrected and insulin causes glucose uptake into cells, potassium shifts back to an intracellular location and serum potassium levels may rapidly decline. Therefore, after the patient has been treated for 3 to 4 h, and provided urine output is adequate, potassium chloride should be added to the IV fluid at a concentration of 40 mEq/L. Serum potassium should be determined every 2 to 4 h. In the interim, electrocardiographic monitoring may reveal signs of high or low potassium.

Cerebral Edema

If severe hyperglycemia is reversed too rapidly, cerebral edema may be precipitated. This is generally irreversible and fatal. Typically, it occurs in a patient who has initially responded to treatment of DKA but then progressively loses consciousness. Neurologic findings include papilledema, elevated CSF pressure, and dilated pupils. Fever may occur. This rare syndrome is believed to be due to continued hyperosmolarity of the brain after the serum osmolarity has declined. The consequences of these differences in osmolarity are fluid shifts into the brain and the occurrence of edema. Mannitol and/or corticosteroids have been used to treat this problem, but successful therapy has not been reported. Cerebral edema should be even less common in obstetrical patients than in nonpregnant individuals, since DKA tends to occur at lower blood glucose levels in pregnancy.

Special Considerations in Pregnancy

Electronic Fetal Monitoring. Because of the high risk of intrauterine fetal death with maternal DKA, continuous electronic fetal monitoring (EFM) is mandatory when this condition occurs. LoBue and Goodlin[18] have described serial monitoring tracings obtained in a class C diabetic in DKA at 35 weeks. The patient was in premature labor, perhaps as a result of diminished uterine blood flow brought about by hypovolemia. At the time of diagnosis, maternal blood glucose was 944 mg/dl, bicarbonate 4.1 mEq/L, pH 7.12, and PCO_2 13 mmHg. External fetal monitoring revealed diminished beat-to-beat variability and recurrent late decelerations. Preparations were made for cesarean section. As the mother was stabilized with insulin, fluids and bicarbonate, the contractions diminished and the decelerations disappeared. By 4½ h after the start of treatment, the maternal glucose was 278 mg/dl, bicarbonate 8 mEq/L, pH 7.26, and PCO_2 18 mmHg. Fetal heart rate monitoring continued to reveal reduced beat-to-beat variability. Unfortunately, the patient left the hospital against medical advice 12 h after admission. She returned 3 days later for an uncomplicated repeat cesarean section and delivered a healthy baby. This case documents the precarious fetal condition that may accompany maternal DKA and also suggests that prompt and aggressive treatment of the maternal problem may reverse fetal distress. It cannot be stated with certainty whether the bicarbonate infusion was responsible for fetal improvement or whether the 160 units of insulin and 3 L of IV fluids infused would have sufficed.

The importance of electronic fetal monitoring during DKA is further underscored by the case reported by Schilthuis and Aarnoudse,[25] in which a diabetic patient slipped into DKA while on IV ritodine. Following a 6-h hiatus in which EFM was not used, the fetal condition went from what was described as "normal" to death in utero. In this case, the DKA was only diagnosed after approximately 24 h of severe hyperglycemia, and aggressive treatment was begun when the maternal pH was 6.97! A continuous EFM record might even have caused a more timely diagnosis of DKA.

There is no large series of fetuses monitored during the course of maternal DKA, but it is certainly reasonable to recommend such monitoring. It is likely that some fetuses will "clear" their fetal distress as the mother "clears" her DKA. Since it would be inadvisable to operate on a mother in DKA, it may well be that in these cases by the time the mother is stable enough for surgery, the fetal condition will have improved enough that immediate delivery is not necessary.

Because hypokalemia may occur during the treatment of DKA, and because maternal hypokalemia has been associated with fetal bradycardia due to heart block,[1] EFM may detect this problem and allow prompt correction of the mother's serum potassium

Fetal Scalp pH. Since DKA may occur during labor (especially in patients being treated with tocolytic agents for premature labor) and because EFM patterns suggestive of fetal distress may occur, scalp sampling must be available as a backup in such cases. The interpretation of fetal scalp pH may be confounded by the presence of maternal alkalosis or acidosis. Seeds[26] has discussed this problem in detail. Because pH is expressed as a log scale, the actual difference in hydrogen ion concentration when the maternal pH is 7.42 and fetal pH is 7.30 is not the same as when the maternal pH is 7.22 and fetal pH is 7.10. Thus, simply studying the difference between maternal and fetal pH (M/F ΔpH) is not satisfactory, since this will vary by different orders of magnitude depending upon the actual pH values.

Base Deficit Determination. The base deficit may be derived from the pH and PCO_2 and represents the loss of buffering capacity of blood from an acidotic individual. The normal base deficit is defined as zero. However, because of the relative anemia and hypoproteinuria of late pregnancy, maternal base deficit is usually +2 to +3 mEq/L despite the respiratory alkalosis which is usually present. In normal labor, the fetal base deficit is lower than that of the mother.[24] When maternal acidosis exists, calculation of the fetal base deficit, which is measured on a linear rather than a logarithmic scale, gives a more reliable estimate of fetal acidosis than does fetal pH alone.

Bicarbonate ion crosses the placenta slowly,[6] with maternal-fetal equilibration occurring over hours, and thus a high fetal base deficit could be caused by long-standing maternal acidosis. If, in addition to maternal acidosis, fetal hypoxia also exists, lactic acid produced in the fetus will be buffered by fetal buffer bases and the fetal base deficit will be increased even further than could be explained by maternal acidosis alone. Thus, acidosis of fetal origin may best be expressed as the maternal-fetal base deficit difference (M/F ΔBD).[3] Normally, the fetal base deficit is less than that of the mother by 2 to 3 mEq/L. In conditions of fetal acidosis secondary to maternal acidosis, this relationship will be maintained. However, if acidosis of fetal origin is superimposed, the M/F ΔBD will reverse its direction, and the fetus will have a higher base deficit than the mother.

Fetal base deficit is derived from measurement of pH and PCO_2, with the Sigaard-Andersen nomogram[27] utilized to derive a value appropriate to the hemoglobin level of the subject (Fig. 15-6). Measuring pH and PCO_2 requires about 120 μl of scalp blood, as opposed to only 50 μl for pH alone. Methods based upon smaller volumes, with direct measurement of pH followed by a second pH measurement after equilibration at a PCO_2 of 40 mmHg, may introduce an error of 4 to 5 mEq/L in fetal base deficit.

Another source of error is the phenomenon of dissolved CO_2 diffusing into red blood cells, where some buffering by hemoglobin occurs, with bicarbonate (a buffer base) being released into plasma. Some of this bicarbonate diffuses into the interstitial fluid, increasing the apparent base deficit. Jacobson and Rooth[15] have suggested correcting for this artifactual change by calculating base deficit on the basis of a hemoglobin concentration of 5 g/dl. This is called the BD_{Hb5} and approximates the base deficit of extracellular fluid. The correction can be easily read on the Sigaard-Anderson nomogram. Thus the M/F ΔBD_{Hb5} is the most useful way of ruling out

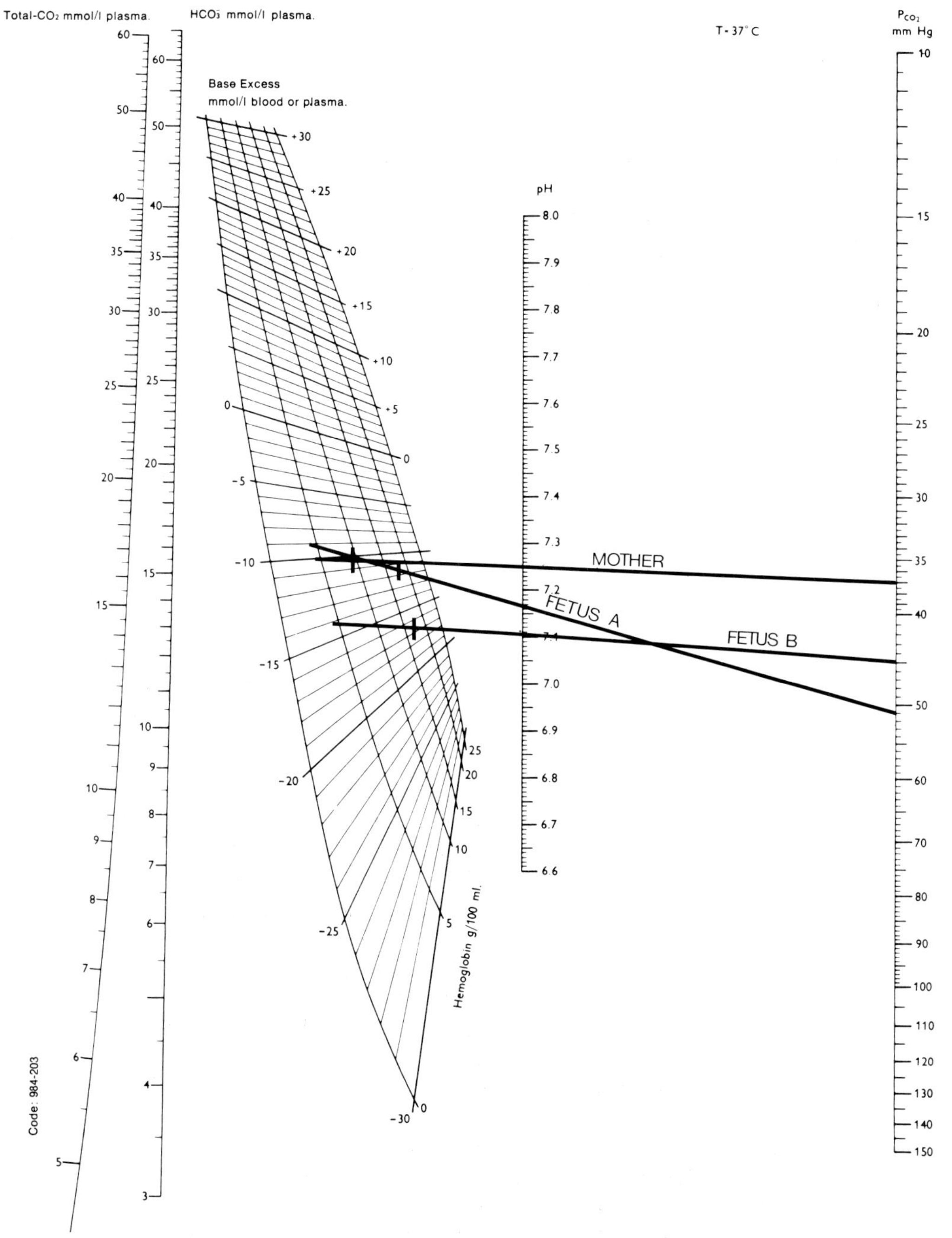

Fig. 15-6 Sigaard-Anderson nomogram. The values have been plotted for examples A and B on page 426.

acidosis of fetal origin in the presence of maternal acidosis. If the fetal BD_{Hb5} is greater than the maternal value, fetal acidosis exists. Two examples will serve to illustrate the value of estimating M/F ΔBD_{Hb5} in clinical situations.

Example A. A diabetic enters the hospital in labor, stating that she has "forgotten" to take her insulin for the past 2 days. Absent beat-to-beat variability and mild late decelerations are revealed by EFM. Maternal venous blood is drawn and found to have pH 7.25, pCO_2 37 mmHg, and hemoglobin 12 g/dl. Calculated maternal base deficit is thus 10 mEq/L. A fetal scalp blood sample is drawn and values of pH 7.17, PCO_2 51 mmHg, and hemoglobin 18 g/dl are determined. Calculated fetal base deficit is thus 12 mEq/L, and M/F ΔBD is −2 mEq/L. When both values are corrected to a hemoglobin of 5 g/dl, maternal BD_{Hb5} is 10 mEq/L and fetal BD_{Hb5} is 9 mEq/L (Fig. 15-6). Thus the M/F ΔBD_{Hb5} is +1 mEq/L, and in this case fetal acidosis is secondary to maternal acidosis.

Example B. The second patient presents with the same clinical history as the first. Maternal venous samples show the same values (pH 7.25, PCO_2 37 mmHg, BD_{Hb12} 10 mEq/L, BD_{HB5} 10 mEq/L). A fetal scalp sample reveals pH 7.10, PCO_2 45 mmHg, and hemoglobin 18 g/dl. Thus fetal BD_{Hb18} is 17 mEq/L and M/F ΔBD is −7 mEq/L; fetal BD_{Hb5} is 14 mEq/L and M/F ΔBD_{Hb5} is −4 mEq/L (Fig. 15-6). Since M/F ΔBD exceeds −3.0 mEq/L (the upper limit of normal at uncorrected hemoglobin), this fetal acidosis is not entirely secondary to maternal acidosis but has a fetal asphyxial origin as well. The M/F ΔBD_{Hb5} of −4 mEq/L is a reversal from the normal situation, in which maternal BD_{Hb5} is greater than the fetal value. This, too, indicates acidosis of fetal origin.

Tocolytic Therapy for the Diabetic. Premature labor not infrequently occurs in pregnant diabetics. This may be even more serious than it is in nondiabetics owing to the possible delay in pulmonic maturation and greater incidence of respiratory distress syndrome in infants of diabetic mothers. The agents commonly used for tocolysis are the $beta_2$ agonists ritodrine, terbutaline, isoxsuprine and, in countries other than the United States, salbutamol. In addition to uterine tocolysis, these agents stimulate other beta receptors throughout the body. Effects include bronchodilation, tachycardia, and, of special concern with diabetic pregnancies, changes in metabolism. Metabolic effects include hyperglycemia (due to glycogenolysis), hyperinsulinemia (probably a primary effect on islet cells),[17] increased lactic acid,[14] and increased FFAs (probably secondary to lipolysis). With the exception of hyperinsulinemia, these changes would be expected to predispose towards hyperglycemia and ketoacidosis. In the overt diabetic, who is unable to increase unsulin output in response to beta stimulation, it is not difficult to understand why DKA has been frequently reported when these agents are administered. The only change that might be worse would be increased glucagon production. This latter effect has been found by some[17] but not by all investigators[29] as a sequel of beta-agonistic therapy.

There are numerous case reports of DKA occurring in patients on betamimetic therapy. As mentioned earlier, Schilthuis and Aarnoudse[25] have reported an intrauterine fetal death in such circumstances. Chapman[7] has reported ketoacidosis occurring in two nondiabetics receiving salbutamol.

Other problems associated with tocolytic therapy include hypokalemia. The explanation for this phenomenon is that high glucose and insulin levels cause potassium to shift to an intracellular location in exchange for hydrogen ions. Thus, the hypokalemia may be accompanied by an acidosis, with lowered serum bicarbonate levels.[13] Transient but severe hypokalemia is almost routinely seen with initiation of betamimetic therapy for tocolysis. Although it is usually self-correcting, this condition may contribute to the cardiac arrhythmias reported in such patients. In the insulinopenic diabetic, it would be anticipated that hypokalemia would not occur until exogenous insulin was administered.

Pulmonary edema has been reported in patients receiving betamimetic tocolytic therapy, both with and without concomitant corticosteroid therapy. A great part of this problem may be fluid overload,[23] but direct cardiac effects, acidosis, and electrolyte imbalance may also be implicated. This complication would be especially worrisome in a severe diabetic with preexisting renal or cardiac problems.

The beta-adrenergic tocolytic agents cross the placenta, with cord blood levels being 50 percent or more of simultaneously measured maternal blood levels.[4,14] Brazy and Pupkin[5] have prospectively studied 43 preterm infants born within 48 h of maternal isoxsuprine administration and 107 whose mothers did not receive the drug. Significant increases in the incidence of neonatal hypotension (63 vs. 43 percent), hypoglycemia (14 vs. 5 percent), and hypocalcemia (59 vs. 31 percent) were reported in the treated group. Neonatal mortality rates were higher for the isoxsuprine-treated patients, especially at younger gestational ages. The severity of the complications was inversely proportional to the interval between loading dose and delivery.

It is clear that significant maternal and fetal risks accompany the use of beta-adrenergic tocolytic agents, and these risks can only be increased when the mother is diabetic. A decision to use these agents in the diabetic must, of course, ultimately depend upon an assessment of the risk/benefit ratio. If one decides to attempt tocolysis in a diabetic, a number of precautions are in order:

1. If the labor is advanced and successful inhibition is highly unlikely, fetal risks contraindicate beta-adrenergic therapy.
2. Close monitoring (every 1 to 2 h for the first 12 h) of blood glucose, potassium, and bicarbonate is mandatory.
3. Strict measurement of intake and output, with the aim of avoiding fluid overload, is critical.
4. Insulin infusion is begun at the same time tocolytic therapy is instituted. Barnett et al.[2] have reported the successful management of 8 out of 10 cases of premature labor in overt diabetics, using an insulin infusion rate of 16 units/h (a very high dose) from the outset. Five percent glucose was also infused if the patient was not eating. The range of insulin infusion necessary to maintain euglycemia was 8 to 32 units/h. When beta-adrenergic agents were discontinued, insulin requirements dropped to 2 to 6 units/h. It should be noted that all these patients were being concomitantly treated with dexamethasone to induce lung maturity. If corticosteroids are not used, I would expect insulin needs to be lower.

Perhaps a starting dose of 5 to 6 units/h would be appropriate. The important point is that aggressive insulin therapy and close attention to glucose levels should obviate the development of DKA in these patients.

5. Continuous electronic fetal monitoring should be maintained while IV tocolytic therapy is administered.

6. Frequent auscultation of the lungs is necessary so that if pulmonary edema occurs, it can be diagnosed early.

REFERENCES

1. Anderson, G.G. and Hanson, T.M.: Chronic fetal bradycardia. Obstet. Gynecol., *44:*896, 1974.
2. Barnett, A.H., Stubbs, S.M., and Mauder, A.M.: Management of premature labour in diabetic pregnancy. Diabetologia, *18:*365, 1980.
3. Beard, R.W., Morris, E.D., and Clayton, S.G.: pH of foetal capillary blood as an indicator of the condition of the foetus. J. Obstet. Gynaecol. Br. Commonw., *74:*812, 1967.
4. Brazy, J.E., Little, V., Grimm, J., and Pupkin, M.: Risk: benefit considerations for the use of isoxsuprine in the treatment of premature labor. Obstet. Gynecol., *58:*297, 1981.
5. Brazy, J.E. and Pupkin, M.J.: Effects of maternal isoxsuprine administration on preterm infants. J. Pediatr., *94:*444, 1979.
6. Caspi, E., Ron-el, R., and Modai, D.: Controlled intravenous bicarbonate and fetal-maternal acid-base balance. Obstet. Gynecol., *54:*615, 1979.
7. Chapman, M.G.: Salbutamol-induced acidosis in pregnant diabetics. Br. Med. J., *1:*639, 1977.
8. Churchill, J.A., Berendes, H.W., and Nemore, J.: Neuropsychological deficits in children of diabetic mothers. Am. J. Obstet. Gynecol., *105:*257, 1969.
9. Drury, M.I., Greene, A.T., and Stronge, J.M.: Pregnancy complicated by clinical diabetes mellitus: a study of 600 pregnancies. Obstet. Gynecol., *49:*519, 1977.
10. Felig, P.: The endocrine pancreas: diabetes mellitus. p. 761, Ch. 19. In Felig, P., Baxter, J.D., Broadus, A., and Frohman, L.A., Eds.: Endocrinology and Metabolism, McGraw-Hill, New York, 1981.
11. Gerich, J.E.: Somatostatin modulation of glucagon secretion and its importance in human glucose homeostasis. Metabolism, *27:*suppl. 1, 1283–1290, 1978.
12. Goodlin, R. and Kaiser, I.: The effect of ammonium chloride induced maternal acidosis on the human fetus at term. Am. J. Med. Sci., *233:*662, 1957.
13. Gross, T.L. and Sokol, R.J.: Severe hypokalemia and acidosis: a potential complication of beta-adrenergic treatment. Am. J. Obstet. Gynecol., *138:*1225, 1980.
14. Ingemarsson, I., Westgren, M., Linberg, C. et al.: Single injection of terbutaline in term labor: placental transfer and effects on maternal and fetal carbohydrate metabolism. Am. J. Obstet. Gynecol., *139:*697, 1981.
15. Jacobson, L. and Rooth, G.: Some aspects of foetal-maternal acid-base and electrolyte balance during labour. Acta Obstet. Gynecol. Scand., *48:*supp. 3, 86–87, 1969.
16. Levy, L.J., Duga, J., Girgis, M., and Gordon, E.E.: Ketoacidosis associated with alcoholism in nondiabetic subjects. Ann. Intern. Med., *78:*213, 1973.
17. Lipshitz, J. and Vinik, A.I.: The effects of hexoprenaline, a β_2-sympathomimetic drug, on maternal glucose, insulin, glucagon, and free fatty acid levels. Am. J. Obstet. Gynecol., *130:*761, 1978.

18. LoBue, C. and Goodlin, R.C.: Treatment of fetal distress during diabetic ketoacidosis. J. Reprod. Med., *20:*101, 1978.
19. McGarry, J.D. and Foster, D.W.: Diabetic ketoacidosis. p. 185, Ch. 21. In Rifkin, H. and Raskin, P., Eds.: Diabetes Mellitus, Vol. 5, Robert J. Brady, Bowie, Md., 1981.
20. Myers, R.E.: Brain damage due to asphyxia: mechanism of causation. J. Perinat. Med., 9:78, 1981.
21. Naeye, R.L. and Chez, R.A.: Effects of maternal acetonuria and low pregnancy weight gain on children's psychomotor development. Am. J. Obstet. Gynecol., *139:*189, 1981.
22. Pedersen, J.: The Pregnant Diabetic and Her Newborn, 2nd Ed. Williams and Wilkins, Baltimore, 1977, p. 202.
23. Philipsen, T., Eriksen, P.S., and Lunggard, F.: Pulmonary edema following ritodrine-saline infusion in premature labor. Obstet. Gynecol., 58:304, 1981.
24. Roversi, G.D., Canussio, V., and Spennacchio, M.: Recognition and significance of maternogenic fetal acidosis during intensive monitoring of labor. J. Perinat. Med., 3:53, 1975.
25. Schilthuis, M.S. and Aarnoudse, S.G.: Fetal death associated with severe ritodrine induced ketoacidosis. Lancet, *1:*1145, 1980.
26. Seeds, A.E.: Maternal-fetal acid-base relationships and fetal scalp-blood analysis. Clin. Obstet. Gynecol., *21:*579, 1978.
27. Sigaard-Andersen, O.: Blood acid-base alignment nomogram. Scand. J. Clin. Lab. Invest., *15:*211, 1963.
28. Smythe, A.R. III and Sakakini, J., Jr.: Maternal metabolic alterations secondary to terbutaline therapy for premature labor. Obstet. Gynecol., 57:566, 1981.
29. Spellacy, W.N., Cruz, A.C., Buhi, W.C., and Birk, S.A.: The acute effects of ritodrine infusion on maternal metabolism: Measurements of levels of glucose, insulin, glucagon, triglycerides, cholesterol, placental lactogen, and chorionic gonadotropin. Am. J. Obstet. Gynecol., *131:*637, 1978.
30. Stehbens, J.A., Baker, G.L., and Kitchell, M.: Outcome at ages 1, 3, and 5 of children born to diabetic women. Am. J. Obstet. Gynecol., *127:*408, 1977.
31. White, P.: Pregnancy and diabetes. p. 583, Ch. 19. In Marble, A., White, P., Bradley, R. and Krall, L., Eds.: Joslin's Diabetes Mellitus. 11th Ed. Lea and Febiger, Philadelphia, 1971.

16

Amniotic Fluid Embolism

Dwight P. Cruikshank, M.D.

Amniotic fluid embolism is an obstetric catastrophe which often leads to maternal death. It has been called the most "unpredictable and largely unpreventable" cause of maternal death[16] and "the most dangerous and untreatable condition in obstetrics."[11] Although that may seem to be a somewhat pessimistic way to introduce a chapter devoted to the treatment of the disorder, it remains true that there is little consensus regarding the etiology and pathogenesis of amniotic fluid embolism and thus therapy is largely empiric. Furthermore, the disorder is uncommon and the mortality rate is high, so no physician has a great deal of experience treating amniotic fluid embolism, and no therapeutic regimen can be claimed to be proven effective.

Amniotic fluid embolism was first described by Meyer in 1926. In 1927 Warden[45] demonstrated serious cardiovascular effects from the intravenous infusion of amniotic fluid into animals, but those experiments were directed toward finding the etiology of preeclampsia, and the clinical significance of the effects was not recognized. Recognition of the importance of amniotic fluid embolism as a clinical entity really began in 1941, with the report of Steiner and Lushbaugh[43] describing the syndrome in eight women who died suddenly in the peripartum period. Since then there have been 278 reported cases in the English language literature, 272 of which have been summarized recently in an excellent review by Morgan.[31] Since that review, six additional cases have been reported.[10,26,29,46]

INCIDENCE AND MORTALITY

The reported incidence of amniotic fluid embolism ranges from 1 in 8,000 births[43] to 1 in 80,000.[24] Peterson[32] states that 10 percent of maternal deaths in this country are due to amniotic fluid embolism, and Lucas and Jackson[25] found it to be the second leading cause of maternal death in U.S. Naval hospitals worldwide. It is probably the most frequent cause of maternal death during labor and delivery, and certainly the mortality rate is extremely high in recognized cases. Among the 272 cases reviewed by Morgan[31] there were only 39 survivors, a mortality rate of 86 percent. In the past, in fact, the diagnosis of amniotic fluid embolism was considered suspect if the patient survived. However, cases of conclusively proven amniotic fluid embolism with survival have been reported[9,37] and it seems likely that the entity is not as rare as previously thought. With modern diagnostic techniques it will probably become apparent that survival is also more frequent than previously stated.

ETIOLOGY

The reason amniotic fluid suddenly enters the maternal circulation is unknown, but it would seem to always be a pathologic event. The studies of Roche and Norris,[38] who autopsied 20 women dying of eclampsia postpartum, could demonstrate no evidence of amniotic fluid debris in the lungs. Likewise Sparr and Pritchard,[42] using radioactive-labeled red cells, could demonstrate no escape of amniotic fluid into the maternal circulation during normal labor and delivery.

In order for amniotic fluid to enter the maternal circulation it is necessary to postulate a tear or defect in the membranes adjacent to open maternal vessels. Two possible sites for this to occur have been proposed. One is the placental implantation site, which Leary and Hertig[23] consider the location of entry. They were able to demonstrate fetal squamous cells in normal placentas between the amnion and chorion, in blood clots along the margin of the placenta, and within decidual sinusoids. This theory necessitates the presence of tears in the membranes near the placental site. Such disruptions have indeed been demonstrated in some[10] but by no means all cases. Furthermore, the high intramyometrial pressures in the contractile portion of the uterus would seem to minimize the chance for entry at this site.[39] The other proposed area of entry is the lower uterine segment or cervix. The intramyometrial pressures in these locations would be more favorable to amniotic fluid entry into the maternal circulation. Certainly endocervical veins are lacerated during labor and some authors[36] feel that these, or small incomplete tears in the lower segment,[4] are the portals of entry of amniotic fluid. Others have associated amniotic fluid embolism with traumatic disruptions of the uterus, including rupture,[6,8,20] cesarean section,[37,41,47] and placenta accreta,[22] as well as minor trauma such as amniotomy[40] or insertion of intrauterine pressure-monitoring catheters.[9]

In the past, numerous clinical factors have been said to predispose to amniotic fluid embolism. These include advanced maternal age, high parity, excessive fetal size, short labor, tumultuous labor, oxytocin stimulation, and intrauterine fetal death. In Morgan's review,[31] 88 percent of the 272 reported patients were multiparous, and the average maternal age was 32 years. However, the youngest patient was a 15-year-old primigravida. Furthermore, short or tumultuous labors were reported in only 28 percent of cases, and uterine stimulation with oxytocin or other drugs in only 22 percent. Morgan concluded that no direct association between amniotic fluid embolism and either duration of labor or oxytocin stimulation could be demonstrated. The average size of neonates in his series was 3,330 grams, and Morgan believes "there would appear to be no justification for the statement" that large babies and traumatic delivery are predisposing factors. Morgan's review also convinced him that the only association between intrauterine fetal death and amniotic fluid embolism is that the effects of the embolism on the physiology of the mother often resulted in death of the fetus.

Nearly all the proposed etiologic factors discussed above involve events occurring during labor or at delivery, but 10 percent of reported cases occur prior to labor.[31] In fact, there has been at least one report of amniotic fluid embolism at 20 weeks of gestation.[48]

In summary, the etiology of amniotic fluid embolism is unknown, and no definite predisposing factors have been identified.

PATHOPHYSIOLOGY

The underlying pathophysiology of the disease remains controversial. However, there seem to be two separate life-threatening processes, which may occur simultaneously or in sequence. These are cardiorespiratory collapse and coagulation failure.

The initial event leading to cardiorespiratory collapse is sudden pulmonary hypertension. This results in acute cor pulmonale, reduction in left atrial pressure, reduced cardiac output, and systemic hypotension. The pulmonary hypertension may be due to pulmonary capillary obstruction by debris from the amniotic fluid, but this is controversial. Autopsy material consistently demonstrates fetal squamae, lanugo hairs, mucin, and occasionally meconium in the small pulmonary vessels of patients dying from amniotic fluid embolism,[43] especially when these elements are searched for with special stains.[3] In sheep, unfiltered amniotic fluid injected intravenously leads to pulmonary hypertension and dyspnea, whereas the changes do not occur with filtered fluid.[18] However, the pathophysiologic picture of amniotic fluid embolism has been produced in dogs with injection of both filtered and unfiltered fluid.[5] MacMillan[27] demonstrated that human amniotic fluid contained an average of 560 cells per milliliter. Extrapolating from experiments in the rabbit, he estimated that an infusion of 7 L of amniotic fluid would be necessary to cause death in the human if blockade of pulmonary vessels by fetal cells were the basic pathophysiologic event.

It has recently been proposed that the pulmonary hypertension might be the result of amniotic fluid prostaglandins.[21,35] In fact, Kitzmiller and Lucas have demonstrated pulmonary hypertension in cats injected with amniotic fluid from laboring women but not in those injected with amniotic fluid from women who were not in labor. The cardiovascular response elicited by fluid from laboring women could be reproduced by injection of prostaglandin F2α, a substance found in human amniotic fluid during labor. Further support for prostaglandins being etiologically important comes from the work of Reeves et al.,[35] who caused pulmonary hypertension in cattle by injecting a lipid extract of amniotic fluid and prevented this effect by treatment with aspirin. If prostaglandins are the final common pathway leading to the cardiovascular effects of amniotic fluid embolism, it would explain some of the marked discrepancies reported in experimental animal studies, since the type and concentration of amniotic fluid prostaglandins vary greatly with duration of gestation and particularly with the presence or absence of labor. If the cardiovascular derangements are due to prostaglandins present in amniotic fluid, treatment with aspirin and other agents which inhibit prostaglandin synthesis should not prove to be especially beneficial. If, however, arachidonic acid or some other prostaglandin precursor in amniotic fluid is converted to prostaglandin after embolization occurs, there might be some usefulness for these agents.

Although it has been stated that part of the pathophysiology of amniotic fluid embolism is anaphylaxis or an "anaphylactoid reaction,"[20,43] there seems to be little evidence to support this. There is little histamine in amniotic fluid,[4] and one of the hallmarks of histamine-related events, namely bronchospasm, rarely occurs with amniotic fluid embolism. Bronchospasm was listed as a symptom in only 3 of the 272 patients reviewed by Morgan.[31]

In summary, the cardiovascular events following amniotic fluid embolism are pulmonary hypertension, whether caused by mechanical obstruction or mediated by prostaglandins, leading to decreased left atrial pressure, decreased cardiac output, and systemic hypotension. Acute cor pulmonale develops and ventilation/perfusion inequalities ensue, leading to hypoxia, cyanosis, tachypnea, and perhaps seizures. Vagus-mediated bradycardia and constriction of coronary arteries may occur simultaneously.

The second major consequence of amniotic fluid embolism is coagulation failure. In 10 to 15 percent of patients, excessive bleeding may be the first indication of this condition, although in most patients it does not become apparent for 30 to 60 min. Up to 50 percent of patients who survive the first hour after amniotic fluid embolism will develop bleeding secondary to disseminated intravascular coagulation[2] and most will develop laboratory evidence of coagulopathy. Amniotic fluid contains an activator of Factor X,[13,33] which might be the trigger for intravascular clotting. Stolte et al.[3] have demonstrated a weak thromboplastin activity in amniotic fluid which renders flowing blood hypercoagulable and causes intravascular clotting if stasis occurs. Amniotic fluid embolism has also been associated with marked activation of the fibrinolytic system,[7] which could certainly contribute to a bleeding diathesis.

CLINICAL FEATURES

The onset of symptoms is sudden and catastrophic. Although not universally true, the patient usually will be in labor or have been recently delivered. Often the onset of symptoms is on the delivery table. There usually is no recognizable prodrome,[2] and although it is often stated that symptoms are ushered in by chills, shivering, or an episode of vomiting, most authors agree that this usually is not the case.[2,31] In over half of the patients the initial indication of amniotic fluid embolism will be respiratory distress—dyspnea, tachypnea, and cyanosis.[31] Chest pain is rare.[39] Another 25 percent of patients will have shock out of proportion to blood loss as the presenting sign, while in 10 to 15 percent a seizure will occur before the onset of other cardiorespiratory symptoms. As previously stated, in 10 to 15 percent of patients the first indication of amniotic fluid embolism will be hemorrhage secondary to coagulation failure. Regardless of the presenting sign or symptom, within minutes of onset all patients will experience cardiorespiratory collapse with dyspnea, cyanosis, and hypotension. The heart rate is inconsistent—there may be supraventricular or ventricular tachycardia, bradycardia, or asystole. The patient may or may not have a seizure, and may or may not become comatose. Pulmonary edema develops in about 25 percent of cases, but some have ascribed this to overly vigorous resuscitative efforts rather than to a primary entity.[31] As previously pointed out, bronchospasm is rare.

The mortality is exceedingly high—25 percent of patients diagnosed as having amniotic fluid embolism die within 1 h of the onset of symptoms. Overall, the reported mortality is 86 percent and the interval from onset of symptoms to death varies between 10 min and 32 h.[2] If the patient survives the first hour she will almost certainly develop laboratory evidence of coagulation failure, and 40 to 50 percent of such patients will have clinically significant bleeding. If the patient is postpartum, the most serious bleeding may be vaginal, originating from the placental site as well as from lacerations of the genital tract.

The provisional clinical diagnosis of amniotic fluid embolism can usually be made with confidence,[31] considering the timing, suddenness, and severity of the major signs and symptoms and the absence of predisposing factors for other conditions in the differential diagnosis. The differential diagnosis includes anything which can produce cardiorespiratory collapse and/or hemorrhage during late pregnancy, labor, delivery, and the immediate puerperium (Table 16-1). Thrombotic pulmonary embolism, air embolism (which has been described with placenta previa), and myocardial infarction are all associated with chest pain, which is rare in amniotic fluid embolism. Acute left ventricular failure will usually be associated with some evidence of preexisting disease. Aspiration of stomach contents (Mendelson's syndrome) is always associated with bronchospasm, which is uncommon in amniotic

Table 16-1. Differential Diagnosis of Amniotic Fluid Embolism

Cardiovascular
Thrombotic pulmonary embolism
Air embolism
Myocardial infarction
Acute left ventricular failure of any cause
Cerebrovascular accident
Respiratory
Aspiration of gastric contents
Bilateral pneumothorax
Obstetric
Eclampsia
Abruptio placentae
Ruptured uterus
Inverted uterus
Hemorrhagic shock
Other
Sepsis
Reaction to local anesthetic agent

fluid embolism. Bilateral pneumothoraces have occurred secondary to bearing down in the second stage of labor, but they are rare, and if large enough to cause cardiorespiratory collapse, should be detectable on physical examination. Eclamptic seizures are usually associated with hypertension, while the patient who suffers convulsions because of amniotic fluid embolism will be hypotensive. Abruptio placentae can be associated with coagulation failure and hemorrhage, but the clinical picture is so different from that of amniotic fluid embolism that confusion of these two diagnoses should not occur. Any patient with shock and hemorrhage immediately after delivery must have a manual exploration of the uterus, which should be sufficient to identify a ruptured or inverted uterus. Gram-negative sepsis can cause cardiorespiratory collapse and coagulation failure, but the onset is usually more gradual than that of amniotic fluid embolism. It is not unusual, however, to see a transient fever spike at the onset of an amniotic fluid embolism.[9] As conduction anesthesia is used with increasing frequency in obstetrics, adverse reaction to local anesthetic drugs must be considered in patients who undergo convulsions during labor or delivery, although these patients will not develop a bleeding diathesis, and usually do not become hypotensive.

Although the provisional clinical diagnosis of amniotic fluid embolism is usually not difficult, it must be stated that most patients who have a cardiovascular, respiratory, or coagulation crisis during labor and delivery probably have *not* had an amniotic fluid embolus. The diagnosis can only be proved by finding fetal squamae, mucin, and lanugo hairs in the small vessels of the lungs at autopsy or by finding these same elements in the blood of the right heart or pulmonary arteries during life. Since in this era any case of cardiorespiratory collapse should be managed with a central venous pressure (CVP) line or Swan-Ganz catheter, a definitive diagnosis should always be attempted. Upon insertion of a line into the right heart or pulmonary vessels, a 10 to 20 ml sample of blood should be aspirated and anticoagulated. After centrifugation, the buffy coat of this blood can be examined for the presence of fetal elements. Since special staining techniques are required for such identification, this will not be useful in the acute situation but it will make a definitive diagnosis possible retrospectively.

MANAGEMENT

Management of Cardiorespiratory Collapse

Oxygen. It is universally agreed[2,12,14,16,29,31,37,39] that oxygen under pressure is the cornerstone of therapy. Upon entertaining the diagnosis of amniotic fluid embolism, positive-pressure ventilation with bag and mask should be begun. As soon as possible a cuffed endotracheal tube should be placed and attached to a mechanical ventilator. Masson et al.[29] treated a patient who survived an amniotic fluid embolism with 70 percent oxygen and 5 cmH_2O positive end-expiratory pressure (PEEP) delivered by ventilator for 48 h. They felt that small amounts of PEEP, as well as appropriate use of diuretics, were the keys to success and survival of their patient. The PEEP made possible the maintenance of higher arterial PO_2 levels than would otherwise have been attainable. The amount and duration of PEEP should be the minimum necessary to maintain the PO_2 around 100 mmHg, and attempts at weaning should be begun as soon as the blood gas values have been stabilized.

Cardiac Resuscitation. If asystole is present, intracardiac epinephrine, 1.0 mg in 10 ml, should be administered and closed-chest cardiac massage begun. If ventricular fibrillation is present, closed cardiac massage should be followed as soon as possible with lidocaine, 100 mg intravenously, and DC cardioversion. Sodium bicarbonate, one ampule (44 mEq) should be given every 5 min until tissue perfusion and ventilation are restored.

General Measures. A large-bore (14 to 16 gauge) intravenous catheter should be placed in a peripheral vein and an intravenous infusion of 5 percent dextrose in water begun. Until more is known about the patient's cardiovascular status, this line should be used to keep a vein open for administration of drugs, and care should be taken to ensure that large quantities of fluid are not administered inadvertently. As the intravenous catheter is inserted, blood should be obtained for type and cross match for 4 to 6 units of fresh whole blood and 4 to 6 units of fresh frozen plasma or cryoprecipitate. Clotting studies (prothrombin time, partial thromboplastin time, fibrinogen concentration, fibrin degradation products, platelet count) and a tube of blood for clot observation should be obtained, as well as a baseline complete blood count. Ideally, a Swan-Ganz catheter should be placed to measure pulmonary wedge pressure. If this is not possible, a CVP line should be placed in the right atrium. If the clot observation test is normal, the CVP line may be placed via the right subclavian vein. However, if there is any evidence of coagulopathy, the internal jugular or antecubital veins offer safer approaches. As soon as one or the other of these central lines is in place, 10 to 20 ml of blood should be withdrawn through it and placed in a tube containing an anticoagulant for later use in confirming the diagnosis by searching for fetal squamae, mucin, and lanugo hairs. An arterial line should be inserted to monitor blood pressure and to allow frequent determination of blood gas values. Most of the subsequent pharmacologic management will depend on the information obtained from the Swan-Ganz catheter and arterial line. A Foley catheter should be placed in the bladder to monitor urine output. The patient should have a cardiac monitor attached.

Drug Therapy. As previously stated, no drug regimen has been proved effective. Minimal data from animal studies support the use of some agents, but many are used on the basis of tradition or anecdotal experience. Often the patient becomes a pharmacologic bouillabaisse, and then if she survives, this result is attributed to whatever agents were used.

Atropine. It has been stated that vagus-mediated constriction of the pulmonary and coronary vessels results from amniotic fluid embolism, perhaps as a reflex secondary to acute dilatation of the proximal pulmonary arterioles.[2] On this basis, it has been recommended that atropine 0.4 mg be given intravenously as soon as the diagnosis is suspected. However, there seems to be no experimental evidence supporting such a pathophysiologic mechanism, and atropine has not been helpful in enhancing survival after experimental amniotic fluid embolism in animals.[15] Furthermore, in some case reports the patient has had marked supraventricular tachycardia[9,28] or even ventricular tachycardia immediately after the insult, and atropine would seem contraindicated in such cases. Likewise, patients with asystole are better managed with intracardiac epinephine and closed-chest cardiac massage. There may be a place for atropine in a patient with bradycardia, but its routine use in the management of amniotic fluid embolism seems difficult to justify.

Digitalis. Some have suggested fast-acting digitalis glycosides in the acute situation,[2] because of the frequency of pulmonary edema after amniotic fluid embolism. However, pulmonary edema is not a universal finding. Digitalis preparations may be indicated by the clinical situation or by elevated pulmonary wedge pressures, but their use in the acute situation, i.e., the first 15 to 20 min after amniotic fluid embolism, probably is unnecessary.

Diuretics. Masson et al.[29] felt that diuretics and PEEP were the keys to success in the survivor they reported. As in the case of digitalis, individualized therapy based on clinical and laboratory parameters may be indicated in some patients who develop pulmonary edema, but diuretics probably are not necessary in the management of the acute episode.

Steroids. Most reported survivors[9,19] have been treated with high-dose glucocorticoid therapy, usually 500 mg to 2.0 g hydrocortisone intravenously as soon as possible after the amniotic fluid embolism. However, the majority of nonsurvivors also were treated with steroids. There is no proof regarding the efficacy of these agents in amniotic fluid embolism, but most authors continue to believe that "hydrocortisone is recommended for its supposed antihistamine reaction and for the overwhelming stress situation."[39] There certainly is no evidence that such therapy is deleterious to these patients' cardiovascular or respiratory status, which is not true of many of the other drugs which have been proposed.

Antihistamines. Animal data[15] show improved survival after pretreatment with promethazine before experimental amniotic fluid embolism, and some authors[14,39] have recommended use of antihistamines such as diphenhydramine hydrochloride (Benadryl). However, there is no evidence that any of the adverse effects of amniotic fluid embolism are histamine-mediated, and these agents probably are unnecessary.

Spasmolytics. In the past, some authors[2,14,39] have recommended intravenous papaverine to reduce bronchial and pulmonary vasospasm. However, this agent can aggravate systemic hypotension and may cause apnea and cardiac arrhythmias. Furthermore, there is no evidence that papaverine is in fact beneficial in these patients. Goodman and Gilman's text,[17] or AMA Drug Evaluations.[1] Thus the use of this agent therapeutic value in any condition." Interestingly, there is no intravenous preparation of papaverine listed in the latest editions of the Physicians Desk Reference,[34]

Goodman and Gilman's text,[17] or AMA Drug Evaluations.[1] Thus the use of this agent in the treatment of amniotic fluid embolism will of necessity be abandoned, and it seems that this will be no great loss. Aminophylline has also been used in the treatment of amniotic fluid embolism, but there is no apparent basis for this.

Vasopressors. If necessary, the beta-adrenergic agonist isoproterenol should be administered to increase cardiac output by its inotropic effect on the heart. The dose is 0.2 mg (1 ml of a 1 : 5,000 solution) by intravenous push, followed by an intravenous infusion of 0.33 μg/kg/min.

Alpha-adrenergic agonists may be necessary to support systemic blood pressure, but their use in amniotic fluid embolism is complicated by the fact that many of these agents also cause pulmonary vasoconstriction, which is undesirable in the face of pulmonary hypertension. Ephedrine causes less pulmonary vasoconstriction than many of the other alpha agonists and may be used in intravenous doses of 25 to 50 mg. If this is not successful, a levarterenol drip may be useful as a last resort to maintain systemic blood pressure, although it definitely causes increased pulmonary vasoconstriction. The usual dose is 4 mg levarterenol in 1,000 ml 5 percent dextrose in water infused at a rate of 0.5 to 1.0 ml/min. The use of mephenteramine, metaraminol, phenylephrine, and methoxamine in the treatment of amniotic fluid embolism have all been described, but when alpha-adrenergic agonists become necessary, these agents offer no advantage over ephedrine or levarterenol.

Alpha-adrenergic agonists should not be used in the treatment of shock when intravascular volume is deficient. If the CVP or pulmonary wedge pressure is low, the appropriate therapy is additional intravenous infusion of crystalloid solutions and/or blood, along with continued treatment with isoproterenol. Only if shock persists in the face of adequate fluid replacement, should alpha-adrenergic agonists be employed.

Management of Coagulation Failure

Heparin. Infusion of amniotic fluid into the circulation leads to disseminated intravascular coagulation. While clinically significant bleeding is the presenting symptom of amniotic fluid embolism in 10 to 15 percent of cases, hemorrhage and/or laboratory evidence of coagulopathy usually does not appear for 30 to 60 min.

Thrombus formation in the small vessels of the pulmonary circulation may be partially responsible for some of the cardiorespiratory manifestations of amniotic fluid embolism. Rapid anticoagulation may reduce the magnitude of the intravascular coagulation and thereby lessen the initial pulmonary and cardiovascular insult. Anticoagulation early in the course of the disease may also prevent the subsequent development of coagulation failure and hemorrhage. Chung and Merkatz[9] and Maki et al.[28] have presented cases in which early heparinization was felt to be the key to survival after amniotic fluid embolism. Opinions are not unanimous, however; Resnik et al.[37] present a case of a survivor who was not treated with heparin, and they argue against the use of this therapy.

Nonetheless, the majority of investigators seem to support early use of heparin if clinically significant bleeding has not already begun. As soon as the diagnosis of amniotic fluid embolism is made, heparin, 10,000 units, should be given intravenously, followed by approximately 5,000 units intravenously every 6 h unless hemorrhage ensues. Heparin therapy is contraindicated, of course, in the presence of active bleeding.

Replacement Therapy. If coagulation failure and hemorrhage ensue despite initial treatment with heparin or if these problems are present from the onset of the disease, the treatment of choice is fresh whole blood. This contains all necessary clotting factors, including platelets. Each unit of fresh blood will raise the patient's serum fibrinogen concentration by approximately 12 to 15 mg/dl. If fresh whole blood is not available, packed red cells and fresh frozen plasma can be used, and will provide all the clotting factors except platelets. If fluid overload is a problem, fibrinogen and factor VIII can be replaced rapidly by using cryoprecipitate. The patient's arterial pressure, pulmonary wedge pressure, and urine output will dictate which of these regimens should be employed. Treatment for coagulation failure should continue until clotting parameters such as fibrinogen concentration and platelet count return to normal. This may occur in as little as 12 h but may not occur for 2 to 3 days.

Management of Uterine Bleeding. Uterine atony may accompany coagulation failure for reasons which are not clear and lead to increased vaginal blood loss. This is best managed with sustained and vigorous bimanual uterine massage and a continuous intravenous infusion of oxytocin. If necessary, methylergonovine maleate (Methergine), 0.2 mg, may be given intravenously every 2 h. If vaginal bleeding persists in the face of adequate therapy for uterine atony and coagulation failure, a careful search for lacerations of the reproductive tract and for retained placental fragments should be made. If all these measures fail to control uterine bleeding, supracervical hysterectomy is indicated. However, surgical therapy should be undertaken only as a last resort, as the precarious status of these patients' respiratory and cardiovascular systems places them at extreme risk during an operative procedure.

SUMMARY OF THERAPY

When the diagnosis of amniotic fluid embolism is considered likely, the following should be done immediately:

1. Oxygen, 100 percent positive pressure, endotracheal tube, ventilator
2. Cardiac resuscitation as indicated
3. Heparin 10,000 units intravenous push
4. Hydrocortisone (Solu-Cortef) 1.0 g intravenous push

These should be followed immediately by the institution of peripheral venous and arterial lines, Swan-Ganz or CVP lines, Foley catheter, and cardiac monitor. Appropriate laboratory studies and type and cross match should be obtained.

Following this, the therapy should be individualized, and the clinical situation should dictate the use of atropine, digitalis preparations, diuretics, isoproterenol infusion, ephedrine or levarterenol, whole blood, fresh frozen plasma, or cryoprecipitate.

REFERENCES

1. AMA Drug Evaluations. 4th Ed. American Medical Association, Chicago, 1980.
2. Anderson, D.G.: Amniotic fluid embolism: a re-evaluation. Am. J. Obstet. Gynecol., *98:*336, 1967.
3. Attwood, H.D.: Fatal pulmonary embolism by amniotic fluid. J. Clin. Pathol., *9:*38, 1956.
4. Attwood, H.D.: Amniotic fluid embolism. Pathol. Annu., *7:*145, 1972.
5. Attwood, H.D. and Downing, S.E.: Experimental amniotic fluid and meconium embolism. Surg. Gynecol. Obstet., *120:*255, 1965.
6. Barno, A. and Freeman, D.W.: Amniotic fluid embolism. Am. J. Obstet. Gynecol., *77:*1199, 1959.
7. Beller, F.K.: Disseminated intravascular coagulation and consumption coagulopathy in obstetrics. Obstet. Gynecol. Annu., *3:*267, 1974.
8. Bouton, S.M. and Saunders, J.R.: Pulmonary embolism by amniotic fluid. Report of a case with review of the literature. Am. J. Clin. Pathol., *21:*566, 1951.
9. Chung, A.F. and Merkatz, I.R.: Survival following amniotic fluid embolism with early heparinization. Obstet. Gynecol., *42:*809, 1973.
10. Corridan, M., Kendall, E.D., and Begg, J.D.: Cord entanglement causing premature placental separation and amniotic fluid embolism. Br. J. Obstet. Gynaecol., *87:*935, 1980.
11. Courtney, L.D.: Amniotic fluid embolism. J. Ir. Med. Assoc., *66:*51, 1973.
12. Courtney, L.D.: Amniotic fluid embolism. Obstet. Gynecol. Surv., *29:*169, 1974.
13. Courtney, L.D. and Allington, M.: Effect of amniotic fluid on blood coagulation. Br. J. Haematol., *22:*353, 1972.
14. Cruikshank, D.P. and Zlatnik, F.J.: Amniotic fluid embolism. p. 44. In Quilligan, E.J., Ed.: Current Therapy in Obstetrics and Gynecology. W.B. Saunders, Philadelphia, 1980.
15. Dutta, D., Bhargava, K.C., Chakravarti, R.N., and Dhall, S.R.: Therapeutic studies in experimental amniotic fluid embolism in rabbits. Am. J. Obstet. Gynecol., *106:*1201, 1970.
16. Editorial. Amniotic-fluid embolism. Lancet, *2:*398, 1979.
17. Gilman, A.G., Goodman, L.S., and Gilman, A. p. 83. Goodman and Gilman's The Pharmacologic Basis of Therapeutics, 6th Ed. Macmillan, New York, 1980.
18. Halmagyi, D.F.J., Starzecki, B., and Shearman, R.P.: Experimental amniotic fluid embolism: Mechanism and treatment. Am. J. Obstet. Gynecol., *84:*251, 1962.
19. Harbison, R.G.: Amniotic fluid embolism. Med. J. Aust., *2:*687, 1973.
20. Kistner, R.W., Graf, W.R., and Johnstone, R.E.: Pulmonary embolism by particulate matter of the amniotic fluid: A report of two cases with a review of the literature. Obstet. Gynecol. Surv., *5:*629, 1950.
21. Kitzmiller, J.L. and Lucas, W.E.: Studies on a model of amniotic fluid embolism. Obstet. Gynecol., *39:*626, 1972.
22. Landing, B.H.: The pathogenesis of amniotic fluid embolism: Uterine factors. N. Engl. J. Med., *243:*590, 1950.
23. Leary, O.C. and Hertig, A.H.: The pathogenesis of amniotic fluid embolism: Possible placental factors. N. Engl. J. Med., *243:*588, 1950.
24. Lewis, T.L.T.: Progress in Clinical Obstetrics and Gynaecology, 2nd ed. Churchill Livingstone, London, p. 48.

25. Lucas, W.E. and Jackson, N.D.: Maternal mortality in U.S. Naval hospitals. Obstet. Gynecol., *32:*60, 1968.
26. Lumley, J., Owen, R., and Morgan, M.: Amniotic fluid embolism: A report of 3 cases. Anaesthesia, *34:*33, 1979.
27. Macmillan, D.: Experimental amniotic fluid infusion. J. Obstet. Gynaecol. Br. Commonw., *75:*849, 1968.
28. Maki, M., Tachita, K., Kawasaki, Y., and Nagasawa, K.: Heparin treatment of amniotic fluid embolism. Tohoku J. Exp. Med., *97:*155, 1969.
29. Masson, R.G., Ruggieri, J., and Siddiqui, M.M.: Amniotic fluid embolism: Definitive diagnosis in a survivor. Am. Rev. Respir. Dis., *120:*187, 1979.
30. Meyer, J.R.: Embolis pulmonar-caseosa. Brazil-Medico, *2:*301, 1926.
31. Morgan, M.: Amniotic fluid embolism. Anaesthesia, *34:*20, 1979.
32. Peterson, E.P. and Taylor, H.B.: Amniotic fluid embolism: An analysis of 40 cases. Obstet. Gynecol., *35:*787, 1970.
33. Phillips, L.L. and Davidson, E.C.: Procoagulant properties of amniotic fluid. Am. J. Obstet. Gynecol., *113:*911, 1972.
34. Physician's Desk Reference. 35th Ed. Medical Economics Co., Oradell, N.J., 1981.
35. Reeves, J.T., Daoud, F.S., Estridge, M. et al.: Pulmonary pressor effects of small amounts of bovine amniotic fluid. Respir. Physiol., *20:*231, 1974.
36. Reid, D.E., Weiner, A.E., and Roby, C.C.: Intravascular clotting and afibrinogenemia. The presumptive lethal factor in the syndrome of amniotic embolism. Am. J. Obstet. Gynecol., *66:*465, 1953.
37. Resnik, R., Swartz, W.H., Plumer, M.H. et al.: Amniotic fluid embolism with survival. Obstet. Gynecol., *47:*295, 1976.
38. Roche, W.D. and Norris, H.J.: Detection and significance of maternal amniotic fluid embolism. Obstet. Gynecol., *43:*729, 1974.
39. Russell, W.S. and Jones, W.N.: Amniotic fluid embolism: A review of the syndrome with a report of 4 cases. Obstet. Gynecol., *26:*476, 1965.
40. Schenken, J.R., Slaughter, G.P., and De May, G.H.: Maternal pulmonary embolism of amniotic fluid. Am. J. Clin. Pathol., *20:*147, 1950.
41. Seto, M. and Gustafson, D.C.: Amniotic fluid embolism with placenta previa and cesarean section: A case report and clinical reviews. Pacific Med. Surg., *73:*258, 1965.
42. Sparr, R.A. and Pritchard, J.A.: Studies to detect the escape of amniotic fluid into the maternal circulation during parturition. Surg. Gynecol. Obstet., *107:*560, 1958.
43. Steiner, P.E. and Lushbaugh, C.C.: Maternal pulmonary embolism by amniotic fluid as a cause of obstetric shock and unexpected deaths in obstetrics. JAMA, *117:*1245, 1340, 1941.
44. Stolte, L.A.M., Lim, H.T., VanArkel, C. et al.: Amniotic fluid embolism. p. 435. In Fairweather, D.V.I. and Eskes, T.K.A.B., Eds.: Amniotic Fluid—Research and Clinical Applications. 2nd Ed. Excerpta Medica, New York, 1978.
45. Warden, R.M.: Amniotic fluid as a possible factor in the etiology of eclampsia. Am. J. Obstet. Gynecol., *14:*292, 1927.
46. Wasser, W.G., Tessler, S., Kamath, C.P., and Sackin, A.J.: Nonfatal amniotic fluid embolism: A case report of post-partum respiratory distress with histopathologic studies. Mt Sinai J. Med. (NY), *46:*388, 1979.
47. Willocks, J., Mone, J.G., and Thompson, W.J.: Amniotic fluid embolism: Case with biochemical findings. Br. Med. J., *2:*1181, 1966.
48. Woodfield, D.G., Galloway, R.K., and Smart, G.E.: Coagulation defect associated with presumed amniotic fluid embolism in the mid trimester of pregnancy. J. Obstet. Gynaecol. Br. Commonw., *78:*423, 1971.

17

Renal Disease during Pregnancy

David J. Hirsch, M.D.
John P. Hayslett, M.D.

Alterations in renal function during pregnancy have important clinical implications because of the possible threat to fetal development as well as to the health of the mother. Since pregnancy is accompanied by significant and unique functional and morphological changes in the kidney and lower urinary tract, this review will provide a summary of the salient features of renal physiology during gestation, as well as a description of the more commonly encountered clinical disorders.

RENAL FUNCTION AND VOLUME HOMEOSTASIS DURING PREGNANCY

Whereas the external balance of water and sodium is maintained within narrow limits in nonpregnant individuals, pregnancy is characterized by a gradual, cumulative retention of 500 to 900 mEq of sodium and 6 to 8 L of water, which are distributed between the maternal extracellular fluid and the products of conception. Plasma volume rises concurrently by 30 to 45 percent; the increment in plasma volume is marked in the second trimester and is sustained to term. Despite the increase in extracellular volume, blood pressure falls owing to a decrease in peripheral vascular resistance.

Changes in renal function during gestation occur against this background of alterations in volume homeostasis. The glomerular filtration rate (GFR) begins to rise immediately after conception and achieves an incremental increase of 30 to 50 percent by the twelfth week of gestation.[23] Recent studies have shown that the elevation in GFR is sustained until term, after which the rate rapidly falls to non-gravid levels[28] (Fig. 17-1). Similar and concurrent increases in effective renal plasma flow have also been demonstrated during pregnancy. The mechanism responsible for these changes in renal physiology has not been elucidated but probably relates to a selective decrease in renal vascular resistance and, at least in part, to a rise in cardiac output. A detailed discussion of the factors which may regulate the change in volume status is given in the monograph by Lindheimer and Katz.[22]

Sodium balance is mediated by the rate of reabsorption of filtered sodium; in the average gravida the filtered amount of sodium is approximately 30,000 mEq/day. The cumulative retention of sodium during gestation is therefore due to an increase in the fraction of filtered sodium that is reabsorbed. This gestational change in renal function appears to reflect a physiologic response to pregnancy, since the reactions to acute volume expansion with sodium salts and to acute restriction in sodium intake are similar to those in nonpregnant women.[22]

The urinary excretion of glucose and amino acids is often increased in pregnancy in the absence of an increase in plasma levels. Reabsorption of these substances by the proximal tubule is governed by the maximal absorptive capacity and by the affinity of tubular transport processes for glucose and amino acids in tubular fluid; it seems likely that one or both of these determinants of proximal reabsorption are altered by pregnancy. Whatever the responsible mechanism for the observed

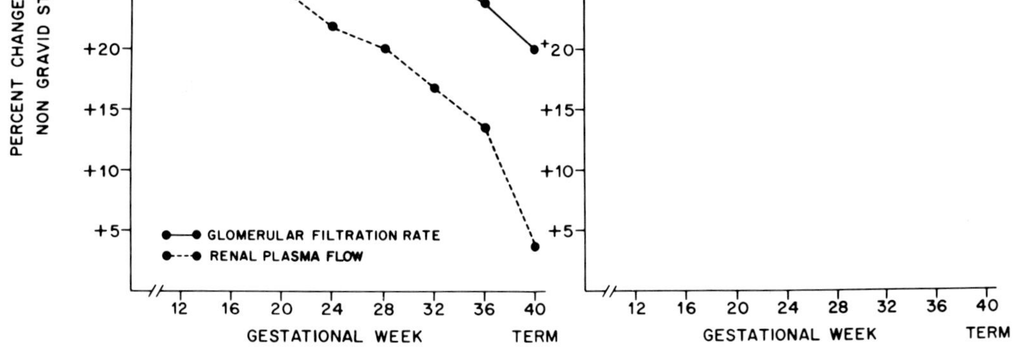

Fig. 17-1 Changes of renal function during pregnancy. There is no decline in renal plasma flow or glomerular filtration during the last trimester if subjects are tested in lateral recumbency. (After Pippig, L., in: Clinical aspects of renal disease in pregnancy, Med. Hyg. *27*:181, 1969, modified by Lindheimer, M.D. and Katz, A.I.: Kidney Function and Disease in Pregnancy, Lea and Febiger, Philadelphia, 1977.)

presence of glucosuria and/or aminoaciduria, these findings are not regarded as representing disease. In the presence of glucosuria, however, a 2-h postprandial blood sugar determination should be performed to exclude the occurrence of diabetes mellitus.

The clearance of uric acid, commonly used as a clinical marker for preeclampsia, is increased in pregnancy. This functional characteristic probably also results from a change in tubular handling of uric acid and is not merely a consequence of the rise in GFR. Since uric acid production is unchanged in pregnancy, the increase in urinary excretion and the dilutional effect caused by the incremental rise in plasma volume result in a fall in plasma levels to 3 to 4 mg/dl. Previous workers have indicated that since many factors affect uric acid levels, it is unwise to rely heavily on this clinical parameter in the diagnostic evaluation of preeclampsia.[22]

In the presence of a normal thirst mechanism, free access to water, and a normal renal mechanism for dilution and concentration of urine, plasma osmolality is maintained at approximately 280 mosm/kg H_2O in nonpregnant individuals. A rise above that level induces a release of antidiuretic hormone, while a fall inhibits hormone release. In pregnancy the plasma osmolality regularly falls to about 270 mosm/kg H_2O. Recent studies in experimental animals have demonstrated that the gestation-induced change in osmolality is secondary to a resetting of the osmostat, the mechanism responsible for release of antidiuretic hormone.[7] The physiologic response to changes below or above the new level is comparable with that in the nonpregnant state.

Finally, plasma bicarbonate levels are reduced in the healthy gravida from 26 to 28 mEq/L to approximately 20 mEq/L owing to a mild respiratory alkalosis. This reduction in plasma bicarbonate is accompanied by an increase in arterial pH from 7.40 to 7.44 and decrease in PCO_2 from 39 to 31 mmHg. The evaluation of acid-base status in pregnant patients with renal disease therefore should take into account these values, which are appropriate during gestation.

Techniques for Measuring Renal Function

The GFR is the most fundamental measure of renal function and reflects the rate at which plasma is ultrafiltered by the renal glomeruli. The rate of elimination of substances that rely primarily on renal filtration for excretion provides an estimate of GFR provided that the production rate (or infusion rate) is constant. In clinical practice the measurement of creatinine clearance (C_{cr}) is commonly used for this purpose, since creatinine is endogenously produced, its rate of production is constant and is not affected by pregnancy, and its determination in plasma and urine is easily performed, widely available, and accurate. The clearance is derived by dividing the quantity excreted into urine per unit time (urine creatinine concentration (U_{cr}) times urine flow rate (V)) by plasma creatinine concentration (P_{cr}), using the formula

$$C_{cr}\ \text{ml/min} = \frac{U_{cr}\ \text{mg/ml} \times V\ \text{ml/min}}{P_{cr}\ \text{mg/ml}}$$

In nonpregnant individuals and in early pregnancy C_{cr} can be measured from 24-h collections of urine. In the latter half of pregnancy and especially in the third trimester, however, accurate clearance measurements are difficult to perform because complete bladder emptying is often impaired and because of the effect of posture on GFR. In late pregnancy when a subject changes from lying on her side to an upright or supine position, there is an immediate fall in renal plasma flow and GFR[28] (Fig. 17-1). Thus, GFR in third-trimester women should be measured with the subject lying on her side after hydration in such a manner that urine flow exceeds 5 to 6 ml/min. Two or three timed collections of urine of at least 30 min are obtained, along with a plasma sample, for the determination of creatinine concentrations. Conventional 24-h collections may result in falsely low clearances.

Although formal estimates of C_{cr} are required in patients with suspected or established renal disease, simple screening techniques for estimating the level of GFR usually rely on measurements of serum levels of urea nitrogen and plasma creatinine. Owing to the physiologic increase in GFR and expansion of extracellular fluid, however, levels of these substances are substantially lower during gestation than in nonpregnant women. Compared with nonpregnant values of 13 ± 3 mg/dl (mean ± SD) of serum urea nitrogen and 0.67 ± 0.14 mg/dl of plasma creatinine, levels fall to 8.7 ± 1.5 mg/dl and 0.46 ± 0.13 mg/dl, respectively. Concentrations of urea nitrogen and creatinine during pregnancy which exceed 13 mg/dl or 0.8 mg/dl should alert the physician to the possibility of renal insufficiency.

The upper level of normal urinary protein excretion is approximately 150 mg/day. Since proteinuria (> 150 mg/day) is a common and sensitive index of renal disease, qualitative and quantitative estimates of protein excretion are routinely employed in antenatal care. Qualitative methods are inexpensive and easy to use and provide a measure of protein concentration. Color-reactive papers respond to the concentration of albumin, while the acid precipitation test measures total protein (albumin plus globulin). It should be recalled that these tests assume a normal daily urine volume of about 1 L and are adjusted to register a positive reaction when the protein concentration exceeds approximately 200 mg/L. Variations in urine volume above or below the arbitrary "normal" urine volume will give false negative or false positive reactions, respectively. A positive reaction greater than 2+, in the absence of clinical evidence of volume contraction, should be evaluated with a quantitative determination of urine protein excretion, measured in a timed 24-h collection of urine.

CLINICAL MANIFESTATIONS OF RENAL DISEASE

Although renal disease may be caused by many different types of tissue injury reactions, the functional consequences of renal injury commonly result in the nephrotic syndrome, due to heavy urinary losses of protein, and/or renal insufficiency, due to a significant fall in GFR. Since alterations in renal function result in characteristic syndromes that are common to different types of renal disease, diagnostic investigations and therapy can be initiated on the basis of these clinical features.

Nephrotic Syndrome

This clinical syndrome is defined as heavy proteinuria, exceeding 3.0 g/1.73 m^2 and a serum albumin level less than 3.0 g/dl. Patients with this complication of renal disease always have a reduced ability to excrete urinary sodium and are prone to develop generalized edema. In addition, and apparently as a consequence of hypoalbuminemia, these patients also usually exhibit hyperlipidemia, with elevations of cholesterol and triglyceride levels. The GFR may also be reduced, depending on the type and severity of the injury reaction.

The cause of heavy proteinuria invariably involves a glomerular lesion, which results in increased glomerular filtration of plasma proteins and subsequent loss of protein into final urine. The glomerulonephropathy may result from primary kidney disease or from a systemic disorder which involes the kidney as well as other organ systems. A classification of renal parenchymal disease is shown in Table 17-1.

Since patients with the nephrotic syndrome tend to have a reduced capacity to excrete sodium, a positive balance of sodium will develop, with expansion of the extracellular fluid volume, unless dietary sodium is significantly reduced. The mechanism for this change in the renal handling of sodium has not been delineated but is thought to involve a reduction in circulating plasma volume. In general, the impairment in sodium excretory capacity correlates inversely with the serum albumin level. Pitting edema initially accumulates in dependent parts and, in the event of a large positive balance for sodium, edema may be manifest clinically as anasarca and ascites. In addition to the cosmetic effects of severe edema, stasis ulcers and thromboembolic phenomena may also result from edema formation. Lastly, since hypertension is volume-dependent in some patients, expansion of the extracellular fluid volume may cause hypertension or aggravate preexisting hypertension. The occur-

Table 17-1. Classification of Renal Parenchymal Disease

- I. Glomerular
  - A. Primary renal disease
    - 1. Epithelial disease
      - a. Minimal-change disease
      - b. Focal glomerulosclerosis
    - 2. Membranous nephropathy
    - 3. Proliferative glomerulonephritis
    - 4. Chronic glomerulonephritis
  - B. Systemic diseases
    - 1. Diabetic glomerulosclerosis
    - 2. Systemic lupus erythematosus
    - 3. Systemic vasculitis
    - 4. Amyloidosis
    - 5. Toxemia of pregnancy
- II. Interstitial
  - A. Acute interstitial nephritis
  - B. Chronic interstitial nephritis
  - C. Pyelonephritis
- III. Vascular
  - A. Arterionephrosclerosis
  - B. Renal artery stenosis
  - C. Renal vein thrombosis

rence of generalized edema in this syndrome may mask the clinical signs of contracted plasma volume caused by hemorrhage, vomiting, diarrhea, and the rapid action of diuretic agents.

Causes of Nephrotic Syndrome. The nephrotic syndrome in pregnancy may be caused by preexisting renal disease, renal disease which first develops during pregnancy, or preeclampsia. The clinical distinction between renal disease and preeclampsia has important implications because of differences in patient management. In patients with established renal disease before conception or in whom proteinuria is documented before the twentieth week of gestation, a diagnosis of renal disease as the cause of nephrotic syndrome is easily made. Uncommon exceptions to this principle include "early preeclampsia" as seen in hydatidiform mole or multiple gestation pregnancies. The onset of proteinuria in the latter part of pregnancy, however, presents certain diagnostic problems because of the similarities in clinical features.

Fisher and associates have recently provided information on the relative incidence of the various causes of proteinuria and hypertension during gestation.[10] An essential feature in their study of 176 patients was the histopathologic diagnosis of all patients by renal biopsy within 6 days of delivery. Amongst primigravidas with some degree of proteinuria and hypertension, the incidence of preeclampsia, primary renal disease, and hypertensive glomerulosclerosis was 83, 12, and 5 percent, respectively. Although the nephrotic syndrome is not a common complication of preeclampsia, preeclampsia was the most common cause of nephrotic syndrome in primigravidas in this series. In multiparous patients, in contrast, preeclampsia occurred in only 38 percent of patients with proteinuria and hypertension, while renal disease accounted for 26 percent of cases and hypertensive renal disease for 24 percent, and 12 percent had normal morphology by biopsy. Not unexpectedly, therefore, preeclampsia was a less frequent cause of proteinuria in multiparous women.

Effect of Nephrotic Syndrome on the Underlying Renal Disease and Pregnancy Outcome. From the standpoint of practical clinical management, important questions raised concerning pregnant women with the nephrotic syndrome include: (1) Does pregnancy adversely affect the course of the underlying renal disease? (2) Is the likelihood of a successful outcome of pregnancy reduced? Recent retrospective analysis of large series of nephrotic women in whom a specific diagnosis was established by renal biopsy have provided some answers to these provocative questions. In the series of cases reported by Studd and Blainey[34] and Strauch and Hayslett[32] with several of the more common types of glomerulonephropathies, the course of renal disease appeared similar to the expected outcome of the underlying renal lesion in nonpregnant patients. Katz et al.[18] recently reported an analysis of 121 pregnancies in 89 women with various primary renal disorders. Increased proteinuria was the most common renal effect of gestation and was manifest in 57 pregnancies in this series, with nephrotic syndrome occurring in 39. In the group as a whole renal function decreased slightly in five and progressed to end-stage renal failure in another five during the mean follow-up of 62 months. The onset of renal insufficiency had no consistent relationship to pregnancy. At the end of follow-up protein excretion exceeded 3.0 g/day in only five patients.

As noted above, heavy proteinuria and nephrotic syndrome may also occur in preeclampsia. Fisher et al.[9] reported a long-term follow-up (mean 36 months) of 23 women with biopsy-proven preeclampsia and nephrotic syndrome. At follow-up only one patient, subsequently proven to have adult polycystic kidney disease, had an elevated serum creatinine level. The 24-h protein excretion was borderline high in only two patients, who also exhibited modest elevations of blood pressure. In summary, therefore, the effect of pregnancy in patients with various types of primary renal disease, including those with nephrotic syndrome during pregnancy, does not appear to influence the natural course of the renal disorder. Moreover, the occurrence of heavy proteinuria in patients with preeclampsia does not indicate a different long-term outlook from that for patients with lesser amounts of proteinuria.

In each of these series the effects of renal disease and heavy proteinuria on the fetus were also considered, but this analysis was complicated by the concurrence of renal insufficiency and hypertension in many patients with nephrotic syndrome. Nevertheless, in spite of multiple factors which are known or may be expected to have an adverse effect on the fetus, perinatal survival was reduced only modestly below expected rates. For example, in the report of Studd and Blainey[34] the incidence of live births was 29 in 30 pregnancies, with 1 stillbirth due to a cord accident and 1 neonatal death. The infant birth weight, apart from being affected by hypertension, was directly related to the maternal albumin level. Excluding therapeutic abortions, the live birth rate reported by Strauch and Hayslett[32] was 91 percent in 34 pregnancies. Among preeclamptics with heavy proteinuria reported by Fisher,[9] however, there were 5 stillbirths in 23 pregnancies, compared with 2 in 44 pregnancies of preeclamptic women with moderate proteinuria. Neither Apgar scores nor mean maternal blood pressures were different in the two groups. This preliminary evidence suggests that the degree of proteinuria may be a prognostic indicator of perinatal outcome in preeclampsia, but this relationship has not been observed in nephrotic syndrome due to other types of renal disease.

Clinical Management of the Nephrotic Syndrome. The tendency for generalized edema formation in patients with nephrotic syndrome results in several management problems. The progressive accumulation of extracellular fluid often causes considerable morbidity because of massive edema, may increase the risk of thromboembolic disease, may aggravate or cause hypertension, and has been reported to complicate vaginal delivery because of vulvar edema. Some authors suggest that prolonged bed rest is the only treatment indicated because of possible hazard associated with diuretic therapy. In our judgment, however, dietary sodium restriction, initiated in the early phase of edema formation, offers both theoretical and practical advantages in management. Since pregnancy is normally associated with an increased reabsorption of filtered sodium and this process is exaggerated in the nephrotic syndrome, reduction in dietary sodium intake from the normal level of 4 to 5 g to about 1 g will blunt the rate of edema formation. Patients with nephrotic syndrome, whether pregnant or not, will not experience a negative sodium balance, with reduction in plasma volume, on this regimen; indeed, most will continue to experience a cumulative positive balance, albeit at a slower rate.

In most patients with nephrotic syndrome, salt restriction and frequent periods of bed rest, especially if the subject lies on her side to promote a higher GFR during the latter phases of gestation, will suffice to prevent the development of anasarca.

Owing to avid sodium retention, however, some women will continue to gain weight rapidly. In these edematous individuals we have employed diuretics on an intermittent basis to avoid excessive edema formation. The minimum dosage of the diuretic agent that induces a natriuretic response should be empirically determined in individual patients. The goal of therapy is to maintain edema at a tolerable level by inducing weight decrements of 2 to 3 lb with each course of treatment. Clinical signs of edema should never be eliminated with this regimen. Daily or prophylactic use of diuretic agents is not employed because of the possibility of inducing volume contraction and/or electrolyte abnormalities. Hypertension, if present, is treated with vasodilating agents, using criteria described in Chapter 11 on hypertensive crises.

The obstetrical management of labor and delivery in patients with nephrotic syndrome due to renal disease does not differ from the usual practice employed in uncomplicated pregnancies, but electronic fetal monitoring is indicated. In preeclamptic patients with the nephrotic syndrome the usual approach to the management of preeclampsia should be employed.

Most patients experience a spontaneous diuresis, associated with a gradual fall in urinary protein and rise in serum albumin within 2 to 6 weeks of delivery. In patients in whom the cause of the nephrotic syndrome has not been established, we advocate renal biopsy within 1 week of delivery. Since clinical criteria alone will not distinguish between preeclampsia, primary renal disease, and hypertensive glomerulosclerosis, a definitive diagnosis depends on renal histopathological criteria, and the diagnostic histologic changes of endotheliosis in preeclampsia are present only in late pregnancy and the immediate postpartum period.

Moderate Renal Insufficiency

Since compensatory renal mechanisms usually preserve external balance for water and electrolytes until GFR is reduced to about 20 percent of normal, the phrase "moderate renal insufficiency" is used to characterize patients with a decreased GFR which, however, is not lower than 25 ml/min. These patients may have elevations of serum urea nitrogen and plasma creatinine as high as 20 to 40 mg/dl and 2 to 3 mg/dl, respectively. Although this level of renal insufficiency is not marked by significant alterations in serum electrolytes or in recognizable neurological symptoms, these patients experience many of the metabolic and hemodynamic consequences of impaired renal function. A GFR level of 25 to 40 ml/min, for example, is usually associated with reduced fertility. As the mass of functional renal tissue shrinks, anemia develops, owing to reduced production of erythropoietin, and hypertension is a common complication. Further, increased production of parathyroid hormone is observed after only modest reductions in renal function, and plasma levels of parathyroid hormone will increase further with additional declines in GFR. Patients with moderate renal insufficiency therefore are prone to renal osteodystrophy, with the usual clinical manifestations of bone and muscle pain, pathological fractures, and bone erosion. Although clinical experience in patients with significant reductions in GFR during pregnancy is limited, there has been a general concern that renal insufficiency impairs fetal development.

Diagnosis of moderate renal insufficiency in obstetric patients will be missed unless it is recalled that the GFR is normally increased above nonpregnant levels by 30 to 40 percent during pregnancy. It is important to emphasize that renal function in the gravida should be related to expected levels during gestation and not to values that are appropriately normal for the nonpregnant individual. Thus, a GFR of 100 ml/min should be considered low in pregnancy, while prior to conception the same level could reflect normal function.

In regard to moderate renal insufficiency, analysis of the literature is complicated by two factors. First, the level of renal function is usually represented by serum creatinine levels, and second, in most series it is not possible to separate the individual effects of reduced renal function from hypertension on pregnancy outcome. The problem of using serum creatinine values as a measure of GFR relates to the fact that the creatinine level is often a poor reflection of renal function at modest but significant reductions of filtration rate. Figure 17-2 demonstrates the relationships of blood urea nitrogen and serum creatinine levels to the rate of glomerular clearance of those substances. This curve, derived from values in the nonpregnant state, indicates that a 50 percent reduction in clearance usually occurs before plasma levels of

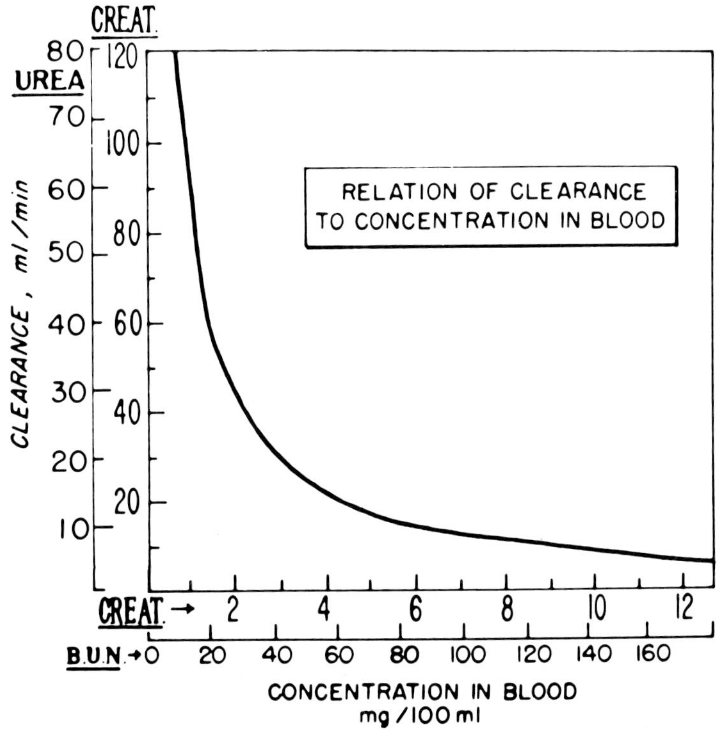

Fig. 17-2 Relation of clearance of urea or creatinine to blood concentrations assuming a constant urea and creatinine production rate. (From Relman, A.S., and Levinsky, N.G.: Clinical examination of renal function. In Strauss, M.B., and Welt, L.G., Eds.: Diseases of the Kidney. 2nd Ed. Little, Brown, Boston. © 1971.)

either urea nitrogen or creatinine rise above values considered to be normal. In pregnancy the curve is shifted toward the left because of the rise in GFR and fall in circulating blood and plasma levels of the index substances. It is apparent, therefore, that the true incidence of significant renal insufficiency in any series of patients may be markedly underestimated when a plasma creatinine of 1.2 or 1.5 mg/dl is used as the criterion.

It is of interest that when serial renal function studies were prospectively performed in patients with renal insufficiency, an increase in both GFR and effective renal plasma flow was found that was similar to that seen in normal pregnancy.[18] In 33 pregnancies of gravidas with a baseline inulin clearance 1 standard deviation or more below that of a normal pregnant woman, the increase in GFR of about 30 percent was essentially the same as that found in women without renal disease.

Effect of Moderate Renal Insufficiency on Pregnancy Outcome. As discussed above, analysis of several large series of patients strongly suggests that the natural course of primary renal disease is not adversely affected by pregnancy. Similarly, the outlook for the fetus seems favorable as long as hypertension is absent and renal function is only minimally or moderately reduced. In an analysis of eight series of pregnancies complicated by renal disease published since 1956, Ferris reported no maternal deaths and a fetal survival rate of 93 percent in 176 normotensive gravidas.[3] In contrast, a fetal death rate of 45 percent was found in women with both renal disease and hypertension. These results compare favorably with rates reported in women with the nephrotic syndrome during pregnancy. In the entire series of 121 pregnancies reported by Katz et al.,[18] there were 7 spontaneous abortions beyond the first trimester and 6 instances of neonatal death. However 20 percent of deliveries were preterm and 27 of 111 infants whose birth weights were known (24.3 percent of all live births) were small for gestational age. These data indicate therefore that although the likelihood of perinatal survival is only slightly reduced by the presence of primary renal disease with normal to moderately reduced renal function, the incidence of preterm delivery and retarded fetal growth is increased. Since significant hypertension was noted in 23 percent of all pregnancies in the Katz report, it is apparent that even in recent large series it is difficult to separate the effects of renal disease from those of hypertension.

Besides primary renal disease the occurrence of renal disease secondary to a systemic disorder is a common management problem in pregnancy. Diabetes mellitus, for example, is one of the most prevalent causes of renal insufficiency and nephrotic syndrome. In an excellent study, Sims[30] found no evidence that pregnancy worsened renal function even in women with severe, long-standing diabetes mellitus. However, since the interval from the first appearance of proteinuria to severe renal failure in diabetic glomerulosclerosis is approximately 2 to 3 years, it is not surprising that a progressive decline during gestation is often observed in women with clinical evidence of proteinuria prior to conception.

Another important systemic disease which often involves the kidney is systemic lupus erythematosus (SLE). A recent study of 65 pregnancies in 47 patients with SLE,[16] indicated that pregnancy probably adversely affects this condition and causes relapses or exacerbations of the underlying disease. The activity of SLE before conception, however, was found to be strongly correlated with the effect of pregnancy on SLE. In the complete absence of SLE activity for at least 6 months prior to conception, there was a relapse rate of 30 percent during the pregnancy. Significant morbidity, however, occurred in only about 10 percent of these women and in most patients there was a complete reversal of symptoms following delivery. The live birth rate in this group was 90 percent. In contrast, among patients with signs of clinical activity through the time of conception, approximately one-half experienced exacerbations, most of which were severe, and the likelihood of a live birth was reduced to 70 percent.

Clinical Management of Patients with Moderate Renal Insufficiency. Since hypertension is a common complication of renal insufficiency and is often exacerbated by pregnancy, the occurrence of hypertension should be anticipated in these patients and should be managed by the usual guidelines for obstetric patients. Anemia, sometimes of significant proportions, may also require direct intervention. Although nonpregnant individuals tend to adapt to hematocrit levels below 30 percent, there is concern that low hematocrit levels may adversely influence fetal development. It is generally advocated therefore that hematocrit levels be maintained above 25 percent with intermittent transfusion of packed cells. As far as we are aware there have been no prospective studies to analyze the effect of this approach. Abnormalities of plasma electrolytes usually do not occur in patients with moderate renal insufficiency, and specific changes in diet and regimes designed to inhibit intestinal phosphate absorption and raise serum levels of bicarbonate are not required.

It should be noted that patients with reduced renal function have a reduced capacity to excrete water and electrolytes. Therefore, they are at increased risk of developing dilutional hyponatremia when large amounts of solute-free water are administered, or hypernatremia, hyperkalemia, and metabolic acidosis after treatment with various types of electrolyte-containing intravenous solutions. Appropriate restrictions in the use of parenterally administered fluids are required during treatment of severe hypertension, prolonged labor, and other conditions requiring intensive therapy.

There is no evidence that the usual treatment offered to nonpregnant patients with primary or systemic diseases involving the kidney should be altered during pregnancy. In patients with moderate renal insufficiency due to diabetes mellitus, clinical management should follow the same general guidelines that apply to pregnant diabetic women without clinical evidence of renal disease. Specific modes of treatment, with proven efficacy, are generally not available for patients with primary renal disease. There is evidence, however, that treatment with glucocorticoids, often used in combination with immunosuppressive agents, is useful in suppressing the underlying disease in patients with systemic necrotizing vasculitis[8,15] and SLE.[12,17] Previous studies in patients with SLE[6,16] and renal transplantation[27] have failed to show teratogenic effects or an adverse influence on fetal development when glucocorticoids were administered in amounts equivalent to 60 to 80 mg of prednisone per day, or after treatment with azathioprine or cyclophosphamide in doses of 1.0 to 1.5 mg/kg/day. Although no long-term follow-up is available on children exposed in utero, these agents appear to be safe to use during pregnancy. The same indications for treatment that are employed in nonpregnant individuals should be used for obstetric patients.

Although renal biopsy has important value in establishing the cause of renal damage and in evaluating the severity of the tissue reaction, limited experience with this technique during gestation should preclude its use until after delivery. Decisions relating to clinical management therefore should be made on the basis of clinical and pathological features of disease, exclusive of renal biopsy.

Since there is no evidence that pregnancy alters the natural course of renal disease, with the possible exception of lupus nephropathy, early delivery does not prevent progressive renal failure. Renal insufficiency has been associated, however, with impaired fetal development, and careful monitoring of fetal growth is indicated in these patients. In addition, since hypertension and the activity of some systemic diseases, such as SLE and systemic vasculitis, result in increased perinatal mortality,[16,21] efforts should be made to control hypertension and suppress systemic disorders. Finally, antepartum electronic fetal monitoring should be performed in women with SLE because cardiac conduction disorders have been reported and may require special care in infants born to these women.[1]

It should also be mentioned that preeclampsia may complicate the course of pregnancy in women with diabetes mellitus and primary renal disease.[10,35] Although in our judgment the incidence of preeclampsia under these conditions is probably greatly overestimated, it is very difficult to rule out this diagnosis because the clinical features of renal disease and preeclampsia are similar, and proteinuria usually increases during pregnancy in women with renal disease from any cause. The obstetrician therefore must weigh the question of delivery in patients with the suspected diagnosis of superimposed preeclampsia and declining renal function against the likelihood of neonatal survival based on gestational age and studies of fetal lung maturity. The factor of parity has important implications since preeclampsia is less common in multiparous women, even with underlying renal disease from other causes.[10]

Severe Renal Failure

This category of renal dysfunction is characterized by a fall in GFR to a level less than 25 ml/min. Since women with severe renal failure are generally infertile, this condition in pregnancy results from either acute renal failure or the rapid progression of renal parenchymal disease acquired prior to conception or during gestation. This complication of pregnancy is associated with a high incidence of intrauterine death and fetal growth retardation.[26] Although maternal death rates remain high in underdeveloped countries, modern intensive care treatment modalities and renal dialysis have substantially improved survival in western nations.

Acute Renal Failure. This is usually defined as a rapid decline in GFR toward a value that approaches zero. Hallmark clinical features include a near linear increase in serum creatinine concentration at a rate of 0.5 to 1.5 mg/dl/day, a progressive rapid rise in serum urea nitrogen, and usually a fall in urine flow rate to less than 400 to 500 ml/day. Sustained severe renal failure beyond a few days results in marked azotemia, metabolic acidosis, hyperkalemia, anemia, and eventually the neurological manifestations of uremia. In the absence of appropriate treatment, death within 1 to 2 weeks will occur. The general classification of acute renal failure is shown in Table 17-2.

Classification. The term *prerenal acute renal failure* implies that GFR is markedly reduced owing to renal hypoperfusion without renal histopathological changes or impaired tubular function. After renal blood flow falls, fractional sodium excretion is reduced to less than 1 percent (calculated as $U_{Na} \times P_{cr}/U_{cr} \times P_{Na}$, where U_{Na} and P_{Na} are the sodium contents of urine and plasma, respectively) and U_{Na} is usually less than 20 mEq/L. Concurrently, filtered water is maximally conserved and urine osmolality rises above 500 mosm/kg H_2O. As noted in Table 17-2, renal hypoperfusion can result from hypotension, volume contraction, and heart failure. Common causes of renal hypoperfusion during pregnancy include hyperemesis gravidarum, septic shock, and preeclampsia, which result in volume contraction, and abruptio placentae, which causes hypotension. Correction of renal hypoperfusion in these conditions promptly restores GFR and reverses the metabolic consequences of renal failure.

Acute tubular necrosis occurs when the renal insult from severe ischemia or the action of nephrotoxins causes severe but reversible damage to renal tubular cells. The histopathological lesion is characterized by interstitial edema and necrotic sloughed tubular cells; glomeruli appear normal by light microscopy, although in disseminated intravascular coagulation (DIC) fragments of red blood cells and fibrin deposits are commonly seen in glomerular capillaries. In contrast to prerenal acute failure, tubular transport function is markedly impaired and results in increased fractional excretion of sodium (greater than 1 to 2 percent), urinary sodium greater than 40 mEq/L, and impaired concentrating ability (urine osmolality <400 mosm/kg H_2O).[24] The same factors which cause prerenal hypoperfusion also cause acute tubular

Table 17-2. Classification of Causes of Acute Renal Failure

Prerenal
Renal hypoperfusion due to:
1. Hypotension
2. Decreased circulating plasma volume
3. Decreased cardiac output
Renal parenchymal
Acute tubular necrosis—reversible
Cortical necrosis—irreversible
Caused by:
1. Renal hypoperfusion due to
a. Hypotension
b. Decreased circulating plasma volume
c. Decreased cardiac output
d. Disseminated intravascular coagulation (DIC)
2. Nephrotoxins
Postrenal
Obstruction of ureters or bladder outlet
Extravasation of urine from urinary collecting system

necrosis in pregnancy. In addition, hemoglobinuria due to hemolysis and DIC in septic patients and the specific nephrotoxic effects of soap and lysol used as chemical abortifacients are sufficient to provoke renal shutdown.

Restoration of renal function usually becomes clinically evident within 10 to 21 days and is dependent, at least in part, on regeneration of tubular epithelial cells and increased renal blood flow. Since the rise in GFR precedes full recovery of tubular function, the early phase of improved renal function is usually marked by a progressive rise in urine flow rate, with a urine sodium concentration of 60 to 90 mEq/L and potassium concentration of 20 to 30 mEq/L. Studies performed several months later have demonstrated normal parameters of renal function.

Renal cortical necrosis is a pathologic entity characterized by tissue death throughout the cortex in a diffuse or patchy pattern, with sparing of the medullary portions of the kidney, and is a form of irreversible acute tubular necrosis. Although cortical necrosis is uncommon in nonpregnant individuals, it is a frequent complication of obstetric conditions. Cortical necrosis is more likely to occur in multigravidas who are beyond 30 years of age[26] and is most commonly associated with abruptio placentae. The reasons for the propensity of pregnant women to develop cortical necrosis are unknown. Previous workers, however, have postulated that the increased reactivity of the renal vasculature to vasoactive amines and the local activation of coagulation may play an important role in the induction of tissue injury leading to cell death. The causes and clinical characteristics of cortical necrosis are the same as those of acute tubular necrosis except for the lack of recovery of renal function.

Lastly, postrenal causes of acute renal failure are listed in Table 17-2, since factors which prevent the external elimination of final urine can result in uremia with clinical features that are indistinguishable from prerenal and renal types of acute renal failure.

Diagnostic Evaluation. The clinical approach to acute renal failure begins by determining the category which most likely explains the cause for the sudden decline in renal function. Bladder outlet obstruction is evaluated by simple catheterization of the urinary bladder. Examination of the urine for fractional excretion of sodium and concentrating ability is useful in distinguishing prerenal from renal causes of acute renal failure. The presence of hypotension or clinically evident cardiac failure or dehydration demands prompt corrective measures with specific therapeutic modalities to maximize renal perfusion. A careful bedside examination to evaluate skin turgor and jugular venous pressure and attention to changes in body weight and a history of vomiting or bleeding will often provide important clues regarding volume status. In cases of abruptio, sufficient occult bleeding has occurred by the time the patient presents to warrant immediate volume replacement. Since effective plasma volume is often difficult to ascertain by physical examination, particularly in edematous patients, Swan-Ganz catheterization to determine pulmonary wedge pressure is the most reliable means for evaluating volume status. In the presence of reduced filling pressures, isotonic fluids, or packed RBCs when hemorrhage has occurred, should be administered until filling pressures are normalized. If the clinical history suggests possible ureteral obstruction, renal ultrasound should be performed to determine the presence of ureteral dilatation. In the absence of such a history, studies to exclude this diagnosis are usually only performed if clinical recovery does not occur with 7 to 10 days.

In the absence of tubular injury, restoration of plasma volume through the administration of colloid and/or isotonic fluids, along with correction of hypotension and/or cardiac output, should increase renal perfusion and GFR. This will be reflected by a rise in urine flow rate and progressive fall in serum creatinine and blood urea nitrogen. The administration of potent diuretics should not be used as a diagnostic test for prerenal acute renal failure or in an attempt to hasten the rate of recovery in acute tubular necrosis. Although large sustained doses of furosemide may result in increased urine volume, such treatment does not stimulate recovery and is associated with a high incidence of ototoxicity.[11,19]

Clinical Management. If the diagnosis of acute tubular necrosis or cortical necrosis seems likely after exclusion of pre- and postrenal factors, therapy is begun to minimize the consequences of severe renal failure. Fluid administration is restricted to replacing the volume of external losses (urine and intestinal fluids) plus insensible losses of water (approximately 400 to 500 ml/day). Intake of substances containing potassium, metabolic acid, and sodium should be eliminated. A caloric intake of at least 2,000 kcal/day can be achieved through the administration of carbohydrates and lipids. The dose of pharmacologic agents that depend on kidney function for external elimination should be adjusted to maintain plasma levels within therapeutic ranges. Excellent reviews are available that provide guidelines for treating patients with renal insufficiency with commonly used drugs.[2]

Hypertension should be treated with vasodilatory agents, hydralazine being the drug of choice in the undelivered patient. Since magnesium levels tend to rise in renal failure and may reach toxic levels, $MgSO_4$ should be avoided in the clinical setting of renal insufficiency. Elevated plasma levels of potassium, above 5.5 mEq/L, should be reduced. The administration of sodium polystyrene sulfonate (Kayexalate) 40 g every 4 to 6 h by retention enema is a useful means by which to increase elimination of potassium. Efforts to correct acidosis are indicated when the serum HCO_3^- level falls to 12 to 14 mEq/L; this is done by the administration of $NaHCO_3$ to raise the level to a range of 18 to 20 mEq/L. In addition to the retention of metabolic acid in patients with severe renal insufficiency, sepsis and hypotension are often associated with lactic acidosis owing to reduction in metabolism of pyruvic acid. Conversion of pyruvic to lactic acid leads to a severe, persistent acidosis, which demands the administration of large amounts of $NaHCO_3$ to maintain the blood pH above 7.3. Dialysis therapy is often required under these conditions to remove the large sodium load. It should also be noted that anemia is a complication of severe renal failure, even in the absence of hemorrhage or DIC. Blood should be administered to maintain the hematocrit value above 25 percent in order to enhance fetal viability.

We believe that dialysis treatment should be established if renal failure persists for more than 3 to 4 days without signs of improvement or if the serum creatinine level rises to above 5.0 mg/dl. In patients with a high catabolic rate due, for example, to sepsis or hemorrhage, dialysis may be indicated even earlier. Early dialysis has the advantage of preventing many of the severe manifestations of uremia and permits the administration of protein and calories in the large amounts that are often required in severely catabolic patients. Specific suggestions for dialysis therapy during pregnancy are discussed below. If the conceptus is mature, it should be delivered as soon as the mother's condition has stabilized.

Recent studies have shown a decreased incidence of acute renal failure during pregnancy in the United States and Europe within the last two decades, attributed to liberalized abortion laws and improvement in prenatal care.[4] In centers where dialysis treatment is available, the incidence of maternal death is reported to be approximately 14 percent, and this is usually attributed to the conditions which cause renal failure rather than to renal insufficiency per se. In these same centers perinatal death averaged 40 percent in patients with acute renal failure.[13]

Severe Progressive Renal Disease. This may occur with any type of glomerular or interstitial renal disease shown in Table 17-1. In contrast to acute renal failure, in which GFR falls suddenly over hours, the decline in GFR in progressive renal disease usually occurs over days, weeks, or months. Reduction in GFR to a level of less than 25 ml/min results in electrolyte disturbances, as well as worsening of the metabolic consequences of moderate renal failure.

The electrolyte alterations include a rise in serum potassium levels to 5.0 mEq/L or greater owing to impaired urinary excretion. Concurrently, serum phosphorus levels also increase to values of 5 to 8 mg/dl because of reduction in the amount of filtered phosphorus. Calcium levels are usually normal or reduced, depending on the action of parathyroid hormone in increasing calcium release from bone. Intestinal absorption of calcium falls below normal levels because of decreased 1,25-dihydroxy vitamin D production. Lastly, metabolic acidosis is a common complication of severe renal failure owing to decreased rates of excretion of metabolic acid as ammonium and titratable acid; urinary acidification (pH), however, remains normal.

Metabolic and hemodynamic complications of severe renal failure include worsening anemia, with hematocrit values commonly less than 25 percent, hypertension, impaired cardiac function, weakness, and anorexia. Manifestations of central nervous system dysfunction cause substantial morbidity in patients with severe renal failure—somnolence, impaired intellectual function, hiccups, and depression.

The final stage in renal failure, reached when GFR levels are below 5 ml/min, is termed *uremia* and is marked by severe toxic symptoms of nausea, vomiting, pruritus, hypothermia, and if dialysis is not initiated, by the terminal events of myoclonus, convulsion, and coma.

Diagnosis. In most patients the specific cause of renal failure will have been established before conception or in early pregnancy or will be evident from the clinical manifestations of a systemic disorder. Changes in the rate of decline of GFR in these patients, however, or the finding of progressive renal insufficiency for the first time during pregnancy requires exclusion of prerenal causes of renal hypoperfusion and postrenal sources of urinary tract obstruction.

The discovery of progressive renal insufficiency after the twentieth week of gestation may present a difficult diagnostic problem because of the lack of specific criteria by which to distinguish preeclampsia from primary renal disease. Since renal biopsy, which can usually provide specific histologic findings of preeclampsia, is not a safe procedure in most centers during the third trimester, the clinician will usually assume that preeclampsia is present and will deliver the fetus if the clinical features are highly suggestive of that disorder.

Clinical Management. Disturbances in acid-base balance and electrolytes can be managed by conservative means before dialysis is instituted. Elevated levels of potassium can be reduced below a level of 5.0 mEq/L by restricting daily dietary intake to about 20 mEq. The complication of hyperphosphatemia can be managed by dietary reductions of phosphorus to 600 to 800 mg/day and by the administration of oral phosphate binding agents such as Basogel to reduce serum phosphorus below 5.0 mg/dl. As in the treatment of acute renal failure, $NaHCO_3$ should be administered to patients with serum HCO_3^- levels below 12 to 14 mEq/L. An oral dose of 1 to 4 g/day is usually sufficient to titrate the daily production of metabolic acid; it should be remembered that each gram of $NaHCO_3$ contains 12 mEq of Na. Recent studies have demonstrated marked alterations in calcium metabolism in patients with renal failure due to low production rates of 1,25-dihydroxycalciferol and high levels of parathyroid hormone. Since fetal bone development utilizes maternal calcium stores, it can be anticipated that the effect of severe renal failure on maternal calcium metabolism may be more severe than in nonpregnant individuals. Despite the lack of experimental studies it seems reasonable to administer 1,25-dihydroxycalciferol in a dose of 0.25 μg/day and supplemental calcium to patients with severe renal failure provided that serum calcium levels are carefully monitored to prevent hypercalcemia and that plasma phosphate levels are maintained below 5.0 mg/dl.

Dialysis therapy should be instituted when the GFR is less than 5 to 10 ml/min to prevent uremic complications. Since urea, creatinine, and probably other metabolites that accumulate in uremia readily cross the placenta, the advantages of early dialysis may have important implications for the fetus.

There is a paucity of data reported on fetal survival in severe renal failure. In small series of patients the live birth rate was approximately 20 percent and growth retardation was common.[13,25] Since there is no evidence that the continuation of pregnancy adversely affects the underlying disease, except in cases of preeclampsia, pregnancy should not be terminated in the absence of fetal distress until fetal maturity has been demonstrated. Because these patients exhibit a reduced capacity to excrete water and sodium, the volume of parenteral fluids should be carefully monitored and restricted during labor and delivery.

DIALYSIS IN PREGNANCY

Both peritoneal dialysis and hemodialysis have been used in pregnant patients with renal failure. Smith et al.[31] have reported their experience with peritoneal dialysis in 10 patients with acute renal failure, occurring in both early and late pregnancy. They advocate initiating early treatment before uremic symptoms are manifest and daily rather than intermittent peritoneal dialysis to avoid removal of large excesses of sodium and water and to provide smooth control of blood chemistry. These authors indicate that neither pelvic peritonitis nor an enlarged uterus is a contraindication to dialysis provided the catheter is inserted high in the abdomen.

We believe that the catheter should be placed surgically under direct vision. The fetal survival in this series of patients was not reported.

In a recent review Nissenson[25] has listed a total of 20 gravid women treated with hemodialysis. In this series there were 2 fetal deaths and 12 preterm deliveries. He reported that hypotension and vaginal bleeding were frequent complications of dialysis and premature contractions or labor often occurred during or immediately after treatment. To optimize the safety of the procedure in the pregnant patient he suggests measures to reduce hypotension, including the use of sequential ultrafiltration. This is a technique which allows fluid removal independently of dialytic solute exchange. In addition, since acidosis may transiently occur with the use of acetate in the dialysate, he suggests employing bicarbonate. Lastly, low-dose heparinization to reduce the likelihood of hemorrhage is advocated rather than full-dose anticoagulation during dialysis.

RENAL STONE DISEASE IN PREGNANCY

Nephrolithiasis has been reported to occur with an incidence of about 1 in 1,500 pregnancies.[33] This condition creates diagnostic problems because of the difficulty of distinguishing ureteral colic from obstetrical causes of abdominal pain. Most patients manifest typical symptoms of flank pain, urgency, and dysuria and are found to have microhematuria. Atypical clinical presentations, however, have been reported,[14] and nephrolithiasis should be considered in patients with urinary tract infection that is refractory to antibiotics and in patients with recurrent pyelonephritis. Some investigators claim that the incidence of acute renal colic in patients with a history of nephrolithiasis is not increased during pregnancy.[5]

The principal causes of nephrolithiasis in this population are similar to those observed in general. Patients who pass stones during pregnancy for the first time should be evaluated, therefore, for hyperparathyroidism with at least three determinations of plasma calcium and for cystinuria by examination of the urine with the nitroprusside test. Although stones are passed spontaneously in most cases, operative intervention may be required to eradicate infection or correct complete ureteral obstruction. The incidence of induction of labor by operative procedures is estimated to be about 5 to 10 percent.[29] To reduce the exposure to radiation of the fetus it has been suggested that a modified intravenous pyelogram should include only a single plain film prior to administration of dye and a repeat film after 20 min.

RENAL TRANSPLANTATION AND PREGNANCY

Penn et al.[27] have recently reviewed the course of 56 pregnancies in 37 women with kidney transplants. They emphasize that these patients should be counseled in family planning after successful transplantation since previously impaired fertility may be restored. Those wishing to become pregnant should be advised to employ contraception for at least 18 months because of the higher incidence of rejection episodes, infection, and permanent loss of graft function in the early postoperative interval. Because of the increased risks of hypertension and thrombosis with use of anovulatory agents and the risk of infection in immunosuppressed hosts with intrauterine devices, the authors favor barrier types of contraception.

In this series, 21 patients had impaired graft function with evidence of renal insufficiency and/or hypertension before conception, and 10 of these developed presumed evidence of preeclampsia during pregnancy. In 5 other transplant recipients, preeclampsia occurred despite normal graft function, and 3 of these patients developed persistent impairment of renal function. Of the 56 pregnancies, there was 1 ectopic pregnancy and 8 abortions, 7 of which were therapeutic. Of the 44 live-born neonates, 70 percent were normal and 30 percent had one or more complications, such as respiratory distress, seizures, and anomalies. Only 6 of the 44 infants were small for gestational age but 4 had congenital abnormalities. These data were interpreted as showing no clear evidence that immunosuppressive agents and glucocorticoids cause congenital abnormalities. Two infants, however, experienced transient adrenal insufficiency after birth and another two developed sepsis. This type of complication should be anticipated in neonates born to immunosuppressed women.

Labor and delivery were uncomplicated. This is not surprising, as the graft is located in the false pelvis and should not cause dystocia. Patients were routinely treated with supplemental doses of glucocorticoids at the time of delivery because of long-term adrenal suppression. In addition, because of the immunosuppressed state sterile precautions were followed during vaginal examinations, and premature rupture of membranes was an indication for early induction of labor.

REFERENCES

1. Barrett, C.T.: Neonatal outcome of maternal systemic lupus erythematosus. p. 674. In Fine, L.G., Moderator: Systemic Lupus Erythematosus in Pregnancy. Ann. Intern. Med., *94*:667, 1981.
2. Bennett, W.M., Muther, R.S., Parker, R.A. et al.: Drug therapy in renal failure: dosing guidelines for adults. Ann. Intern. Med., 93(Part 1):62; 93:286, 1980.
3. Burrow, A.N. and Ferris, T.F.: Medical complications during pregnancy. W.B. Saunders, Philadelphia, 1975.
4. Chapman, A. and Legrain, M.: Acute tubular necrosis and interstitial nephritis. p. 386. In Hamburger, J., Crosnier, J., and Grunfeld, J.P., Eds.: Nephrology. John Wiley & Sons, New York, 1979.
5. Coe, F.L., Parker, J.H., and Lindheimer, M.D.: Nephrolithiasis during pregnancy. N. Engl. J. Med., *298*:324, 1978.
6. Conolly, M.E.: The pharmacologic management of systemic lupus erythematosus in pregnancy. p. 671. In Fine, L.G., Moderator: Systemic Lupus Erythematosus in Pregnancy. Ann. Intern. Med., *94*:667, 1981.
7. Davison, J.M., Vallotton, M.B., and Lindheimer, M.D.: Alterations in plasma osmolality during human pregnancy. Clin. Res., *28*:442A, 1980.
8. Fauci, A.S., Katz, P., Haynes, B.F., and Wolff, S.M.: Cyclophosphamide therapy of severe systemic necrotizing vasculitis. N. Engl. J. Med., *301*:235, 1979.
9. Fisher, K.A., Ahuja, S., Luger, A. et al.: Nephrotic proteinuria with pre-eclampsia. Am. J. Obstet. Gynecol., *129*:643, 1977.

10. Fisher, K.A., Luger, A., Spargo, B.H., and Lindheimer, M.D.: Hypertension in pregnancy: clinical-pathological correlations and remote prognosis. Medicine (Baltimore), *60:*267, 1981.
11. Gallagher, K.L. and Jones, J.K.: Furosemide-induced ototoxicity. Ann. Intern. Med., *91:*744, 1979.
12. Ginzler, E.M., Bollet, A.J., and Friedman, E.A.: The natural history and response to therapy of lupus nephritis. Ann. Rev. Med., *31:*463, 1980.
13. Grunfeld, J.P., Ganeval, D., and Bounerias, F.: Acute renal failure in pregnancy. Kidney Int., *18:*179, 1980.
14. Harris, R.E. and Dunnihoo, D.R.: The incidence and significance of urinary calculi in pregnancy. Am. J. Obstet. Gynecol., *99:*237, 1967.
15. Haynes, B.F.: Treatment of the granulomatous vasculitides. p. 671. In Fauci, A.S., Moderator: The Spectrum of Vasculitis. Ann. Intern. Med., *89*(Part I):660, 1978.
16. Hayslett, J.P. and Lynn, R.I.: Effect of pregnancy in patients with lupus nephropathy. Kidney Int., *18:*207, 1980.
17. Hayslett, J.P. and Siegel, N.J.: Treatment of lupus nephropathy. Nephron, *19:*193, 1977.
18. Katz, A.I., Davison, J.M., Hayslett, J.P. et al.: Pregnancy in women with kidney disease. Kidney Int., *18:*192, 1980.
19. Kleinknecht, D., Ganeval, D., Gonzalez-Duque, L.A., and Fermanian, J.: Furosemide in acute oliguric renal failure—a controlled trial. Nephron, *17:*51, 1976.
20. Kreisberg, R.A.: Lactate homeostasis and lactic acidosis. Ann. Intern. Med., *92:*(Part 1):227, 1980.
21. Lieb, S.M.: The effect of systemic lupus erythematosus on fetal survival. p. 672. In Fine, L.G., Moderator: Systemic Lupus Erythematosus in Pregnancy. Ann. Intern. Med., *94:*667, 1981.
22. Lindheimer, M.D. and Katz, A.I.: Kidney function and disease in Pregnancy. Lea & Febiger, Philadelphia, 1977.
23. Lindheimer, M.D. and Katz, A.I.: The renal response to pregnancy. p. 1762. In Brenner and Rector, Eds.: The Kidney. 2nd Ed., W.B. Saunders, Philadelphia, 1981.
24. Miller, T.R., Anderson, R.J., Linas, S.L. et al.: Urinary diagnostic indices in acute renal failure. Ann. Intern. Med., *89:*47, 1978.
25. Nissenson, A.R.: The use of hemodialysis to treat end-stage renal failure during pregnancy. p. 670. In Fine, L.G., Moderator: Systemic Lupus Erythematosus in Pregnancy. Ann. Intern. Med., *94:*667, 1981.
26. Ober, W.E., Reid, D.E., Romney, S.L., and Merrill, J.P.: Renal lesions and acute renal failure in pregnancy. Am. J. Med., *21:*781, 1956.
27. Penn, I., Makowski, E.L., and Harris, P.: Parenthood following renal transplantation. Kidney Int., *18:*221, 1980.
28. Pippig, L.: Clinical aspects of renal disease during pregnancy. Med. Hyg., *27:*181, 1969.
29. Shnider, S.M. and Webster, A.M.: Maternal and fetal hazards of surgery during pregnancy. Am. J. Obstet. Gynecol., *92:*891, 1965.
30. Sims, E.A.H.: Serial studies of renal function in pregnancy complicated by diabetes mellitus. Diabetes, *10:*190, 1961.
31. Smith, K., Browne, J.C., Schackman, R., and Wrong, O.M.: Renal failure of obstetric origin. Br. Med. Bull., *24:*49, 1968.
32. Strauch, B.S. and Hayslett, J.P.: Kidney disease and pregnancy. Br. Med. J., *2:*578, 1974.
33. Strong, D.W., Murchison, R.J., and Lynch, D.F.: The management of ureteral calculi during pregnancy. Surg. Gynecol. Obstet., *146:*604, 1978.
34. Studd, J.W.W. and Blainey, J.D.: Pregnancy and the nephrotic syndrome. Br. Med. J., *1:*276, 1969.
35. White, P.: Pregnancy and diabetes, medical aspects. Med. Clin. North Am., *49:*1015, 1965.

18

Management of Hepatic Failure in Pregnancy

Denis Miller, M.D.
Roberto Romero, M.D.

Hepatic failure is a syndrome produced by acute or chronic hepatocellular necrosis. It is clinically characterized by the presence of encephalopathy, hemostatic failure, hypoglycemia, hypoalbuminemia, and/or portal hypertension. The extent of hepatocellular injury necessary to cause hepatic failure varies and is dependent upon many factors, including the type of injury and the regenerative response of the liver.

DIAGNOSIS OF HEPATIC FAILURE IN PREGNANCY

Acute Hepatic Failure

Hepatic failure in obstetric patients is caused either by conditions which are associated with and peculiar to pregnancy or conditions which are unrelated to pregnancy. Causes of liver failure specifically related to pregnancy include acute fatty liver of pregnancy and toxemia (preeclampsia and eclampsia). The most common cause of liver failure unrelated to pregnancy is viral hepatitis. Drug-associated hepatitis secondary to halothane, isoniazid, or methyldopa and a variety of other conditions may be responsible for this disorder.

It is imperative to differentiate pregnancy-related from unrelated causes of hepatic failure as early as possible, since rational therapy is contingent on this distinction. Both acute fatty liver of pregnancy and toxemia-related liver injury occur almost exclusively in the third trimester.

Acute Fatty Liver. Acute fatty liver of pregnancy is a rare disease of unknown etiology, unique to the gravidopuerperal state and histologically characterized by the accumulation of microvesicular fat in the hepatic parenchyma. Although only fewer than 100 cases have been reported in the English language literature, the prevalence of this disease is likely to be higher than that inferred from the number of reported cases. It is not uncommon for a tertiary perinatal center to see one or more cases of this disease per year.

The disorder carries a serious prognosis, and high fetal (85 percent) and maternal (75 percent) mortality rates have been reported.[41] In the authors' institution, no maternal deaths due to acute fatty liver of pregnancy have occurred in the last 7 years in six biopsy-proven cases of the disease.[34]

Patients usually present in the third trimester of pregnancy or in the postpartum period with abdominal pain, nausea, vomiting, and varying degrees of jaundice. Pruritus is rare. Although hypotension can be observed when the patient is in hepatic failure, hypertension is usually present at the onset of the disease. The course of acute fatty liver of pregnancy is characterized by the rapid development of acute hepatic failure, with coagulation disturbances[14] and encephalopathy. In contrast to hepatitis, the disease has a short prodomal period and abdominal pain is a predominant feature. Complications frequently reported include hypoglycemia,[30] gastrointestinal bleeding, renal failure, and metabolic acidosis.[19]

The etiology and pathogenesis are unknown. Histopathologic features resemble those found in Reye's syndrome. It has been hypothesized that in both conditions an unidentified injurious agent[19] causes hepatic mitochondrial and ribosomal dysfunction.[37,43] Mitochondrial dysfunction can lead to reduced activity of the mitochondrial urea cycle enzymes and, consequently to hyperammonemia.[43] Ribosomal dysfunction can result in depressed glucose 6-phosphatase activity and lipoprotein synthesis. The former may lead to hypoglycemia and the latter to impaired fat export from the liver and its accumulation in the hepatocyte.[37]

The biochemical abnormalities include mild to moderate jaundice (serum bilirubin usually less than 10 mg %) and only mild to moderate increases in transaminases. This is in contrast to hepatic failure associated with viral hepatitis, in which the bilirubin may be markedly elevated and the transaminase levels are invariably higher than 1,000 I.U./ml. The differentiation of acute fatty liver from pregnancy-unrelated causes thus is usually not difficult.

The liver biopsy characteristically shows microvesicular fat in the hepatocytes with sparing of the periportal areas. Inflammation is minimal, in contrast to acute hepatitis. Demonstration of the presence of microvesicular fat requires special stains, such as oil red O.

Remission of the disease is frequently observed after termination of the pregnancy. Although delivery by cesarean section has been recommended, there is no evidence to suggest that this is superior to vaginal delivery. The latter is actually preferable, in our opinion, since it imposes less stress on the hemostatic system.

Toxemia of Pregnancy. Toxemia is a multisystem disease which is clinically characterized by the development of hypertension and proteinuria. Liver dysfunction has been detected in approximately 18 percent of patients.[35]

The etiology and pathogenesis of toxemia remain to be established. It has been suggested that impaired prostacyclin activity, with resultant excessive intravascular platelet aggregation, activation of the coagulation system, and fibrin deposition in different organs accounts for the multisystem nature of this disease.[35] If this is true, the liver dysfunction results from ischemia and is related to the intensity of activation of the hemostatic systems. This hypothesis is supported by the immunofluorescent demonstration of fibrin deposits in the hepatic sinusoids of toxemic women with liver dysfunction[1] and a higher prevalence of hepatic involvement in patients with thrombocytopenia.

Liver dysfunction is usually subclinical in toxemia but nausea, vomiting, and abdominal pain are strongly associated with its occurrence. The mechanism for abdominal pain has not been established. Right upper quadrant discomfort could be due to hepatic edema and hemorrhage, with distension of Glisson's capsule. Epigastric pain may result from ischemic pancreatitis or gastritis. It must be stressed that the occurrence of abdominal pain, liver dysfunction, and thrombocytopenia can precede the development of hypertension and proteinuria by one or more days. Pruritus is not generally observed and its presence should suggest another diagnosis. The most sensitive test to detect hepatocellular involvement in this disease is an abnormality of serum transaminase activity. Usually, the elevations are mild, i.e., in the range of 50 to 300 I.U., although elevations up to 2,000 units have been observed. Abnormalities in other liver function tests occur less frequently. Bilirubin elevations are usually mild and reflect both hepatic injury and intravascular hemolysis. Lactic dehydrogenase isoenzyme determinations can be helpful in establishing the hepatic contribution to the elevation of this enzyme. 5′-nucleotidase is usually normal but can be elevated when there is a cholestatic component.

Liver biopsy findings are similar to the histopathologic features of toxemia in other organs. Fibrin deposition can be observed in the hepatic sinusoids and periportal areas.[1] Hepatocellular injury can vary from lobular disarray and cellular pleomorphism to frank focal hepatocyte necrosis. If shock has complicated the process, massive centrizonal necrosis can be observed at autopsy. Inflammation is conspicuously absent. Hemorrhage can be present in severe cases.

The course of the liver dysfunction generally parallels that of the pregnancy-induced hypertension. If hepatic dysfunction has been detected in the antepartum period, resolution invariably occurs after delivery, usually within the first 3 to 5 postpartum days. Spontaneous resolution of the abdominal pain, liver dysfunction, and thrombocytopenia may occur prior to delivery, and on rare occasions the onset of this triad takes place in the immediate postpartum period. Infants born to mothers with toxemia, liver dysfunction, and thrombocytopenia have a higher incidence of intrauterine growth retardation than the infants of toxemic patients who do not have these findings. Liver dysfunction should therefore be considered a sign of severe toxemia. The hepatic abnormalities of toxemia rarely progress to frank liver failure.

The differentiation between hepatic failure caused by toxemia of pregnancy and acute fatty liver of pregnancy is very difficult because both diseases affect primigravidas and have multisystemic involvement. Liver biopsies frequently cannot be performed because these patients have coagulopathies. Furthermore, it has been suggested that acute fatty liver of pregnancy is the severe end of the spectrum of the liver dysfunction seen with toxemia of pregnancy.

Hepatic Rupture is a rare but life-threatening event. Outside of pregnancy, this condition is usually due to trauma. In pregnancy, however, spontaneous hepatic rupture may occur in women with severe toxemia gravidarum. It has been proposed that the vasoconstriction present in toxemia can produce hepatic ischemia, necrosis, and hemorrhage and that the latter can eventually dissect peripherally and rupture Glisson's capsule. Contributing factors could be the presence of disseminated intravascular coagulation with hemostatic failure and the sudden increases in intra-abdominal pressure associated with nausea and vomiting, seizures, and parturition. The typical history is that of a toxemic patient complaining of nausea, vomiting, and abdominal pain in the right upper quadrant or epigastric area who suddenly becomes anemic and develops hypovolemic shock. On occasion, the preoperative diagnosis is abruptio placentae and the patient is found unexpectedly to have massive hemoperitoneum when the abdomen is entered at the time of emergency cesarean section.

The most frequent localizations of hepatic hematomas are the anterior and superior aspects of the right lobe and the rupture site is usually on the inferior margin. A definitive diagnosis prior to the development of hypovolemic shock is difficult to make. A high index of suspicion should therefore be maintained in cases of toxemic patients complaining of right upper quadrant pain. Sonographic examination of the abdomen and selective angiography can be ancillary tools to detect an intrahepatic hematoma prior to rupture.

Although rupture of the liver is not a cause of hepatic failure, it is a serious catastrophe. Bis and Waxman[3] have recently reviewed the literature and reported a maternal mortality of 35 percent in 91 obstetrical cases. Intraoperative management is obviously directed at arresting the bleeding from the lacerated liver. Temporary intraoperative hemostasis can be accomplished by intermittent digital compression of the hepatic pedicle. Surgical repair can then be accomplished with atraumatic sutures on needles. When this is not possible because of the multiplicity and irregularity of the lacerations, packing of the liver with hemostatic materials such as gel foam can be tried. Drainage of the hepatorenal pouch has been recommended as part of the surgical management of this condition. When the lacerations involve the intraparenchymal portion of the vena cava or the hepatic veins, the condition is especially serious and a vascular surgeon should be consulted. In this situation temporary cannulation and occlusion of the vena cava or portal vein may be necessary prior to the repair of the injured vessel.[27]

Viral Hepatitis. The diagnosis of viral hepatitis is usually not difficult. The classic presentation of malaise, anorexia, nausea, jaundice, and right upper quadrant discomfort is well known. In patients with hepatitis B infection there is frequently a prodrome of arthralgia, occasionally urticaria, and other manifestations of immune complex disease. Hepatitis A may have a prodrome of gastrointestinal symptoms, general "flulike" manifestations, and even low-grade fever. Non-A, non-B hepatitis most often does not have a prodrome other than malaise and anorexia. The epidemiological setting in which these three forms of hepatitis occur is outlined in Table 18-1.

Biochemically, patients with viral hepatitis have high transaminases, with serum glutamic pyruvic transaminase higher than serum glutamic oxaloacetic transaminase, and varying bilirubin and alkaline phosphatase levels. Use of serological markers in the diagnosis of the type of viral hepatitis is summarized in Table 18-1.

Signs that a patient with viral hepatitis is developing liver failure include: (1) encephalopathy, which initially may present as a reversed sleep pattern and subtle

Table 18-1. Profile of Hepatitis A, B, and Non-A, Non-B

Parameter	Hepatitis A	Hepatitis B	Non-A, Non-B
Infectious agent	27-nm RNA virus (enterovirus-like)	42-nm DNA virus	Unknown
Antigen/Antibody	Antigen excreted in stool during incubation period until onset of jaundice	HBsAg in serum during acute disease, followed by anti-HBs after recovery	Unknown
	Anti-HA IgM in serum for 12–16 weeks	Anti-HBc in serum shortly after HBsAg; may persist as long as anti-HBs	
	Anti-HA IgG in serum for years	HBeAg in serum shortly after HBsAg; disappears before HBsAg does; never found in absence of HBsAg	
Transmission	Oral-fecal route	Parenteral, enteral, venereal, maternofetal	Parenteral, ?enteral, ?venereal, ?maternofetal
Factors that increase risk	Shellfish ingestion, food handling by infected person, poor hygiene, contaminated water supply	Drug addiction, hemophilia, dialysis (patients and personnel), homosexuality in males	Transfusion, drug addiction, hemophilia, dialysis, ?homosexual males
Factors that do not increase risk	Venereal or perenteral exposure to virus, blood transfusion, hemophilia	Food handling by infected person, shellfish ingestion	Unknown
Prognosis	Very good, short-term	Variable	Variable
Chronic hepatitis	Not observed	10% patients with acute hepatitis B	20–50% patients with acute hepatitis
Chronic carrier state	Not observed	< 0.5% of U.S. population	Probable
Prophylaxis	0.06 ml/kg immune serum globulin (effective in 80% of patients if given within 2 weeks of contact)	0.06 ml/kg of Hepatitis B immune globulin after needle stick or mucosal contact with HBsAg-positive blood or in sexual partners of patients with acute hepatitis B	10 ml Isg empiric contacts as in B
Isolation	In acute case until jaundice peaks; stool precautions until that time	Not necessary unless frank bleeding is present; otherwise only needle precautions	As in B

Anti-HA, antibody to hepatitis A antigen; HBsAg/Anti-HBs, hepatitis B surface antigen/antibody; HBcAg/anti-HBc, hepatitis B core antigen/antibody; HBeAg/anti-HBe, hepatitis B e antigen/antibody.

mental changes (such as inability to perform serial 7s), followed by the onset of confusion, drowsiness, tremors with asterixis, and then stupor and coma; (2) diminution of liver size detected by daily percussion and measurement; (3) edema and ascites, which are obviously difficult to detect in the pregnant patient but can be confirmed by ultrasound; and (4) bleeding diathesis, which is a late sign. The most sensitive biochemical index of fulminant hepatic failure is a prolonged prothrombin time, which correlates better with the histologic lesion of severe hepatitis with underlying necrosis than any other biochemical study.[5] A prothrombin time more than 3 s over control which does not correct with the administration of vitamin K_1, 10 mg daily for 3 days, is an ominous sign and should suggest severe liver injury. Any of the above features occurring in a pregnant patient with viral hepatitis should be absolute indications for admission to the hospital.

Budd-Chiari Syndrome. The Budd-Chiari syndrome is a disorder caused by obstruction of the hepatic venous outflow tract at any point between the sublobar veins and the entry of the inferior vena cava into the right atrium.[16,36] The obstruction can be caused by intravascular membranes in the hepatovenous tract or by extravascular compression of the hepatic venous drainage by a cyst, abscess, or neoplasm. This condition has occurred during pregnancy[16] and particularly in the postpartum period. The existence of a hypercoagulable state has been linked to the increased predisposition of pregnant and puerperal patients to develop generalized venous thrombosis.

The obstruction to venous flow can cause acute congestion and hypoxic hepatocellular damage. The hepatocyte injury is typically centrizonal. The increased venous pressure is transmitted to the portal system and results in portal hypertension.

The Budd-Chiari syndrome is characterized by the clinical triad of abdominal pain, hepatomegaly, and ascites. Patients with this syndrome have ascites as an early and prominent finding and lack the multisystem involvement seen in acute fatty liver of pregnancy. A definitive diagnosis depends on demonstrating venous obstruction on hepatic venography. If this is negative, a liver biopsy should be performed since it may show evidence of microvascular occlusion, a rare cause of the syndrome. The Budd-Chiari syndrome typically occurs in the puerperal period and the prognosis is poor. Khuroo and Datta[16] have recently reported that 8 of 16 patients with puerperal Budd-Chiari syndrome died within 1 year of the onset of disease.

Anticoagulant and thrombolytic therapy have been used for the treatment of this condition with uncertain results. Some advocate as the treatment of choice a side-to-side shunt, which decompresses the liver but has the notorious complications of central portosystemic shunts, namely encephalopathy, decreased hepatic blood flow, and hepatic failure. When a diaphragm or web is present in the inferior vena cava, surgical treatment is more helpful.[20]

Chronic Hepatic Failure

It is rare to encounter this problem in pregnancy, simply because patients with cirrhosis and borderline liver function are usually not able to conceive. However, occasionally this can occur. The problems presented by a patient with chronic liver disease and hepatic failure in pregnancy are usually those of: (1) complications of portal hypertension, particularly bleeding from esophageal varices and hemorrhoids; and (2) overt hepatic failure with encephalopathy, bleeding, and ascites. Ascites is rare in pregnancy and the complications of this, such as spontaneous bacterial peritonitis, are even rarer. The second syndrome is much less common than the first, since it is possible to have severe portal hypertension with good liver function and still conceive.

It is unusual for the diagnosis of chronic liver failure to be made initially in pregnancy. The patient has usually been seen before conception and the diagnosis is known. However, in a few rare instances this is not the case and the patient presents *de novo* in pregnancy with features of chronic liver failure.

In females of childbearing age there are six important causes of chronic liver disease, which are described below.

"Autoimmune" (Lupoid) Chronic Active Hepatitis. This condition[26] usually occurs in either young or perimenopausal women. Amenorrhea is frequent and pregnancy occurring in a patient with this disease is rare. The diagnosis should be suspected if the biochemical pattern is one of hepatocellular injury with marked elevation (> 10-fold) of transaminases and moderate hyperbilirubinemia. The hallmarks of the disease are marked hypergammaglobulinemia (usually > 3 g %) and the presence of autoantibodies, notably smooth muscle antibody, in a titer exceeding 1:32, and high titers of antinuclear antibody. Fifteen percent of patients have lupus erythematosus (LE) cells in their peripheral blood, hence the name lupoid hepatitis.[15] It should be stressed, however, that this is the only common denominator with systemic lupus erythematosus (SLE); liver involvement with SLE is rare and when it does occur is *not* chronic active hepatitis but mild focal hepatitis or aspirin hepatotoxicity.

Viral Hepatitis. Hepatitis B and non-A, non-B hepatitis cause chronic hepatitis in 10 percent and 30 to 50 percent, respectively, of patients with acute hepatitis. Approximately one-third of the patients with chronic hepatitis B infection will develop significant chronic active hepatitis and, potentially, cirrhosis with liver failure.[32] It is unknown how many of the patients with chronic non-A, non-B hepatitis develop a significant degree of liver damage, but it is generally accepted that the severity of the disease and the frequency of liver failure is less in non-A, non-B hepatitis.[2] Part of the diagnostic evaluation of a patient with chronic hepatitis is therefore a careful history, evaluating risk factors for viral hepatitis, particularly blood transfusions, previous parenteral drug abuse, tattoos, and other form of parenteral exposure. Serological screening for hepatitis B surface antigen (HBsAg) is essential. Chronic hepatitis in the absence of HBsAg excludes hepatitis B in the majority of cases.[32] Unfortunately, there is currently no marker for non-A, non-B hepatitis and the diagnosis is one of exclusion.

It should be stressed that hepatitis A does *not* cause chronic hepatitis and thus is not a consideration in such patients. Hepatitis A is an acute, self-limited disease.

Alcoholic Hepatitis and Cirrhosis. Females are more susceptible than males to the adverse affects of alcohol on the liver; nevertheless, at least 80 g of ethanol per day for many years is generally necessary to produce this lesion.[23] It is exceedingly uncommon in pregnancy. The classic histology on liver biopsy confirms the diagnosis but it is not advisable to perform this procedure during pregnancy.

Cirrhosis of Undetermined Etiology with Portal Hypertension. So-called cryptogenic cirrhosis, or cirrhosis without any known cause, may present during pregnancy. Although cirrhosis and pregnancy do not commonly occur together, patients with well-compensated hepatic function and severe portal hypertension may indeed conceive and continue to term. Many cirrhotic patients are asymptomatic and because of good hepatic reserve do not manifest features of hepatic failure such as generalized bleeding or hepatic encephalopathy. Those patients may remain undetected until they present with complications of portal hypertension such as bleeding hemorrhoids, gastrointestinal bleeding, or the onset of ascites early in pregnancy. Examination of the abdominal wall may show superficial abdominal collateral vessels, and ultrasound can demonstrate free intra-abdominal fluid late in pregnancy.

Wilson's Disease. Hepatolenticular degeneration or Wilson's disease is an inborn error of copper metabolism transmitted in an autosomal recessive pattern. Although the precise nature of the metabolic disturbance has not been established, the disorder can be viewed as a copper storage disease. It has been suggested that the basic problem is a hepatic defect in copper metabolism that leads to an impaired biliary excretion of copper and a decreased synthesis of ceruloplasmin. The defective biliary excretion of copper leads to hepatocyte accumulation of this metal and hepatotoxicity. The intrahepatic copper can be released to the peripheral circulation and then stored in other organs such as brain, cornea, kidneys, and red blood cells. This process is responsible for the clinical manifestations of the disease, namely, neurologic dysfunction, the corneal Kayser-Fleischer ring, renal dysfunction, and hemolytic anemia. *The disease should be suspected in any patient under the age of 40 with chronic liver disease or cirrhosis of unknown etiology*. The diagnosis can be made by the demonstration of a low ceruloplasmin level and elevation of both serum copper and urinary copper excretion. The definitive diagnosis is made by liver biopsy with quantitative determination of tissue copper. The Kayser-Fleischer ring can be present despite the absence of active liver disease. Furthermore, it is not diagnostic of Wilson's disease since patients with primary biliary cirrhosis may have a similar lesion.

Untreated patients have been considered to have impaired fertility due to anovulation. An increased incidence of early pregnancy loss has been reported, particularly in patients with overt clinical cirrhosis.[39] Deterioration of the disease does not generally occur during pregnancy, however, and remission has been observed in approximately half of the reported cases. The phenomenon has been attributed to a physiologic transplacental transfer of copper in the later part of pregnancy.

Therapeutic goals are to decrease the dietary intake of copper and to promote its excretion. D-Penicillamine is the agent of choice to achieve the latter objective. Although this drug crosses the placenta, no adverse fetal side effects have been associated with its use in Wilson's disease and the medication should probably be continued during pregnancy. A reduction of the dose of D-penicillamine is probably safe in the latter part of pregnancy, as the disease tends to improve prior to term.

Congenital Hepatic Fibrosis. This congenital disease is manifested histologically as presinusoidal fibrosis, dilatation of the extrahepatic duct system, or even hepatic cysts. When far advanced, it produces portal hypertension, but good hepatic function is usually maintained. The diagnosis can often only be made by liver biopsy. In patients with portal hypertension who have bled, porta-caval shunts are well tolerated, and it is thus important to make the diagnosis as soon as possible.

TREATMENT

Despite a plethora of literature over the past two decades evaluating new forms of therapy for acute hepatic failure, the mortality rate remains appallingly high, and controlled studies have shown no benefit from either exchange transfusion[29] or corticosteroids.[13] The mainstay of treatment remains extremely fastidious, supportive general medical therapy. A well-coordinated approach involving subspecialists in the areas of perinatology, hematology, nephrology, infectious disease, and gastroenterology-hepatology is usually necessary and this should occur in an intensive care setting in a tertiary medical facility. It is always essential to have a coordinating physician who makes clinical decisions regarding the appropriateness of certain treatment regimes and modalities, such as renal dialysis and Swan-Ganz monitoring. This individual must also make decisions regarding diagnostic workups which may be superfluous and even harmful, such as studies of the biliary tree or liver biopsy. Treatment of the patient with hepatic failure can conveniently be considered in relation to the conditions discussed below.

Hepatic Encephalopathy

While the pathophysiology of hepatic encephalopathy has not been clearly defined, certain facts are well established:

1. Factors responsible for hepatic encephalopathy are related to the bacterial colonic flora, and alteration of the bacterial content of the gut has become the cornerstone of therapy.
2. Products of nitrogenous metabolism are important in the production of coma, since this clinical state is frequently produced by the increased availability of proteins of exogenous (dietary) or endogenous (bleeding) origin to the colonic bacteria. Blood ammonia levels are related to the degree of hepatic encephalopathy, albeit in an inexact nonlinear fashion.

A cardinal principal in the treatment of hepatic encephalopathy is to reduce ammonia production in the colon. This can be accomplished by reducing the pH of the colon, decreasing intestinal transit time, and decreasing the population of colonic bacteria.

Lactulose is a nonabsorbable disaccharide which has been demonstrated in controlled trials to be effective in the treatment of hepatic encephalopathy. Its administration produces an acid diarrhea. The increased intestinal motility can reduce ammonia production in the colon by decreasing the exposure time of nitrogenous compounds in the stool to colonic bacteria. Reducing the pH of the colon will also decrease the ammonia flux. Lactulose can be administered orally or rectally. The dose for rectal administration is 250 ml in 250 ml of tap water, and this is given by retention enema for 30 to 45 min every 6 to 8 h. Lactulose by mouth is given in a dose of 15 to 60 ml, 3 to 4 times a day. Unlike neomycin, lactulose does not decrease the colonic bacterial count. Recent evidence suggests that these two medications are synergistic when administered together.[8]

Neomycin is an aminoglycoside that is poorly absorbed from the gastrointestinal tract. It reduces the population of urease-producing bacteria in the colon and thereby diminishes the total amount of ammonium generated. This antibiotic can be administered either orally or rectally. The total oral dose is 4 to 6 g/day. The rectal dose is 1 to 2 g in 100 to 200 ml of isotonic saline given twice or three times a day. It must be stressed that approximately 1 percent of the administered neomycin may be absorbed, and this amount can be nephrotoxic in the presence of renal failure.[6]

Protein restriction is also an important part of therapy. It is believed that the products of protein catabolism are responsible for the encephalopathy associated with hepatic failure. Protein sources can be exogenous (diet) or endogenous (gastrointestinal blood). Exogenous protein intake must be eliminated in the initial phase of the treatment of hepatic failure. Mixtures containing a large amount of branched-chained amino acids[28] may allow the administration of additional protein without increasing the risk of encephalopathy.[11]

The administration of *L-dopa* has recently been proposed for the treatment of hepatic encephalopathy.[31] Its mechanism of action is postulated to be competition by false neurotransmitters with the toxic amines produced in hepatic failure. This therapy, however, does not seem to be as effective as more conventional treatments and the reports of its success are anecdotal. For this reason, the use of L-dopa cannot be recommended.

Cerebral Edema

Cerebral edema may be an important cause of death in fulminant hepatic failure. Most of the data in this regard have been obtained from children with Reye's syndrome. Loss of doll's-eye movements and pupillary or ciliary-spinal reflexes may indicate cerebral edema and herniation. Papilledema is a late sign. Dexamethasone is the treatment of choice, but is rarely successful. In patients with Reye's syndrome, ventricular pressure measurements with vigorous use of mannitol in addition to dexamethasone have been advocated. However, there are no data to support the effectiveness of this therapy in the adult patient with fulminant hepatic failure.

General Management. Fluid and electrolyte balance, along with the general nutritional status of the patient, are crucial aspects in the management of this disorder. Early placement of CVP lines is recommended. In the presence of ascites a Swan-Ganz catheter provides more accurate information about volume-pressure status.

Adequate caloric intake is important in encephalopathic patients. While the patient is conscious and able to swallow and while adequate bowel sounds are present, oral feeding is obviously employed. In the intubated unconscious patient, feeding by a nasogastric tube is preferable to parenteral feeding. However, if the patient has a paralytic ileus, intravenous feeding of a minimum of 1,500 calories a day is recommended. This should be given in the form of carbohydrate and fat, since amino acids will increase the blood ammonia and also have an adverse effect on hepatic function.

Bleeding

The most life-threatening complication of hepatic failure in the pregnant patient is that of bleeding. The major cause of this problem is impaired hepatic synthesis of clotting factors. Vitamin K is rarely effective in this situation, since substrate is present but the liver is unable to perform its synthetic function. Factor repletion may be accomplished by frequent transfusion of fresh frozen plasma. There is no consensus as to what constitutes a safe prothrombin level in a patient who has not yet bled. It is not uncommon to find a prothrombin time which is more than 30 s prolonged, and an empiric rule of thumb is not to allow the prothrombin time to exceed 20 s over control values in a pregnant patient. This has to be balanced, however, against the effects on central venous pressure (CVP) of infusing large volumes of colloid, which is inherent in replacement of factors with fresh frozen plasma.

Hypoprothrombinemia and bleeding secondary to hepatic failure must be distinguished from disseminated intravascular coagulation. Fibrinogen levels may fall in liver failure and the partial thromboplastin time can rise; however, a fall in factor VIII, thrombocytopenia, and an increase in fibrin-split products over 40 μg/ml suggest the diagnosis of intravascular coagulation.

There should be an increased awareness of the propensity for gastrointestinal bleeding in these patients since this is one of the commonest sites of massive bleeding in hepatic failure. There are data indicating that cimetidine, while it may not affect overall survival, decreases the incidence of significant gastric bleeding in hepatic failure.[25] It is recommended that this be used intravenously as a prophylactic measure.

Respiratory Failure

Patients in hepatic failure typically have a respiratory alkalosis with a low PCO_2. This may have a protective effect since the hypocapnia may reduce the amount of cerebral edema. Attempts to correct the hypocapnia by adding dead space or by hypoventilation can increase cerebral edema and cerebral metabolic rate. Later in the course of hepatic failure, usually in the presence of thrombocytopenia, hemorrhage, and renal failure, the adult respiratory distress syndrome can occur.

Endotracheal intubation is an important part of the management of hepatic encephalopathy. This should be done in all patients who are in stage 4 coma to prevent aspiration, since paralytic ileus and gastric atony are so common and predispose to this problem. When hypoxemia occurs, intubation is mandatory. Most patients should be aggressively treated, if necessary with positive end-expiratory pressure. It should be added that patients with chronic liver disease are particularly prone to hypoxemia due to intrapulmonary shunting.

Sepsis

Sepsis is extremely common in hepatic failure and is a major cause of mortality. There are data to suggest that white cell function is impaired in this syndrome. The sources of sepsis are multiple in comatose patients. Aspiration pneumonia must be considered. Spontaneous bacterial peritonitis should always be suspected in the presence of ascites, and patients in hepatic failure with ascites should have frequent diagnostic paracenteses to rule out this complication. Spontaneous bacterial peritonitis does not occur only in the late stage of alcoholic cirrhosis, as may be the impression of readers of textbooks; it *does* occur in acute and subacute hepatic failure due to other causes and should always be considered a prime source of sepsis of unknown origin. Urinary tract sepsis secondary to indwelling catheters and bacteremia secondary to the use of intravenous catheters, CVP lines, and arterial lines also occur. Venous access routes may be infected with fungi. Biliary tract sepsis is always a possibility, particularly in patients with chronic liver disease, in whom the incidence of gallstones is higher than in the general population.[4] However, endoscopic retrograde cholangiography, which is often the only way of making the diagnosis of choledocholithiasis, is not a benign procedure as these patients may also have pancreatitis. Clinical judgment in this situation becomes paramount. Because of the risk of bleeding, a spinal tap should not be a routine procedure in patients with sepsis, and meningeal signs or focal neurologic deficit should be present before this diagnostic procedure is done. A further complication of lumbar puncture is the possibility of uncal herniation if intracranial pressure is elevated.

Use of Antibiotics. Since sepsis frequently complicates hepatic failure, antibiotic treatment is often employed early. The need for prophylactic antibiotics has not been established, and systemic antibiotics should only be used once clinical evidence of sepsis has been established. If the offending organism is identified, sensitivity disks should be used in the selection of antibiotics. However, in the patient with spontaneous bacterial peritonitis, in whom no organisms are found on gram stain or on culture, and when there are more than 500 neutrophils per square millimeter in the ascitic fluid, ampicillin and gentamicin should be administered. This should provide adequate coverage since the most common offending organism is *Escherichia coli*. If, however, after 48 h of therapy repeat aspiration of peritoneal fluid reveals no diminution in the numbers of bacteria or cells, clindamycin should be added to cover anaerobes, particularly Bacteroides fragilis. In the patient with obvious sepsis but without a definitive source of infection, ampicillin, gentamicin, and clindamycin are the drugs of choice. Although there is no adequate documentation of the potentiation of gentamicin toxicity in patients in liver failure, it is the authors' experience that gentamicin is more likely to precipitate and worsen preexisting renal failure than in the non–liver-compromised patient. It is strongly urged that gentamicin levels be assiduously checked and that if renal function is shown to deteriorate, a non-aminoglycoside be substituted for gentamicin. Cefoxitin is an acceptable alternative since this drug covers *B. fragilis;* the continued use of clindamycin is then not necessary.

Nystatin should be administered orally or down the nasogastric tube in patients receiving broad-spectrum antibiotics, in an attempt to prevent oral thrush and intestinal candidiasis.

Renal Failure

Renal failure complicating acute hepatic failure is ominous and a poor prognostic sign, particularly when it is due to the hepatorenal syndome. A high urine osmolality, low urinary sodium (< 10 mEq/L), and oliguria in the absence of hypovolemia are very suggestive of hepatorenal syndrome. It is frequently a terminal event in hepatic failure. The etiology is unclear, and there are no associated structural renal abnormalities. This syndrome may be due to vascular redistribution in the kidney, with blood being shunted from the cortex to the medulla. The major differentiation is from prerenal hypoperfusion, since the urine electrolytes and osmolality are similar in both disorders. The only way to distinguish between them is by measurement of wedged pulmonary pressures or CVP. Management of the underlying liver disease is the only treatment for hepatorenal syndrome. Acute tubular necrosis secondary to systemic complications is the other important cause of renal failure.

Hypokalemia

Hypokalemia may occur both as a consequence of the respiratory alkalosis and as a result of the use of diuretics. This is particularly true in patients in *chronic* liver failure. Adequate replacement of potassium chloride is obviously mandatory to correct this problem.

Additional Forms of Therapy

Since patients with hepatic failure frequently succumb from the complications of this disorder, the ideal of therapy is to provide support during the acute episode in the hope that the liver will regenerate and resume its prior function. Various modalities have been employed in an attempt to provide this support. Exchange transfusion[40] was the first of these modalities to give rise to optimism. However, controlled prospective studies have not shown this procedure to prolong life in patients with hepatic failure. Pig-liver perfusion,[9] charcoal-column perfusion,[43] asanguineous total body washout[18]—and even plasmapheresis[24]—have all been tried unsuccessfully in this regard. The last-named technique has not been utilized to any significant extent but there is no rationale to suggest that it would work better than exchange transfusions or total body washout. Unfortunately, there is currently no suitable form of therapy for hepatic failure other than fastidious general medical care, general support, and attention to the numerous complications of this disorder.

Obstetric Considerations

Delivery is indicated when hepatic failure is due to acute fatty liver of pregnancy or toxemia gravidarum since empirical evidence suggests that termination of pregnancy can induce remission of the hepatic dysfunction in these conditions. There is no solid evidence to suggest, however, that the course of hepatic failure induced by diseases other than acute fatty liver of pregnancy and toxemia gravidarum would be improved by delivery. Although the frequency of hepatic failure due to non-A non-B viral hepatitis has been reported to be increased in obstetric patients in India,[17] termination of the pregnancy in the acute or fulminant phase has not been shown to accelerate remission. Termination of the pregnancy should therefore only be performed for obstetric indications.

If hepatic failure occurs in the first or second trimester, the goal should be to provide supportive care for the acutely ill mother. Abortion could create additional serious problems in a patient with hemostatic failure or encephalopathy. The main risks are excessive bleeding, aspiration pneumonitis, and the introduction of a new source of infection. Hemorrhage complicating the termination of pregnancy could aggravate preexisting hypotension and renal failure. When hepatic failure occurs after viability has been achieved, however, delivery of the infant is indicated because of the considerable risk of intrauterine fetal death in a patient with hypotension and multiple organ failure. Induction of labor and vaginal delivery is preferable to cesarean section because it imposes a less severe demand on an already compromised hemostatic system. Local anesthesia is ideal for vaginal delivery in a woman with hepatic failure because of the fear of central nervous system bleeding with any of the techniques for regional block. If cesarean section is indicated, general anesthesia will be necessary. A discussion of the agents of choice is presented in Chapter 5.

Portal Hypertension and Esophageal Varices

Normal portal vein pressure is 5 to 10 mmHg. If portal vein pressures measured at surgery exceed 30 cm of saline and wedge hepatic vein pressures are greater than 4 mmHg above inferior vena caval pressures, portal hypertension is present.[32] A gradient of more than 12 mmHg between wedge hepatic vein pressure and inferior vena caval pressure indicates a significant risk of bleeding from varices.

When there is increased pressure in the portal system, collateral vessels develop in areas where veins draining the portovenous system are contiguous with those draining the caval system. The submucosa of the esophagus is clearly the most important of these sites as it is the most likely to bleed. Anastomoses form between the coronary vein and the azygos system, which gives rise to large collaterals in the esophagus and upper stomach.

Diagnosis. Traditionally, esophageal varices can be seen on a barium swallow. However, since barium esophagograms may miss at least half of the patients with varices and they involve the use of ionizing radiation, esophagoscopy is the method of choice for demonstrating these veins during pregnancy. This should be performed, however, only when bleeding has occurred. Even under these circumstances, it is often difficult to demonstrate that the varices are the source of bleeding. However, it is very important to attempt to identify the source of bleeding since gastritis and peptic ulceration occur frequently in patients with cirrhosis.

Portal hypertension is a troublesome complication of chronic liver disease in obstetric patients since portal pressure increases in late pregnancy and the pressure of the gravid uterus increases shunting through the azygos system. This results in increased blood flow through preexisting varices connected to the azygos system and an increased pressure in these varices. The risk of bleeding in late pregnancy is therefore enhanced.

A secondary problem is the morbidity associated with hemorrhoids. Since dilatation of the rectal veins is common during pregnancy, portal hypertension serves only to make the situation worse and to increase the likelihood of annoying rectal bleeding. The lower portion of the rectum normally drains into the inferior vena cava via the inferior hemorrhoidal veins, while the upper portion drains into the portal system via the superior hemorrhoidal veins. Anastomosis between these venous systems results in hemorrhoids. Collaterals in unusual sites, including the vagina, have been reported in a patient with severe portal hypertension and it is possible that significant bleeding can occur at any site.

The risk of pregnancy to a woman with portal hypertension has not been clearly defined. The traditional view has been that pregnancy increases the risk of bleeding from esophageal varices because of the increase in blood volume throughout gestation and the elevation of intra-abdominal pressure resulting from nausea and vomiting in the first trimester and from the second stage of labor. This view has been recently challenged by a retrospective study that has reported no increase in the incidence of variceal bleeding in obstetrical patients when compared with nonpregnant women.[7] This study also failed to demonstrate an increased incidence of bleeding in the peripartum period. Nevertheless, maternal mortality associated with portal hypertension and variceal bleeding remains significant and has been reported to be 18 percent in cirrhotic and 2 percent in noncirrhotic pregnant women.

Treatment of Bleeding Varices. Prophylactic. The best way to prevent variceal bleeding in a patient with prenatal hypertension is to reduce the portal pressure. In obstetric patients it seems prudent to prevent a prolonged second stage since this is likely to increase intra-abdominal and portal pressures. One therapeutic maneuver that has been shown to reduce the gradient between wedge hepatic vein pressure and inferior vena caval pressure is the administration of propranolol in a dose that reduces the pulse rate by 25 percent.[22] When this agent is used during pregnancy, intrauterine growth retardation and neonatal apnea, bradycardia, and hypoglycemia may occur. The decision to administer propranolol to an obstetric patient should therefore be made after an empirical assessment of the risk of gastrointestinal bleeding. Candidates for this therapy are patients who have bled prior to or during pregnancy. If propranolol is administered, fetal growth should be monitored with serial sonographic examinations. Furthermore, the neonatologists should be told that propranolol was given to the mother so that they will be aware of the possible need for resuscitation following delivery and for monitoring glucose levels in the neonatal period.[12]

Therapeutic. The mainstay of therapy is to arrest the bleeding. This can be done by pharmacologic or mechanical means. The mechanical method of choice is the use of a Sengstaken-Blakemore tube. Pharmacologic treatment consists of the intravenous administration of Pitressin. The use of a Sengstaken-Blakemore tube should be carried out in an intensive care setting and is preferable to the administration of Pitressin because of concerns about uterine vasoconstriction and irritability.

Although patients who have portocaval shunts have been successfully carried through pregnancies, an emergency shunt in a pregnant patient is very dangerous and not advisable. Treatment with a Sengstaken-Blakemore tube until stabilization has been achieved is preferable.

REFERENCES

1. Arias, F., Mancilla, and Jimenez, R.: Hepatic fibrinogen deposits in preeclampsia. N. Engl. J. Med., *295:*570, 1976.
2. Berman, M., Alter, H.J., Ishak, K.G. et al.: The chronic sequelae of non-A, non-B hepatitis. Ann. Intern. Med., *91:*1, 1979.
3. Bis, K.A. and Waxman, B.: Rupture of the liver associated with pregnancy: A review of the literature and report of 2 cases. Obstet. Gynecol. Surv., *31:*763, 1976.
4. Bouchier, I.A.D.: Postmortem study of the frequency of gallstones in patients with cirrhosis of the liver. Gut, *10:*705, 1969.
5. Boyer, J.L. and Klatskin, G.: Pattern of necrosis in acute viral hepatitis. Prognostic value of bridging (subacute hepatic necrosis). N. Engl. J. Med., *283:*1063, 1970.
6. Breen, K.J., Bryant, R.E., and Levinson, J.D.: Neomycin absorption in man. Studies of oral and enema administration and effect of intestinal tubation. Ann. Intern. Med., *76:*211, 1972.
7. Birtton, R.C.: Pregnancy and esophageal varices. Am. J. Surg., *143:*421, 1982.
8. Conn, H.O., Leevy, C.M., and Maddrey, W.C.: Lactulose in the treatment of chronic portal systemic encephalopathy. A prospective double-blind cooperative comparison of lactulose with neomycin. Gastroenterology, *67:*784, 1974 (Abstract).

9. Eiseman, B., Liem, D.S., and Rattucci, F.: Heterozygous liver perfusion in treatment of hepatic failure. Ann. Surg., *162:*329, 1965.
10. Erlik, D., Shramek, A., Brandstretter, and Bassan, H.: Surgical cure of primary hepatic vein occlusion syndrome by side-to-side postcaval shunt. Surg. Gynecol. Obstet., *114:*368, 1962.
11. Fischer, J.E. and Baldesarini, R.J.: Pathogenesis and therapy of hepatic coma. p. 386. In Popper, H., Schaffner, F. Eds.: Progress in Liver Diseases. Vol. 5, Grune & Stratton, New York, 1976.
12. Gladstone, G.R., Hordof, A., and Gersony, W.N.: Propanolol administration during pregnancy: effects on the fetus. J. Pediatr., *86:*962, 1975.
13. Gregory, P.B., Knauer, C.M., Kempson, R.L., and Thier, R.: Steroid therapy in severe viral hepatitis. A double-blind randomized trial of methylprednisone versus placebo. N. Engl. J. Med., *294:*681, 1976.
14. Holzbach, R.T.: Acute fatty liver of pregnancy with disseminated intravascular coagulation. Obstet. Gynecol., *43:*740, 1974.
15. Joske, R.A. and King, W.E.: The L.E. cell phenomenon in active chronic viral hepatitis. Lancet, *2:*477, 1955.
16. Khuroo, M.S. and Datta, D.V.: Budd-Chiari syndrome following pregnancy. Am. J. Med., *68:*113, 1956.
17. Khuroo, M.S., Teli, M.R., Skedmore, S. et al.: Incidence and severity of viral hepatitis in pregnancy. Am. J. Med., *70:*252, 1981.
18. Klebanof, G.: Early experience with total body washout for hepatic coma (Abstract). Gastroenterology, *64:*156, 1973.
19. Krejs, G.J. and Haemmerli, U.P.: p. 1572. In Schiff, L. Ed.: Diseases of the Liver, 5th Ed., J.B. Lippincott, Philadelphia, Toronto, 1982.
20. Lam, C.R., Gate, H., and Green, E.: Transcardiac membranotomy for obstruction of the hepatic portion of the inferior vena cava. Circulation, suppl., *31*, *32:*1, 1965.
21. Langer, B., Stone, R.M., Colapinto, R.F. et al.: Clinical spectrum of the Budd-Chiari syndrome and its surgical management. Am. J. Surg., *129:*137, 1975.
22. Lebrec, D., Poynard, T., Hillon, P., and Benhamou, J.P.: Propranolol for prevention of recurrent gastrointestinal bleeding in patients with cirrhosis. N. Engl. J. Med., *305:*1371, 1981.
23. Lelbach, W.K.: Organic pathology related to volume and pattern of ethanol use. In Gibbons, R.J. et al., Eds.: Research Advances in Alcohol and Drug Problems. Vol. 1. John Wiley & Sons, New York, 1974.
24. Lepore, M.J., McKenna, P.J., Martinez, D.B. et al.: Fulminant hepatitis with coma successfully treated by plasmapheresis and hyperimmune Australia-antibody-rich plasma. Am. J. Gastroenterol., *58:*381, 1972.
25. Macdougall, B.R.D., Bailey, R.J., and Williams, R.: H_2-receptor antagonists and antacids in the prevention of acute gastrointestinal hemorrhage in pulmonary hepatic failure: two controlled trials. Lancet, *1:*617, 1977.
26. Mackay, I.R., Taft, L.T., and Cowling, D.C.: Lupoid hepatitis Lancet, *2:*1323, 1956.
27. Madden, J.L.: Surgery of the liver and bile system in pregnancy. In Barber, H.R.K. and Graber, E.A., Eds.: Surgical Disease in Pregnancy. W.B. Saunders, Philadelphia, 1974.
28. Mattson, W.J. Jr., Iob, V., and Sloan, M.: Alterations of individual free amino acids in brain during acute hepatic coma. Surg. Gynecol. Obstet., *130:*263, 1970.
29. Miller, D.J., Saunders, S.J., Hickman, R., and Terblanche, J.: Acute hepatic necrosis: A review of causes and management of fulminant hepatic failure. p. 64. In A. Read, ed.: Gastroenterology, Butterworth, 1975.
30. O'Loughlin, S., Sweeney, E.C., Keelan, P.: Persistent hypoglycemia and severe hyponatremia in a case of acute fatty liver of pregnancy. J. Indian Med. Assoc., *64:*45, 1971.

31. Parkes, J.D., Sharpstone, P., and Williams, R.: Levodopa in hepatic coma. Lancet, *2:*1341, 1970.
32. Redeker, A.G.: Viral hepatitis: Clinical aspects. Am. J. Med. Sci., *270:*9, 1975.
33. Reynolds, T.B.: Portal hyptertension in disease of the liver. p. 394. In Schiff, L., Ed.: J.B. Linppincott, Philadelphia, Toronto, 1982.
34. Romero, R. and Riely, C.A.: The changing prognosis of acute fatty liver of pregnancy. (In preparation.)
35. Romero, R., Synder, E., Rickles, F. et al.: The clinical significance and mechanism of thrombocytopenia in pregnancy-induced hypertension. (Abstract.) Society of Gynecological Investigation Meeting, March 1982.
36. Sherlock, S.: Classification of functional aspects of portal hypertension. Am. J. Surg., *127:*121, 1974.
37. Sherlock, S.: Patterns of hepatocyte injury in man. Lancet, *1:*782, 1982.
38. Speroff, L.: Prostaglandin and Reproduction. Fertility and Sterility. (Submitted for publication.)
39. Toaff, R., Toaff, M.E., Peyser, M.R., and Streifler, M.: Hepatolenticular degeneration (Wilson's disease) and pregnancy. Obstet. Gynecol. Surv., *32:*497, 1977.
40. Trey, C., Burns, D.G., and Saunders, S.J.: Treatment of hepatic coma by exchange blood transfusions. N. Engl. J. Med., *274:*473, 1966.
41. Varner, M. and Rinderknecht, N.K.: Acute fatty metamorphosis of pregnancy. J. Reprod. Med., *24:*177, 1980.
42. Warren, R.L., Schlant, R.C., Wenger, N.K., and Galambos, J.T.: Treatment of Budd-Chiari syndrome with streptokinase. (Abstract.) Gastroenterology, *62:*200, 1972.
43. Weber, F.L. Jr., Snodgrass, P.J., Powell, D.E. et al.: Abnormalities of hepatic mitochondral urea-cycle enzyme activities and hepatic ultrastructure in acute fatty liver of pregnancy. J. Lab. Clin. Med., *94:*27, 1979.
44. Willson, R.A., Winch, J., Thompson, R.P.H., and Williams, R.: Rapid removal of paracetamol by hemoperfusion through coated charcoal. Lancet, *1:*77, 1973.

19

Cardiac Failure and Arrhythmias during Pregnancy

Steven J. Mason, M.D.

Pregnancy imposes a significant hemodynamic burden on the cardiovascular system, and many healthy women develop symptoms and signs of cardiopulmonary overload during pregnancy. Previously undetected or only mildly symptomatic cardiac disease may deteriorate during pregnancy, with life-threatening or fatal results. The incidence of heart disease in obstetric patients is quite high, averaging 2 percent in the United States (range 1.2 to 3.7 percent).[1] Furthermore, cardiac disease is the leading nonobstetrical cause of maternal death in the United States[35] and the British Isles.[5,85] The etiology of the cardiac disease in Hibbard's[35] series of maternal fatalities was 36 percent rheumatic, 23 percent congenital, 17 percent myocarditis or cardiomyopathy, and 13 percent myocardial infarction. The causes of death in those cases in which it could be determined were congestive heart failure (CHF) (61 percent), myocardial infarction (13 percent), Eisenmenger's syndrome or primary pulmonary hypertension with hemodynamic collapse (8 percent), bacterial endocarditis (8 percent), embolization (6 percent), and ventricular arrhythmia (4 percent). The most likely cardiac disease to be encountered, therefore, is rheumatic heart disease, and its most likely complication is CHF.

HEMODYNAMIC CHANGES DURING NORMAL PREGNANCY AND LABOR

In order to anticipate and manage cardiac problems in obstetrical patients with heart disease, it is important to understand the course of development and magnitude of hemodynamic alterations during normal pregnancy. Plasma volume begins to increase during the first trimester, averaging one-third greater than nonpregnant values at 21 to 24 weeks and reaching a peak 50 percent greater than baseline in the middle of the third trimester.[72] There is considerable individual variation in this increase, and the percentage gain is highest for the smallest women.[38] The gain is greater for multigravidae and for twin and triplet pregnancies.[73] In addition, there is an increase in red cell volume and hemoglobin, which averages 28 to 32 percent.[65,72] Since plasma volume rises more than red cell mass, the hematocrit will decrease. Hemoglobin levels and the oxygen-carrying capacity of maternal blood may be maintained, however, if iron and folic acid supplements are given to the mother.[12] This is of particular significance to the patient with cardiac disease. Since plasma volume and red cell volume both increase, there is a parallel expansion of whole blood volume.

Cardiac output also increases markedly, beginning in the first trimester and reaching a peak at the end of the second trimester of 27 to 64 percent greater than nonpregnant values.[44,97] During the last trimester, cardiac output remains the same or diminishes slightly if measured in the left lateral position. It diminishes markedly, however, when measured in the supine position in the third trimester, owing to the weight of the gravid uterus compressing the inferior vena cava and diminishing venous return.[45,58,99] During the first half of pregnancy the increased cardiac output is primarily achieved by an increase in stroke volume, while in the last trimester it is due to an increase in heart rate with a slight fall in stroke volume.[73,97]

Resting oxygen consumption increases during pregnancy, although not as much as the increase in cardiac output; consequently the arteriovenous oxygen gradient narrows. In normal pregnant women, exercise produces a greater increase in cardiac output than a similar amount of exercise in nonpregnant women; however in the presence of heart disease cardiac output cannot increase as much during pregnancy, the arteriovenous oxygen gradient widens, and there is reduced oxygen delivery to the periphery.[96] This is paricularly true for patients with mitral stenosis, even to a mild degree.

With the onset of labor, cardiac output increases progressively between contractions, by approximately 10 percent over prelabor levels early in the first stage and by 20 percent late in the first stage.[93] In the left lateral position cardiac output and stroke volume have higher average values between contractions than in the supine position; further increases during contractions are minimal in the lateral position but significant in the supine position.[93] This is due to positional differences in venous return, depending on the relationship of the gravid uterus to the inferior vena cava, as well as the "milking" of up to 500 ml of blood from the uterine circulation with each contraction.[2] Cardiac output reaches its peak just after delivery, with values as much as 80 percent higher than those prior to labor when delivery is performed vaginally under local anesthesia. This peak increase can be reduced to 59 percent with caudal and to 52 percent with spinal anesthesia.[92,93] With continuous epidural analgesia the gradual cumulative rise in cardiac output occurring between contractions during the late first and second stages of labor, thought to be related to pain and apprehension, can be prevented. However the peak postpartum rise in cardiac output, which is related to increased venous return from the emptying uterine blood pool, is not prevented.[94]

The immediate postpartum rise in cardiac output abates significantly by 1 h postpartum and disappears in a day or two. It is frequently accompanied by mild maternal bradycardia. The blood loss associated with uncomplicated vaginal delivery is 500 to 600 ml, and that for a cesarean section is 900 to 1,000 ml.[67,95]

CARDIOPULMONARY SYMPTOMS AND SIGNS IN NORMAL PREGNANCY

Certain complaints and physical findings frequently associated with cardiac disease in the nonpregnant patient may be common findings in the healthy pregnant woman. Dyspnea is one of the most frequent subjective sensations during pregnancy, found in up to three-fourths of patients by the thirtieth week.[57] It is due to physiological hyperventilation, which lowers maternal PCO_2 and augments fetal gas exchange, as well as to progressive elevation of the diaphragm secondary to the enlarging uterus. For the latter reason, orthopnea and paroxysmal nocturnal dyspnea may also develop. Fatigue and decreased exercise tolerance are almost universal and are related in part to the weight gain of pregnancy and in part to the greater cardiac output than is required by nonpregnant women for the same external work.[96] Lightheadedness, especially upon abrupt standing, and even syncope, are not unusual. Syncope may also occur in the supine position owing to obstruction to venous return by the gravid uterus.[44]

One of the most frequent developments towards the end of normal pregnancy is the appearance of peripheral edema. This has been estimated to occur during pregnancy in 50 to 83 percent of women without antecedent renal or cardiac disease; the incidence increases with age.[39,68] Bibasilar rales may occur in the absence of CHF presumably because an elevated diaphragm causes compression of the lower lungs and atelectasis. Elevation of the diaphragm similarly displaces the cardiac apex upward and laterally and, with the increased cardiac output associated with pregnancy, the apical impulse may be quite forceful as well as leftwardly displaced. A right ventricular lift may also be a normal finding. When pregnant women are studied carefully and serially by auscultation and phonocardiography, loud wide-splitting of the first sound may be found in 88 percent, systolic flow murmurs along the left sternal border in 96 percent, an S3 in 84 percent, and an S4 in 16 percent.[18] Continuous murmurs may appear during pregnancy. In the neck the increased cardiac output may cause a venous hum, which can be eliminated by moving the head forward or using light pressure over the jugular vein.[32] Another continuous murmur may appear during the last half of pregnancy or during lactation over either breast. This mammary *souffle* may be obliterated by pressure and arises from increased venous or internal mammary arterial flow.[32] Diastolic murmurs are distinctly unusual in healthy obstetric patients; indeed, the murmur of aortic insufficiency present prior to conception may disappear during pregnancy, presumably owing to decreased peripheral vascular resistance (decreased afterload).[48]

DETECTION OF CARDIAC DISEASE AND CONGESTIVE HEART FAILURE IN PREGNANCY

Some women will be aware of the diagnosis of cardiac disease and their physicians of the risk of CHF prior to the onset of pregnancy. However, as many as half of the patients who are found to have cardiac disease during pregnancy are previously unaware of the condition. In the presence of the above-mentioned normally developing cardiopulmonary symptoms and signs, the diagnosis of heart disease and the detection of CHF may be difficult. Burwell and Metcalfe[11] have suggested that unless at least one of the following four findings is present, maternal cardiac disease can be excluded: a diastolic murmur, significant cardiac enlargement by x-ray, a grade III/VI or more intense systolic murmur, or a severe arrhythmia (e.g., sustained atrial fibrillation or flutter, or complete heart block). More recently McAnulty et al.[50] have suggested that attention also be paid to the occurrence of hemoptysis, syncope, or anginal chest pain on exertion; cyanosis; clubbing; and the development of severe or progressive dyspnea, orthopnea, or paroxysmal nocturnal dyspnea. Szekeley and Snaith[89] differentiated three types of heart failure with distinct clinical manifestations and prognosis: right heart failure, pulmonary congestion, and acute pulmonary edema. The diagnosis of right heart failure was based on abnormal jugular venous distension and excessive peripheral edema without other obvious causes. Pulmonary congestion was present when there was undue exertional dyspnea in the presence of pulmonary rales and/or x-ray signs of interstitial edema. Pulmonary edema was diagnosed when there was acute dyspnea with cough, frothy sputum, pulmonary congestion, and intra-alveolar edema. Over the last half century the incidence and mortality of right heart failure, particularly that due to rheumatic heart disease, have declined owing to better management and earlier surgical intervention.[89] In older series, when pulmonary congestion worsened to frank pulmonary edema, maternal mortality was as high as 30 to 41 percent.[41,89] The decreased incidence of pulmonary edema in recent years and consequent decreasing mortality from CHF[85,89] relates in part to the decreasing incidence of rheumatic fever, earlier surgical intervention, and, hopefully, better medical management.

Heart failure of any type has its onset in approximately 4 percent of cases in the first trimester; 20 percent in the second trimester; 17, 20, and 32 percent in the seventh, eighth, and ninth months respectively; and 9 percent in the puerperal period.[89] Failure is more likely to occur with mitral stenosis than with any other valvular lesion, with increasing age of the mother, and with increasing degree of cardiac enlargement as measured by cardiothoracic ratio on chest x-ray. Women with paroxysmal atrial tachycardia, even in the presence of rheumatic heart disease, are no more likely to develop heart failure than women who maintain sinus rhythm, but women with paroxysmal or established atrial fibrillation before the onset of pregnancy have a higher incidence of CHF. The risk of developing failure is 3 times as high if atrial fibrillation begins during pregnancy.[89]

Aside from paroxysmal arrhythmias, CHF may be precipitated by physical exertion, toxemia, embolism, transfusion, emotional distress, and miscarriage.[89] In the absence of paroxysmal arrhythmia, it is unusual for heart failure to develop during labor in a patient who is fully compensated prior to its onset.[89] This is one argument for early hospitalization of patients with significant cardiac disease near term.

ETIOLOGY OF CONGESTIVE HEART FAILURE IN PREGNANCY

In Table 19-1 the etiologies of CHF developing in pregnancy are listed. These have been divided into disease states present prior to conception and those arising during pregnancy or as a consequence of it. The ratio of rheumatic heart disease to congenital heart disease in pregnancy has been falling. This is due both to the decreasing incidence of acute rheumatic fever and to increasing surgical success in treating previously inoperable congenital heart disease so that more of these patients are reaching the childbearing age. Nevertheless, even in recent series, rheumatic heart disease comprises at least 80 percent of heart disease in pregnancy.[85] The most likely cause of CHF in a pregnant woman, therefore, is mitral stenosis since it is the most common rheumatic lesion in young women and has a higher risk than other valvular lesions of causing CHF during pregnancy.[89] The particular risk of CHF in pregnancy complicated by mitral stenosis is due to the fact that the pressure gradient across the mitral valve is directly proportional to cardiac output and heart rate, both of which increase significantly in pregnancy. Moreover, if the patient develops atrial fibrillation, with its attendant marked rise in heart rate and loss of atrial "kick," the

Table 19-1. Etiology of Congestive Heart Failure in Pregnancy

I. Cardiovascular disease present prior to pregnancy
    A. Rheumatic heart disease
    B. Congenital heart disease
        1. Pressure overload: aortic stenosis, idiopathic hypertrophic subaortic stenosis, coarctation of the aorta, pulmonic stenosis
        2. Volume overload: left-to-right shunts
        3. Cyanotic congenital lesions: right-to-left shunts
    C. Hypertension
    D. Endocarditis
    E. Arrhythmia
II. Diseases arising during or as a result of pregnancy
    A. Peripartum cardiomyopathy
    B. Toxemia of pregnancy
    C. Myocardial infarction
    D. Pheochromocytoma

risk is even higher. In Szekeley and Snaith's series,[89] 23 percent of patients with mitral stenosis developed CHF, in contrast to 7 percent with aortic regurgitation and 5.5 percent of patients with mitral regurgitation. Patients with rheumatic aortic stenosis are unlikely to develop CHF during pregnancy, primarily because this lesion does not generally become hemodynamically significant until later in life. The largest reviews in the presurgical era reported no cases of heart failure or other complications of rheumatic aortic stenosis in pregnancy.[54,89] The overall incidence of CHF in pregnant women with rheumatic heart disease in Szekeley and Snaith's large series[89] was 20 percent in the years from 1942 to 1971, with a progressive fall with each passing decade. In the more recent series of Sugrue,[85] covering the decade ending in 1978, the incidence of heart failure was only 12 percent for rheumatic heart disease. The functional class of the patient prior to conception, particularly in the presence of mitral stenosis, is no guide to either the risk of developing CHF or of dying during pregnancy. A woman who was functional class III or IV (New York Heart Association classification) prior to pregnancy or during a previous pregnancy is likely to have severe problems with CHF in the absence of operative intervention. However, a woman in class I or II prior to pregnancy may also be at risk. Sugrue et al.[85] found that 39 percent of patients developing heart failure had been in functional class I prior to the onset of failure.

The incidence of CHF in pregnancy complicated by congenital heart disease is also falling. Mendelson[54] in his extensive review found the following risks of congestive heart failure: tetralogy of Fallot 40 percent, congenital aortic stenosis 25 percent, Lutembacher's syndrome (atrial septal defect with mitral stenosis) 20 percent, atrial septal defect 10 percent, coarctation 9 percent, ventricular septal defect 8 percent, and patent ductus arteriosus 6 percent. Most recently Whittemore et al.[100] have reported no maternal mortalities and an incidence of failure of only 7 percent in 233 mothers with congenital heart disease. The risk was only 1 percent for women in functional class I prior to the onset of pregnancy while it was 25 percent for women in poorer functional classes. Congenital aortic stenosis and cyanotic congenital heart disease carried the highest risks, 19 and 11 percent, respectively. Importantly, in the group with "excellent" or "good" results from surgical repair of cyanotic congenital heart disease, there were no cases of CHF, while two out of the three patients who were only "fair" or "poor" following partial or complete repair did develop CHF.[100]

The high risk of heart failure as well as fetal and maternal death in congenital aortic stenosis deserves further comment. Arias and Pineda[4] carefully reviewed 23 patients reported in the literature and found documented severe aortic stenosis to be present in only 7. In those 7 there were 4 maternal and 7 fetal mortalities in a total of 12 pregnancies. Consideration should be given, therefore, to termination of pregnancy or elective operative intervention if an obstetric patient has severe aortic stenosis. Oxytocin has been reported to cause ventricular fibrillation in one case,[69] but intra-aortic balloon pumping proved beneficial for cesarean delivery of another.[4]

Patients with left-to-right shunts in the absence of pulmonary hypertension rarely develop difficulty during pregnancy because the increased hemodynamic burden is well tolerated by a compliant pulmonary vascular bed. The combination of a left-to-right shunt and pulmonary hypertension at or near systemic levels comprises Eisenmenger's syndrome. Obstetrical patients with this syndrome have a very high mortality rate due, not to CHF, but to hemodynamic collapse and reversed shunting across the defect. This complication will be discussed later.

As indicated in Table 19-1, bacterial endocarditis and arrhythmias may aggravate the hemodynamic burden of preexisting rheumatic or congenital heart disease and precipitate congestive heart failure. Both these complications are extremely rare causes of CHF in women without preexisting heart disease. The occurrence of a fever should always raise the question of endocarditis, particularly when CHF begins more than 1 day postpartum. Sugrue et al.[86] found a 4 percent incidence of maternal bacteremia in the peripartum period and reviewed 27 cases of endocarditis following an uncomplicated vaginal delivery. Antibiotic prophylaxis of all women with a pathological heart murmur using ampicillin and gentamicin is recommended beginning at the onset of labor or 1 h prior to cesarean section and continued for 48 h postpartum. In a patient with a borderline-compensated hemodynamic state, not only will profound tachycardia or bradycardia precipitate CHF but very frequent atrial or ventricular ectopic beats may also be detrimental. Appropriate treatment should be undertaken promptly, as outlined in the section on arrhythmias.

Peripartum cardiomyopathy refers to a congestive cardiomyopathy or myocarditis beginning during the last trimester of pregnancy or during the 6 months following delivery, for which no other etiology can be found. There is considerable disagreement as to whether this is a specific entity arising as a consequence of pregnancy, whether pregnancy precipitates preexisting latent left ventricular failure, or whether myocarditis develops coincidentally during the course of pregnancy. The clinical picture is that of a diffusely dilated left ventricle with poor contractility and characteristic signs and symptoms of left ventricular failure with associated arrhythmias and pulmonary and systemic emboli. There is a significant mortality, and the long-term prognosis is variable. If the cardiomegaly resolves within 6 months following delivery, later difficulty is unusual. However, if cardiomegaly persists, subsequent pregnancy is associated with high maternal mortality, and even without pregnancy there is a significantly shortened life span.[19,20]

Toxemia of pregnancy is dealt with in detail in Chapter 11. Dyspnea and even pulmonary edema may develop as complications in a small percentage of cases. In those cases that have been hemodynamically monitored there is disagreement as to whether pulmonary edema is due to leaky capillaries with normal left heart pressures or due to left ventricular failure.[67,83]

Myocardial infarction is a rare complication of pregnancy. The etiology may be atherosclerosis; however, some patients have had normal coronary arteriograms shortly thereafter, which raises the possibility of embolism with subsequent recanalization or coronary spasm.[74] Eclampsia may predispose to coronary spasm.[7] Occasionally the infarction is due to dissection arising in the aorta or limited to the coronary arteries themselves. If premature labor begins soon after a myocardial infarction, terbutaline should be avoided since angina has been reported during its use.[90]

Pheochromoctyoma is also very rare during pregnancy but carries a maternal mortality of almost 50 percent.[25] Persistent or intermittent hypertension, arrhythmias, and CHF are the usual manifestations. Clinical management involves use of alpha- and beta-blocking agents and has been reviewed by Smith[77] and in Chapter 14.

TREATMENT OF CONGESTIVE HEART FAILURE IN PREGNANCY

The principles of management of CHF developing in pregnancy are similar to those of heart failure developing at any other time. They are summarized in Table 19-2 and include measures to increase peripheral oxygen delivery, decrease circulatory demand, augment myocardial contractility, decrease intravascular volume, and decrease left ventricular afterload.

Increasing peripheral oxygen supply is of only modest benefit in improving CHF in most patients. In more advanced states, such as pulmonary edema or severe cyanotic congenital heart disease, this assumes an important role. Supplemental oxygen by nasal cannula or face mask should be administered if CHF is severe enough to warrant hospitalization. If the hematocrit is less than 30 percent, transfusion of packed red blood cells is appropriate after initiating diuresis. Transfusion both improves oxygen-carrying capacity and decreases the high cardiac output of anemia. Supplemental iron and possibly folic acid are important to minimize the "physiological anemia" of pregnancy. In the patient who develops CHF at a high altitude, consideration occasionally must be given to persistent oxygen supplementation or to removing her from the high altitude for the duration of pregnancy. Finally, carbon monoxide exposure through heavy cigarette smoking, prolonged exposure to automobile fumes, or occupational exposure causes irreversible deoxygenation of hemoglobin. This is avoidable.

Decreasing peripheral circulatory demand is likewise important in the control of CHF. Prompt attention to arrhythmias (see below) and pharmacological suppression, if necessary, improve cardiac output and decrease myocardial demand. Suffi-

Table 19-2. Management of Congestive Heart Failure in Pregnancy

I. Increase oxygen supply
   A. Supplemental oxygen
   B. Correct anemia (transfusion, iron supplements)
   C. Avoid high altitudes and carbon monoxide exposure
II. Decrease peripheral demand
   A. Control arrhythmias
   B. Rest, especially after meals
   C. Control fever and treat infection
   D. Avoid extremes of temperature and humidity
   E. Avoid psychological stress
   F. Correct polycythemia (hyperviscosity)
   G. Treat high-output states (thyrotoxicosis, beriberi)
   H. Avoid certain drugs and additives (thyroid hormone, caffeine and theophylline compounds, sympathomimetics, bronchodilators, ritadrine, and terbutaline)
III. Augment myocardial contractility
   A. Digitalis
   B. Avoid myocardial depressants: beta blockers, disopyramide, alcohol
IV. Decrease intravascular volume
   A. Diuresis
   B. Restrict salt and fluid intake
   C. Avoid intravenous overload from fluids or rapid transfusion
V. Decrease left ventricular afterload
   A. Control hypertension
   B. Vasodilators (hydralazine)

cient rest is important, especially following meals, as pregnant women with cardiac disease cannot adequately increase their cardiac output with exercise. Bed rest at home for prolonged periods or hospitalization to enforce bed rest may be necessary. Fever should be promptly suppressed with antipyretics and the source of infection aggressively sought and treated. Extremes of temperature and humidity increase cardiac output and can be controlled. Psychological stress should be avoided wherever possible. Patients with cyanotic congenital heart disease have a tendency to develop compensatory polycythemia. Above a hematocrit of 55 percent the increasing viscosity adds more to cardiac work load than the benefit from increased peripheral oxygen-carrying capacity. Consideration may be given to periodic phlebotomies in such patients. In addition to anemia, thyrotoxicosis and beriberi rarely may complicate pregnancy and cause a further increase in cardiac output. These conditions are medically correctable. Finally, certain drugs and food additives may increase cardiac output and precipitate or aggravate CHF. These include thyroid hormone, caffeine (in coffee, tea, or cola beverages) theophylline compounds in bronchodilators, and sympathomimetic compounds in over-the-counter cold and sinus remedies. Occasional patients with underlying cardiac disease who have been given ritadrine or terbutaline to suppress premature labor have had CHF precipitated.[22,84]

Myocardial contractility may be increased by digitalis compounds. Digoxin is the most frequently used of these preparations and modestly increases contractility. Although digoxin readily crosses the placenta, there is no associated fetal toxicity or report of its teratogenicity. In fact, maternal serum digoxin concentrations are lower than usual during pregnancy and quite high doses may be necessary in order to attain therapeutic blood levels.[71] Other drugs may suppress myocardial contractility and should be avoided in the presence of CHF. These include beta blockers, disopyramide, and alcohol.

The cornerstone of treatment of heart failure is reduction of intravascular volume. This is achieved through restricting salt use and, when failure is florid, restricting fluid intake. Intravenous overload from fluid administration or aggressive transfusion should be avoided. In more severe forms of congestive failure, diuretics are necessary despite the fact that they may potentially decrease placental perfusion.[26] Electronic fetal heart rate monitoring should be performed whenever maternal CHF is treated in the third trimester. Thiazides or furosemide may be administered with appropriate caution to avoid hypokalemia. Rare cases of neonatal juandice[17] and thrombocytopenia[70] have been reported when thiazides were administered prior to delivery.

Finally, decreasing left ventricular afterload in the presence of CHF may improve placental blood flow and augment cardiac output. Hypertension should be controlled (see Ch. 11) and even in the presence of normal blood pressure, vasodilators such as hydralazine are beneficial in improving cardiac output.[14] The more potent vasodilator nitroprusside has been associated with reports of fetal cyanide poisoning.[60] Thiocyanate is a known metabolic breakdown product of the drug. Some authors restrict the use of nitroprusside to less than 30 min in the prepartum state. Hydralazine may be given, if necessary, parenterally, with similar hemodynamic effects and no known toxicity.

Patients with severe heart failure who do not respond promptly to the conventional treatment modalities outlined above or in whom the etiology is not clear, are candidates for invasive hemodynamic monitoring. The safety and usefulness of this technique in pregnant women have been demonstrated.[67,83] If the heart failure does not resolve promptly or if significant failure recurs despite an aggressive medical regimen, then consideration must be given to operative intervention. The experience with cardiac surgery during pregnancy has been reviewed.[91,102] In patients with mitral stenosis, closed mitral valvotomy can be accomplished with little maternal or fetal morbidity. Closure of a patent ductus arteriosus is the only other major cardiac operation which does not require cardiopulmonary bypass and can be accomplished with little risk. Operative interventions that require extracorporeal circulation, such as replacement of the mitral or aortic valve and closure of intracardiac left-to-right shunts, are associated with significant fetal wastage, especially during the first trimester. This subject has been discussed at length in Chapter 4.

In certain situations termination of pregnancy should be seriously considered. These include severe aortic stenosis and uncorrected cyanotic congenital heart disease in which medical management or surgical repair during pregnancy carries high maternal and/or fetal risk.[4,100] In these patients, however, subsequent operative repair may allow a full-term pregnancy with little risk to either the mother or fetus. In addition, uncorrectable maternal diseases, including Eisenmenger's syndrome and primary pulmonary hypertension, both of which carry maternal mortalities greater than 30 percent for each pregnancy,[28,51] should be considered strong indications for termination.

EISENMENGER'S SYNDROME

Eisenmenger's syndrome may be defined as the occurrence of pulmonary hypertension equal to, or nearly equal to, systemic blood pressure, in the presence of a congenital cardiovascular lesion that allows shunting from the right to the left side of the heart. The shunt may occur at the aortopulmonary, ventricular, or atrial level and is usually caused by a patent ductus arteriosus, ventricular septal defect, or atrial septal defect, respectively. Wood[101] originally described the 12 different congenital lesions tht may produce Eisenmenger's syndrome. It may develop in 3 percent of patients with congenital heart disease;[13] however, with its intrinsically high morbidity and mortality, as well as its potential preventability with early aggressive corrective cardiac surgery, the true incidence in the childbearing population with congenital heart disease is probably lower.

Eisenmenger's syndrome in pregnancy has an extremely high maternal mortality rate. In women with Eisenmenger's syndrome, 30 percent of all pregnancies result in the death of the mother,[28] and despite its rarity amongst cases of congenital heart disease, it is responsible for 55 percent of all maternal deaths due to congenital cardiac disorders.[5]

An appreciation of the pathophysiology of Eisenmenger's syndrome is important in understanding the risks as well as the treatment of complications in the crucial peripartal period. Pulmonary hypertension, which is the sine qua non of Eisenmenger's syndrome, arises over a period of years as a consequence of high flow through the pulmonary circulation. The congenital defects associated with Eisenmenger's syndrome all initially produce left-to-right shunting, with much higher flow rates through the pulmonary than the systemic circulation. In some patients this leads to progressive irreversible pathological changes in the pulmonary microvasculature,[33] which in turn result in increased pulmonary vascular resistance and pulmonary hypertension. As pulmonary vascular resistance rises in relation to systemic resistance, shunt flow from left to right gradually decreases and eventually there may be bidirectional shunting or predominantly right-to-left shunting with cyanosis. Once pulmonary vascular changes occur, they are irreversible, and if the pulmonary pressure and resistance reach near-systemic levels, the patient is inoperable because although the shunt may be closed, the severe pulmonary hypertension leads to rapid death from right ventricular failure and hypoxia. If the congenital lesion is not detected and corrected in childhood, it may be too late. While many patients with Eisenmenger's syndrome have had the diagnosis established before adulthood and may have had CHF, arrhythmis, cyanosis, or syncope, a few patients are entirely asymptomatic, even through pregnancy.[40] Many women with Eisenmenger's syndrome go through the antepartum period without aggravation of their symptoms, but the immediate postpartum period carries a high risk of syncope, systemic hypotension with shock, severe cyanosis, and death. The final common denominator is increasing right-to-left shunt across the congenital defect with increasing hypoxia and cyanosis leading to pulmonary vasoconstriction and further right-to-left shunting. The exact precipitant of this catastrophic cycle is frequently impossible to define. Any factor which increases pulmonary resistance or pressure or decreases systemic resistance or pressure can initiate the cycle. Specific precipitants that have been cited include pulmonary thromboemboli, volume loss secondary to postpartum bleeding (particularly in association with cesarean section, tubal ligation, or abortion after 20 weeks), and toxemia.[28]

In counseling and caring for the woman with Eisenmenger's syndrome who is considering pregnancy or has become pregnant, it is important to understand the risks to the unborn child as well as to the mother. Slightly more than half of pregnancies will result in living children, as there is a high incidence of fetal wastage due to spontaneous abortion and death in utero.[28,42] The maternal functional classification has no prognostic value for fetal outcome since half of the patients in functional class I will spontaneously abort.[42] Likewise, this classification system is not correlated with maternal survival. The risk of maternal mortality is no less in asymptomatic or minimally symptomatic women than in their more symptomatic counterparts.[28] Moreover, a previously uncomplicated pregnancy offers no assurance of maternal survival in a subsequent pregnancy, the maternal mortality rates being identical for first, second, and third pregnancies.[28]

Only 32 percent of pregnancies in women with Eisenmenger's syndrome in whom gestational age is known will proceed to term (greater than 38 weeks), while 68 percent will be delivered prematurely. Even accounting for prematurity, a third of the babies show growth retardation for gestational age. The overall perinatal mortality is 28 percent and is primarily proportional to the degree of prematurity. The total fetal wastage (including spontaneous abortion) is 42 percent.[28]

Gleicher et al.[28] reviewed 115 cases reported in the literature and excluded all those patients in whom the diagnosis of Eisenmenger's syndrome was not definitely documented by catheterization before pregnancy or within 1 year or at autopsy.

They found that 30 percent of all pregnancies in patients with documented Eisenmenger's syndrome led to maternal death. When every pregnancy experienced by this group was considered, it was found that 52 percent of the women died of pregnancy-related complications.

The logical recommendation for women with Eisenmenger's syndrome is that they do not become pregnant or if pregnant, seek an early abortion. Abortions performed earlier than 20 weeks are much safer than any type of delivery after that time.[28] If, despite knowing these sobering facts, a woman chooses to proceed with pregnancy, there are a number of recommendations that can be made for optimal care during pregnancy, delivery, and the immediate postpartum period.

A coordinated management plan between perinatologist and cardiologist is necessary throughout pregnancy. The usual attention to maternal nutrition, vitamins, and iron supplements is essential. In order to avoid hypoxia it is important for the mother to have prolonged periods of rest. Some patients with Eisenmenger's syndrome will have established right-to-left shunting with cyanosis and compensatory polycythemia. Since the viscosity of blood doubles when the hematocrit increases from 50 to 70 percent,[49] with consequent significant increases in pulmonary vascular resistance, consideration should be given to phlebotomizing such patients if it can be shown to improve their hemodynamics. Supplemental oxygen at home may be recommended in some instances. The increased work load of pregnancy may precipitate CHF and arrhythmias; digitalis, diuretics, and antiarrhythmics may be required. Special care must be given to avoid situations in which the systemic resistance falls, thereby leading to increased right-to-left shunting. Respiratory and urinary infection should be detected early and treated aggressively. The risk of toxemia was reported to be 18 percent, which is higher than for uncomplicated pregnancies, in the review of Gleicher et al.[28] It is not clear, however, that pregnancies complicated by toxemia carry a higher maternal mortality. Although it has not been proven to affect outcome, it is prudent to recommend elective hospitalization for the duration of the pregnancy at approximately 20 weeks of gestation. This will allow for optimal treatment of CHF and hypoxia as well as for concerted planning by perinatologist, cardiologist, and anesthesiologist.

The role of anticoagulation before delivery is controversial. Forty-four percent of maternal deaths have been associated with thromboembolic phenomena,[28] and postmortem examination in some but not all patients has shown disseminated thromboemboli in the pulmonary microcirculation.[59] Pitts et al.[64] argue that anticoagulation was of no benefit in preventing five deaths among seven patients with Eisenmenger's syndrome. However, in none of these patients was anticoagulation started before delivery and as pointed out by Gleicher et al.,[28] only one of the patients was adequately anticoagulated postpartum. In view of the high risk of embolization it would seem prudent to initiate anticoagulation in the second trimester. Heparin should be administered intravenously if the patient is hospitalized or subcutaneously if she resists this recommendation. Heparin is preferable to warfarin (see below). If, however, warfarin is used, the patient should be switched to heparin at the beginning of the third trimester since premature labor is likely to occur and warfarin increases the risk of peripartal fetal hemorrhage.[31,82] Heparin should be stopped at the onset of labor, restarted 6 h following delivery, and continued until 10 days postpartum.

The final complication of Eisenmenger's syndrome in pregnancy is that of syncopal spells, frequently associated with cyanosis. In the published case reports these are more likely to occur in the last half of pregnancy,[16,42] and this is another reason to advise early hospitalization. The exact precipitant is not clearly documented, but cyanosis, systemic hypotension, and tachycardia are frequently reported. Crawford et al.[16] were successful in treating two such episodes with leg elevation and 0.25 mg phenylephrine intravenously, although in view of the decreased uteroplacental flow caused by most pressors, ephedrine might be a preferable agent.[76] High-concentration face-mask oxygen and intravenous atropine should also be available since syncope may be a manifestation of the same phenomenon that causes hemodynamic collapse postpartum.

Planning for delivery begins early. Cesarean section is reported to be associated with a very high mortality rate. Gleicher et al.[28] found a 74 percent maternal mortality for abdominal delivery of either living or stillborn infants compared with a 34 percent maternal mortality for vaginal delivery. These figures may be somewhat skewed because of emergency cesareans performed on the sickest patients in the process of hemodynamic deterioration. The anticipated blood loss for a cesarean section is usually larger than for a vaginal delivery, potentially causing hypotension and increased right-to-left shunting. Nevertheless, in patients in whom a very prolonged labor is anticipated because of cephalopelvic disproportion or other reasons, an elective operative delivery might be considered. With careful hemodynamic monitoring a successful elective cesarean section despite several episodes of postoperative hypoxia and cyanosis has been reported.[80]

Spontaneous vaginal delivery is recommended rather than cesarean section for most patients. Elective induction with an unfavorable cervix, however, carries the risk of a long labor as well as an increased risk of needing to perform a cesarean section.

Once labor has begun, intensive hemodynamic monitoring is suggested. Systemic arterial and triple-lumen pulmonary arterial catheters should be inserted in order to monitor systemic and pulmonary arterial pressures, systemic arterial oxygen saturation, and the magnitude of shunt.[56,80] Maternal EKG and fetal heart rate monitoring should be continuously employed. Detailed hemodynamic studies in two patients during labor showed no significant difference in arterial oxygen concentration, systemic blood pressure, or shunt flow between the supine and lateral decubitus positions.[56,80] Oxygen should be administered by face mask in the maximum concentration available since this may increase pulmonary blood flow and decrease right-to-left shunting; high oxygen concentration is much more effective than low oxygen concentration.[56] Nevertheless, in some patients even high inspired oxygen concentrations may have no effect on the elevated pulmonary vascular resistance. In one study[56] oxytocin infusion (dose unspecified) produced no change in shunt flow or arterial oxygen saturation, while uterine contractions were associated with increased systemic and pulmonary pressure, decreased pulmonary/systemic flow ratio, and increased right-to-left shunting. The administration of epidural anesthesia was not associated with any change in shunt flow or oxygenation,[56,80] but measurements during a contraction after application of low forceps in the second stage of labor showed slightly more right-to-left shunting and arterial hypoxia.[56] Caridac output roughly doubles at the time of delivery.[80] If oxytocin is needed, a dilute solution should be used since intravenous administration of large amounts of concentrated oxytocin may produce systemic hypotension,[34] thereby aggravating right-to-left shunting. Immediately following delivery, if blood loss is appreciable, prompt transfusion should be carried out with whole blood that has been typed and cross matched beforehand.

Despite the increased cardiac demands, right-to-left shunting, and fall in oxygen saturation described above with labor and delivery, complications do not develop in many patients until the hours and days following delivery. The majority of maternal deaths have occurred within 8 days after delivery although pregnancy-related death up to 22 days postpartum has been reported.[28] Therefore, arterial and Swan-Ganz catheters should remain in place for several days and the patient should be monitored in the intensive care unit for 1 week postpartum. In the initial hours following delivery, the patient should not be allowed to sit up since this may elevate pulmonary arterial pressure; one carefully monitored patient arrested upon sitting up for a portable chest x-ray.[3] In those monitored patients who have developed hemodynamic collapse, the primary event appears to be a spontaneous rise in pulmonary artery pressure.[3,80] Presumably this represents pulmonary vasoconstriction, perhaps in response to changing hormonal balance in the postpartum period. As a consequence of this, cyanosis from right-to-left shunting, systemic hypotension, and bradycardia may result. In one carefully studied patient, phenylephrine and atropine administration proved useless, but the prompt administration of a high concentration of inhaled oxygen reversed an acute rise in pulmonary arterial pressure. In this patient, 48 h postpartum a decrease in inspired oxygen concentration still led to a significant rise in pulmonary artery pressure; consequently sustained high-concentration oxygen inhalation is recommended for several days postpartum. Aside from oxygen administration, no other agent has been of proven value. Midwall et al.[56] suggest the use of tolazoline or nifedipine as pulmonary vasodilators, but DeWitt and Noble[21] point out that isoproterenol, nitroprusside, and phentolamine may decrease systemic vascular resistance more than pulmonary vascular resistance, thereby producing more right-to-left shunting. Captopril has been shown to cause similar effects.[23] Dopamine may increase pulmonary artery pressure more than systemic pressure,[55] with similar results. Arias[3] suggests administering phenylephrine or levarterenol for hypotensive spells. With patients being hemodynamically monitored, these spells should be detectable early, pharmacologic intervention undertaken, and a better outcome obtained.

The best overall treatment would be prevention of Eisenmenger's syndrome by corrective operations upon children with large left-to-right shunts long before they reach childbearing age. Although this is increasingly being done, a few women will nevertheless present already pregnant. For these patients termination during the first trimester is unquestionably the safest recommendation.

Primary pulmonary hypertension is a condition of unknown etiology in which there is high pulmonary vascular resistance and pulmonary artery pressure, and like Eisenmenger's syndrome, a very high risk of maternal death related to pregnancy. Unlike patients with Eisenmenger's, those with primary pulmonary hypertension do not have any intracardiac shunt. Jones and Howitt[42] reviewed 8 deaths in 15 reported cases (53 percent). McCaffrey and Dunn[51] had earlier reviewed many of the same histories, however, and found 9 deaths in a total of 23 pregnancies, giving a true mortality based on total pregnancies of 39 percent, which is higher than that of

Eisenmenger's syndrome. Death in primary pulmonary hypertension is usually from spells of hypotension, cyanosis, and low cardiac output that occur in the immediate postpartum hours and days. It is possible that the slightly lower mortality of Eisenmenger's syndrome is due to a small protective advantage of the right-to-left shunt, which may contribute to systemic blood flow when pulmonary hypertension (presumably mediated by vasospasm) becomes severe.

Careful monitoring and analysis of the hemodynamic events at the time of these spells in the peripartum period has not been reported for patients with primary pulmonary hypertension; thus specific recommendations for therapy cannot be based on experience. It is prudent to strongly recommend avoidance of pregnancy, or if pregnancy occurs, early termination. That failing, recommendations similar to those for Eisenmenger's syndrome are logical: early and prolonged hospitalization with restricted activity, heparin anticoagulation long before delivery, supplemental oxygen, invasive monitoring of pulmonary and systemic pressure during and for several days after labor and delivery, vigorous treatment of blood loss, and early use of potent pulmonary vasodilators if low output pulmonary vasospastic spells occur.

MANAGEMENT OF CARDIAC ARRHYTHMIAS DURING PREGNANCY

Many women become aware of cardiac pulsations during pregnancy becasue of the faster heart rate and higher stroke volume and perhaps also because the heart is displaced upward and laterally by the elevated diaphragm. Awareness is therefore enhanced of all irregularities of cardiac rhythm, many of which are common in patients with entirely normal cardiac function. Atrial and ventricular premature contractions (occasionally in a bigeminal rhythm), wandering atrial pacemaker, and junctional rhythms all may occur.[89] In women with no evidence of organic heart disease, reassurance is generally all that is necessary.

First-degree atrioventricular (AV) block (P–R interval > 0.20 s) occurs rarely. It is usually an indication of active rheumatic fever or chronic rheumatic heart disease; less frequently it may be due to digitalis toxicity or toxemia.[54] In itself it does not adversely influence the outcome of pregnancy. Second-degree AV block, in which some P waves are not conducted into the ventricles, is always a sign of acquired heart disease. Possible etiologies include active or chronic rheumatic heart disease, syphilis, endocarditis, coronary artery disease, diphtheria, or polio. Occasional cases in the older literature were associated with maternal fatality due to heart failure.[54] Treatment is directed towards the underlying condition, and a pacemaker is rarely required. Third-degree AV block may occur in acquired cardiac disease or as a congenital abnormality. Congenital complete heart block is more likely to be well tolerated than acquired block.[54] Occasionally complete heart block will lead to CHF or syncopal episodes.[8,75] Insertion of a pacemaker is curative.[27]

Labor and delivery are a time of particular cardiac stress even in the normal patient. In one series of 13 healthy women without cardiac disease, *all* patients had arrhythmias when continuously monitored during labor, most of them asymptomatic.[98] Wandering pacemaker, atrial premature contractions (APCs), and ventricular premature contractions (VPCs) were reported, as well as sinus tachycardia up to a rate of 176 and asymptomatic supraventricular tachycardia. Spritzer et al.[81] reported that serious arrhythmias are more frequent in women with heart disease, but in their cases the potential effects of digitalis and general anesthesia could not be separated from the effects of the maternal heart disease.

Paroxysmal atrial tachycardia (PAT) is characterized by a rapid atrial rate, usually between 160 and 240 per minute, frequently with 1 : 1 ventricular conduction. Some authors believe that pregnancy increases the susceptibility of normal hearts to PAT.[88] In women with episodes of PAT prior to pregnancy, the arrhythmia tends to occur more frequently and with greater duration and severity during pregnancy.[53] The arrhythmia is most likely to occur in the last trimester[89] after cardiac output has reached its peak. In three-fourths of the patients who develop their first attack when pregnant, recurrences happen only during that or a subsequent pregnancy and not in the nonpregnant state.[89] This was found to be true even after a mean follow-up of 10 years.[87] Slightly more than half of patients with PAT complicating pregnancy have organic heart disease.[54] In those without cardiac disorders the arrhythmia does not affect fetal or maternal health. In the presence of organic heart disease, however, the rhythm may precipitate CHF, particularly if sustained for more than 6 h,[89] and, rarely, may lead to maternal death.[54] Of patients with PAT and rheumatic heart disease, 22 percent will develop atrial fibrillation in the same or a subsequent pregnancy.[89]

The differentiation of PAT from atrial flutter with 2 : 1 block is beyond the scope of this chapter, and the interested reader is referred to recent reviews on this subject.[43,62] Aside from CHF there is usually no clear-cut precipitating event, but hypoxia, anemia, electrolyte disturbance, and physical or emotional stress should be considered. Carotid sinus pressure may cause AV block and allow differentiation of the underlying rate and morphology of the atrial waves. This should not be undertaken without EKG monitoring and an intravenous line since fatal ventricular fibrillation has been reported to occur after carotid sinus stimulation.[36] Carotid sinus massage or other vagal stimulation such as the Valsalva maneuver or gagging may terminate PAT in as many as 80 percent of cases.[43] Edrophonium (Tensilon) is sometimes successful in terminating PAT because of its vagotonic effects but may cause hypotension and is therefore probably best avoided in pregnancy. Alpha-adreergic agents, such as phenylephrine, are also used in nonpregnant patients and work by raising the blood pressure through vasoconstriction and reflex increase of vagal tone. The vasoconstriction would reduce placental blood flow and these agents should therefore also be avoided. Digitalis compounds have long been the mainstay for treatment of PAT. Digoxin is given as an initial dose of 0.5 mg intravenously followed by two further doses of 0.25 mg at hourly intervals. Carotid sinus massage is repeated periodically since it may be efficacious with the additional vagotonic action of digoxin. Digoxin crosses the placenta, achieving equal levels in fetal and maternal serum,[71] but the fetus is quite tolerant of therapeutic levels of digoxin, and teratogenesis has not been reported.[9,94] Despite earlier beliefs to the contrary, digoxin therapy does not cause earlier or shorter labor in normal women.[61]

If digitalization and repeat carotid massage fail to convert the arrhythmia, there are two choices, propranolol or cardioversion. Propranolol is quite effective in terminating the arrhythmia because it slows conduction through the AV node and interrupts the reentrant cycle that is usually the cause of PAT. However, maternal and fetal morbidity have been reported. Propranolol has oxytoxic effects and may initiate preterm labor.[6] In patients with underlying CHF not due to tachyrhythmia, propranolol decreases myocardial contractility and may aggravate the failure. Intrauterine growth retardation has been reported as well as neonatal bradycardia, respiratory depression, and hypoglycemia.[9,15,29,94] These problems are more serious in patients receiving at least 160 mg/day of chronic oral propranolol but have been reported in patients receiving as little as 20 to 40 mg daily. It is likely that propranolol administered intravenously for a brief period of time will not be associated with these side effects, unless given near to term or during labor. Accordingly, the usual dosage is 1 mg administered intravenously every 5 min up to a total of 8 to 10 mg, while watching carefully for evidence of bronchospasm, hypotension, or CHF. Propranolol is contraindicated in patients with asthma and should be used with caution in women with diabetes.

Ueland et al.[94] have reviewed the use of cardioversion during pregnancy and concluded that it is generally a safe procedure. The only maternal complications were related to severe CHF and not the cardioversion itself. The one fetal complication was related to the loss of normal beat-to-beat variability in fetal heart rate following a cardioversion with 300 W · s for atrial fibrillation at 37 weeks of gestation. An emergency cesarean section was performed without complication. Only small amounts of electricity are necessary for cardioversion of PAT, frequently 20 W · s or less. Recent experience has shown that overdrive temporary pacing may also be used for termination of PAT.[43] In experienced hands this may be offered as an alternative when drug therapy has failed. The temporary wire has to be positioned under fluoroscopic control, but x-ray exposure to the fetus can be minimized by abdominal shielding.

Long-term prophylaxis against recurrence of PAT is most efficaciously achieved with digoxin. Propranolol is effective, but long-term administration is best avoided during pregnancy. Quinidine and procainamide are less efficacious.

Atrial fibrillation is the most common hazardous arrhythmia developing during pregnancy in patients with organic heart disease. When atrial fibrillation has occurred paroxysmally or has been established before pregnancy, 22 percent of patients will develop CHF; if the arrhythmia develops during pregnancy or the puerperium, the incidence of CHF is 62 percent.[89] Atrial fibrillation rarely develops in a normal heart and is usually associated with rheumatic mitral vavular disease, developing in the second or third trimester when blood volume and cardiac demand are maximal. In addition to the risk of CHF, atrial fibrillation carries a significant risk of pulmonary or systemic embolism, occurring in 13 to 23 percent of cases, usually within the first month or two of development of arrhythmia.[54,89] The risk of embolization can be reduced by anticoagulation. The morbid significance of the development of atrial fibrillation is indicated by the fact that in older series the maternal mortality in patients who developed this arrhythmia was 17 percent.[54]

Atrial fibrillation is recognized by the irregular nature of the pulse and R-R intervals on the EKG, a fact which may be less noticeable with rapid ventricular rates of response, and the undulating baseline of the EKG. The initial treatment of atrial fibrillation is directed at slowing conduction through the AV node and therefore controlling heart rate. This is usually readily accomplished with the use of intravenous digoxin in the same doses as used for the control of PAT. If necessary on a short-term basis, small doses of propranolol may also be administered to slow ventricular response. Verapamil has not had widespread use during pregnancy and is best avoided until more is known about its effects in obstetric patients.

The causative factor in the development of atrial fibrillation is usually the underlying cardiac disease and the added stress of pregnancy, but CHF, electrolyte disturbance, unnecessary cardiac stimulating substances, and thyrotoxicosis should be considered. In a certain number of patients, treatment with digoxin with or without propranolol will cause reversion to sinus rhythm. If this does not occur, further efforts should be devoted to restoring sinus rhythm if this is the first epidsode of atrial fibrillation. A return to sinus rhythm will significantly increase cardiac output and decrease the risk of heart failure and embolization. If the onset of atrial fibrillation can be accurately timed and is more than 2 weeks prior to the planned pharmacological or electrical cardioversion, the patient should be anticoagulated, since this will significantly reduce the frequency of embolization associated with conversion to sinus rhythm.[10] If atrial fibrillation is recent in onset and rheumatic in etiology, the chances of restoring sinus rhythm and maintaining it for a significant period of time may be as high as 90 percent.[87]

Following conversion to sinus rhythm, the patient should be maintained on quinidine to help prevent recurrence of the fibrillation.[78] Digoxin should also be continued in order to prevent rapid conduction of atrial fibrillation, should it recur. Serum levels of digoxin and quinidine must be carefully monitored during the remainder of pregnancy and reevaluated following childbirth. Quinidine tends to increase serum digoxin concentrations,[30] and digoxin levels in maternal serum rise significantly following delivery without change in the administered dose.[71] Quinidine is felt to be safe to use during pregnancy.[9,94] It does cross the placenta, achieving nearly the same level in the fetus as in maternal serum,[37] but adverse effects are rare. Thrombocytopenia has been reported in the newborn,[94] an effect which is known to occur rarely in adults taking quinidine.

Conversion is frequently successful pharmacologically. When anticoagulation is desirable prior to an attempt at conversion, the regimen described below should be followed. After the establishment of adequate levels of anticoagulation for 2 weeks, conversion is attempted using quinidine. Digoxin is withheld for 24 h and quinidine is instituted in a dosage of 300 mg PO every 6h. The digoxin is restarted at one-half the previous dosage. If conversion has not occurred after 48 h of quinidine therapy, the dosage may be increased to 400 mg every 6 h if the EKG does not show an increase in the QRS duration or QT interval more than 50 percent of the baseline. Trough serum levels should be checked 30 to 60 min before the sixth scheduled dose of the drug and the dosage adjusted accordingly. If conversion with quinidine is not successful, digoxin is withheld for 24 h while quinidine is continued, and the patient is scheduled for electrical cardioversion. Digoxin is restarted and quinidine therapy maintained following cardioversion.

If cardioversion fails to establish normal sinus rhythm or if atrial fibrillation recurs, further attempts at cardioversion should not be undertaken during pregnancy. Quinidine should be discontinued and the dosage of digoxin increased appropriately. Chronic atrial fibrillation, particularly in the presence of rheumatic mitral valve disease, is an indication for long-term anticoagulation in order to reduce the risk of pulmonary and systemic embolization. Anticoagulation clearly increases the risk of hemorrhagic complications to both the mother and the fetus, but in certain situations in which the risk of embolization in the unanticoagulated state is high, the benefits outweigh the risks. There is some controversy about the relative risk of heparin as opposed to warfarin anticoagulation.[31,94] Warfarin crosses the placental barrier and when administered during the first trimester, is well recognized as a cause of a specific embryopathy, with nasal hypoplasia and stippled epiphyses.[82] In addition, if administered near term, warfarin may lead to severe, even fatal, hemorrhagic complications in the fetus during delivery. Heparin, on the other hand, does not cross the placental barrier and therefore does not cause teratogenic effects or fetal or neonatal bleeding.[9] It may cause maternal hemorrhage, osteoporosis and fractures, and, rarely, transient alopecia or thrombocytopenia. It must be administered parenterally, either subcutaneously or intravenously, and is therefore both uncomfortable and inconvenient. Hall et al.[31] maintain that heparin is no safer than warfarin, but as pointed out by Ueland et al.,[94] Hall's series contains a large number of patients given heparin experimentally for severe preeclampsia, a condition known to be associated with significant maternal and fetal morbidity. Spearing et al.[79] have demonstrated the safety of long-term subcutaneous heparin administration, and this appears to be the method of choice. Dosages of 5,000 to 15,000 units subcutaneously every 12 h have been reported to be effective,[79] but more careful control can be achieved by administering smaller doses intravenously at 4-h intervals. Indwelling "butterfly" cannulae can be maintained long-term and changed every several days. Periodic monitoring of the activated partial thromboplastin time (PTT) is mandatory, and the dosage usually must be increased as pregnancy proceeds.[79] An alternative, but much less preferable, approach is to use heparin parenterally during the first trimester when organogenesis takes place, switch to oral warfarin for the second trimester, and return to heparin during the third trimester 6 weeks or more before term in order to anticipate a premature delivery. If premature labor occurs earlier than this, however, the effects of the warfarin on the fetus cannot be quickly reversed.

Atrial flutter is an unusual rhythm disturbance in pregnancy. When it occurs, it is usually due to rheumatic or congenital heart disease, myocarditis, or hyperthyroidism.[54] Electrocardiographically the rhythm is very regular, usually with a ventricular rate of 150 since the predominant atrial rate is 300 and 2:1 AV block is almost universal. If the ventricular rate is more than 180 per minute, PAT is much more likely. Atrial flutter is more difficult to control pharmacologically than PAT or atrial fibrillation. Carotid sinus massage and other vagal maneuvers may increase the degree of AV block, allowing a diagnosis, but is unlikely to break the arrhythmia. Digoxin should be administered in the same doses as in PAT, and short-term propranolol therapy may be instituted intravenously in order to control the maternal ventricular rate. If there are signs of hypotension or CHF, prompt cardioversion should be undertaken. If, on the other hand, the rhythm is reasonably well tolerated and does not convert with digoxin, quinidine should be administered 300 mg PO every 6 h, further doses of digoxin withheld, and cardioversion undertaken electrically 24 h later if sinus rhythm has still not been pharmacologically restored.

Although premature ventricular contractions are common in pregnancy, ventricular tachycardia and fibrillation are very rare. Ventricular tachycardia has been reported in two pregnant patients without evidence of cardiac disease.[52,63] For the acute management of life-threatening ventricular arrhythmias, intravenous lidocaine is the drug of choice. Lidocaine does cross the placenta, and very high serum maternal levels have been associated with neonatal depression, which may last for several days.[24,47] It appears to be safe for use in emergency situations, especially prior to labor,[9] but doses should be held to the necessary minimum. The usual dosage is 1 mg/kg intravenously, slowly, followed by a second similar bolus in 15 to 30 min, after which a continuous intravenous infusion at 2 mg/min should be administered. If the underlying situation precipitating the ventricular arrhythmia cannot be successfully corrected and the lidocaine discontinued in several hours, long-term suppression should be undertaken with quinidine administered orally, or if necessary, intramuscularly. There has not been much experience during pregnancy with other ventricular antiarrhythmic drugs. Procainamide is largely untested. Disopyramide should be avoided since it has been reported to reproducibly stimulate uterine contractions.[46] Phenytoin is a second-line ventricular antiarrhythmic with limited efficacy. It should be avoided during pregnancy if possible because of its teratogenicity and potential for causing intrauterine growth retardation.[9]

REFERENCES

1. Adams, J.Q.: Management of the pregnant cardiac patient. Clin. Obstet. Gynecol., *11*:910, 1968.
2. Adams, J.Q. and Alexander, A.M., Jr.: Alterations in cardiovascular physiology during labour. Obstet. Gynecol., *12*:542, 1958.
3. Arias, F.: Maternal death in a patient with Eisenmenger's syndrome. Obstet. Gynecol., *50*:76, 1977.
4. Arias, F. and Pineda, J.: Aortic stenosis and pregnancy. J. Reprod. Med., *20*:229, 1978.
5. Arthure, H., Tomkinson, J., Organe, G. et al.: Report on confidential enquiries into maternal deaths in England and Wales, 1967–1969. H. M. Stationery Office, Department of Health and Social Security, London, 1972.
6. Barden, T.P. and Stander, R.W.: Myometrial and cardiovascular effects of an adrenergic blocking drug in human pregnancy. Am. J. Obstet. Gynecol., *101*:91, 1968.
7. Bauer, T.W., Moore, G.W., and Hutchins, G.H.: Morphologic evidence for coronary artery spasm in eclampsia. Circulation, *65*:255, 1982.
8. Begg, T.B. and Thompson, W.R.: Stokes-Adams attacks in pregnancy. Br. Heart J., *23*:729, 1961.
9. Berkowitz, R.L., Coustan, D.R., and Mochizuki, T.K.: Handbook for Prescribing Medications During Pregnancy. Little, Brown, Boston, 1981.
10. Bjerkelund, C.J. and Orning, O.M.: The efficacy of anticoagulant therapy in preventing embolism related to D.C. electrical conversion of atrial fibrillation. Am. J. Cardiol., *23*:208, 1969.
11. Burwell, C.S. and Metcalfe, J.: Heart Disease and Pregnancy. Little, Brown, Boston, 1958.
12. Butler, E.B.: The effect of iron and folic acid on red cell and plasma volume in pregnancy. J. Obstet. Gynaecol. Br. Commonw., *75*:497, 1968.
13. Campbell, M.: Incidence of cardiac malformations at birth and later, and neonatal mortality. Br. Heart J., *35*:189, 1973.

14. Chatterjee, K., Ports, T.A., Brundage, B.H. et al.: Oral hydralazine in chronic heart failure: sustained beneficial hemodynamic effects. Ann. Intern. Med., *92:*600, 1980.
15. Cottrill, C.M., McAllister, R.G., Jr., Gelles, L. et al.: Propranolol therapy during pregnancy, labour and delivery. Evidence for transplacental drug transfer and impaired neonatal drug disposition. J. Pediatr., *91:*812, 1977.
16. Crawford, J.S., Mills, W.G., and Pentecost, B.L.: A pregnant patient with Eisenmenger's syndrome. Br. J. Anaesth., *43:*1091, 1971.
17. Crosland, D.M. and Flowers, C.E., Jr.: Chlorothiazide and its relationship to neonatal jaundice. Obstet. Gynecol., *22:*500, 1963.
18. Cutforth, R. and MacDonald, C.B.: Heart sounds and murmurs in pregnancy. Am. Heart J., *71:*741, 1966.
19. Demakis, J.G. and Rahimtoola, S.H.: Peripartum cardiomyopathy. Circulation, *44:*964, 1971.
20. Demakis, J.G., Rahimtoola, S.H., Sutton, G.C. et al.: Natural course of peripartum cardiomyopathy. Circulation, *44:*1053, 1971.
21. Devitt, H.J. and Noble, W.H.: Eisenmenger's syndrome and pregnancy. N. Engl. J. Med., *302:*751, 1980.
22. Elliot, H.R. and Abdulla, U.: Pulmonary edema associated with ritadrine infusion and betamethasone administration in premature labour. Br. Med. J., *2:*799, 1978.
23. Fagard, R., Bulpitt, C., Lijnen, P. et al.: Response of the systemic and pulmonary circulation to converting-enzyme inhibition (Captropril) at rest and during exercise in hypertensive patients. Circulation, *65:*33, 1982.
24. Finster, M., Morishima, H.O., Boyes, R.N. et al.: The placental transfer of lidocaine and its uptake by fetal tissues. Anesthesiology, *36:*159, 1972.
25. Fox, L.P., Grandi, J., Johnson, A.H. et al.: Pheochromocytoma associated with pregnancy: specialty team management and review. Am. J. Obstet. Gynecol., *104:*288, 1969.
26. Gant, N.F., Madden, J.D., Siiteri, P.K., and Macdonald, P.C.: The metabolic clearance rate of dihydroisoandrosterone sulfate. III. The effect of thiazide diuretics in normal and future pre-eclampic pregnancies. Am. J. Obstet. Gynecol., *123:*159, 1975.
27. Ginns, H.M. and Hollinrake, K.: Complete heart block in pregnancy treated with an internal cardiac pacemaker. J. Obstet. Gynaecol. Br. Commonw., *77:*710, 1970.
28. Gleicher, N., Midwall, J., Hochberger, D., and Jaffin, H.: Eisenmenger's syndrome and pregnancy. Obstet. Gynecol. Surv., *34:*721, 1979.
29. Habib, A. and McCarthy, J.S.: Effects on the neonate of propranolol administered during pregnancy. J. Pediatr., *91:*808, 1977.
30. Hager, W.D., Fenster, P., Mayersohn, M. et al.: Digoxin-quinidine interaction. Pharmacokinetic evaluation. N. Engl. J. Med., *300:*1238, 1979.
31. Hall, J.G., Pauli, R.M., and Wilson, K.M.: Maternal and fetal sequelae of anticoagulation during pregnancy. Am. J. Med., *68:*122, 1980.
32. Harvey, W.P.: Alterations of the cardiac physical examination in normal pregnancy. Clin. Obstet. Gynecol., *18:*51, 1975.
33. Heath, D. and Edwards, J.E.: The pathology of hypertensive pulmonary vascular disease. Circulation, *18:*533, 1958.
34. Hendricks, C.H. and Brenner, W.E.: Cardiovascular effects of oxytocic drugs used postpartum. Am. J. Obstet. Gynecol., *108:*751, 1970.
35. Hibbard, L.T.: Maternal mortality due to cardiac disease. Clin. Obstet. Gynecol., *18:*27, 1975.
36. Hilal, H. and Massumi, R.: Fatal ventricular fibrillation after carotid-sinus stimulation. N. Engl. J. Med., *275:*157, 1966.
37. Hill, L.M. and Malkasian, G.D.: The use of quinidine sulfate throughout pregnancy. Obstet. Gynecol., *54:*366, 1979.

38. Hytten, F.E. and Paintin, D.B.: Increase in plasma volume during pregnancy. J. Obstet. Gynaecol. Br. Commonw., *70:*402, 1963.
39. Hytten, F.E., Thomson, A.M., and Taggart, N.: Total body water in normal pregnancy. J. Obstet. Gynaecol. Br. Commonw., *73:*553, 1966.
40. Jewett, J.F.: Patent ductus arteriosus and pulmonary hyptertension. N. Engl. J. Med., *285:*1085, 1971.
41. Jones, A.M.: Heart disease in pregnancy. Proc. R. Soc. Lond. [Med.], *52:*767, 1959.
42. Jones, A.M. and Howitt, G.: Eisenmenger's syndrome in pregnancy. Br. Med. J., *1:*1627, 1965.
43. Josephson, M.E. and Kastor, J.A.: Supraventricular tachycardia: Mechanisms and management. Ann. Intern. Med., *87:*346, 1977.
44. Kerr, M.G.: Cardiovascular dynamics in pregnancy and labour. Br. Med. Bull., *24:*19, 1968.
45. Lees, M.M., Taylor, S.H., Scott, D., and Kerr, M.G.: A study of cardiac output at rest throughout pregnancy. J. Obstet. Gynaecol. Br. Commonw., *74:*319, 1967.
46. Leonard, R.F., Braun, T.E., and Levy, A.M.: Initiation of uterine contractions by disopyramide during pregnancy. N. Engl. J. Med., *299:*84, 1978.
47. Mann, L.I., Bailey, C., Carmichael, A. et al.: Effect of lidocaine on fetal heart rate and fetal brain metabolism and function. Am. J. Obstet. Gynecol., *112:*781, 1972.
48. Marcus, F.I., Ewy, G.A., O'Rourke, R.A. et al.: The effect of pregnancy on the murmurs of mitral and aortic regurgitation. Circulation, *41:*795, 1970.
49. Mair, D.D.: Effect of markedly elevated hematocrit level on blood viscosity and assessment of pulmonary vascular resistance. J. Thorac. Cardiovasc. Surg., *77:*682, 1979.
50. McAnulty, J.H., Metcalfe, J. and Ueland, K.: General guidelines in the management of cardiac disease. Clin. Obstet. Gynecol., *24:*773, 1981.
51. McCaffrey, R.M. and Dunn, L.H.: Primary pulmonary hypertension in pregnancy. Obstet. Gynecol. Surv., *19:*567, 1964.
52. McMillan, T.M. and Bellett, S.: Ventricular paroxysmal tachycardia: report of a case in pregnant girl of sixteen years with apparently normal heart. Am. Heart J., *7:*70, 1931.
53. Mendelson, C.L.: Disorders of the heart beat during pregnancy. Am. J. Obstet. Gynecol., *72:*1268, 1956.
54. Mendelson, C.L.: Cardiac Disease in Pregnancy. F.A. Davis, Philadelphia, 1960.
55. Mentzer, R.M. Jr., Alegre, C.A., and Nolan, S.P.: The effects of dopamine and isoproterenol on the pulmonary circulation. J. Thorac. Cardiovasc. Surg., *71:*807, 1976.
56. Midwall, J., Jaffin, H., Herman, M.V., and Kupersmith, J.: Shunt flow and pulmonary hemodynamics during labor and delivery in Eisenmenger's syndrome. Am. J. Cardiol., *42:*299, 1978.
57. Milne, J.A., Howie, A.D. and Pack, A.T.: Dyspnea during normal pregnancy. Br. J. Obstet. Gynaecol., *85:*260, 1978.
58. Mulholland, H.C. and Boyle, D. McD.: The effect of posture on the cardiac output during the last six weeks of pregnancy. Am. Heart J., *76:*291, 1968.
59. Naeye, R.L., Hagstrom, H.W., and Talmadge, B.A.: Postpartum death with maternal congenital heart disease. Circulation, *36:*304, 1967.
60. Naulty, J.C., Cefalo, R., and Rodkey, F.L.: Placental transfer and fetal toxicity of sodium nitroprusside. (Abstr. 543). Presented at the Annual Meeting of the American Society of Anaesthesiology, San Francisco, 1976.
61. Norris, P.R.: The action of cardiac glycosides on the human uterus. J. Obstet. Gynaecol. Br. Commonw., *68:*916, 1961.
62. Peters, R.W. and Scheinman, M.M.: Emergency treatment of supraventricular tachycardia. Med. Clin. North Am., *63:*73, 1979.

63. Pine, H.L., Fox, L., and Shook, D.M.: Paroxysmal ventricular tachycardia complicating pregnancy. Am. J. Cardiol., *15:*732, 1965.
64. Pitts, J.A., Crosby, W.M., and Basta, L.L.: Eisenmenger's syndrome in pregnancy. Am. Heart J., *93:*321, 1977.
65. Pritchard, J.A.: Changes in the blood volume during pregnancy and delivery. Anaesthesiology, *26:*393, 1965.
66. Pritchard, J.A., Baldwin, R.M., Dickey, J.C., and Wiggins, K.M.: Blood volume changes in pregnancy and the puerperium. II. Red blood cell loss and changes in apparent blood volume during and following vaginal delivery, cesarean section and cesarean section plus total hysterectomy. Am. J. Obstet. Gynecol., *84:*1271, 1962.
67. Rafferty, T.D. and Berkowitz, R.L.: Hemodynamics in patients with severe toxemia during labour and delivery. Am. J. Obstet. Gynecol., *138:*263, 1980.
68. Robertson, E.G.: The natural history of oedema during pregnancy. J. Obstet. Gynaecol. Br. Commonw., *78:*520, 1971.
69. Robinson, M., Newman, N., Creery, D.C. et al.: Congenital aortic stenosis in pregnancy; ventricular fibrillation induced by oxytocin. JAMA, *200:*378, 1967.
70. Rodriquez, S.U., Leikin, S.L., and Hiller, M.C.: Neonatal thromboctyopenia associated with antepartum administration of thiazide drugs. N. Engl. J. Med., *270:*881, 1964.
71. Rogers, M.C., Willerson, J.T., Goldblatt, A. et al.: Serum digoxin concentrations in the human fetus, neonate and infant. N. Engl. J. Med., *287:*1010, 1972.
72. Rovinsky, J.J. and Jaffin, H.: Cardiovascular hemodynamics in pregnancy. I. Blood and plasma volumes in multiple pregnancy. Am. J. Obstet. Gynecol., *93:*1, 1965.
73. Rovinsky, J.J. and Jaffin, H.: Cardiovascular hemodynamics in pregnancy. III. Cardiac rate, stroke volume, total peripheral resistance and central blood volume in multiple pregnancy: Synthesis of results. Am. J. Obstet. Gynecol., *95:*787, 1966.
74. Sasse, L., Wagner, R., and Murray, F.E.: Transmural myocardial infarction during pregnancy. Am. J. Cardiol., *35:*448, 1975.
75. Schonbrun, M., Roland, W., and Castro-Quiroz, A.: Complete heart block in pregnancy. Obstet. Gynecol., *27:*243, 1966.
76. Shnider, S.M., deLorimier, A.A., Holl, J.W. et al.: Vasopressors in obstetrics. I. Correction of fetal acidosis with ephedrine during spinal hypotension. Am. J. Obstet. Gynecol., *102:*911, 1968.
77. Smith, A.M.: Phaeochromocytoma in pregnancy. J. Obstet. Gynaecol. Br. Commonw., *80:*848, 1973.
78. Södermark, T., Johnsson, B., Olsson, A. et al.: Effects of quinidine on maintaining sinus rhythm after conversion of atrial fibrillation or flutter. Br. Heart J., *37:*486, 1975.
79. Spearing, G., Fraser, I., Turner, G. et al.: Long term self-administered subcutaneous heparin in pregnancy. Br. Med. J., *1:*1457, 1978.
80. Spinnato, J.A., Kraynack, B.J., and Cooper, M.W.: Eisenmenger's syndrome in pregnancy. Epidural anaesthesia for elective cesarean section. N. Engl. J. Med., *304:*1215, 1981.
81. Spritzer, R.C., Seldon, M., Mattes, L.M. et al.: Serious arrhythmias during labour and delivery in women with heart disease. JAMA, *211:*1005, 1970.
82. Stevenson, R.E., Burton, O.M., Ferlanto, G.J., and Taylor, H.A.: Hazards of oral anticoagulants during pregnancy. JAMA, *243:*1549, 1980.
83. Strauss, R.G., Keefer, R., Burke, T. et al.: Hemodynamic monitoring of cardiogenic pulmonary edema complicating toxemia of pregnancy. Obstet. Gynecol., *55:*170, 1980.
84. Stubblefield, P.G.: Pulmonary edema occurring after therapy with dexamethasone and terbutaline for premature labor: a case report. Am. J. Obstet. Gynecol., *132:*341, 1978.
85. Sugrue, D., Blake, S. and MacDonald, D.: Pregnancy complicated by maternal heart

disease at the National Maternity Hospital, Dublin, Ireland, 1969–1978. Am. J. Obstet. Gynecol., *139:*1, 1981.
86. Sugrue, D., Blake, S., Troy, P., and MacDonald, D.: Antibiotic prophylaxis against infective endocarditis after normal delivery—is it necessary? Br. Heart J., *44:*499, 1980.
87. Szekely, P. and Julian, D.G.: Heart disease and pregnancy. Curr. Probl. Cardiol., *4:*No. 6, 1979.
88. Szekely, P. and Snaith, L.: Paroxysmal tachycardia in pregnancy. Br. Heart J., *15:*195, 1953.
89. Szekely, P. and Snaith, L.: Heart Disease and Pregnancy. Churchill Livingstone, Edinburgh, 1974.
90. Tye, K-H., Desser, K.B., and Benchimol, A.: Angina pectoris associated with use of terbutaline for premature labor. JAMA, *244:*692, 1980.
91. Ueland, K.: Cardiac surgery and pregnancy. Am. J. Obstet. Gynecol., *92:*148, 1965.
92. Ueland, K., Gills, R.E., and Hansen, J.M.: Maternal cardiovascular dynamics. I. Cesarean section under subarachnoid block anaesthesia. Am. J. Obstet. Gynecol., *100:*42, 1968.
93. Ueland, K. and Hansen, J.M.: Maternal cardiovascular dynamics. III. Labor and delivery under local and caudal analgesia. Am. J. Obstet. Gynecol., *103:*8, 1969.
94. Ueland, K., McAnulty, J.H., Ueland, F.R. et al.: Special considerations in the use of cardiovascular drugs. Clin. Obstet. Gynecol., *24:*809, 1981.
95. Ueland, K. and Metcalfe, J.: Circulation changes in pregnancy. Clin. Obstet. Gynecol., *18:*41, 1975.
96. Ueland, K., Novy, M.J. and Metcalfe, J.: Cardiorespiratory responses to pregnancy and exercise in normal women and patients with heart disease. Am. J. Obstet. Gynecol., *115:*4, 1973.
97. Ueland, K., Novy, M.J., Peterson, E.W. et al.: Maternal cardiovascular dynamics. IV. The influence of gestational age on the maternal cardiovascular response to posture and exercise. Am. J. Obstet. Gynecol., *104:*856, 1969.
98. Upshaw, C.B.: A study of maternal electrocardiograms recorded during labor and delivery. Am. J. Obstet. Gynecol., *107:*17, 1970.
99. Vorys, N., Ullery, J.C., and Hanusek, G.E.: The cardiac output changes in various positions in pregnancy. Am. J. Obstet. Gynecol., *82:*1312, 1961.
100. Whittemore, R., Hobbins, J.C., and Engle, M.A.: Pregnancy and its outcome in women with and without surgical treatment of congenital heart disease. Am. J. Cardiol. *50:*641, 1982.
101. Wood, P.: The Eisenmenger syndrome or pulmonary hypertension with reversed central shunt. Br. Med. J., *2:*701, 1958.
102. Zitnik, R.S., Brandenburg, R.O., Sheldon, R., and Wallace, R.B.: Pregnancy and open-heart surgery. Circulation, *39:*suppl. I, I257–I262, 1969.

20

Cardiopulmonary Complications Associated with Beta-Adrenergic Tocolytic Therapy

Mark M. Jacobs, M.D.
Fernando Arias, M.D., Ph.D.

The introduction of beta-adrenergic drugs into the obstetric pharmacopeia represented a significant advance in our ability to effectively treat patients in preterm labor. The initial enthusiasm with the use of these compounds has been tempered, however, with the finding of frequent and occasionally severe adverse maternal cardiopulmonary effects occurring during their administration. Because of its potential for fetal and maternal death, pulmonary edema is the most important of these side effects. This complication was described first in the North American literature in 1978 by Stubblefield.[57] Other reports from the United States[31,35,47] and from Europe,[1,21,33] have enlarged the literature on this subject. Much of the existing information is confusing and the etiology of pulmonary edema in these patients is unclear.

In this chapter we will review some aspects of the clinical pharmacology of beta-adrenergic agents, the pathophysiologic changes of pregnancy and the effects of these agents that would predispose to pulmonary edema, the diagnosis of cardiovascular complications, and finally, their prevention and treatment. It should be clear, however, that our efforts are best directed toward prevention of preterm labor and not to the management of the adverse effects of its treatment.

CLINICAL PHARMACOLOGY OF BETA-ADRENERGIC TOCOLYTIC AGENTS

Beta-adrenergic agonists, long recognized as potent smooth muscle relaxants, are logical choices as tocolytic agents. Early attempts to utilize this type of drug included isoxsuprine hydrochloride,[27] a nonspecific beta-adrenergic agonist. Isoxsuprine's lack of specificity for uterine $beta_2$ adrenoceptors resulted in stimulation of cardiac $beta_1$ receptors, which caused unacceptable maternal tachycardia in as many as 30 percent of patients.[19] In addition, this agent has an alpha-adrenergic sympatholytic effect, which causes profound hypotension in many patients. To address these difficulties, more selective agents, capable of stimulating uterine $beta_2$ adrenoceptors with resultant tocolysis and with fewer cardiovascular side effects, were developed. Although all selective $beta_2$ agents have been shown to be efficacious as tocolytic agents, we will focus our discussion on ritodrine hydrochloride, a noncatecholamine $beta_2$-adrenergic agonist, which was approved for use as a tocolytic agent in the United States in 1980.[6,42]

In sheep studies,[53] beta- but not alpha-adrenergic blockade prevented both the uterine relaxation and the hemodynamic effects of ritodrine, suggesting specific beta-adrenergic activity. In humans, the pharmacokinetics of ritodrine have been studied in pregnant and nonpregnant patients by using a specific radioimmunoassay:[24] a serum level of 40 ng/ml was necessary to cause an increase of 20 percent in the heart rate of healthy volunteers, and this concentration was associated with tocolysis in pregnant patients. An intravenous infusion rate of 140 μg/min was required to achieve this serum level. The kinetics of intravenously administered ritodrine was complex and three half-lives (6 to 9 min, 1.7 to 2.6 h, and 3 h) were calculated. When 10 mg of ritodrine was administered intramuscularly, the peak serum concentration was 20 ng/ml, and one 20-mg oral dose resulted in a peak serum level of 10 ng/ml. Intramuscular administration resulted in peak serum concentrations in 10 min and a half-life of 2 h, while oral administration resulted in a serum peak at 20 to 40 min and a half-life of 1.3 h.

Tritium-labeled ritodrine is excreted in the urine promptly, maximum excretion rate is reached in 1 h, and ultimately 90 percent of the absorbed oral or intravenous dose is excreted in the urine. Excretion products consist of either unconjugated ritodrine or its glucuronide. In the rabbit, which was the most sensitive animal studied, the lethal dose (LD_{50}) of ritodrine was 64 mg/kg intravenously. This is nearly 200 times the intravenous dose that is administered hourly to humans. The cause of death in these rabbits was pulmonary edema and cardiovascular collapse.[44]

Multiple maternal cardiovascular and metabolic effects have been reported with ritodrine therapy. Cardiovascular effects include increased heart rate, decreased diastolic and increased systolic blood pressure, decreased total peripheral vascular resistance, increased velocity of myocardial fiber shortening, increased stroke volume, and increased cardiac output.[7,10,53] These cardiovascular effects are consistent with stimulation of cardiac $beta_1$ adrenoceptors by ritodrine, demonstrating a nonselective beta-agonist effect.

Metabolic effects include increased plasma levels of glucose, insulin, renin activity, aldosterone, lactate, and free fatty acids.[40,52] The effects on carbohydrate and lipid metabolism are exaggerated in diabetic patients.[40] A decrease in serum potassium during intravenous infusion has been consistently observed[29,38,40] and some studies have found increased urinary potassium and decreased body potassium stores,[29] while others have failed to show increased urinary potassium excretion.[39]

Several studies have failed to show alterations in maternal pH, $PaCO_2$, or PaO_2 during ritodrine infusion.[40,54] Maternal plasma renin activity is increased during ritodrine infusion[22] and serum aldosterone concentration is significantly raised by salbutamol,[39] another $beta_2$-adrenergic agonist.

Fetal effects of beta-adrenergic tocolytic agents can be expected since these drugs readily cross the placenta. In the case of ritodrine four of eight subjects who had simultaneous maternal and fetal serum concentration measurements exhibited approximately equal levels, while in the remaining patients maternal levels exceeded those in the fetus.[24] No teratogenic effects have been demonstrated[44] and, in general the fetal effects parallel those seen in the mother although the magnitude of cardiovascular and metabolic changes is usually less. However, in some cases these changes may be exaggerated and there are reports of fetal hypoglycemia, hypotension, hypocalcemia, and death.[11,51,59] Also, there is preliminary evidence that isoxsuprine may cause fetal cardiac septal hypertrophy[17] and increased liver, kidney, and heart weight in fetal rats.[16] Effects of beta-adrenergic agents on the fetal lung include evidence that short-term treatment may improve[62] and long-term treatment may harm[20,59] neonatal respiratory function.

PATHOPHYSIOLOGY OF PULMONARY EDEMA

The precise mechanism leading to the production of pulmonary edema, the most feared and important complication of beta-adrenergic tocolytic therapy, is not presently known. However, prevention, recognition, management, and the search for the eventual answer to this problem all require an understanding of the basic mechanisms of pulmonary edema.

About 10 to 15 percent of the total intravascular volume is contained within the pulmonary arteries, veins, and capillaries. Of the blood present in the pulmonary circulation, about 60 percent is in the pulmonary veins and the rest is almost equally divided between the pulmonary arteries and the capillaries. This blood flows through the lungs at a rate equal to the cardiac output. Under normal circumstances blood remains within the pulmonary vascular system because of the balance among several factors that regulate fluid exchange between the capillaries and the interstitial space, factors that are described by Starling's equation:

$$Fl = k(Pc - Pt) - d(p - t)$$

where
- Fl = movement of fluid
- k = permeability factor
- Pc = capillary hydrostatic pressure
- Pt = interstitial tissue hydrostatic pressure
- d = reflection coefficient
- p = plasma osmotic pressure
- t = interstitial tissue oncotic pressure

A representation of the relationships among the different variables described in this equation is shown in Fig. 20-1. Under normal conditions Starling's equation results in a small positive value (0.5 to 1.0 mmHg). This means that there is a constant movement of fluid from the intravascular into the interstitial space of the lung, which is efficiently removed by the pulmonary lymphatics and returned to the systemic circulation.[56] When one or more of these variables are altered and the Starling equation results in a large positive value, fluid will move from the intravascular into the interstitial space of the lung in amounts that exceed the capacity of the lymphatics to remove fluid, and pulmonary edema will develop.

Obviously, a derangement of any of the factors involved in Starling's equation may lead to pulmonary edema. In practice, decreased plasma colloid osmotic pressure and alterations of interstitial tissue pressure are rare primary causes of pulmonary edema. They are, however, factors which frequently contribute to the severity of the problem and alter the response to therapy. For example, intravenous fluid overload may produce pulmonary edema, primarily by elevating the capillary hydrostatic pressure. However, if the intravascular volume expansion causes a significant decrease in plasma colloid osmotic pressure, pulmonary edema may develop despite relatively small alterations in capillary hydrostatic pressure.[55] Similarly, alterations in the lymphatic circulation interfering with fluid removal from the interstitial space may modify the clinical characteristics and the response to therapy in some patients with pulmonary edema. For example, patients with pulmonary silicosis causing chronic obstructive lymphangitis may develop pulmonary edema of extreme severity with only minimal or moderate increases in pulmonary capillary hydrostatic pressures.[18]

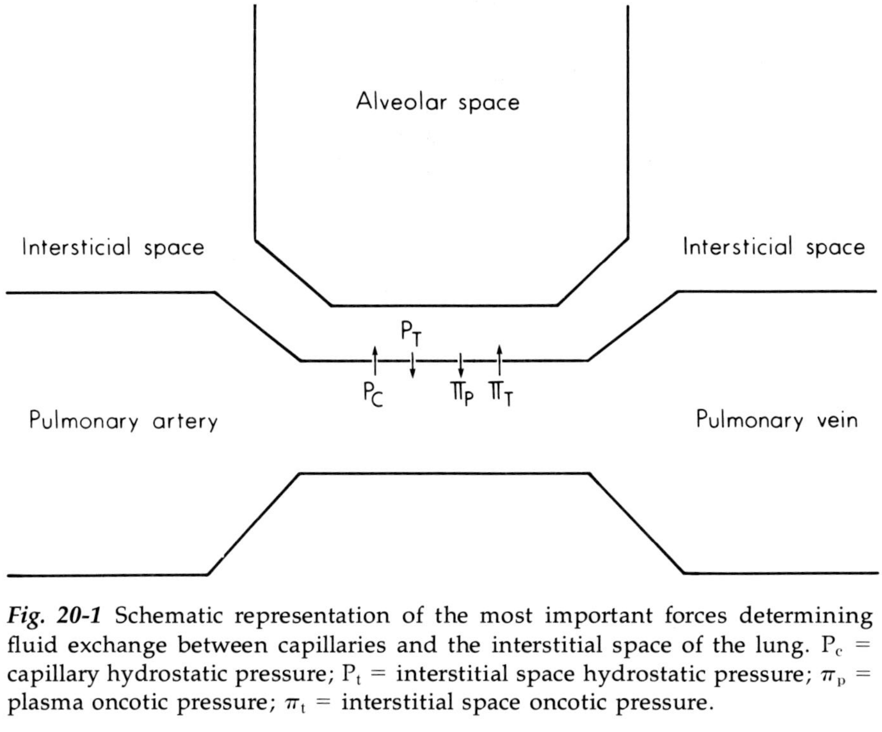

Fig. 20-1 Schematic representation of the most important forces determining fluid exchange between capillaries and the interstitial space of the lung. P_c = capillary hydrostatic pressure; P_t = interstitial space hydrostatic pressure; π_p = plasma oncotic pressure; π_t = interstitial space oncotic pressure.

The above examples typify situations in which the origin of pulmonary edema is multifactorial and the contribution of factors other than increased capillary permeability and increased capillary hydrostatic pressure is of significant pathophysiologic importance. Similar situations occur in the case of high-altitude pulmonary edema,[30] heroin overdose,[37] and preeclampsia.[13] In the majority of patients with pulmonary edema, however, an increase in capillary pressure due to heart failure (high-pressure pulmonary edema, cardiogenic pulmonary edema) or an alteration in capillary permeability (low-pressure pulmonary edema, noncardiogenic pulmonary edema, adult respiratory distress syndrome) will be clearly identified as the cause of the problem.

CARDIOPULMONARY ALTERATIONS IN NORMAL PREGNANCY FAVORING THE DEVELOPMENT OF PULMONARY EDEMA

The rarity of the occurrence of pulmonary edema during pregnancy is a tribute to the adaptative capacity of the cardiovascular system. In fact, several of the hemodynamic changes that occur during pregnancy facilitate the production of pulmonary edema. These changes are discussed below.

Increased Intravascular Volume. A normal pregnant woman increases her intravascular volume 40 to 60 percent during pregnancy,[46] and as a result her pulmonary vasculature will be filled with 800 to 1,200 ml of blood rather than the nonpregnant levels of 500 to 750 ml. Since the increase in plasma volume is larger than the increase in red cell mass, 60 to 70 percent of the intravascular volume will be plasma volume. Fortunately, the vascular tree of the pregnant woman can undergo marked vasodilation and accept this physiologic volume overload without deleterious effects. However, the high frequency of pulmonary edema in twin gestations treated with beta-adrenergic agents,[35] in which intravascular volume expansion is greatest, suggests that the volume expansion of pregnancy heavily taxes cardiac reserve and places pregnant patients with marked volume expansion at high risk for the development of pulmonary edema.

Decreased Peripheral Vascular Resistance. The development of the large placental shunt causes a marked decrease in peripheral vascular resistance during pregnancy that is only partially compensated by increased sympathetic vascular tone.[5] When this sympathetic tone is reduced, as during regional block anesthesia, hypotension and decreased cardiac output are produced unless special precautions, such as volume loading, are taken.

Low Blood Viscosity. An important factor contributing to the high cardiac output of pregnancy is reduced blood viscosity resulting from the proportionally greater expansion of plasma volume than of red cell mass. It is not generally appreciated that the tachycardia which accompanies anemia is due more to altered blood viscosity than to decreased oxygen-carrying capacity. This has been demonstrated in experiments in which one group of dogs had half of their red cell mass replaced with erythrocytes exposed to carbon monoxide and unable to carry oxygen. A second group of animals had a similar amount of their red cell mass removed and the volume replaced with plasma. Both groups of animals had decreased oxygen-carrying capacity but only the second group had decreased blood viscosity. The result of this experiment was that only the animals with low viscosity developed tachycardia.[45]

Increased Heart Rate. There is an elevation of the resting heart rate in pregnancy. It is difficult to determine if this merely reflects the high output stimuli previously mentioned or if it represents an additional and independent factor. Alterations in basal metabolic rate and thyroid function may explain this observation.

The net effect of the high output stimuli which are operative during normal pregnancy is an increase in cardiac output resulting from increases in both heart rate and end-diastolic ventricular volume.[36] Further increases in either of these two variables may lead to decompensation: stimuli which further increase heart rate will result in decreased time of diastolic filling and decreased stroke volume; stimuli which increase end-diastolic ventricular volume will result in increased stroke volume to a point, but this adaptive response may eventually be overwhelmed and then the stroke volume will fall. Many pregnant patients may be near the "top" of their Starling curve and have little cardiac reserve as a consequence of the hemodynamic changes just described (Fig. 20-2).

Decreased Plasma Colloid Osmotic Pressure. Plasma albumin concentration decreases progressively during gestation and by the end of pregnancy reaches levels barely compatible with the maintenance of a normal colloid osmotic pres-

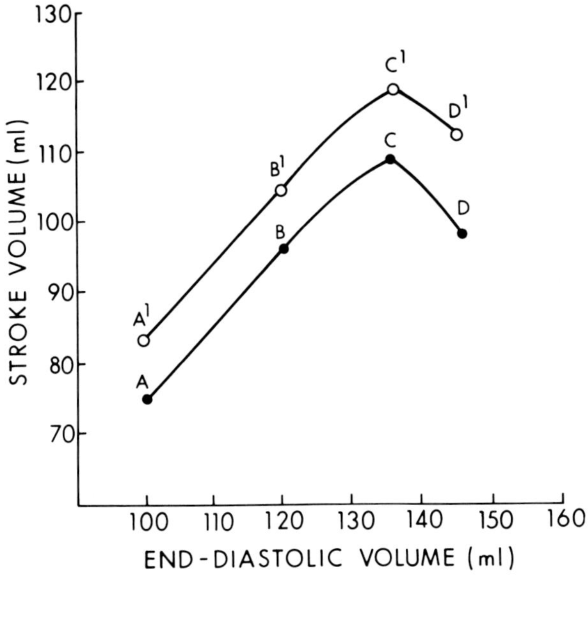

Fig. 20-2 Effect of pregnancy and beta-adrenergic tocolytic agents on stroke volume. As ventricular end-diastolic volume increases from the nonpregnant state (A) to the pregnant state (B), so does stroke volume. Administration of beta-adrenergic drugs causes further increase in end-diastolic volume (C) and stroke volume. However, past a certain point further increases in end-diastolic volume will cause a decrease in stroke volume (D). Drugs which increase the force of myocardial contraction (ephedrine, dopamine) shift the curve to the left (A'B'C'D'), resulting in a greater increase in stroke volume for each increase in end-diastolic volume.

sure.[50] This factor favors the movement of fluid out of the intravascular space and contributes to the tendency to peripheral edema of pregnant women.

Permeability Factor. There is no direct evidence that pregnancy per se alters the permeability of the endothelial membranes. However, it can be seen from the foregoing discussion that with increased intravascular volume and decreased plasma colloid osmotic pressure, any stimulus that alters permeability will result in relatively large fluid shifts from the intravascular into the interstitial space. In the lung this will result in pulmonary edema.

Intrapartum Volume Shifts. At the time of placental separation there is an increase in both systemic and pulmonary pressures. This is caused by increased preload secondary to an acute transfer of blood from the uteroplacental bed into the systemic circulation and increased afterload secondary to the closure of the placental shunt. These phenomena have been most clearly documented in patients with preeclampsia[49] but probably also occur in patients without hypertension. In addition to this internal transfusion, pregnant women, especially those delivering by cesarean section under epidural anesthesia, frequently receive rather impressive amounts of crystalloid solutions at the time of delivery. These factors increase the risk for pulmonary edema during the intrapartum and immediate postpartum periods.[48]

EFFECTS OF BETA-ADRENERGIC TOCOLYTIC THERAPY RELEVANT TO THE DEVELOPMENT OF PULMONARY EDEMA

Although the precise mechanism of pulmonary edema associated with beta-adrenergic tocolytic therapy is not presently known, most patients display signs and symptoms of acute high-output left ventricular failure. Thus, it is possible that these agents produce pulmonary edema by directly exaggerating the high-output cardiac state of pregnancy or by impairing compensatory mechanisms. However, a recent case report describes a patient monitored with a Swan-Ganz catheter during an episode of pulmonary edema associated with beta-adrenergic treatment in whom the presence of low-pressure, noncardiogenic pulmonary edema was demonstrated.[7] More observations are obviously necessary.

As reviewed in the discussion of the clinical pharmacology of beta-adrenergic tocolytic agents, these drugs produce a series of alterations secondary to the stimulation of $beta_2$ adrenoceptors (in blood vessels and the bronchial tree), and $beta_1$ adrenoceptors (in myocardium, liver, adipose tissue, and other organs), in addition to their effect upon myometrial contractility. In fact, even the most selective $beta_2$ agents have some degree of $beta_1$ activity, and every time they are used a series of metabolic and cardiovascular changes will be produced that may be significant in the production of pulmonary edema. These changes will be discussed below.

Expansion of Intravascular Volume. Shortly after initiation of intravenous beta-adrenergic therapy it is possible to observe that the hemoglobin/hematocrit values decrease as a consequence of plasma volume expansion, and after 24 h there is a mean drop of 6 percent in hematocrit.[38] This expansion of intravascular volume is a significant factor in the production of increased cardiac output by beta-adrenergic agents. The expansion of plasma volume is simultaneous with a marked decrease in urinary output, which occurs immediately after initiation of therapy and is clearly apparent after 2 h of infusion. The study of Grospietsch et al.[25] indicates that this retention of water and electrolytes may be due to excessive secretion of antidiuretic hormone (ADH). It is interesting, however, that ADH plasma concentration returns to normal levels 6 h after initiation of beta-adrenergic treatment, while the reduction in urinary volume persists for the duration of the intravenous phase of treatment. Plasma renin activity also increases markedly after beta-adrenergic treatment but, as mentioned before, aldosterone concentration decreases to nonpregnant levels, which suggests that the retention of water and electrolytes is not dependent on that hormone. The sensitivity of patients to the sodium-retaining effects of beta agonists varies widely, but it is safe to assume that most of any administered sodium will be retained. The antidiuretic effect disappears shortly after discontinuation of intravenous therapy. In most patients diuresis begins within 1 h of stopping treatment, and it often takes a day or more to eliminate the excess of water and ions.

Decreased Peripheral Vascular Resistance. Beta-adrenergic agents cause a marked drop in arterial vascular resistance. The consequence of this is a decrease in diastolic blood pressure that is apparent within 30 min after initiation of treatment. Since the systolic blood pressure increases, the overall result is a widening of the pulse pressure.[9] Indirectly, peripheral vascular resistance will be further lowered because the hemodilution secondary to fluid retention will cause decreased blood viscosity. The reduction in vascular resistance is another important factor in the production of high cardiac output by beta-adrenergic agents. Cardiac output increases not only as a consequence of decreased afterload but also because the impedance to venous return is decreased, which results in increased preload.

Direct Cardiac Effects. Beta-adrenergic agents have positive inotropic and chronotropic effects on the heart.[9] When these direct myocardial effects are added to decreased peripheral vascular resistance and increased intravascular volume, the overall result is a 50 to 60 percent increase in cardiac output.[10,61] This increase is superimposed on the 40 percent increase already caused by pregnancy and it is not unusual for cardiac output to be 10 L/min or more in pregnant women receiving beta-adrenergic tocolytic treatment.[10] Figure 20-3 is a representation of the changes induced by beta-adrenergic agents on left ventricular function in pregnant women.

Decreased Plasma Colloid Osmotic Pressure. The large and sudden increase in intravascular volume associated with intravenous beta-adrenergic therapy

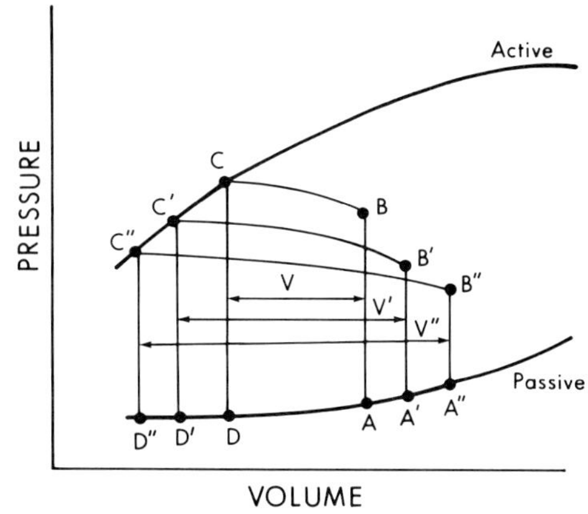

Fig. 20-3 Changes induced by pregnancy and by beta-adrenergic agents on left ventricular function. A normal left ventricular contraction commences at the end of diastole (A) and is isovolumetric until the onset of ejection (B). The end of ejection (C) is followed by isovolumetric relaxation (C to D) and by ventricular filling (D to A). V represents the stroke volume during the normal cycle ABCD. Pregnancy causes reduction in afterload (mainly because of decreased peripheral vascular resistance) and increase in preload (mainly because of increased blood volume), and the cardiac effects of this situation are represented by cycle A′B′C′D′ and its corresponding increased stroke volume V′. Beta adrenergic tocolytic agents (cycle A″B″C″D″) will magnify the changes induced by pregnancy, causing further increase in stroke volume (V″). High output failure may occur when the stroke volume is increased beyond the point of peak efficiency on any of these curves.

will tend to dilute the plasma concentration of albumin and consequently the colloid osmotic pressure.[15] The presence of hyperglycemia and the usual generous administration of crystalloid solutions to patients treated for preterm labor will accentuate the problem. Also, it should be remembered that pregnancy itself is associated with low plasma albumin concentration.[50] Thus, the superimposition of forces tending to expand the blood volume may dilute the already low plasma protein concentration to a level not capable of maintaining adequate colloid osmotic pressure.

Increased Vascular Permeability. Although the commonly utilized beta-adrenergic tocolytic agents are not chemically classified as catecholamines, their clinical pharmacology is similar enough so that consideration should be given to potential toxic effects of these drugs on the pulmonary endothelium. The toxicity of catecholamines has been well described in patients dying of pheochromocytoma who have obliterative endarteritis of the pulmonary vessels.[32] The time course of these changes is not known but they appear to represent chronic toxicity. However, acute endothelial injury as a prelude to the more chronic changes is likely to occur. The clinical course and hemodynamic profile of some patients with pulmonary edema during beta-adrenergic tocolytic therapy is best explained by direct pulmonary capillary toxicity. However, in only one case reported thus far in the literature is there strong evidence suggesting that capillary damage was the most likely pathophysiologic mechanism.[7]

Myocardial Toxicity. With the caveats applied above, there is suggestive evidence that, like the catecholamines, beta-adrenergic tocolytic agents may have cardiotoxic effects. There is a well-characterized cardiomyopathy described in patients with pheochromocytoma who have subendocardial ischemia and fibrosis.[60] Isoproterenol injected into rats produces subendocardial ischemia and necrosis in several days, presumably by causing intracellular adenosine monophosphate depletion.[63] Other beta-adrenergic agents may cause similar problems. Patients receiving beta-adrenergic tocolytic agents have been reported to have electrocardiographic changes suggesting ischemia,[58] and chest pain is not an uncommon historical feature in patients who develop pulmonary edema during tocolytic therapy. However, several investigators have been unable to detect elevated creatine phosphokinase of myocardial origin in patients receiving long-term beta-adrenergic tocolytic therapy.[41]

Metabolic Changes. As reviewed earlier, beta-adrenergic agonists cause hyperglycemia, hyperinsulinemia, accelerated lipolysis, hyper-lactic acidemia, and hypokalemia. The relationship between these changes and the appearance of pulmonary edema in pregnant patients treated with these drugs is tenuous, perhaps with the exception of hyperglycemia and hypokalemia.

Myocardial function may be indirectly impaired by beta-adrenergic agents as a result of reduction in intracellular potassium concentration. A significant decrease in plasma potassium concentration is seen within the first 30 min of intravenous beta-adrenergic treatment and will persist for the duration of treatment if it is not corrected. The potassium level will return quickly to a normal range, however, after beta agonists are discontinued. Many patients who develop pulmonary edema during tocolytic treatment are found to have marked hypokalemia, but this association may merely reflect increased sensitivity of the renin-aldosterone system to beta agonists in these patients.

Serum glucose increases markedly 30 min after starting an intravenous infusion of beta-adrenergic agents and this high concentration of glucose is another factor favoring mobilization of fluids into the intravascular compartment. Also, the metabolic degradation of large amounts of glucose generates lactic acid, which contributes to a decrease in the peripheral vascular resistance.[26]

DIAGNOSIS

Physical Signs and Symptoms. Established severe pulmonary edema is not difficult to recognize, but early signs and symptoms are subtle and may be missed. For this reason obstetric patients receiving beta-adrenergic tocolytic therapy must be carefully observed. Tachycardia and tachypnea unaccompanied by subjective shortness of breath may be the earliest signs. Auscultation of the lungs may reveal scattered rales and ronchi. However, in many cases, this examination is unremarkable. In the initial stages of pulmonary edema most patients do not report shortness of breath because the process may be so insidious in its onset that they do not fully recognize the source of their discomfort. These patients may only manifest agitation as a sign of their hypoxia. When shortness of breath is noticeable to both the physician and the patient, pulmonary edema is well established.

It is important not to rely on cyanosis as an indicator of hypoxia. At least 5 g of reduced hemoglobin must be present in peripheral venous blood before cyanosis becomes manifest. Since venous oxygen saturation is rarely less than 40 percent, the 5 g of reduced hemoglobin necessary to produce clinically evident cyanosis will not be present if the hemoglobin concentration is 12 g/dl or less.

Chest Radiograph. A chest radiograph should be obtained if the degree of respiratory distress is more than mild. Initially, the chest radiograph may appear normal but as pulmonary edema progresses, patchy infiltrates will become apparent. When the disease becomes more severe, total opacification of the lung fields may occur. Patients receiving increased inspiratory pressures by endotracheal tube may have x-rays which appear less opaque than they might otherwise, giving a lessened impression of the severity of the problem.

Arterial Blood Gases. An interpretation of arterial blood gas values requires an understanding of factors affecting pH, PaO_2, and $PaCO_2$ and the delivery of oxygen to the tissues. Cardiac output and the relationship of hemoglobin saturation and tissue oxygenation must also be evaluated.

The normal PaO_2 is 90 mmHg; however, it is frequently reduced by 10 to 15 mmHg in the supine position during pregnancy. Therefore, pregnant patients should be sitting or in the left lateral decubitus position when blood gas determinations are made. Since oxygen is much less soluble in tissues than carbon dioxide, when pulmonary injury occurs it is relatively easier for the lung to eliminate CO_2 than to take up O_2. Therefore, in early pulmonary edema there will be hypoxemia in the face of normal or reduced CO_2 tension. Under normal circumstances, O_2 tension will rise 1 mmHg above 90 mmHg for each mmHg fall in $PaCO_2$ below 40 mmHg. For example, with normal lungs if hyperventilation lowers the $PaCO_2$ to 25 mmHg, the PaO_2 should increase to 105 mmHg. The PaO_2 is also raised by increasing the O_2 concentration in inspired air (FIO_2). If the inspired O_2 concentration is above 30 percent, the PaO_2 should be approximately 6 times the FIO_2.

$$PaO_2 = 6 \times FIO_2$$

For example, if the FIO_2 is 40 percent, PaO_2 should be 240 mmHg. If the actual PaO_2 is significantly lower than the expected value, a large O_2 gradient exists between the alveolus and the capillary. A more direct measurement of the lung's ability to move O_2 from the alveolus to the arterial blood is the alveolar-arterial oxygen difference, which is discussed in Chapter 12.

Because CO_2 diffuses so readily across the lung, the $PaCO_2$ reflects ventilation and the amount of respiratory effort that is being made. A $PaCO_2$ greater than 45 mmHg in a patient with respiratory distress is markedly abnormal and signifies that many alveoli are not being ventilated or perfused. The pH reflects the ability of the lungs to compensate for the metabolic acidosis often seen in pulmonary edema. Shifts in pH, along with changes in temperature and erythrocyte 2,3-diphosphoglyceric acid (2,3-DPG) content also have a major effect on the amount of O_2 that hemoglobin will carry at any given PaO_2 (oxyhemoglobin dissociation curve). Cold, acidosis, and reduced red-blood-cell 2,3-DPG concentration, as seen in patients who have received a large transfusion of banked blood, cause the curve to shift to the right, resulting in a higher PaO_2 for any given hemoglobin saturation. The effect of this shift will be that hemoglobin will release O_2 more easily to the tissues but the total O_2-carrying capacity of the blood will be reduced. Alkalosis has the opposite effect and it will increase the affinity of hemoglobin for oxygen, which reduces the PaO_2 at each hemoglobin saturation. The effect of this shift to the left is to decrease the ability of hemoglobin to release its O_2 to the tissues, but the total O_2-carrying capacity of the blood is increased. Although neither alkalosis nor acidosis is desirable, the net effect of alkalosis seems to be worse because it causes poor O_2 delivery at the tissue level and concomitantly depresses the ventilatory drive.

Lung Volume. The appearance of interstitial pulmonary fluid, an early change in the development of pulmonary edema, may be detected by a decrease in functional lung volume. In fact, there is evidence that serial measurements of the vital capacity in pregnant patients receiving beta-adrenergic tocolytic agents may be a simple and sensitive method for detecting the development of pulmonary edema before it reaches full clinical expression.[8] This, of course, allows time for the institution of preventive measures.

Protein Measurement of Pulmonary Edema Fluid. Although of little help in immediate management, establishing the differential diagnosis of cardiogenic vs. noncardiogenic pulmonary edema is important in predicting the clinical course, in guiding therapy, and in helping to better understand the pathophysiology of this disorder. Measurement of the protein content of the airway fluid and its relationship to that of simultaneously obtained plasma can differentiate noncardiogenic from cardiogenic pulmonary edema.[23] If the airway fluid has a protein content which is 80 percent or more of the plasma value, pulmonary capillary leak and noncardiogenic pulmonary edema can be diagnosed. If the value is 60 percent or less, the fluid is a transudate and the etiology of the pulmonary edema must be cardiogenic. Unfortunately, airway fluid can be obtained only from patients with severe enough pulmonary edema to require endotracheal intubation and mechanical ventilation.

PREVENTION

Prevention of cardiopulmonary complications of beta-adrenergic tocolytic therapy should be a primary consideration whenever these drugs are used. This is because established pulmonary edema places both mother and fetus at grave risk, in most cases at much greater risk than if preterm delivery were allowed to occur. Also, these complications are almost totally preventable. We have noted a decrease of almost 100 percent in the incidence of cardiopulmonary problems following the institution of a set of simple principles.[3] Prevention rests on three factors: identification of patients at high risk for cardiopulmonary complications, rational use of beta-adrenergic agents, and avoidance of iatrogenic exacerbation of the high-output cardiac state of pregnancy.

Identification of Patients at High Risk for Cardiopulmonary Complications of Beta-Adrenergic Tocolytic Therapy

Patients at high risk include those in whom an identifiable obstetric or medical condition may contribute to the development of cardiopulmonary problems (Table 20-1). Women with ventricular outflow obstruction, specifically pulmonic stenosis or hypertrophic infundibular subaortic stenosis, are at high risk for sudden death if given beta agonists. It is crucial that a thorough history and physical examination be performed to rule out heart disease, thyroid disease, severe preeclampsia, pulmonary disease or other contraindications to therapy. In addition, it is important to obtain a complete blood count, urinalysis, serum electrolytes, glucose concentration, and any other information needed to assure that occult cardiac or pulmonary disease does not exist. Since gallop rhythm, basilar rales, jugular venous distention, peripheral edema, tachycardia and tachypnea may be all associated with normal pregnancy, cardiopulmonary problems may be very hard to detect if marked decompensation has not occurred. Chest x-ray, arterial blood gases, electrocardiography, and echocardiography should all be performed as needed before or as early as possible during the course of beta-adrenergic tocolytic therapy. Also, fetal distress should be carefully ruled out with electronic fetal heart rate monitoring.

Rational Use of Beta-Adrenergic Tocolytic Agents

All patients receiving intravenous beta-adrenergic treatment for preterm labor, and particularly those belonging to the high-risk groups identified above, should be

Table 20-1. Contraindications to Beta-adrenergic Tocolytic Therapy

Absolute
Severe preeclampsia
Thyrotoxicosis
Structural heart disease
Ventricular outflow obstruction
Valvular disease
Cardiac arrhythmia
Wolff-Parkinson-White syndrome
Hypervolemia
Severe anemia
Severe asthma already on beta-adrenergic therapy
Diabetic ketoacidosis
Relative
Diabetes
Fetal distress
Hypertension
Vaginal bleeding
Multiple gestation

under a rigid protocol for the administration of these medications, which should include the points discussed below.

Careful Patient Monitoring. While the patient is on intravenous therapy, maternal weight, fluid input and output, serum electrolytes, glucose, hematocrit, vital signs, fetal well-being, and signs and symptoms of pulmonary congestion should be evaluated frequently, preferably every 12 h or less.

Fluid Balance. Most cases of pulmonary edema appear to be associated with iatrogenic hypervolemia. Positive fluid balance should be no greater than 500 ml/24 h during intravenous therapy. Increasing maternal weight or decreasing hematocrit should be regarded as early signs of hypervolemia and treated with fluid restriction as well as reduction in the dose of the tocolytic agent being administered. Under special circumstances, small doses of a parental diuretic, such as furosemide, may be indicated.

Duration of Therapy. The intravenous phase of therapy *must not last more than 24 to 48 h*. The risk of cardiorespiratory complications increases with the duration of the intravenous phase of tocolytic treatment. The large majority of patients with beta-adrenergic-associated pulmonary edema reported thus far in the literature have developed this complication while in the intravenous phase of their treatment. Occasionally it may appear convenient to continue intravenous therapy for more than 48 h in patients who are hemodynamically stable and still have what seems to be significant uterine irritability. This is a temptation which must be avoided, especially since a relatively large number of patients with uterine contractions after several hours of intravenous beta-adrenergic therapy show no significant cervical changes in spite of their uterine activity. In many of these cases, when contractions are not producing cervical dilatation, oral therapy can be initiated without worsening the situation.

Indications for Discontinuation of Therapy. Therapy must be discontinued if the patient develops chest pain, shortness of breath, or auscultatory signs of pulmonary congestion. It cannot be overemphasized that subtle, early signs of impending pulmonary edema must be sought if this complication is to be avoided. Do not ascribe chest pain or air hunger to "reflux esophagitis" or "anxiety." If it is wished to continue therapy in the presence of these early signs or symptoms, then a complete evaluation of cardiopulmonary function, including Swan-Ganz catheterization to assess cardiac filling pressures and output, must be immediately performed.[14] This invasive maternal diagnostic workup is rarely warranted unless extreme prematurity is present and the risk of delivery to the fetus is very high.

Maternal Pulse. The maternal pulse must not exceed 120 beats per minute (bpm). The cardiovascular toxicity of beta-adrenergic agents is dose-related, and the correlation between maternal pulse and blood levels of the medication is excellent. Therefore, maternal pulse between 100 and 120 bpm is indicative of therapeutic blood levels and is associated with a low probability for the development of cardiorespiratory problems. A pulse rate persistently above 120 bpm indicates the need for decreasing the dose to a safer level.

Special Precautions. Patients with multiple gestation must be observed very closely. Not only do these women comprise a higher than expected proportion of cases of preterm labor, but they also run a higher than anticipated risk of pulmonary edema while on beta-adrenergic therapy.[35] These patients have up to twice the expansion of intravascular volume that is experienced by patients with singleton pregnancies and have exaggeration of several other high-output stimuli.

Patients receiving glucocorticoids to accelerate fetal pulmonary maturity may have their risk for developing pulmonary edema compounded, especially if a steroid with a large mineralocorticoid effect, such as hydrocortisone, is used. Additionally, there is evidence that glucocorticoids may increase beta-adrenergic responsiveness and adverse effects directly by increasing beta-receptor concentration in several tissues, including the lungs.[12] Some investigators, however, have not noted that glucocorticoids increase the risk of pulmonary edema during beta-adrenergic tocolytic therapy.[34]

Patients with anemia and hypokalemia should have these problems corrected, but it should be established that the anemia is not a dilutional effect of the beta agonist.

TREATMENT

Immediate recognition and adequate therapy can ameliorate the course of the respiratory insufficiency in patients who develop pulmonary edema during tocolytic treatment. Therapy involves discontinuing the medication, ensuring adequate ventilation and oxygenation, correcting fluid imbalance and hypotension, and maintaining adequate cardiac output. Continuous assessment of the fetus must be performed simultaneously with the maternal treatment because the need to intervene for fetal reasons may occur at any time.

Discontinuation of the Medication. The development of pulmonary edema in the course of beta-adrenergic treatment for preterm labor is an indication for discontinuing the treatment and either switching to a different type of labor-inhibiting drug or terminating all efforts to prevent preterm delivery. In the majority of cases, a course of no interference with preterm labor should be chosen. Agents such as intravenous alcohol, diazoxide, magnesium sulfate, progestins, and calcium channel blockers may not be effective, are not used extensively, or produce side effects which may worsen the pulmonary edema.

Ensuring Adequate Ventilation and Oxygenation. A previously healthy obstetric patient manifesting clinically *severe* respiratory distress at any time during the intravenous or the oral phase of tocolytic treatment with beta-adrenergic drugs must be assumed to have pulmonary edema and immediately intubated, preferably in an awake, blind, nasotracheal fashion. There should be no delay for blood gases, chest x-ray, or other studies. In most cases, affected patients exhibit a less severe degree of respiratory distress and can be evaluated in a somewhat less hurried fashion. Chest x-ray and arterial blood gases should be quickly obtained. A previously healthy patient with respiratory distress, a PaO_2 less than 60 mmHg, and/or a $PaCO_2$ greater than 45 mmHg on room air should be immediately intubated. Patients with better blood gas values should receive oxygen by Venturi mask.

Since the pathophysiology of pulmonary edema involves alveolar congestion and collapse, adequate ventilation and oxygenation will not occur until ventilatory pressures are high enough to overcome the increased lung "stiffness." Appropriate end-expiratory or positive airway pressures cannot be adequately maintained through endotracheal tubes with anesthesia machines or bagging devices. Patients in severe pulmonary distress can be much more readily oxygenated if they are placed on ventilators immediately. It is far better to bring the ventilator to the place where the patient is being stabilized than to move an unstable patient to an intensive care unit.

Correction of Fluid Imbalances. This is, perhaps, the most important single step in the treatment of pulmonary edema associated with beta-adrenergic tocolytic therapy. As mentioned before, most of these patients have a large positive fluid balance caused by the beta-adrenergic drugs and by excessive administration of crystalloid solutions.

If blood volume is high, and it will be in most instances of pulmonary edema complicating tocolytic therapy, volume contraction by furosemide is crucial. The intravenous injection of 20 mg of furosemide at the time of diagnosis should be followed by repeated doses of the diuretic at least every 4 h until the intravascular volume is adequately reduced. Furosemide will cause an immediate fall in effective circulating blood volume by increasing venous capacitance in addition to its diuretic effect. The reduction in blood volume should ideally be accompanied with central venous pressure or Swan-Ganz monitoring so that overshoot with resulting hypovolemia does not ensue. Also, careful measurement of the hourly fluid input and output along with serial determinations of the hematocrit must be carried out. We consider that it is safe to decrease the expanded intravascular volume to a point at which the hematocrit is similar to that obtained prior to initiation of beta-adrenergic therapy.

The amount of oral and intravenous fluids given to the patient in pulmonary edema associated with beta-adrenergic therapy must be restricted to no more than 50 to 75 ml/h (daily total of 1,500 to 1,800 ml) until the symptoms of respiratory embarassment disappear. Concern has been raised about the eventual effects of diuretic therapy plus fluid restriction on the uteroplacental circulation and on the fetal status. This is logical in view of evidence showing a direct relationship between maternal intravascular volume and fetal outcome in pregnant patients with hypertension.[2] It should be remembered, however, that in the case of pregnant hypertensive patients a lack of intravascular volume expansion exists which may be aggravated by diuretics and fluid restriction. In the case of patients under beta-adrenergic tocolytic therapy, on the other hand, the problem is one of excessive intravascular volume expansion, and diuretic therapy should be beneficial in this situation.

Treatment of Hypotension. Hypoxemic patients tolerate hypotension poorly. The treatment of hypotension in patients with pulmonary edema requires a knowledge of the circulating blood volume and ventricular filling pressures. If Swan-Ganz catheterization is not immediately available, a central venous catheter should be placed. If the blood volume is high or normal, a drug which will raise blood pressure by increasing the force of myocardial contractions should be used. Dopamine and dobutamine, two drugs which increase cardiac output in this fashion, are effective in the treatment of pulmonary edema complicated by hypotension.[28] Should the blood volume be low, the treatment is rapid intravascular expansion, preferably with fresh whole blood if immediately available. This will increase the patient's oxygen-carrying capacity, colloid osmotic pressure, and 2,3-DPG.

Maternal Monitoring. In literature reports of pulmonary edema associated with beta-adrenergic therapy, most patients have been managed without Swan-Ganz catheterization. In most cases this is appropriate since the diagnosis is usually clear on the basis of clinical, laboratory, and radiology findings and the therapy (furosemide, fluid restriction, oxygen by mask) does not require sophisticated monitoring. In our opinion Swan-Ganz catheterization is indicated in: (1) situations in which there is reasonable evidence of the possibility of underlying heart disease precipitating or aggravating the pulmonary edema; (2) patients who do not respond to conventional therapy in 1 to 2 h; (3) patients who require administration of intravenous fluids at doses substantially greater than those recommended (1,500 to 1,800 ml/24 h); (4) cases complicated by hypoxia and hypotension or requiring mechanical ventilation; and (5) cases in which the presence of intravascular volume expansion is not clear. In patients who do not fulfill these conditions, maternal monitoring should be limited to observations of the vital signs, blood gases, input and output, serial hematocrit determinations, and daily chest radiographs. With improvement the tachypnea and tachycardia will decrease, blood gases will reflect better oxygenation and decreased CO_2 retention, the hematocrit will rise, and the infiltrates present in the chest x-ray will decrease and finally disappear.

Fetal Considerations. There is little reason to believe that termination of pregnancy will significantly improve the respiratory status of a patient who develops pulmonary edema during tocolytic therapy. Vaginal delivery may increase O_2 requirements because of increased cardiac and uterine work.[43] Cesarean section adds all the risks of anesthesia and surgery to a critical situation. It is far better to stabilize the patient and deliver her only for standard obstetric and medical indications. The ideal setting for such a patient is in an institution with facilities for both intensive maternal and fetal care, and if she is not in such a place she should be transported to one as soon as her condition allows her to be moved.

There should be concern for the fetus of a hypoxic gravida although the fetus is well adapted to exist in such an environment. If the maternal hemoglobin concentration is 10 g/dl or more and the maternal PaO_2 is 65 mmHg or greater, fetal oxygenation will probably be adequate. The maternal $PaCO_2$ is of great concern. The fetus eliminates H^+ ions by producing CO_2 that is transferred to the mother through the placenta. When the maternal $PaCO_2$ reaches a level close to the fetal $PaCO_2$ (about 40 mmHg), the diffusion of CO_2 from fetus to mother is impaired and this is followed by fetal acidosis and eventually death. This is an important reason for treating an elevated $PaCO_2$ in pregnancy with assisted ventilation.

Evidence of fetal distress in the pregnant patient with beta adrenergic–associated pulmonary edema must be interpreted within the context of the maternal condition. If maternal hypoxemia and acidosis are present when fetal distress is detected and the maternal problems are correctable, it is much better to treat them first than to perform a delivery which may not be necessary after successful maternal therapy. If the maternal prognosis is poor, the decision to deliver involves many nonmedical factors. In these cases, if an attempt is to be made to salvage the fetus, delivery should not be delayed. It is best if the possibility of maternal death is discussed beforehand and a plan devised which can be rapidly implemented.[4]

REFERENCES

1. Abramovici, H., Lewin, A., Lissak A., et al.: Maternal pulmonary edema occurring after therapy with ritodrine for premature uterine contractions. Acta Obstet. Gynecol. Scand., 59:555, 1980.
2. Arias, F.: Expansion of intravascular volume and fetal outcome in patients with chronic hypertension and pregnancy. Am. J. Obstet. Gynecol., *123:*610, 1975.
3. Arias, F. and Knight, A.B.: Beta adrenergic therapy in the management of preterm labor. In Zuspan, F. and Christian, D., Eds.: Controversy in Obstetrics and Gynecology. Vol. 3. W. B. Saunders, Philadelphia, 1983. pp. 31–43.
4. Arthur, R.K.: Postmortem cesarean section. Am. J. Obstet. Gynecol., *130:*596, 1978.
5. Assali, N.S. and Brinkman, C.R.: Disorders of maternal circulatory and respiratory adjustments. p. 283. In Assali, N.S., Ed.: Pathophysiology of Gestation. Academic Press, New York, 1972.
6. Barden, T.P., Peter, J.B., and Merkatz, I.R.: Ritodrine hydrochloride: a betamimetic agent for use in preterm labor: I. Pharmacology, clinical history, administration, side effects and safety. Obstet. Gynecol., *56:*1, 1980.
7. Benedetti, T.J., Hargrove, J.C., and Rosene, K.A.: Maternal pulmonary edema during premature labor inhibition. Obstet. Gynecol., suppl., 56:33, 1981.
8. Benedetti, T., Johansen, T., Luthey, D.: Prediction of respiratory insufficiency during premature labor inhibition with betasympathomimetics (Abstr.) p. 69. In: Proc. Soc. Perinat. Obstet., San Antonio, 1962.
9. Bieniarz, J.: Cardiovascular effects of beta adrenergic agonists. p. 188. In: Anderson, A., Beard, R., Brudenell, J.M. et al., Eds.: Pre-term Labor. Royal College of Obstetricians and Gynecologists. London, 1977.
10. Bieniarz, J., Ivankovich, A., and Scommegma, A.: Cardiac output during ritodrine treatment in premature labor. Am. J. Obstet. Gynecol., *118:*910, 1974.
11. Brazy, J.E. and Pupkin, M.: Effects of maternal isoxsuprine administration on preterm infants. J. Pediatr., *94:*444, 1979.

12. Cheng, J.B., Goldfein, A., Ballard, P.L. et al.: Glucocorticoids increase pulmonary beta adrenergic receptors in the fetal rabbits. Endocrinology, *107:*1646, 1982.
13. Chesley, L.: Hypertensive Disorders of Pregnancy. Appleton-Century-Crofts, Norwalk, Conn., 1978, p. 363.
14. Cotton, D.B. and Benedetti, T.J.: Use of Swan-Ganz catheter in obstetrics and gynecology. Obstet. Gynecol., *56:*641, 1980.
15. Cotton, D.B., Strassner, H.Z., Lipson, C.G. et al.: The effects of terbutaline on acid-base, serum electrolytes, and glucose homeostasis during the management of preterm labor. Am. J. Obstet. Gynecol., *141:*617, 1981.
16. Crawford, C., Boggs, S., and Neff, C.: In utero isoxsuprine exposure: anatomical and biochemical changes in neonatal rats (Abstr.) Pediatr. Res., *15:*493, 1981.
17. Crawford, C., Bowen, F., Bhutani, V., et al.: Echocardiographic effects of intrauterine isoxsuprine exposure (Abstr.). Pediatr. Res., *15:*493, 1981.
18. Cross, C.E., Shaver, J.A., Wilson, R.J. et al.: Mitral stenosis and pulmonary fibrosis: special reference to pulmonary edema and lung lymphatic function. Arch. Intern. Med., *125:*248, 1970.
19. Csapo, A.I. and Herczeg, J.: Arrest of premature labor by isoxsuprine. Am. J. Obstet. Gynecol., *129:*482, 1977.
20. Dudenhausen, J.W., Kyrast, G., Lange-Lindberg, A. et al.: Influence of long-term betamimetic therapy on the lecithin content of amniotic fluid. Gynecol. Obstet. Invest., *9:*205, 1978.
21. Elliott, H.R., Abdulla, U., and Hayes, P.J.: Pulmonary edema associated with ritrodrine infusion and betamethasone administration in premature labor. Br. Med. J., *1:*799, 1978.
22. Erkkola, R., Lammintausta, R., and Liukko, P.: Maternal and fetal plasma renin activity during ritodrine infusion to the mother. Biol. Neonate *35:*268, 1979.
23. Fein, A., Grossman, R., and James, J.: The value of edema fluid protein measurement in patients with pulmonary edema. Am. J. Med., *67:*32, 1979.
24. Gandar, R., de Zoeten, L.W., and Vanden Schoote, B.: Serum levels of ritodrine in man. Eur. J. Clin. Pharmacol., *17:*117, 1980.
25. Grospietsch, G., Fenske, M., Girndt, J. et al.: The renin-angiotensin-aldosterone system, antidiuretic hormone levels and water balance under tocolytic therapy with fenoterol and verapamil. Int. J. Gynaecol. Obstet., *17:*590, 1980.
26. Haddy, F.J. and Scott, J.B.: Metabolic factors in peripheral circulatory regulation. Fed. Proc., *34:*2006, 1975.
27. Hendricks, C.H.: The use of isoxsuprine for the arrest of premature labor. Clin. Obstet. Gynecol., *7:*687, 1964.
28. Herbert, P. and Tinker, J.: Inotropic drugs in circulatory failure. Intensive Care Med., *6:*101, 1980.
29. Hondros, K. and Schaller, A.: The influence of beta mimetic ritodrine on the potassium balance during tocolytic therapy (German). Geburtshilfe Perinat., *184:*17, 1980.
30. Hultgren, H.N., Lopez, C.E., Jundberg, E. et al.: Physiologic studies of pulmonary edema at high altitude. Circulation, *29:*393, 1964.
31. Jacobs, M.M., Knight, A.B., and Arias, F.: Maternal pulmonary edema resulting from betamimetic and glucocorticoid therapy. Obstet. Gynecol., *56:*56, 1980.
32. James, T.N.: On the cause of sudden death in pheochromocytoma, with special reference to the pulmonary arteries, the cardiac conduction system and the aggregation of platelets. Circulation, *54:*348, 1976.
33. Jorgensen-Niebuhr, U.: Pulmonary edema following treatment with ritodrine and betamethasone in pre-term labor. Dan. Med. Bull., *27:*99, 1980.

34. Katz, M. and Creasy, R.K.: Effect of glucocorticoids on pulmonary edema during terbutaline tocolysis. Am. J. Obstet. Gynecol., *141:*233, 1982.
35. Katz, M., Robertson, P.A., and Creasy, R.K.: Cardiovascular complications associated with terbutaline treatment for preterm labor. Am. J. Obstet. Gynecol., *139:*605, 1981.
36. Katz, R., Karliner, J., and Resnik, R.: Effects of a natural volume overload state (pregnancy) on left ventricular performance in normal human subjects. Circulation, *58:*434, 1978.
37. Katz, S., Aberman, A., Frand, U.I. et al.: Heroin pulmonary edema. Am. Rev. Respir. Dis., *106:*472, 1972.
38. Kirpatrick, C., Quenon, M., and Desir, D.: Blood anions and electrolytes during ritodrine infusion in preterm labor. Am. J. Obstet. Gynecol., *138:*523, 1980.
39. Lammintausta, R. and Erkkola, R.: Effect of long term salbutamol treatment on renin-aldosterone system in twin pregnancy. Acta Obstet. Gynecol. Scand., *58:*447, 1979.
40. Lenz, S., Kuhl, C., and Wang, P. et al.: The effect of ritodrine on carbohydrate and lipid metabolism in normal and diabetic pregnant women. Acta Endocrinol., *92:*669, 1979.
41. Meinen, K.: Radioimmunoassay procedure of serum myoglobulin in case of long-term tocolysis with betasympathomimetics. Gynecol. Obstet. Invest., *12:*37, 1981.
42. Markatz, I.R., Peter, J.B., and Barden, T.P.: Ritodrine hydrochloride: a betamimetic agent for use in preterm labor. II. Evidence of efficacy. Obstet. Gynecol., *56:*7, 1980.
43. Metcalfe, J. and Ueland, K.: Maternal cardiovascular adjustments to pregnancy. Prog. Cardiovasc. Dis., *16:*363, 1974.
44. Midwest Medical Research, Inc. New drug application, Number 18280, for ritodrine hydrochloride. Submitted to the FDA on March 8, 1979 by Midwest Medical Research Inc. Columbus, Ohio, on behalf of Philips-Duphar.
45. Murray, J.F. and Escobar, E.: Circulatory effects of blood viscosity: Comparison of metehemoglobinemia and anemia. J. Appl. Physiol., *25:*594, 1968.
46. Peck, T.M. and Arias, F.: Hematologic changes associated with pregnancy, Clin. Obstet. Gynecol., *22:*785, 1979.
47. Philipsen, T., Eriksen, P.S., and Lynggard, F.: Pulmonary edema following ritodrine-saline infusion in premature labor. Obstet. Gynecol., *58:*304, 1981.
48. Pou-Martinez, A., Kelly, S.H., Newell, F.D. et al.: Postpartum pulmonary edema after ritodrine and betamethasone use. J. Reprod. Med., *27:*428, 1982.
49. Rafferty, T.D. and Berkowitz, R.L.: Hemodynamics in patients with severe toxemia during labor and delivery. Am. J. Obstet. Gynecol., *138:*263, 1980.
50. Robertson, E.G. and Cheyne, G.A.: Plasma biochemistry in relation to oedema of pregnancy. J. Obstet. Gynaecol. Br. Commonw., *79:*769, 1972.
51. Schilthuis, M.S. and Aarnoudse, J.G.: Fetal death associated with severe ritodrine induced ketoacidosis. Lancet, *1:*1145, 1980.
52. Schreyer, P., Caspi, E., Arieli, S. et al.: Metabolic effect of intravenous ritodrine infusion in pregnancy. Acta Obstet. Gynecol. Scand., *59:*197, 1980.
53. Siimes, A.S. and Creasy, R.K.: Effect of ritodrine on uterine activity, heart rate, and blood pressure in the pregnant sheep: Combined use of alpha or beta blockade. Am. J. Obstet. Gynecol., *126:*1003, 1976.
54. Siimes, A.S. and Creasy, R.K.: Maternal and fetal metabolic response to ritodrine in sheep. Acta Obstet. Gynecol. Scand., *59:*181, 1980.
55. Stein, L., Beraud, J.J., Morisette, M. et al.: Pulmonary edema during volume infusion. Circulation, *52:*483, 1975.
56. Straub, N.C.: Steady state pulmonary transvascular water filtration in unanesthetized sheep. Circ. Res., *28:*suppl. 1, 135, 1971.
57. Stubblefield, P.G.: Pulmonary edema occurring after therapy with dexamethasone and terbutaline for premature labor. Am. J. Obstet. Gynecol., *132:*341, 1978.

58. Tye, K., Desser, K., and Benchimal, A.: Angina pectoris associated with the use of terbutaline for premature labor. JAMA, *244*:692, 1980.
59. Unbehaun, U.: Effects of sympathomimetic tocolytic agents on the fetus. J. Perinat. Med., *2*:2, 1974.
60. Van Vliet, P.D., Burchell, H.B., and Titus, J.L.: Focal myocarditis associated with pheochromocytoma. N. Engl. J. Med., *274*:1102, 1966.
61. Wagner, J.M., Morton, M.J., Johnson, K.A. et al.: Terbutaline and maternal cardiac function. JAMA, *246*:2697, 1981.
62. Wyszogrodoski, I., Taeusch, H.W., and Avery, M.E.: Isoxsuprine-induced alterations of pulmonary pressure-volume relationships in premature rabbit. Am. J. Obstet. Gynecol., *119*:1107, 1974.
63. Zimmer, H., Ibel, H., Steinkopff, G. et al.: Reduction of the isoproterenol-induced alterations in cardiac adenosine nucleotides and morphology by ribose. Science, *207*:319, 1980.

21

Drug Intoxication and Anaphylactic Shock in the Obstetric Patient

Frank R. Witter, M.D.
Jennifer R. Niebyl, M.D.

The incidence of drug intoxications in pregnant women is difficult to obtain. According to data from the National Poison Network, Computer System for Documenting Data on Poison Exposures, 46.6 percent of the total of 190,074 reported poisonings in 1980 were in women. However, only 8.1 percent of the total were in women in the reproductive age group. Of all poisonings, 85.4 percent were accidental and only 0.3 percent were by injection. Of events involving women, 85 percent were accidental, 6.1 were suicidal gestures, 3.2 percent were suicides, and 1.4 percent were drug "trips." Unfortunately, the suicidal gestures, suicides, and drug trips concentrated in the reproductive age group. Of all events, 79.3 percent were handled by telephone alone, 10 percent were treated in an emergency room, and only 4.6 percent required hospital admission. The majority of the admissions were in the reproductive age group.

It has been estimated that there are 100,000 to 200,000 narcotic addicts nationwide, of whom 25 to 50 percent are women, 80 percent of female addicts are in the reproductive age group.[18] In New York City, 1 percent of addicts die of overdose each year and the majority of addicts experience overdose at least once.[17] These rough estimates correlate well with the observed total incidence of drug trips in the National Poison Center Network data. Therefore, data from that source can be considered fairly indicative of the national pattern for narcotic abuse and probably for drug intoxications in general. It would seem, then, that the vast majority of drug intoxications in women in the reproductive age group can be handled on an outpatient basis with only a small minority requiring admission; however, in the case of pregnant patients the clinician must be aware of the special risks for the fetus in drug overdose, which will be detailed in this chapter.

GENERAL TREATMENT FOR DRUG INTOXICATION IN PREGNANCY

The nonspecific treatment for drug intoxication consists of (1) maintenance of vital functions, (2) removal of drug, and (3) delay of drug absorption.[8] The first priorities of vital function maintenance in the patient suffering from poisoning are to secure the airway, support the circulation, and if indicated, control seizures.[9]

The fetus normally has an O_2 tension of 20 to 30 mmHg and total maternal asphyxia for as little as 7 min may lead to fetal brain damage.[14] It is therefore important to maintain the maternal arterial PO_2 within an acceptable range. Data from fetal sheep indicate that a maternal arterial PO_2 of 40 to 50 mmHg is the lowest at which the fetus can survive.[7,12,16] In view of this, in clinical practice one should try to keep the maternal arterial PO_2 above 60 mmHg.

Hypotension is a feature of many drug intoxications and should be treated promptly. Although a marked reduction in uterine perfusion can result in death in utero, fetal survival may occur even when uterine blood flow has been decreased by more than 50 percent.[11] It is advisable to correct hypotension as quickly as possible and to maintain the maternal systolic blood pressure above 90 mmHg. Maintenance of blood pressure is best achieved by fluid expansion with Ringer's lactate or normal saline while carefully monitoring the central venous pressure, which should not be permitted to exceed 15 cm H_2O. In addition, the patient should be placed on her left side to avoid supine hypotension secondary to compression by the gravid uterus of the inferior vena cava. If these measures fail, ephedrine (10 to 15 mg) may be given intravenously for careful titration of the patient's blood pressure.

Following initial maintenance of vital functions, the next priority in the nonspecific treatment of drug intoxication should be removal of the drug or delay of its absorption. If, as in most cases, the drug has been ingested, emesis is possibly the most effective means of drug removal.[8] Emesis is contraindicated in the patient with stupor or coma, in the presence of convulsions, or when drugs which may produce convulsions have been ingested. In the latter instance vomiting may induce seizures. The agent of choice to induce emesis is syrup of ipecac in a maximum dose of 30 to 60 ml.[9] The initial dose should be 10 to 30 ml, followed by several large glasses of tepid water. If no vomiting has occurred, this dose may be repeated once in 20 to 30 min. Ipecac has not been shown to increase the risk of congenital malformations when given in pregnancy in humans.[13]

If ipecac fails to induce emesis or if emesis is contraindicated, one should then proceed to gastric lavage. Gastric lavage is most effective against easily absorbed drugs if ingestion occurred within 4 h; however, if the patient is in coma or shock and no bowel sounds are audible, substantial amounts of drug may be removed at any time.[8] The patient should be in the head-down, left lateral decubitus position, and if unconscious, should have the airway protected by a cuffed endotracheal tube. Gavage should be done with a large tube such as a 30 to 36 French Ewald tube, as some intact pills may be removed through a tube of this size. Gavage should be performed with 0.5 N NaCl in 100- to 200-ml aliquots until clear. The quantity of fluid given at any one time should not exceed 50 ml per 10 kg body weight.[8] Large volumes of fluids administered by gavage may force stomach contents through the pylorus and thereby enhance absorption.

After removal of as much drug as possible by either emesis or gavage, delay of absorption may be achieved by giving activated charcoal. It is less effective against water-insoluble drugs. Activated charcoal should be given as a slurry with water in a dose of 1.0 g/kg body weight, or if the quantity of ingested agent is known, 5 to 10 times the quantity of ingestant.[9]

When the patient is transported to the hospital, the drug in its original container should be brought along for identification. Vomitus, urine, and blood may also be used to identify the agent if a history is not obtainable. If the drug was injected, one should apply a tourniquet and cold packs to the extremity where the injection occurred and immobilize the patient. If the drug was taken per rectum, a sodium phosphate enema may be administered. If the drug is known and a specific antidote is available, it should be given while proceeding with drug removal. In addition, while proceeding with drug removal, baseline studies should be obtained consisting of arterial blood gases, electrolytes, creatinine, blood urea nitrogen, liver function tests, electrocardiogram, and chest x-ray. These will make it possible to follow the course of potential pulmonary, renal, cardiac, and liver complications from drug intoxication. The fetal heart rate should be periodically monitored during the treatment but no intervention for the fetus should be considered until the maternal status is stabilized. Following the initial treatment outlined above, supportive therapy is indicated as the patient recovers from her overdose.

TREATMENT FOR SPECIFIC DRUG INTOXICATIONS

Aminophylline and Theophylline

Aminophylline-theophylline intoxication may be either acute or chronic. Acute intoxication with intravenous administration may result in sudden collapse and death within 1 to 2 min.[8] Acute intoxication may also occur following repeated rectal administration or by oral administration. Either route of administration may result in gastric irritation, vomiting, and convulsions. Chronic intoxication by any method of administration results in restlessness, nausea, vomiting, epigastric pain, headache, agitation, tachycardia, arrhythmias, hyperventilation, fever, convulsions, and respiratory failure.[10]

In a large prospective study, theophylline was not shown to be a human teratogen.[13] However, it readily crosses the placenta and has a prolonged half-life and decreased protein binding in the neonate, producing increased toxicity at lower serum levels.[2] Therefore, if delivery occurs at the time of acute intoxication, the infant must be closely observed for signs of toxicity.

Treatment of maternal theophylline intoxication consists of administration of oxygen to maintain the arterial PO_2 above 60 mm Hg, maintenance of blood pressure as described above under general treatment (Table 21-1), discontinuation of theophylline administration, and removal of any rectally administered theophylline by enema. Dehydration secondary to vomiting should be corrected with intravenous normal saline, with potassium replacement based on potassium blood levels. Convulsions if present may be controlled with intravenous diazepam 2 to 10 mg at 1 mg/min if delivery is not anticipated. If delivery is anticipated, it is wiser to avoid diazepam because of its prolonged half-life in the neonate and the increased risk of hyperbilirubinemia.[19] If delivery is anticipated, intravenous magnesium sulfate with a loading dose of 4 g followed by 1 to 2 g/h by continuous infusion is a better choice for the management of seizures. In patients with inadequate urinary output, maternal serum magnesium levels must be carefully followed and administration of $MgSO_4$ adjusted accordingly.

Table 21-1. Treatment of Hypotension, Hypertension, Convulsions, Hyperexcitability, and Coma

Hypotension
Maintain diastolic blood pressure above 90 mmHg.
Initially use fluid expansion with Ringer's lactate or 1 N saline while carefully monitoring the central venous pressure, which should not exceed 15 cm H_2O.
Place the patient on her left side.
If the above measures fail, ephedrine (10 to 15 mg) may be given intravenously.
Hypertension
Treat if the diastolic is greater than 110 mmHg.
Do not lower the diastolic below 90 mmHg.
Treatment of choice: intravenous hydralazine.
Test dose: 5 mg as a bolus
May repeat in 20 to 30 min, twice
If hypertension recurs after test dose, treat with continuous intravenous infusion with lowest effective dose; begin with 2 to 4 mg/h. Dose may be increased by 2 mg every 30 min.
Convulsions
If delivery not anticipated:
Diazepam 2 to 10 mg at 1 mg/min intravenously
If delivery anticipated:
Magnesium sulfate: Loading dose 4 g
Maintenance dose 1 to 2 g/h by continuous infusion in patients with urine output > 30 ml/h.
Follow serum magnesium levels in patients with reduced urine output.
Hyperexcitability
Phenobarbital 30 to 90 mg every 6 h.
Coma
Endotracheal intubation with cuffed endotracheal tube.
Maintain maternal PO_2 between 70 and 100 mmHg.
Maintain maternal PCO_2 at least below 40 mmHg and preferably between 27 and 32 mmHg.
Mechanical ventilation may be required to maintain gas exchange listed above.
Arterial line for frequent blood gas monitoring is indicated.

Amphetamines and Psychotomimetic Agents

This group of agents includes amphetamine, lysergic acid diethylamide (LSD), 2,5-dimethoxy-4-tryptamine (DMT), diethyltryptamine (DET), methylenedioxyamphetamine (MDA), psilocybin, psilocin, bufotenin, ibogaine, harmine, harmaline, ditran, marijuana, and mescaline. Overdose with this class of agents results in hyperexcitability, uncontrollability, hypertension or hypotension, ataxia, hyperreflexia, convulsions, coma, increased suicidal or homicidal tendencies, and prolonged psychotic states.[8] In addition, LSD, although not conclusively demonstrated to be a teratogen, does increase the risk of spontaneous abortion. Mescaline has been associated with central nervous system anomalies following a single intravenous injection in experimental animals.[22]

Treatment should consist of maintenance of vital functions as outlined above, with maternal arterial PO_2 above 60 mmHg and maternal systolic blood pressure above 90 mmHg. If coma is present, intubation is essential to protect the airway. The maternal arterial PCO_2 should at least be kept below 40 mmHg and ideally values within the normal range for pregnancy (27 to 32 mmHg) should be sought in order to facilitate fetal CO_2 transfer. If hypertension is present with a diastolic pressure greater than 110 mmHg, it should be treated with intravenous hydralazine. The initial test dose should be 5 mg and may be repeated twice in 20 to 30 min. Following the test dose if hypertension recurs, continuous hydralazine infusions should be used, starting with as low a dose as possible and titrating the dose upwards. The usual starting dose is 2 to 4 mg/h and may be increased by 2 mg every 30 min. (See Table 21-1). The diastolic blood pressure should not be lowered below 90 mmHg by antihypertensive agents. If amphetamines are the implicated drug, the urine should be acidified and diuresis forced to enhance elimination. Treatment of convulsions should be as described above under Aminophylline and Theophylline (Table 21-1). Excitement may be treated with phenobarbital 30 to 90 mg every 6 h. (Table 21-1). The patient should have suicide precautions and supportive therapy.

Anticholinergic Agents

Common agents in this group are belladonna, atropine, and scopolamine. Symptoms of intoxication include dry mouth, difficulty in swallowing and talking, blurred vision, photophobia, flushed skin, hyperthermia, hypertension, tachycardia, cardiac dysrhythmias, agitation, hallucinations, convulsions, and coma.[10] Atropine and scopolamine have not been shown to be teratogenic; however, belladonna is associated in humans with malformations in general, and specifically with eye and ear defects.[13] As these agents cross the placenta easily, if delivery occurs at the time of maternal intoxication, the newborn will also need treatment.

The specific antidote for anticholinergic intoxication is physostigmine salicylate.[9] The initial dose should be 2 mg intravenously injected slowly at 1 mg/min, with a second dose of 1 to 2 mg given at 20 min if no response is seen. As physostigmine is rapidly destroyed, the patient may relapse within 1 to 2 h and repeat doses of 1 to 4 mg may be required.[10] Repeat administration is risky, however, as it may produce cholinergic crisis. Excessive physostigmine administration may be reversed by half the dose of atropine.[9] If hyperthermia is present with a temperature of 39°C or greater, the patient's temperature should be decreased by a cooling blanket. Hypertension should be treated as described under Amphetamines and Psychotomimetic Agents (Table 21-1), convulsions as described under Aminophylline and Theophylline (Table 21-1), and coma as under Barbiturates (Table 21-1). Supportive therapy is indicated until the patient recovers from her intoxication.

Barbiturates and Methaqualone (Quaalude)

The effects of and therapy for methaqualone intoxication are the same as in the case of those for barbiturate overdose. The major danger to both the mother and the fetus from acute intoxication with any of these agents is respiratory depression with tissue anoxia.[8] Pathologically, one may see pulmonary edema, pneumonia, and cerebral edema. The initial symptoms of barbiturate overdose are sleepiness and mental confusion and, with larger doses, shallow respirations. Atelectasis or aspiration pneumonia with significant pulmonary consolidation may complicate the situation. With larger overdoses, coma, hypotension, and hypothermia[9] may be seen.

Coma, if present, should be treated by intubation with a cuffed endotracheal tube to maintain airway patency, to avoid aspiration, and to allow adequate gas exchange. An arterial line is indicated for frequent follow-up of blood gas determinations. As noted under General Treatment, maternal arterial PO_2 should not fall below 60 mmHg and in the comatose patient requiring intubation, a range of 70 to 100 mmHg is suggested.[8] The maternal arterial PCO_2 should at least be kept below 40 mmHg and ideally values within the normal range for pregnancy should be sought (27 to 32 mmHg) in order to facilitate fetal CO_2 transfer. Mechanical ventilation may be required to maintain these ranges. In the presence of phenobarbital, fetal cerebral damage due to asphyxia is lessened;[14] nevertheless, vigorous efforts should be used to keep maternal oxygenation adequate.

Efforts should be made to remove as much drug as possible by emesis if the patient is alert, or by gavage if she is not. Best results are achieved if removal is attempted within 2 h of ingestion.[8] Drug may also be removed by catharsis, using 15 to 60 ml of Fleet's phosphosoda diluted 1:4 with water and given by mouth. Following removal of drug, activated charcoal should be given as indicated under General Treatment.

Hypotension from barbiturate overdose is best treated with intravenous fluid administration. Because anoxic damage may produce pulmonary edema, careful monitoring of the central venous or pulmonary wedge pressure is necessary when administering fluids. Hypothermia, if present, should be treated by application of warming blankets. If delivery is anticipated soon after intoxication has occurred, consideration must be made for the treatment of neonatal respiratory depression.

Barbiturates have not been shown to be teratogenic in humans when taken for indications other than epilepsy. When they are given for epilepsy, there may be a teratogenic effect, but the evidence is not clear.[22] As barbiturate use may result in nonreactive, nonstress tests,[1] lack of fetal reactivity should not be considered an indication of fetal distress in these patients. However, the oxytocin challenge test should remain effective as a means of diagnosing fetal distress.

Chronic barbiturate use in pregnancy is associated with neonatal withdrawal. This withdrawal consists of hyperexcitability, tremors, restlessness, and increased appetite. It begins at a mean of 7 days of life, peaks at about 2 to 6 weeks of age, and may last for up to 6 months.[6] For this reason, if chronic ingestion is suspected, prolonged follow-up of the neonate is indicated.

If the patient is taking barbiturates chronically but the total dose is less than 400 mg/day, physical dependence is unlikely.[15] If doses in excess of this are taken, physical dependence may be present. In this situation, the patient begins to develop tremulousness, anxiety, weakness, and insomnia and, in severe cases, grand mal seizures and delirium as she emerges from her intoxication.[10] The withdrawal should be treated with paraldehyde 0.2 mg/kg body weight rectally in oil.[8]

During the recovery period, supportive measures are indicated. These should include careful monitoring of electrolytes and intake and output.

Cocaine

Estimates of the lethal dose of cocaine vary from 1.2 g to 30 mg,[8,10] and as little as 20 mg may produce severe toxic effects.[10] In toxic doses, cocaine first excites and then depresses the central nervous system. Death may occur immediately or be delayed for 1 to 3 h. Symptoms and signs of cocaine intoxication include restlessness, excitability, sensory aberrations, hallucinations, tachycardia, dilated pupils, chills and fever, abdominal pain, vomiting, numbness and muscle spasms, irregular or Cheyne-Stokes respirations, circulatory failure, convulsions, and coma.[8] As cocaine has not been shown to be teratogenic,[22] the major risk to the fetus is anoxia due to maternal circulatory failure and convulsions interfering with respirations. If these symptoms follow intoxication which occurred within 30 min of the patient being seen, the drug may be removed by induction of emesis or lavage and by giving activated charcoal.[8] Beyond this point, or when cocaine has been injected, removal measures are ineffective. If injection has occurred in an extremity, application of a tourniquet may delay absorption.

Treatment is supportive. First priority should be given to protecting the airway and maintaining respiration. Coma should be treated as discussed under Barbiturates (Table 21-5). Convulsions should be treated as described under Aminophylline-Theophylline (Table 21-1). If convulsions are refractory to therapy and interfere with respiration, the patient should be treated with paralyzing doses of succinylcholine, endotracheal intubation, and artificial ventilation. Tachycardia and other cardiac arrhythmias induced by cocaine may be treated with propranolol given in a 1-mg slow intravenous injection.[8] This may be repeated up to a total dose of 8 mg. If hypotension is present, it should be treated with intravenous fluid therapy. If the patient can be stabilized during the acute episode, the prognosis is good, as cocaine is destroyed fairly rapidly.[10]

Diazepam and Related Compounds

Diazepam is a frequently used drug and may be utilized in suicide attempts. Intoxication with diazepam results in tinnitus, drowsiness, weakness, nystagmus, diplopia, incoordination, hallucinations, and respiratory depression with cyanosis and coma.[8] Severe toxicity appears rare, since doses from 0.2 to 2.25 g have not resulted in significant respiratory depression or coma. These patients were sedated but arousable.[10]

Treatment consists of removal of as much drug as possible by emesis with ipecac or gavage, followed by giving activated charcoal. Coma should be treated as described above under Barbiturates (Table 21-1). If blood pressure is depressed, it should be treated as described under General Treatment (Table 21-1).

Major risks to the fetus resulting from maternal diazepam overdose include direct effects of the drug and asphyxia from maternal respiratory depression or reduced uterine perfusion secondary to hypotension. The use of diazepam in the first trimester has been associated with increased oral clefts in humans.[22] In the neonate, respiratory depression, excessive drowsiness, and hyperbilirubinemia may occur.[19] Careful maintenance of maternal arterial PO_2 and blood pressure should minimize the first of these risks. If delivery is anticipated at the time of intoxication, provision should be made for supportive therapy and bilirubin monitoring for the infant.

Epinephrine and Ephedrine

Epinephrine and ephedrine intoxication result in nausea, vomiting, chills, cyanosis, nervousness, irritability, fever, opisthotonos, spasms, convulsions, pulmonary edema, gasping respirations, respiratory failure, and coma.[8] In the first trimester, exposure to epinephrine but not ephedrine has been associated with a significant increase in congenital anomalies.[13] In cases of intoxication, however, the major risk to the fetus is from the maternal conditions of hypoxemia, hypotension, and hypertension.

Treatment consists of maintenance of adequate respirations and gas exchange as described under General Treatment. Removal of as much ingested drug as possible should be attempted by use of ipecac to induce emesis or by gavage followed by administration of activated charcoal. Coma should be treated as described under Barbiturates (Table 21-1). Convulsions should be treated as suggested under Aminophylline and Theophylline (Table 21-1). Hypertension should be treated as described under Amphetamines and Psychotomimetic Agents (Table 21-1). If hypotension occurs, vasopressors are contraindicated, as they may produce extreme hypertension.[8] Reduction in blood pressure should therefore be treated by fluid administration while monitoring the central venous pressure. Supportive therapy is indicated until recovery occurs.

Monoamine Oxidase Inhibitors

Monoamine oxidase inhibitors are used in the treatment of serious depression and as might be expected from this use, intoxication may be seen in the context of suicide attempts. Intoxication may result in a number of signs and symptoms, including dry mouth, ataxia, stupor, hypotension, hypertension, fever, tachycardia, precordial pain, acidosis, central nervous system stimulation, excitement, hallucinations, convulsions, and, rarely, jaundice due to acute liver necrosis.[8] Major fetal risks are from asphyxia due to maternal respiratory depression and maternal hypotension. Maternal hypertension also presents a risk to the fetus of abruptio placentae. In addition, monoamine oxidase inhibitors may be potential teratogens in humans. In one study exposure to monoamine oxidase inhibitor was found to be associated with a significant increase in all malformations.[13]

As maternal and fetal death may occur from maternal respiratory and circulatory failure, the first priority is treatment of these problems. Following initial stabilization, as much drug as possible should be removed by emesis or gastric lavage. With severe respiratory depression and stupor or coma, endotracheal intubation and artificial respiration as described under Barbiturates (Table 21-1) are indicated. Hypotension should be treated as described under General Treatment (Table 21-1), convulsions as described under Aminophylline-Theophylline (Table 21-1), and hypertension and hyperexcitability as described under Amphetamines and Psychotomimetic Agents (Table 21-1). Great caution should be exercised in the use of pharmacologic agents for the treatment of these conditions, as additive effects from the antidotal drugs may be expected.[10] Central nervous system depression may be increased with the use of depressants and antihypertensive agents. Furthermore, both vasopressors and hypotensive agents may have exaggerated effects. In general, therefore, pharmacologic treatment should be avoided, if possible. Conservative therapy aimed at maintaining normal temperature, respiration, blood pressure, and good fluid and electrolyte balance is usually all that is required.

Narcotic Analgesics

Narcotic analgesics may account for 10,000 deaths per year in the United States.[8] Street heroin usually contains 1 to 3 percent per bag, and if more than 20 percent is present, lethal overdose is likely.[18] Many narcotic addicts tend to keep their habit at a minimum during pregnancy and these women are most likely to overdose in the postpartum period when they resume their customary habit.[20] A major problem which arises is that 64 to 73 percent of female addicts are oligomenorrheic, but fertility is unaffected.[18] They may not know that they are pregnant and continue with their habit as usual.

Symptoms and signs of narcotic overdose include stupor; coma; pinpoint pupils (dilated with anoxia); gastrointestinal and biliary spasm; irregular, slow, shallow respirations; cyanosis; respiratory arrest; weak pulse; hypotension; pulmonary edema; spasticity and twitching of the musculature; and hypothermia.[8,9,17] Death may occur instantaneously owing to allergic reaction[18] or within 2 to 4 h from respiratory failure.[8]

Although narcotics cross the placenta readily,[15] there is no evidence that they are teratogenic in humans.[22] However, the fetus is at risk from two other conditions. Fetal asphyxia may occur owing to maternal respiratory depression. This may result in considerable asphyxic brain damage when it occurs in the third trimester.[20] The second problem faced by the fetus is withdrawal produced by the treatment of the overdose. Fetal distress from acute withdrawal may result in meconium staining[4] and increased levels of epinephrine and norephinephrine in the amniotic fluid.[24] If delivery occurs at the time of or shortly after overdosage, the infant must be carefully followed for respiratory depression in addition to the usual precautions taken for infants of addicts.

Treatment of the mother consists of maintenance of respirations, if depressed. Naloxone hydrochloride (Narcan) is the specific antagonist of choice and is both diagnostic and therapeutic. The initial dose should be 0.01 mg/kg body weight given intravenously.[8] Naloxone works within 2 min and has its maximum effect shortly thereafter, and its effect is gone in 15 to 30 min.[9] If the initial dose is ineffective, it may be repeated once in 2 to 3 min. After the diagnosis of narcotic overdose is established by response to naloxone, two approaches are possible. The first is to add 4 mg of naloxone to 1 L of 5 percent dextrose in water, which is infused at 100 ml/h, and at the same time to give 2 mg naloxone intramuscularly.[9] It should be noted that naloxone may produce exaggerated withdrawal in the addict.[17] Since maternal withdrawal adversely effects the fetus, an alternative approach to management would be to treat women who responded to a test dose of naloxone with respirator support until adequate spontaneous respirations occurred without the use of additional naloxone. Coma should be treated as described under Barbiturates (Table 21-1), and respiratory and blood pressure support should be provided as described under General Treatment (Table 21-1). Chest x-ray is indicated since the pulmonary edema which accompanies narcotic overdose may occur without physical signs.[21] This complication usually clears with supportive therapy in 24 to 48 h. If overdosage has occurred by mouth and it is within 2 h of the ingestion, significant drug may be removed by ipecac-induced emesis or by gavage. With subcutaneously injected narcotic, absorption may be delayed by tourniquet application. As 90 percent of narcotic overdosages involve more than one drug, careful toxicological screening should be done on urine, blood, and vomitus.[9] Consideration should be made to placing the patient who is a pregnant addict on methadone maintenance during the rest of her pregnancy once she has recovered from her acute overdose.

Phenacetin and Acetominophen

Products containing phenacetin and acetominophen are becoming increasingly popular as analgesics. Medical misuse is the most frequent cause of acute intoxication.[10] Intoxication from these drugs results in cyanosis due to methemoglobin and sulfhemoglobin formation, along with hepatic and renal damage. Cardiac toxicity may occur as well as central nervous system stimulation with delirium, followed by depression, stupor, and coma with circulatory collapse.[10] Neither phenacetin nor acetominophen has been shown to be a human teratogen.[13] Direct toxicity due to hypoxia induced by methemoglobinemia is the major risk to the fetus. The toxic effects of methemoglobinemia are potentiated by maternal anemia. If at 4 h following ingestion the blood levels of acetaminophen exceed 200 μg/ml, death is likely, while levels below 120 μg/ml are nontoxic.[8] The degree of liver damage may be ascertained by initial laboratory testing. If the prothrombin time is above 1.3 times control, plasma bilirubin is above 17 μmol/L, or serum aspartate or alanine aminotransferase is above 40 IU/L,[8] significant hepatic dysfunction is present.

Removal of as much drug as possible by ipecac-induced emesis or gavage is indicated if ingestion has occurred within 4 h. Because of its rapid absorption, attempts to remove the drug after this time are ineffective. If the maternal serum level of acetominophen is greater than 200 μg/ml, N-acetylcysteine should be given orally.[8] The loading dose is 140 mg per kilogram of body weight of 20 percent solution followed by 70 mg/kg every 4 h for 3 days. In the presence of cyanosis, respiratory difficulty, or air hunger, 100 percent oxygen should be given and the patient treated with methylene blue for her methemoglobinemia. The dosage for methylene blue is 0.1 mg/kg of 1 percent solution given intravenously over a 10-min period.[8] Care should be taken to maintain adequate oxygenation to prevent fetal damage. The patient should be observed and kept warm and dry. If she lives 4 days, she will probably recover.[8] For the first 48 h the patient should receive 5 percent dextrose in water intravenously. Her electrolytes, blood urea nitrogen, liver function tests, and prothrombin time should be followed carefully, and if the prothrombin time exceeds 3 times control, phytonadione, 1 to 10 mg intramuscularly, should be given. Fresh frozen plasma or clotting factor concentrates may be needed to treat bleeding and fresh blood may be necessary to treat the methemoglobinemia.

Phencyclidine (PCP, "Angel Dust")

Phencyclidine is a substance of abuse which produces dose-dependent toxic symptoms.[8] At 5 mg or less, hyperactivity, rigidity, peripheral anesthesia, nystagmus, incoordination, and wild movements occur. At higher doses between 5 and 10 mg, salivation, fever, muscle rigidity, and stupor and coma appear. At doses above 10 mg, sweating, hyperthermia, hypertension, laryngeal stridor, decreased or absent reflexes, respiratory depression, convulsions, and acute rhabdomyolysis may occur. The last may release myglobin and result in renal shutdown. Fatalities have occurred with blood levels in excess of 2 μg/ml.[8] Phencyclidine is an animal teratogen,[22] and the human fetus may be at risk for anomalies if this drug is taken during the first trimester. The major fetal risk during intoxication, however, comes from the convulsions, respiratory depression, and hypertension induced in the mother.

Treatment consists of maintaining respiration and treating coma, if present, as described under Barbiturates (Table 21-1). Convulsions should be treated as described under Aminophylline and Theophylline (Table 21-1) and hypertension as stated under Amphetamines and Psychotomimetic Agents (Table 21-1). Hyperthermia with temperatures above 39°C should be treated with a cooling blanket. As much drug as possible should be removed. This can be achieved by ipecac-induced emesis or gastric lavage followed by a saline cathartic consisting of 30 ml of Fleet's phospho-soda diluted to 200 ml and given by mouth. The patient should be on continuous gastric suction except for 1 h following administration of oral medications. Acidification of the urine and diuresis will enhance phencyclidine removal.[8] In noncomatose patients, this may be done by giving 1 to 2 g of ascorbic acid in cranberry juice four times a day. In comatose patients NH_4Cl, 3 mmol/kg diluted 1 : 4, is given by nasogastric tube every 6 h. Ascorbic acid should also be given intravenously 2 g per 500 ml of intravenous fluid every 6 h. The urine pH should be lowered to 5.0 or less, and then 20 mg of furosemide given intravenously to enhance phencyclidine elimination. The urine may need to be acidified for up to a week for complete removal. The blood gases, blood urea nitrogen, and electrolytes should be carefully monitored. The patient should have restricted sensory input and precautions to prevent injury should be taken. Complete recovery from the psychotic state may require up to 2 weeks. Fetal jeopardy can be minimized by scrupulous attention to maintaining maternal oxygenation.

Phenothiazine Drugs

The phenothiazine drugs are used as antiemetics, major tranquilizers, and potentiators of analgesic drugs. They may produce agranulocytosis and liver damage presenting as leukopenia and jaundice. Additional toxic manifestations include hypotension, hypothermia, tachycardia, dry mouth, fever, urinary retention, constipation, nausea, blurred vision, ataxia, stiff muscles, drowsiness, and coma.[8] They have not been shown to be human teratogens[22] but are associated with neonatal Parkinsonian symptoms when given to the mother antenatally.[5]

Treatment for intoxication includes discontinuation of drug administration. Coma and respiratory depression should be treated as described under Barbiturates (Table 21-1). Hypotension should be treated with intravenous Ringer's lactate and hypothermia by warming blankets. Induced emesis or gastric lavage should be used to remove orally ingested drug. Diphenhydramine should be given in a dose of 1 to 5 mg/kg to reverse extrapyramidal signs.[8] The electrocardiogram should be carefully monitored and if ventricular arrhythmias occur, they should be treated with phenytoin 1 mg/kg by slow intravenous injection, not to exceed 50 mg/min.[8] Phenytoin may be repeated every 5 min up to a total dose of 10 mg/kg. If convulsions are present, the agent of choice is pentobarbital[8] in a dose of 5 mg/kg body weight intravenously as a 2.5 percent solution at a rate not to exceed 1 mg/min until convulsions are controlled. Lidocaine is contraindicated in phenothiazine overdose because of profound drug interactions.

Recovery from agranulocytosis is likely if the patient survives 2 weeks. Hepatic recovery following discontinuation of drug takes 4 to 8 weeks. The major fetal risk is from hypoxia and can be minimized by prompt treatment of maternal hypotension and respiratory depression.

Salicylates

Salicylates, especially acetylsalicylic acid (aspirin), are common pain medications. The lethal dose of aspirin is 0.2 to 0.5 g/kg while toxic effects are uncommon at blood levels below 30 mg/dl.[8] Symptoms and signs of salicylate intoxication vary with the degree of intoxication.[10] Mild intoxication results in headache, dizziness, tinnitus, difficulty in hearing, dimness of vision, stupor, mental confusion, sweating, thirst, hyperventilation, nausea, vomiting, and diarrhea. With more severe intoxication, in addition to the above signs and symptoms the patient may have pustular acneform skin eruptions, metabolic acidosis, restlessness, garrulity, incoherent speech, apprehension, vertigo, tremor, maniacal delirium, hallucinations, generalized convulsions, and coma. In addition, hyper- or hypoglycemia, fever, prolonged prothrombin time, gastrointestinal blood loss, and pulmonary and cerebral edema may be present. The risk to the mother is primarily from metabolic acidosis, pulmonary edema, and cerebral edema. As salicylates have not been shown to be human teratogens,[22] the fetus is at risk primarily because of the maternal metabolic derangements in acid-base balance and from hyperthermia if present. Furthermore, fetal platelet aggregation is significantly diminished following maternal salicylate exposure. This could predispose the fetus to bleeding in utero, although that has not yet been reported in association with acute salicylate intoxication.

Salicylate blood levels are very useful in determining the extent of intoxication. The relationship between serum salicylate levels (mg/dl) in the first 6 h after ingestion and the degree of intoxication is as follows: less than 45, not intoxicated; 45 to 65, mild intoxication; 65 to 90, moderate intoxication; 90 to 120, severe intoxication; above 120, usually lethal.[8]

Treatment consists of removal by ipecac-induced emesis or gavage and is best accomplished within 4 h of ingestion; however, some drug may be removed up to 24 h.[9] Following this, activated charcoal and a saline cathartic consisting of 30 ml of Fleet's phosphosoda diluted to 200 ml should be given by mouth. Careful monitoring of electrolytes, glucose, prothrombin time, blood gases, and central venous pressure is indicated, as well as a chest x-ray. If convulsions or coma are present, a trial of 50 to 100 ml of 50 percent dextrose in water given over 1 to 2 min is indicated after a blood sample has been drawn for blood glucose determination. If this is ineffective and the glucose level is normal, coma should be treated as described under Barbiturates (Table 21-1). If coma persists after the blood salicylate levels has returned to normal, cerebral edema may be present. This should be treated with an osmotic diuretic such as manitol. Central nervous system depressants are contraindicated and convulsions not due to hypoglycemia should be treated with succinylcholine administration followed by intubation and artificial respiration.[8] Priority should be given to close monitoring of maternal arterial PO_2, which should be maintained above 60 mmHg. If pulmonary edema is present, positive end-expiratory pressure may be necessary to maintain optimal oxygenation.[9] Adequate hydration is essential, with replacement of water, sodium, and potassium losses. Hyperthermia should not be permitted to continue if present and should be treated by cooling blanket application. Metabolic acidosis should only be treated with alkali if the pH is below 7.0. Salicylates are eliminated by the renal route, and this is enhanced by forced diuresis with an alkalizing solution. Administration of alkali, however, should be limited to those patients with severe intoxication because of the risk of iatrogenic metabolic alkalosis. When alkali is given, the pH should not be raised above 7.5, and in addition potassium should be supplemented in order to avoid further potassium depletion.

Tricyclic Antidepressants

The tricyclic antidepressants include imipramine, amitriptyline, desipramine, protriptyline, cyclobenzaprine, doxepin, and nortriptyline. Agents of this class most frequently produce intoxication due to their anticholinergic properties. Symptoms and signs of intoxication include dry mouth; constipation; dizziness; palpitations; blurred vision; urinary retention; hypotension; hypertension; hypothermia; hyperthermia; tremor; increased intraocular pressure; sweating; mydriasis; respiratory depression; clonic movements or convulsions; coma; cardiac ischemia up to and including myocardial infarction; and cardiac arrhythmias, including sinus tachycardia, multifocal extrasystoles, wandering pacemaker, and atrioventricular or intraventricular block.[10] With these agents ventricular fibrillation usually precedes death.[8] Toxicity is potentiated by concurrent administration of monoamine oxidase inhibitors.[10] As tricyclic antidepressants are probably not human teratogens,[22] the major risks to the fetus are due to maternal hypotension, respiratory depression, and hyperthermia.

Treatment should begin by establishment and maintenance of respirations as described under Barbiturates (Table 21-1). The electrocardiogram should be carefully monitored from onset of therapy until the patients is free of arrhythmias for 24 h. After initial stabilization gastric lavage should be followed by the administration of activated charcoal to remove as much drug as possible. Systolic blood pressure should be maintained at 90 mmHg or greater by infusion of fluids. Care should be taken to avoid fluid overload by carefully monitoring the central venous pressure. Vasoconstrictor agents should be avoided.[8] Hypertension should be treated as described under Amphetamines and Psychotomimetic Agents (Table 21-2). Convulsions may be treated by pentobarbital 5 mg/kg intravenously given as a 2.5 percent solution at a rate not to exceed 1 mg/min until convulsions are controlled.[8] Anticholinergic symptoms such as sinus tachycardia, arrhythmias, and convulsions should be treated as described under Anticholinergic Agents with intravenous physostigmine, 0.03 mg/kg, diluted in 5 ml of saline and injected over 2 min. This dose may be repeated in 5 to 10 min but atropine must be available in the event of "overcorrection." Physostigmine administration is contraindicated in the presence of hypotension because it may aggravate that condition in tricyclic antidepressant overdosage. Hypotension, tachycardia, and arrhythmias may be controlled by slowly administering a 7.5 percent solution of $NaHCO_3$ (44.6 mEq/50 ml) intravenously with electrocardiographic monitoring until the arterial pH is 7.5.[8] This dose may be repeated or a 0.17 *M* solution given as an intravenous drip after the arrhythmias are controlled. Great care must be taken with alkali administration to avoid creating an iatrogenic metabolic alkalosis. Blood gases must be closely followed to monitor acid-base balance. In the presence of refractory arrhythmias, phenytoin, 0.5 to 1.0 mg/kg, may be given intravenously over 3 to 5 min and be repeated up to a total dose of

10 mg/kg in 24 h.[8] Lidocaine is contraindicated in tricyclic antidepressant overdosage because it may cause a lethal drug interaction. Hyperthermia of 39°C or greater should be promptly treated with a cooling blanket.

ANAPHYLAXIS IN PREGNANCY

Anaphylaxis is an acute allergic phenomena which occurs in sensitized individuals and is mediated by immunoglobulin E (IgE).[3] It may be life-threatening and is characterized by rapid onset; pruritis and urticaria with or without angioedema; respiratory distress produced by laryngeal edema and/or bronchospasm; vascular collapse; and shock. It may be produced by a number of substances, usually by injection but occasionally by ingestion. Materials capable of producing anaphylaxis include heterologous proteins in the form of antiserum, hormones, enzymes, hymenoptera venum, pollen extracts, foods, polysaccharides such as iron dextran, diagnostic agents, and drugs, including antibiotics and vitamins.[3] Anaphylaxis due to drug administration is rare. In one review an incidence of 8 cases of anaphylaxis in 11,000 drug administrations was cited, with a fatality rate of 1 to 2 per 100,000 drug administrations.[23] The most common agents to cause anaphylaxis when used therapeutically are xenogenic sera, allergenic extracts, dextrans, therapeutic enzymes, penicillins, and cephalosporins.[23]

The placenta only allows very minimal amounts of IgE to cross from the maternal circulation into the fetal circulation, and thus the fetus is protected from the effects of maternal IgE sensitization, including anaphylaxis.[19] However, maternal anaphylaxis is a threat to the fetus because of hypotension and asphyxia.

Treatment depends on the severity of the reaction. For mild symptoms of pruritis and urticaria, treatment should be 0.2 to 0.5 ml of 1:1,000 epinephrine subcutaneously. Alternatively, diphenhydramine, 50 to 80 mg, may be administered intramuscularly or intravenously. This regimen can also be used for angioedema. While epinephrine is a potential human teratogen,[13] its use is justified in cases of anaphylaxis because of its benefit to the patient. Diphenhydramine does not appear to carry a teratogenic risk in humans.[13] If antigenic material has been injected in an extremity, absorption can be delayed by application of a tourniquet, injection of 0.2 ml of 1:1,000 epinephrine at the injection site, and removal of an insect stinger without compression if one is present.[3] If a severe reaction has occurred, the initial 0.2 to 0.5 ml of 1:1,000 epinephrine may be repeated every 3 min with careful monitoring of the cardiac rhythm. An intravenous line is essential to treat hypotension by expanding intravascular volume with Ringer's lactate or normal saline. The systolic blood pressure should be maintained above 90 mmHg in order to protect the fetus from the adverse effects of maternal hypotension.

If epinephrine administration has not caused cardiac arrhythmias and has failed to improve respiratory distress, hypoxemia secondary to airway obstruction must be considered the cause. The fetus is endangered by low maternal oxygen levels, and consequently the maternal arterial PO_2 should be kept above 60 mmHg. Oxygen by nasal cannula or intermittent positive pressure breathing with 0.5 ml of isoproterenol diluted 1:200 with saline may be sufficient. However, if this is not adequate or if laryngeal edema is present, intubation or tracheostomy may be necessary. Aminophylline in a dose of 0.25 to 0.5 g intravenously over 15 to 30 min may be beneficial for bronchospasm not fully relieved by epinephrine. Aminophylline is relatively safe for the fetus; however, if delivery occurs shortly after high doses are given to the mother, the infant may experience theophylline toxicity in the neonatal period.[2] Corticosteroids are of no benefit for acute anaphylaxis but may be considered in cases of persistent bronchospasm and hypotension.

REFERENCES

1. Aeegan, K.A., Paul, R.H., Broussand, P.M. et al.: Antepartum fetal heart rate testing. Am. J. Obstet. Gynecol., *113:*579, 1979.
2. Arwood, L.L., Dasta, J.F., and Friedman, C.: Placental transfer of theophylline: two case reports. Pediatrics, *63:*844, 1979.
3. Austen, K.F.: Diseases of immediate type hypersensitivity. p. 391. In Adams, R.D., Braunwald, E., Isselbacher, K.J. et al., Eds.: Harrison's Principles of Internal Medicine. 8th Ed. McGraw-Hill, New York, 1977.
4. Blinick, G.: Fertility of narcotics addicts and effects of addiction on the offspring. Soc. Biol., *18:*s34, 1971.
5. Collins, I.S.: Hazards of drug therapy. Med. J. Aust., *1:*222, 1964.
6. Desmond, M.M., Schwanecke, R.P., Wilson, G.S. et al.: Maternal barbiturate utilization and neonatal withdrawal symptomatology. J. Pediatr., *80:*190, 1972.
7. Dilts, P.V., Brinkman, C.R., Kirschbaum, T.H. et al.: Uterine and systemic hemodynamic interrelationships and their response to hypoxia. Am. J. Obstet. Gynecol., *103:*138, 1969.
8. Dreisbach, R.H.: Handbook of Poisoning: Prevention, Diagnosis and Treatment. Lange Medical Publications, Los Altos, Calif., 1980.
9. Goldfrank, L.R. and Kirstein, R.: Toxicologic Emergencies, a Handbook in Problem Solving. Appleton Century Crofts, Norwalk, Conn., 1978.
10. Goodman, L.S. and Gilman, A., Eds.: The Pharmacological Basis of Therapeutics. 6th Ed., MacMillan, New York, 1980.
11. Greiss, F.C.: A clinical concept of uterine blood flow during pregnancy. Obstet. Gynecol., *30:*595, 1967.
12. Greiss, F.C., Anderson, S.G., and King, L.C.: Uterine vascular bed: effects of acute hypoxia. Am. J. Obstet. Gynecol., *113:*1057, 1972.
13. Heinonen, O.P., Slone, D., and Shaprio, S.: Defects and Drugs in Pregnancy. Publishing Sciences Group, Inc., Littleton, MA., 1977.
14. James, L.S.: Intrauterine asphyxia and brain damage. p. 194. In Shnider, S.M. and Moya, F., Eds.: The Anesthesiologist, Mother and Newborn. Williams and Wilkins, Baltimore, 1974.
15. Langer, A. and Caghan, E.N.: Drug and alcohol abuse during pregnancy. p. 543. In Iffy, L. and Kaminetzky, H.A., Eds.: Principles and Practice of Obstetrics and Perinatology. John Wiley & Sons, New York, 1981.
16. Longo, L.D., Hill, E.P., and Power, G.G.: Factors affecting placental oxygen transfer. p. 345. In Longo, L.D. and Bartels, H., Eds.: Respiratory Gas Exchange and Blood Flow in the Placenta. Dept. of Health, Education, and Welfare Publication No. (NIH) 73-361, 1973.
17. Louria, D.B., Hensle, T., and Rose, S.: The major medical complications of heroin addiction. Ann. Intern. Med., *67:*1, 1967.

18. Perlmutter, J.F.: Heroin addiction and pregnancy. Obstet. Gynecol. Surv., *29*:439, 1974.
19. Quilligan, E.J. and Kretchmer, N., Eds.: Fetal and Maternal Medicine. John Wiley & Sons, New York, 1980.
20. Rementeria, J.L., Ed.: Drug Abuse in Pregnancy and Neonatal Effects. C.V. Mosby, St. Louis, 1977.
21. Saba, G.P., James, A.E., Johnson, B.A. et al.: Pulmonary complications of narcotic abuse. Am. J. Roentgenol. Radium Ther. Nucl. Med., *122*:733, 1974.
22. Sheppard, T.H.: Catalog of Teratogenic Agents. 3rd Ed. Johns Hopkins University Press, Baltimore, 1980.
23. van Arsdel, P.P.: Drug allergy, an update. Med. Clin. North Am., *65*:1089, 1981.
24. Zuspan, F.P., Gumpel, J.A., Mejia-Zelayn, A. et al.: Fetal stress from methadone withdrawal. Am. J. Obstet. Gynecol., *122*:43, 1975.

Index

Page numbers followed by f indicate figures; page numbers followed by t indicate tables.